History of Allergy

Chemical Immunology and Allergy

Vol. 100

Series Editors

History of Allergy

Volume Editors

Karl-Christian Bergmann Berlin
Johannes Ring Munich

257 figures, 127 in color and 20 tables, 2014

KARGER Basel • Freiburg • Paris • London • New York • Chennai • New Delhi • Bangkok • Beijing • Shanghai • Tokyo • Kuala Lumpur • Singapore • Sydney

Chemical Immunology and Allergy

Formerly published as 'Progress in Allergy' (Founded 1939), continued 1990–2002 as 'Chemical Immunology'

Edited by Paul Kallós 1939–1988, Byron H. Waksman 1962–2002

Karl-Christian Bergmann

Allergie-Centrum-Charité
Charité – Universitätsmedizin Berlin
Berlin (Germany)

Johannes Ring

Klinik und Poliklinik für Dermatologie und Allergologie am Biederstein
Munich (Germany)

Bibliographic Indices. This publication is listed in bibliographic services, including Current Contents® and PubMed/MEDLINE.

www.karger.com
Printed in Germany on acid-free and non-aging paper (ISO 9706) by Kraft Druck GmbH, Ettlingen
ISSN 1660–2242
e-ISSN 1662–2898
ISBN 978–3–318–02194–3
e-ISBN 978–3–318–02195–0

Contents

3 Mechanisms of Allergy: Important Discoveries

4 Detection of Environmental Influences and Allergens

Contributors

Editors

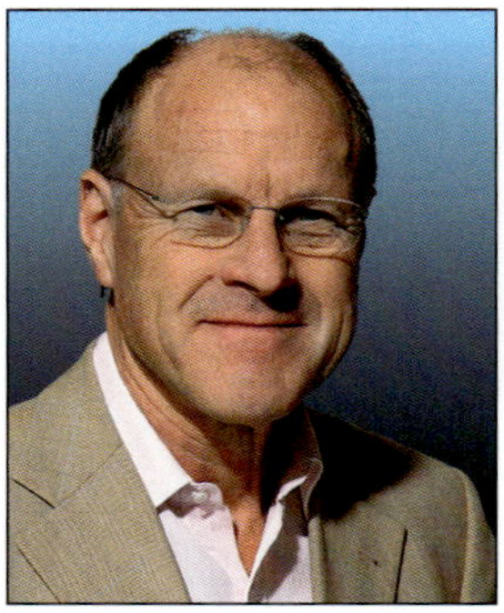

K.-C. Bergmann
Berlin

pp. XVIII, 27, 54, 69, 228, 410

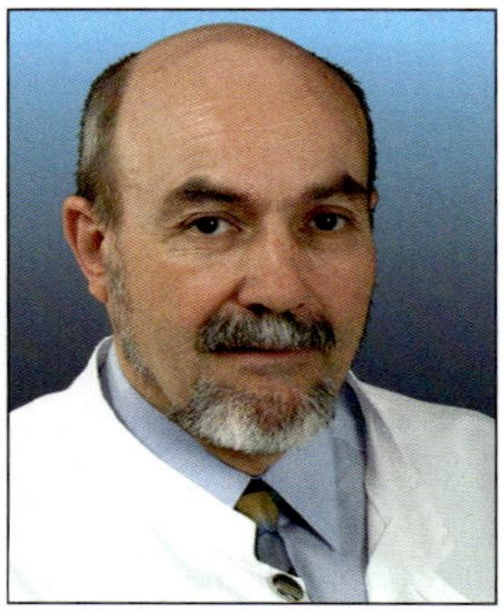

J. Ring
Munich

pp. XVIII, 2, 15, 46, 54, 268, 411

Authors

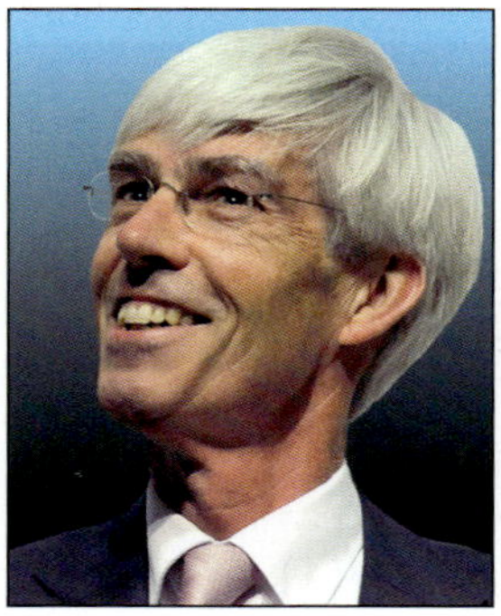

R.C. Aalberse
Amsterdam

p. 243

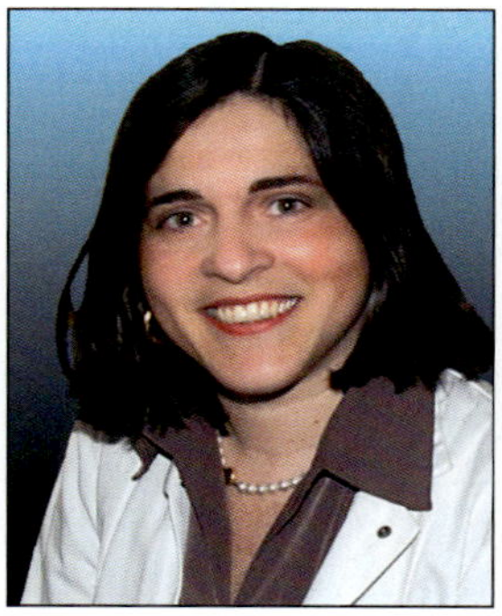

F. Alessandrini
Munich

p. 268

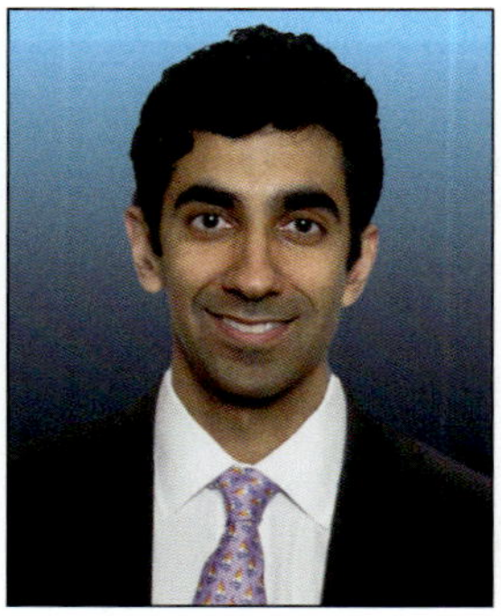

A. Alikhan
Rochester, Minn.

p. 97

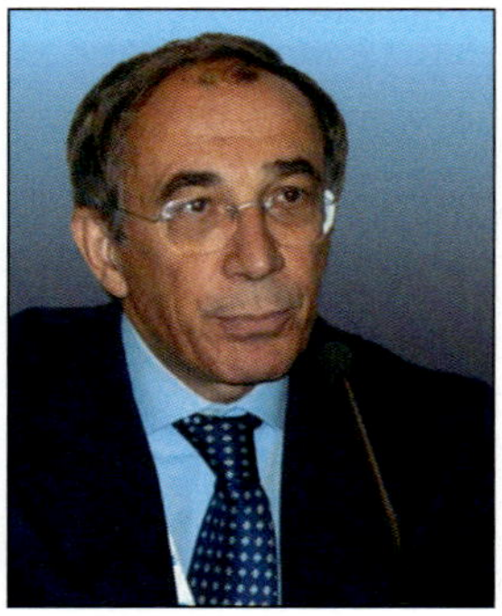

L. Annunziato
Naples

p. 214

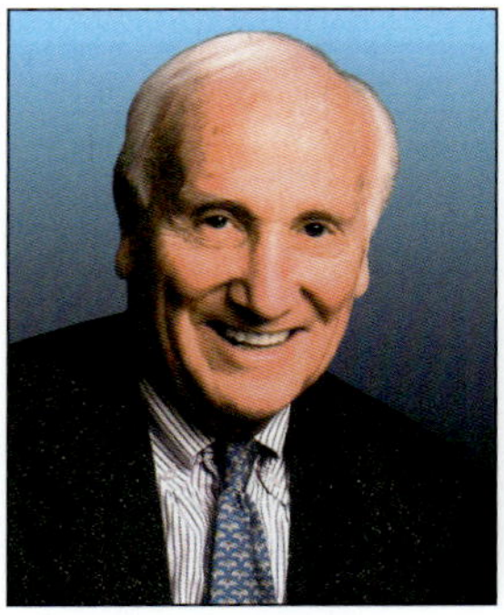

K.F. Austen
Boston, Mass.

p. 340

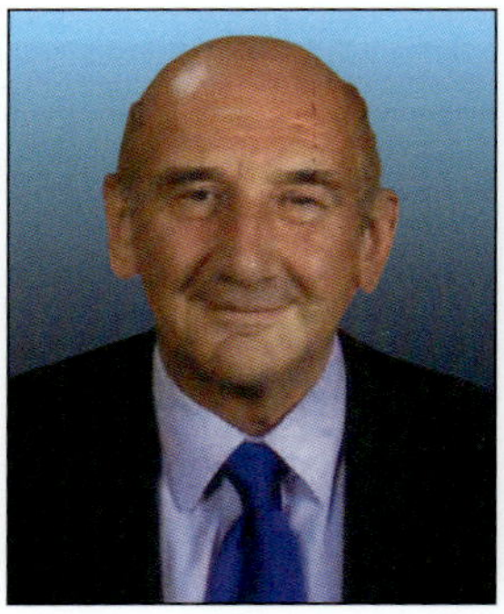

P.J. Barnes
London

p. 311

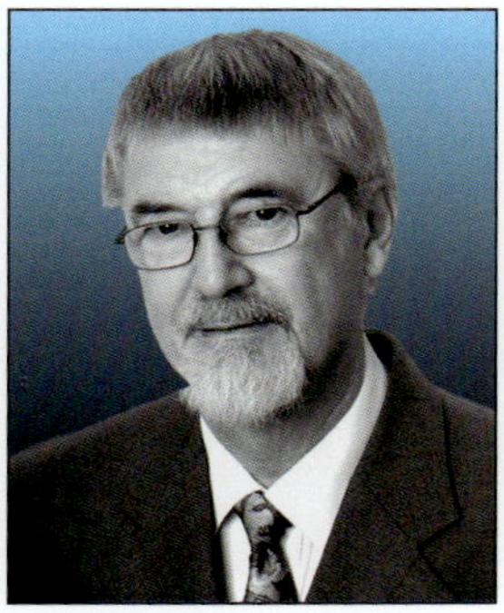

W.M. Becker
Borstel

p. 256

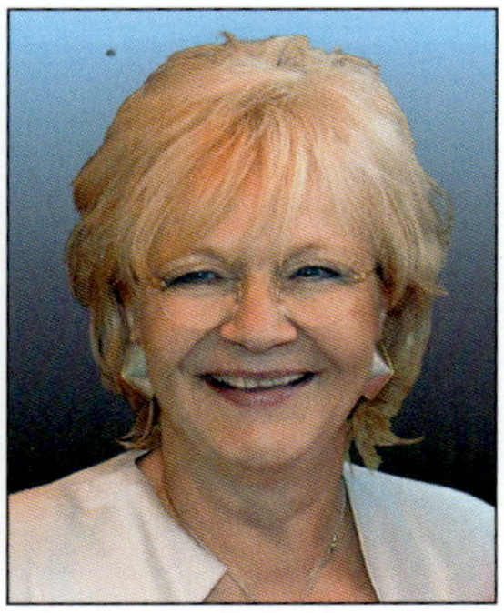

H. Behrendt
Munich

pp. 228, 268

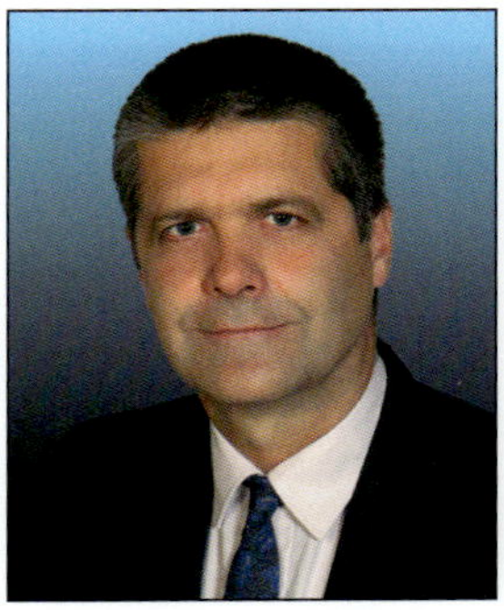

U. Berger
Vienna

p. 228

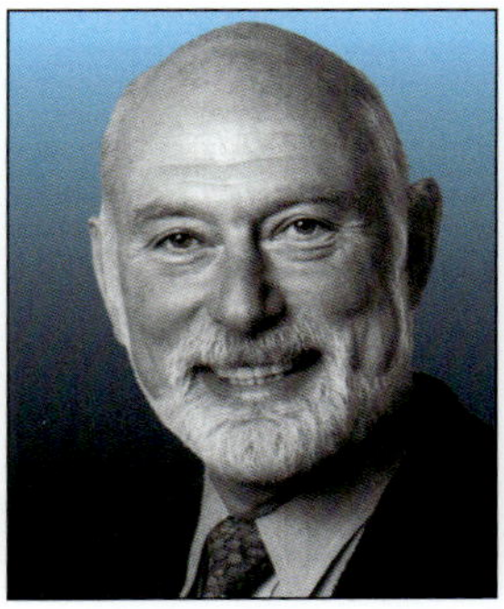

J. Bienenstock
Hamilton, Ont.

p. 342

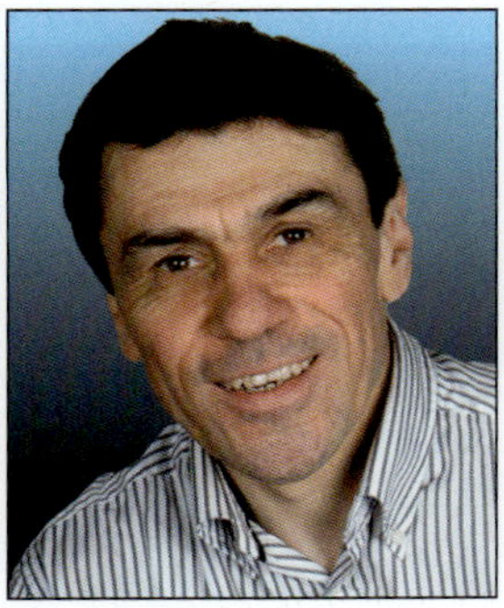

A.J. Bircher
Basel

p. 120

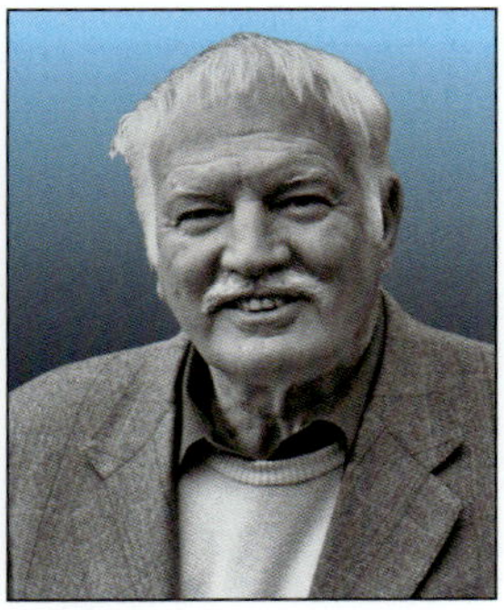

K. Blaser
Davos

p. 344

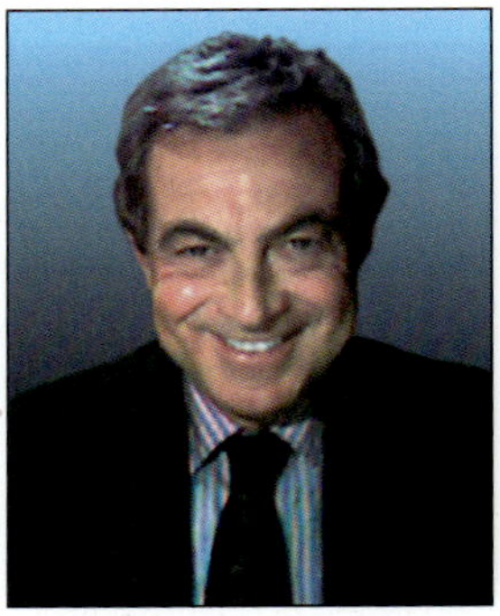

S. Bonini
Rome

p. 105

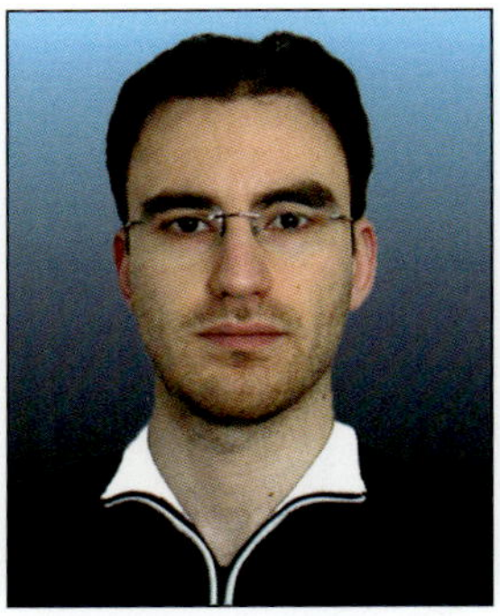

F. Borriello
Naples

pp. 172, 214

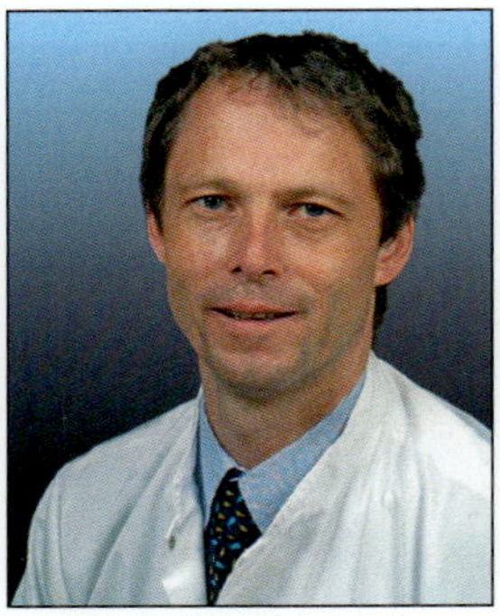

K. Brockow
Munich

p. 54

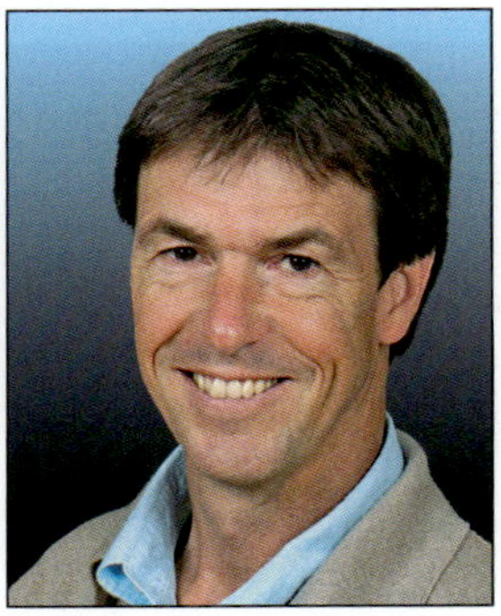

J. Buters
Munich

p. 268

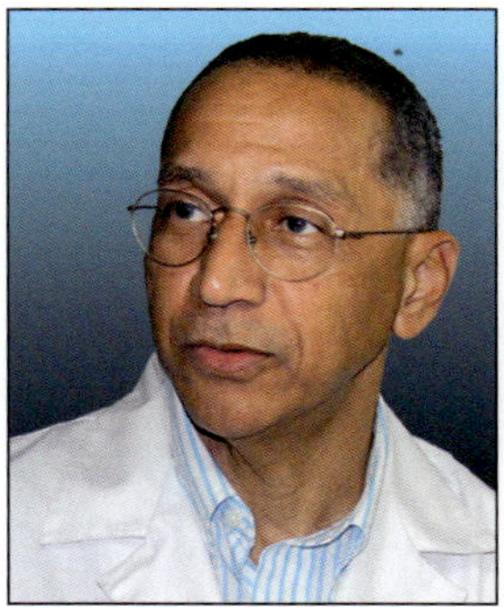

L. Caraballo
Cartagena (Colombia)

p. 234

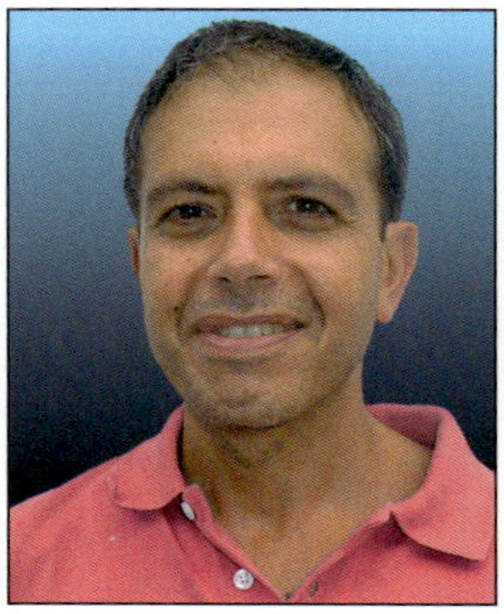

M. Cataldi
Naples

p. 214

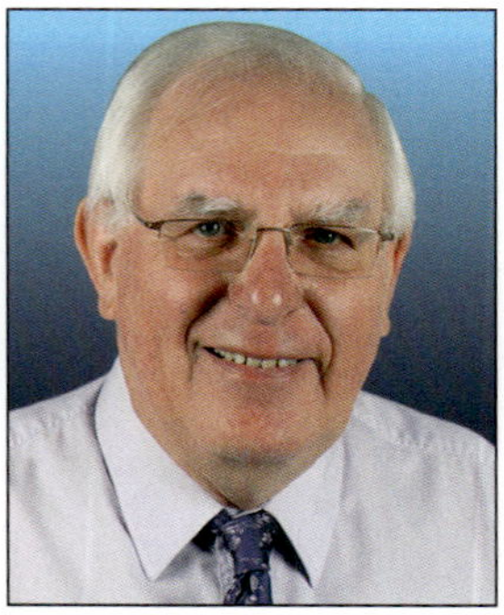

M.K. Church
Berlin

p. 302

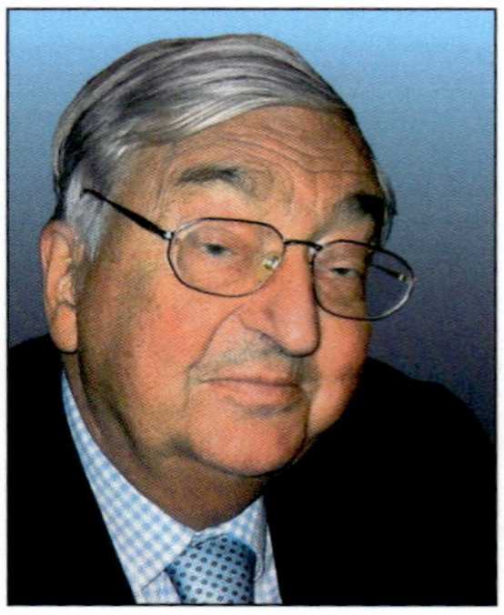

A. de Weck†
Fribourg

p. 346

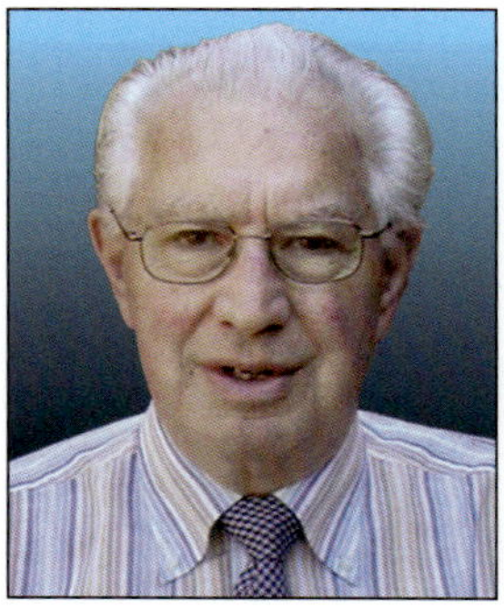

A.M. Edwards
Newport

p. 317

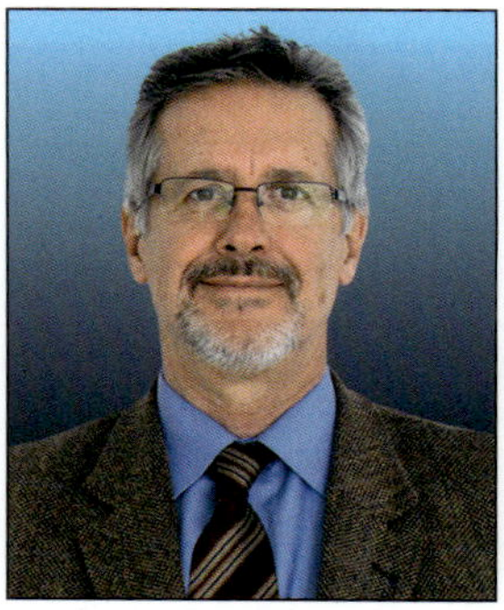

E. Fernández-Caldas
Madrid/Tampa, Fla.

p. 234

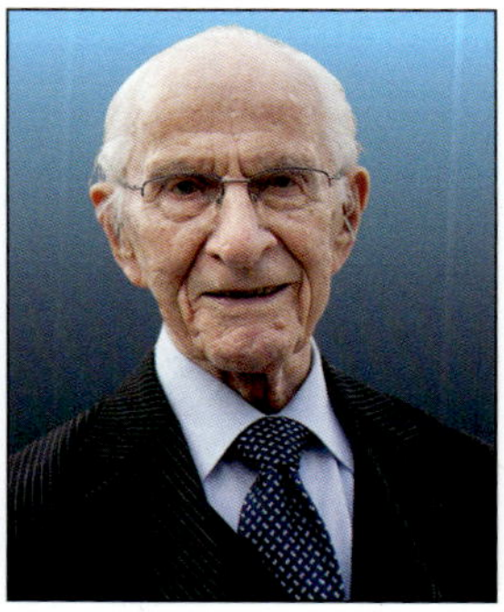

A.W. Frankland
London

p. 350

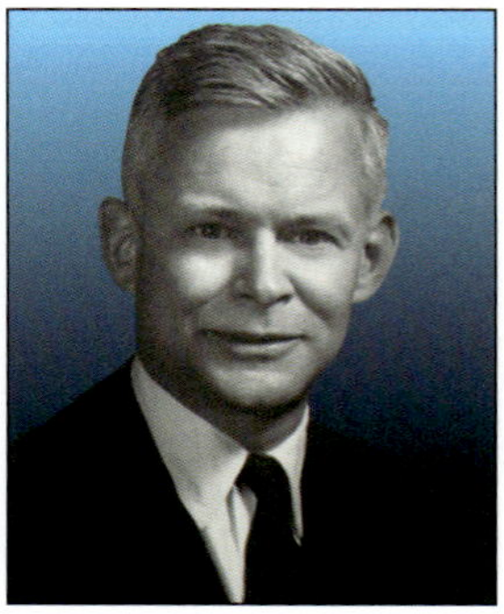

O.L. Frick
San Francisco, Calif.

p. 353

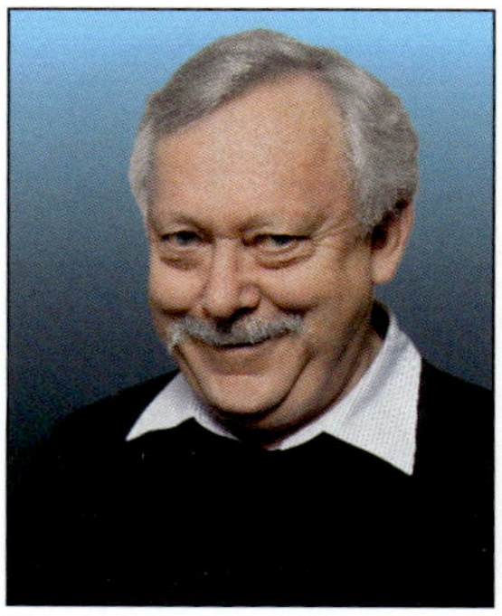

M. Gassner
Zurich

p. 278

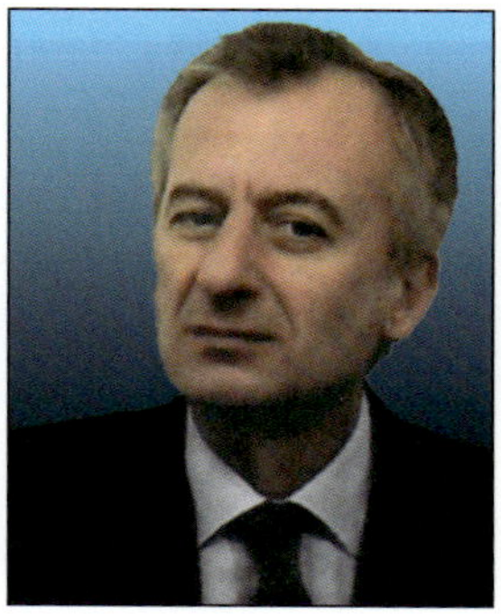

A. Genovese
Naples

p. 172

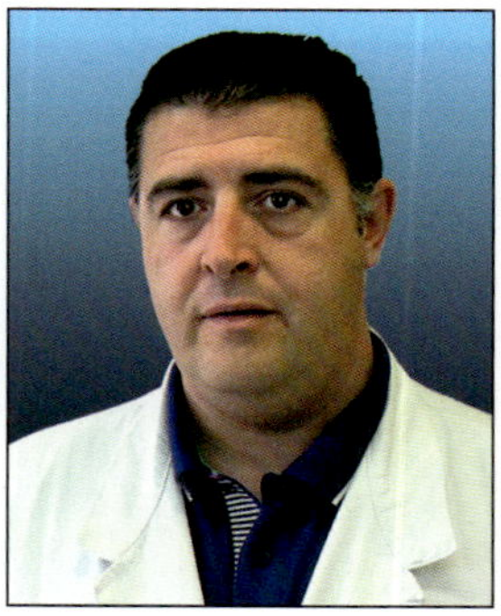

F. Granata
Naples

pp. 172, 214

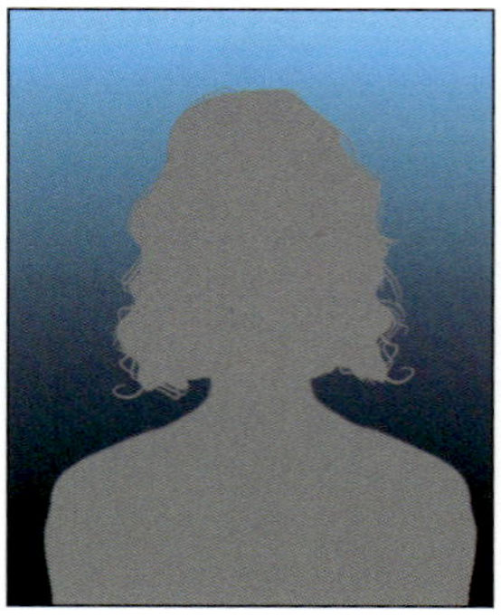

M. Grosber
Munich

p. 54

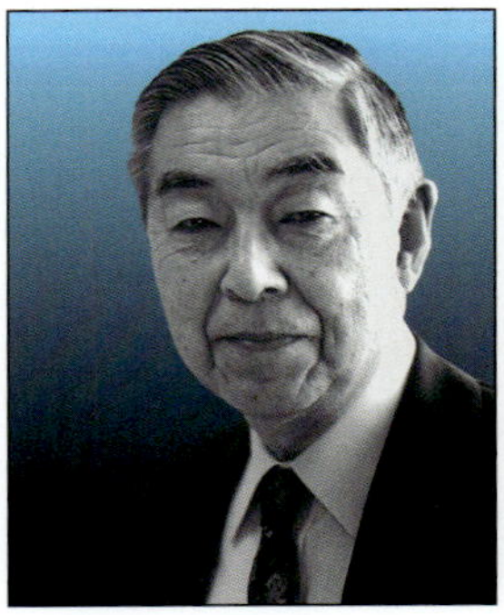

K. Ishizaka
Tokyo

p. 356

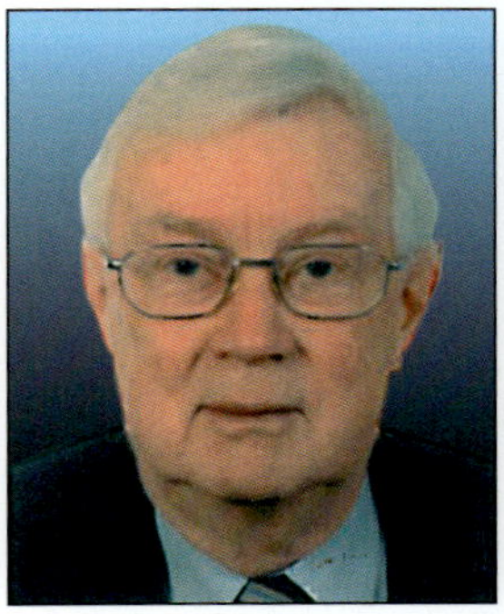

L. Jäger
Jena

p. 361

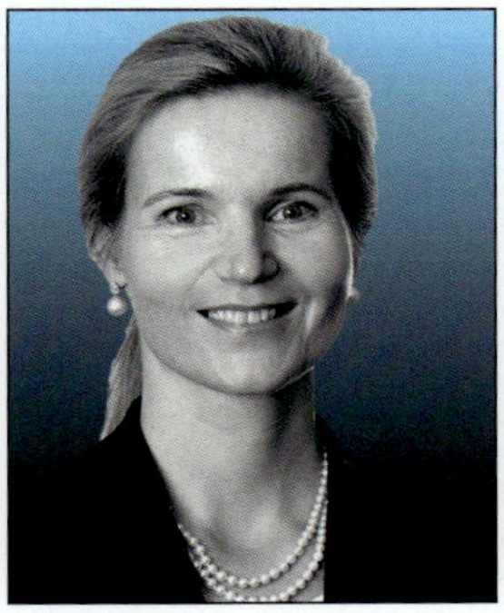

U. Jappe
Borstel/Lübeck

p. 256

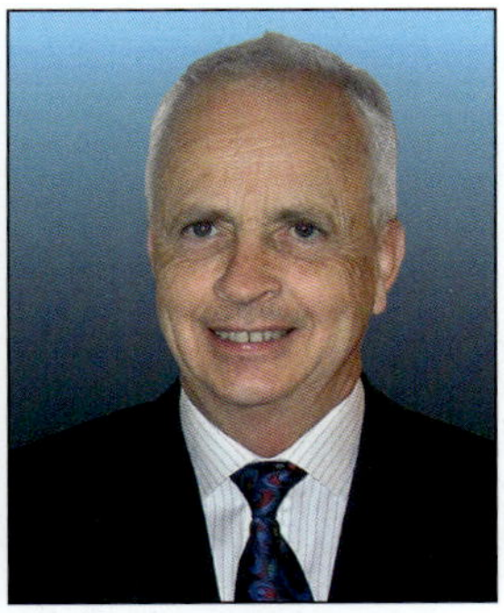

S.G.O. Johansson
Stockholm

p. 150

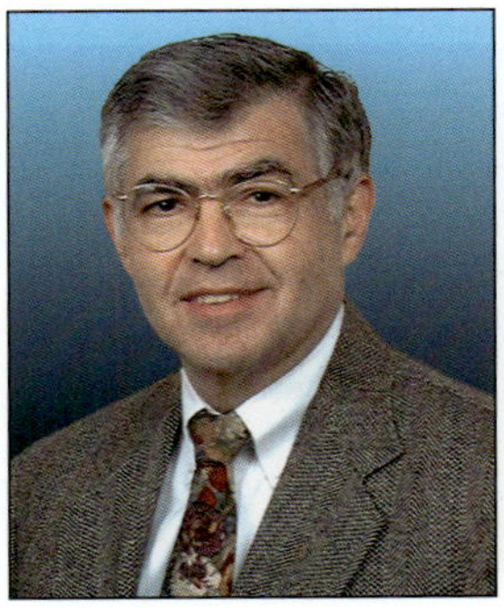

A.P. Kaplan
Charleston, S.C.

pp. 140, 205

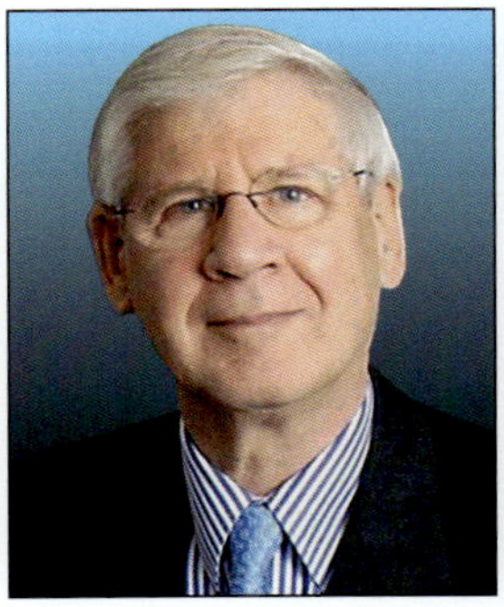

A.B. Kay
London

p. 21

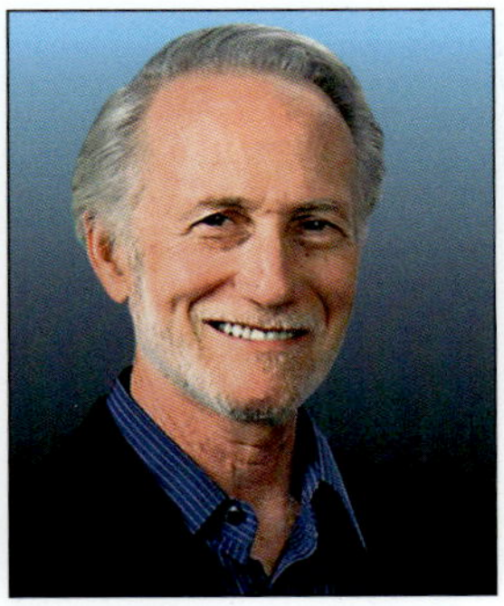

H. Koren,
Durham, N.C.

p. 268

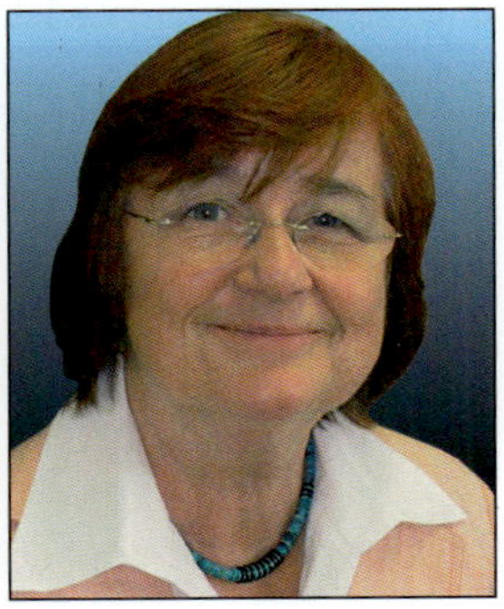

U. Krämer
Düsseldorf

p. 268

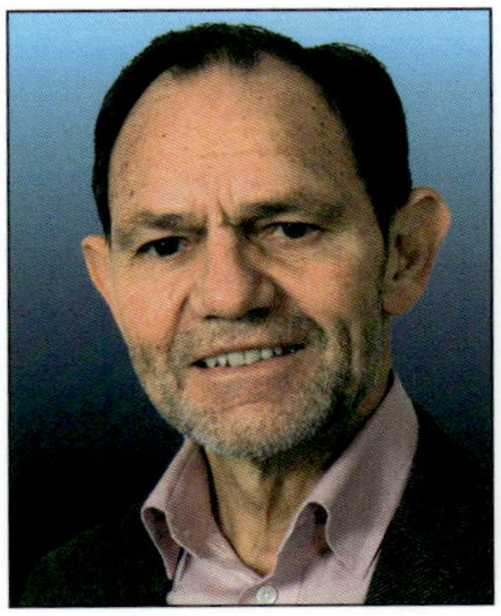

H. Løwenstein
Nødebo

p. 323

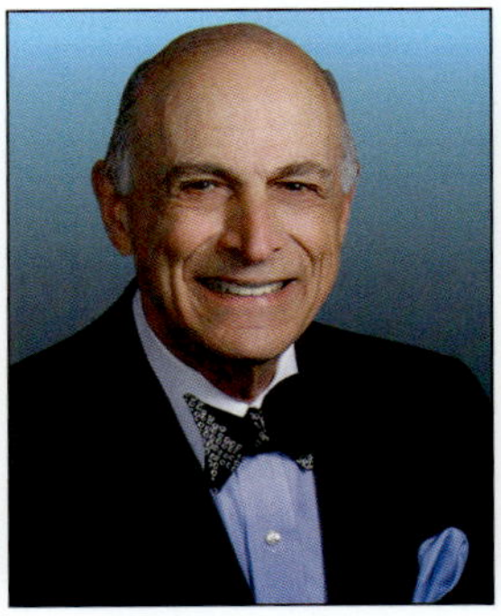

H.I. Maibach
San Francisco, Calif.

p. 97

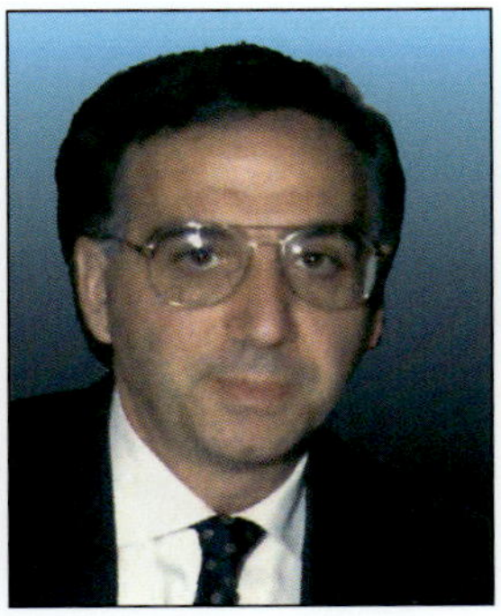

G. Marone
Naples

pp. 172, 214

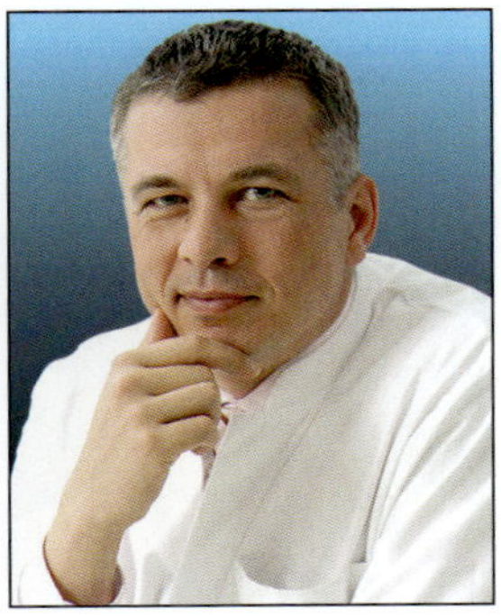

M. Maurer
Berlin

pp. 101, 302

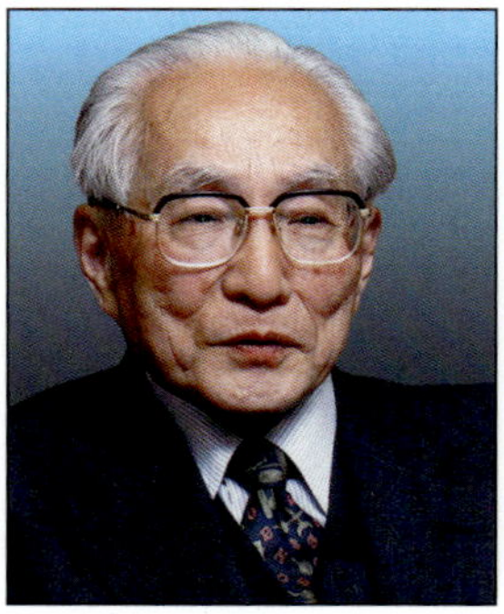

T. Miyamoto
Tokyo

p. 363

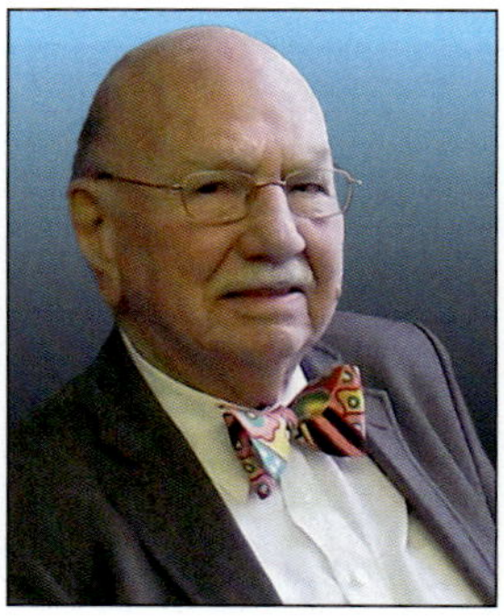

H. Morrow Brown†
Derby

p. 365

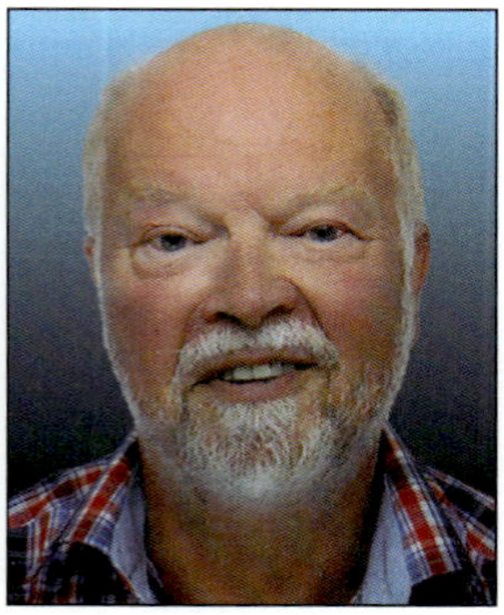

N. Mygind
Copenhagen

p. 62

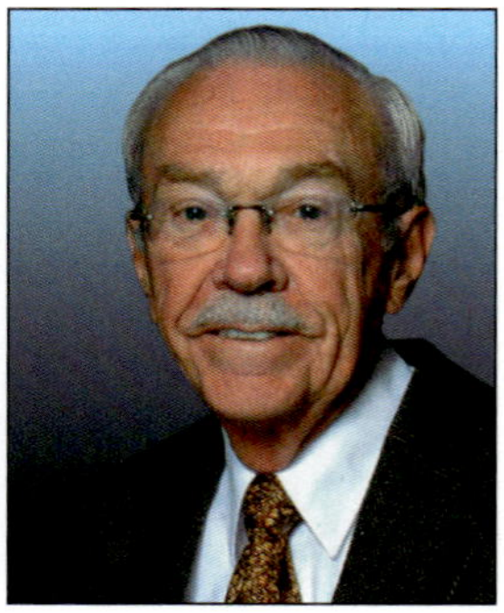

H.S. Nelson
Denver, Colo.

p. 333

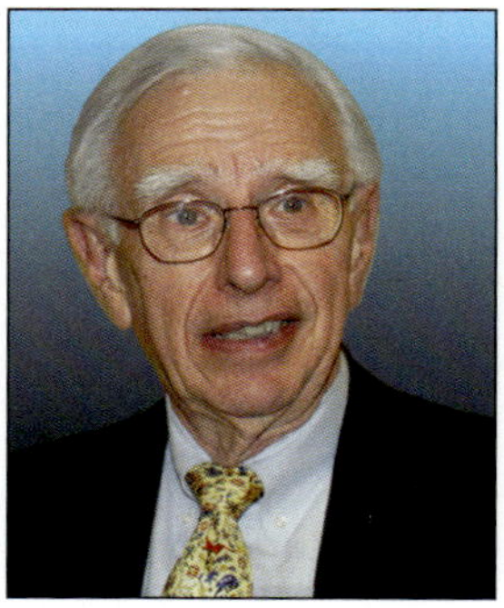

P.S. Norman
Baltimore, Md.

p. 333

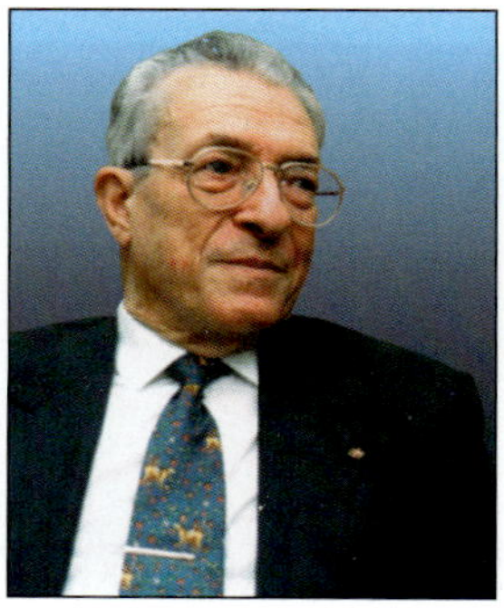

A.K. Oehling
Navaleno

p. 368

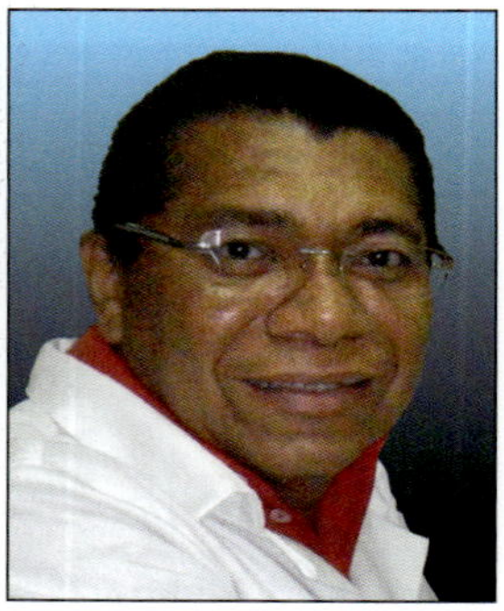

L. Puerta
Cartagena (Colombia)

p. 234

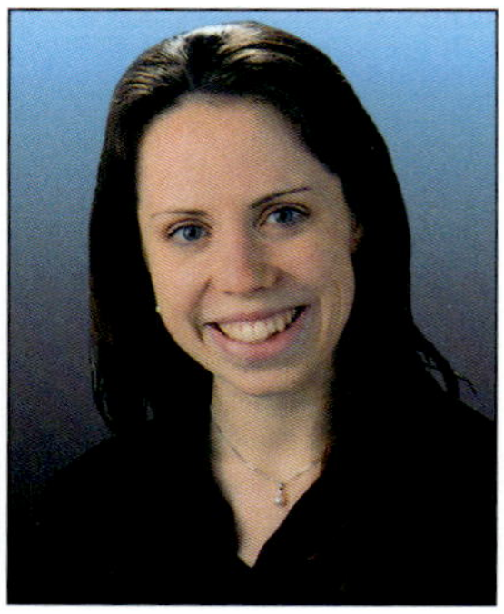

S. Radonjic-Hösli
Bern

p. 193

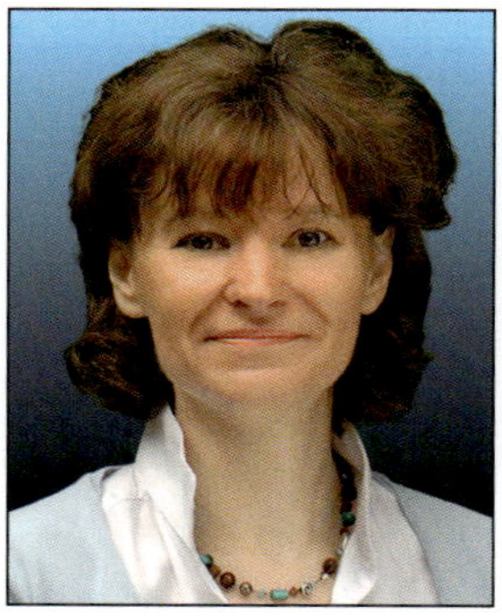

M. Raulf
Bochum

p. 248

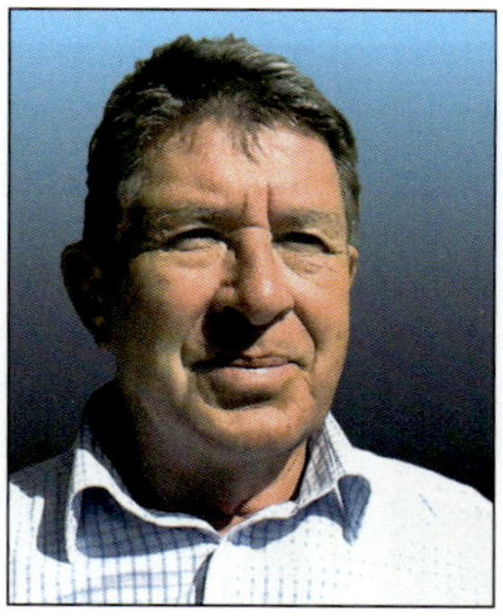

H. Reulecke
Iffeldorf

p. 371

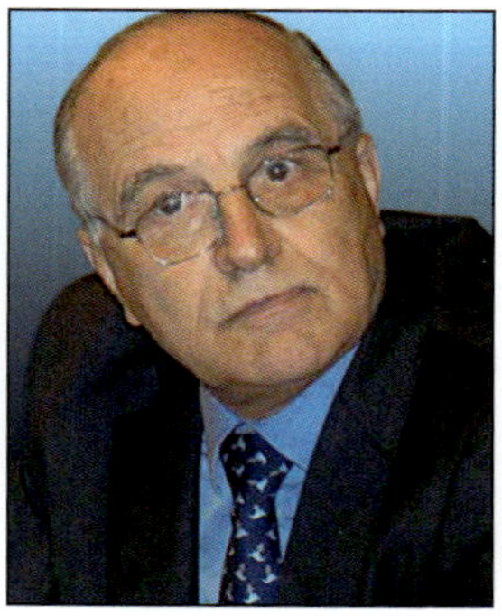

S. Romagnani
Florence

p. 155

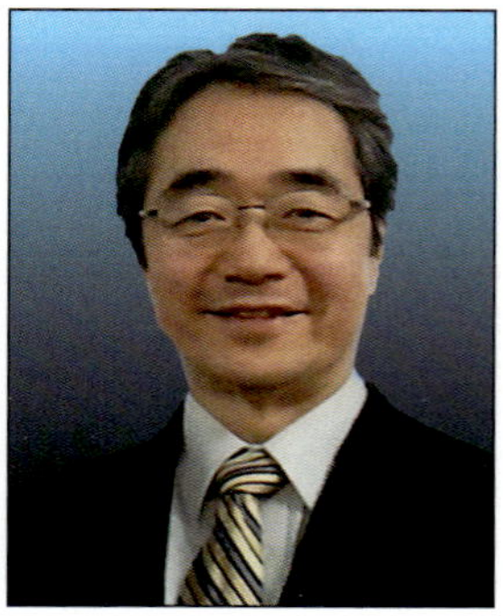

H. Saito
Tokyo

p. 165

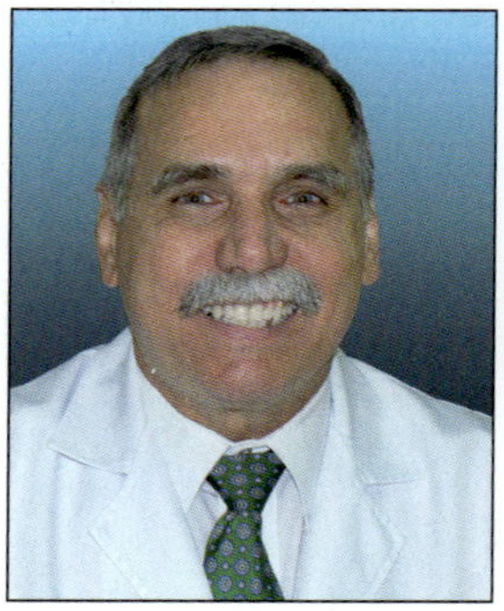

M. Sánchez-Borges
Caracas

p. 132

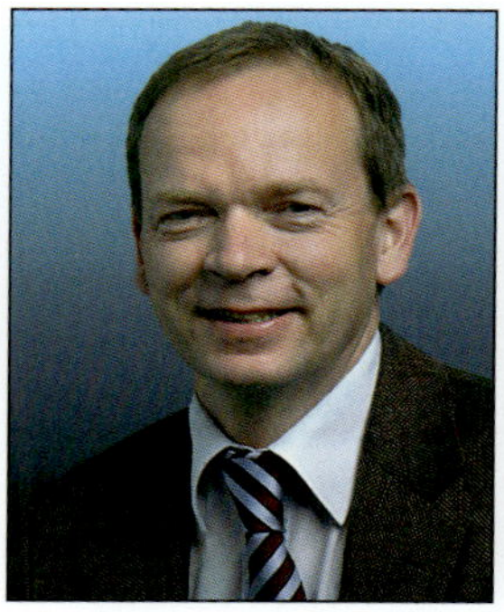

H.-U. Simon
Bern

p. 193

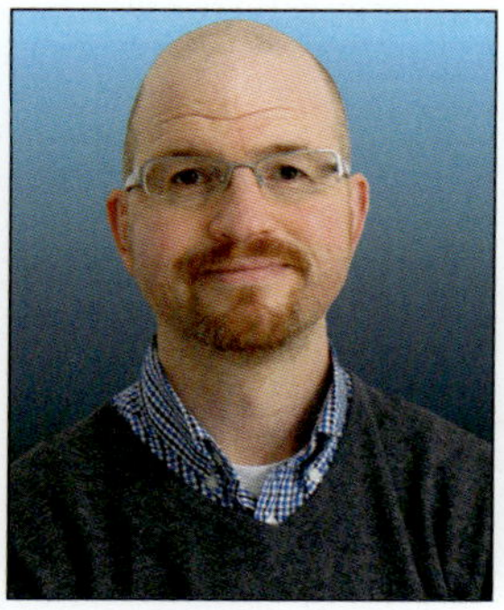

M. Smith
Vienna

p. 228

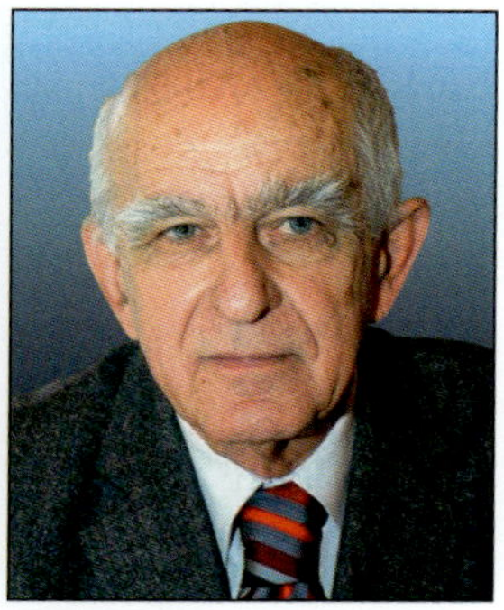

V. Špičák
Prague

p. 373

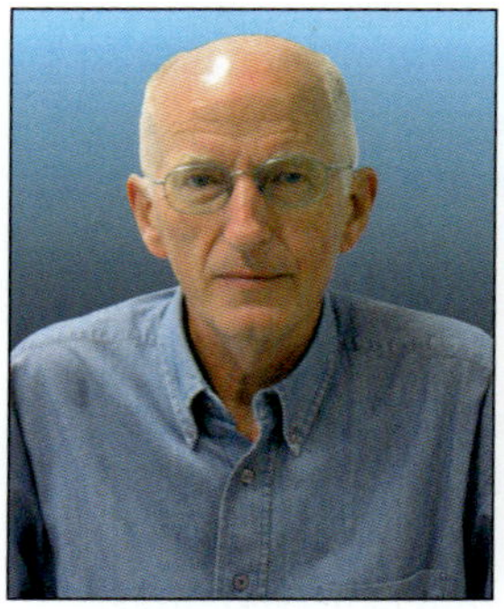

K. Starke
Freiburg

p. 288

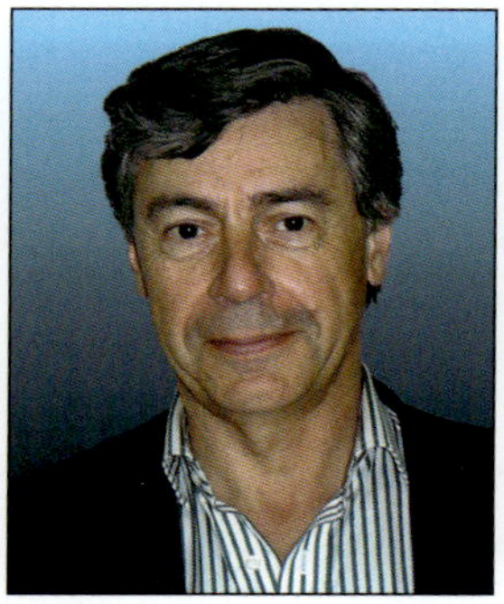

A. Taïeb
Bordeaux

p. 81

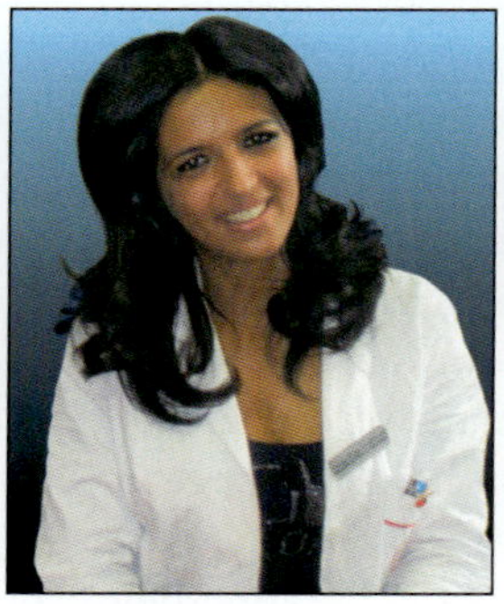

G. Varricchi
Naples

p. 172

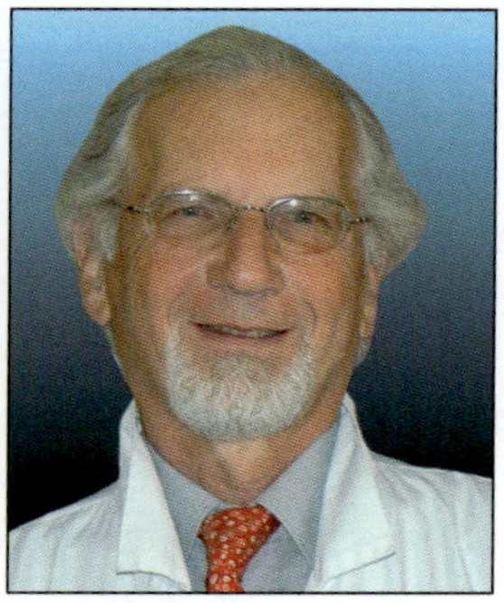

D. Wallach
Paris

p. 81

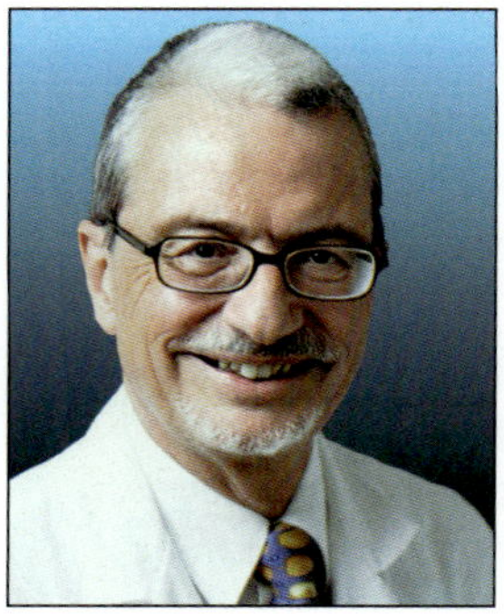

B. Wüthrich
Zurich

p. 109

Preface

Allergies are not new diseases; they have been around for probably 1,000 years or more. However, they have increased in prevalence in a dramatic way over recent decades, leading them to be called by some 'the epidemics of the 21st century'. The questions of how they looked in clinical manifestations, what they were called and how they were treated becomes more and more difficult to answer the farther back in history we go. This is a common challenge in the history of medicine; yet there is an unusual dimension in the case of allergic diseases because they have only been understood in their pathophysiological entity since the beginning of the 20th century. Therefore, terminology may be more difficult in this field than in other disciplines of medicine.

The number of sufferers and the number of allergies is rising all over the world. Additionally, the field of allergology, although relatively young in comparison to others, such as surgery or internal medicine, is growing rapidly. It unites thousands of doctors at world congresses, who devote themselves to the recognition and treatment of allergic illnesses.

It follows a good tradition when a publisher selects a special topic for the 100th volume of a series. Therefore, what could be more appropriate than this book, *History of Allergy*, for the 100th volume of the proud series 'Chemical Immunology and Allergy'?

There are different ways to approach the history of a medical discipline. The purely historical approach deals with the facts, the characters, the lives of 'heroes', the great discoveries and the famous patients. The philosophic approach digs deep into the understanding of diseases and symptoms at different times in the past, often connected with general philosophical attitudes and sometimes also religious beliefs. In this context, terminology also becomes very important since it illustrates the philosophical attitudes of certain times and of great thinkers. At the center of the natural-scientific approach are the great discoveries and progress made in the understanding of natural phenomena, be they physiologic or pathologic in nature. It is in essence the pathophysiological approach trying to find causes for and mechanisms of diseases – progress which only occurred in the field of allergy in the 20th century (with limited exceptions in the 19th century). Finally, the clinical-medical approach refers to the description of symptoms, the hard work of classification, and the art of diagnosis and therapy.

This book represents a mixture of all these approaches. The editors did not want to limit the dialogue to merely the famous stories of great researchers and physicians in this field, and some of their great discoveries. The further we go back in time, the more important the historical approach becomes, in which we have to rely totally upon old scriptures. The philosophical approach is also important in order to understand the thinking of our ancestors. The more recent the period in history we are covering, the more natural science oriented and medical-clinical the text will be. Historical reflection is also given to recent decades, such as in review articles focused on the state of the art in a certain field.

In such a multi-authored book that deals with facts and events and lives that passed many years or centuries ago, it is natural that there are discrepancies with regard to certain events – personal recollections may differ from historical reality even in the life of a Nobel laureate. Great discoveries will also be remembered differently by different researchers, considering that they might be made in different parts of the world using quite different approaches and methods.

The editors gave the authors absolute freedom in the way they wanted to approach the subject. They did not interfere – as they maybe would have done in a textbook of clinical medicine – when they found discrepancies between different chapters. It is left to the reader to decide and form his or her own opinion on the events of the past.

There have been several treatises and essays about the history of allergology, why then one more? The reason for this is that we, the authors and the publisher, were inspired by the task 'not only to protect the cinder but to fan the glow', as was so appropriately expressed by Benjamin Franklin, following the belief of St. Thomas More (1477/78–1535) that 'tradition is not the holds of the cinder, but transmitting the flame'. With this book we weave together hope not only to transmit the flame of enthusiasm for allergology, but also to fan the glow. We all have a passion for the field of allergology, we treat our patients with real enthusiasm, and we look with admiration and pride at the achievements of our medical predecessors, the early allergists. In ancient times they diagnosed and treated based on sense and feeling, and certainly sometimes on need. Even in the Middle Ages, cause and effect was recognized in isolated cases. Since then, new diagnostic and therapeutic methods have been developed with ever greater frequency and rapidity up to present, modern times. In this book we intend to show this development of allergologic science over time, and to remind of its successes as well as its failures.

This is not a pantheon of allergology with biographic representation of all essential allergists and scientists, but we have asked the still living 'pioneers' in the field to participate in a personal reflection. Our special thanks and recognition go to them. The editors are aware that there are many additional dignified personalities worthy of inclusion in the 'pioneers of allergy' section! One criterion was that they should be retired from ordinary daily work in their profession in order to express their view with a certain distance to past events. Unfortunately, one of the pioneers recently passed away before the book was finished: Alain de Weck sent us his reflections as always with his typical precise descriptions and a sharp sense of humor. He also fostered the history of our specialty by producing the marvelous book, *Ancestors of Allergy*, edited by E. Simons, as well as the movie on the history and many facets of allergy presented at the World Allergy Congress (then International Congress of Allergology and Clinical Immunology; IAACI) in Stockholm in 1994 [see www.karger.com/chial100_movie2 and this vol., pp. 411–412]. OSM

In Germany, no one did more to promote the history of allergy than Hans Schadewaldt (1923–2009), to whom the editors are greatly thankful. His book *Geschichte der Allergie* in 4 volumes is an infinite treasure box.

This book is dedicated to all allergists all over the world, and to their patients. Together, they form the basis for this work. There can be no history without researchers and their pioneering inventions, nor without patients, who have served to understand this illness together with their doctors, enabling case reports and participating in studies to determine the effects of new drugs. To all of you, and for all your help with this book, we thank you.

The editors want to thank several individuals, without whom this work would not have been finished. First of all we want to mention Thomas Karger the publisher, who generously supported this project from the beginning. In the publishing house – without the enthusiasm and help of Thomas Nold, Miriam Schulz and Ruedi Jappert – we could not have handled such a large volume of manuscripts of so different character. We also want to thank Dr. Antonia Todorova and Dr. Tanja Müller for their help in providing literature, references and permission to reprint figures.

Two personalities in particular have influenced, motivated and helped both of us over the past decades in the strive to look back on our history in order to better understand what is going on right now, and what will possibly occur in the future. They are Prof. Dr. Dr. Hans Schadewaldt (Düsseldorf), as a historian dedicated to allergy, and Prof. Dr. Alain de Weck (Bern), as the number one allergist and such a formative character over so many decades!

Finally, we ask our readers for constructive criticism if mistakes should have crept into the book. All authors and the publishing company have tried to appreciate the international rules of copyright. We would therefore like to apologize if any errors have been made.

With this book we hope to encourage not only allergists and allergic patients to reflect upon these diseases, but also young scientists and physicians to become enthusiastic for this exciting field, with its interdisciplinary character and its interface between genetics and the environment. May this book help to increase the understanding of so many cumbersome diseases and, thereby, be helpful to millions of patients suffering from allergies!

Karl-Christian Bergmann, Berlin
Johannes Ring, Munich

1 Allergy through 20 Centuries

Bergmann K-C, Ring J (eds): History of Allergy. Chem Immunol Allergy. Basel, Karger, 2014, vol 100, pp 2–14
DOI: 10.1159/000358422

History of Allergy in Antiquity

Johannes Ring

Department of Dermatology and Allergy Biederstein, Christine Kuehne Center for Allergy Research and Education (CK-CARE), Technical University of Munich, Munich, Germany

Abstract

Allergic diseases are not new. They have been described in the early medical literature in various cultures like Egypt, China, indigenous America and in the Greco-Roman tradition. The terms 'idiosyncrasy', 'asthma' and 'eczema' are still in use today. The most famous allergic individual of antiquity with the whole triad of atopic diseases and a positive family history of atopy probably was Emperor Octavianus Augustus.

Today allergic diseases represent one of the major health problems in most countries of the world [1]. They are often regarded as typical diseases of civilization. The impression can be gained that these diseases did not exist in the past and have developed as totally new entities. In this article we want to show that – although probably much rarer – the actual symptoms and clinical conditions of allergic diseases already existed 2,000 years ago.

This is not a scientific historical investigation – the analysis is difficult because there are no classical 'publications'. The descriptions in the literature are often imprecise and we do not have photographs or pictures. However, from the description of symptoms as well as the information regarding therapeutic strategies, conclusions can be drawn with regard to suspected diseases.

This article is based on the excellent work of the chairman of the Institute for History of Medicine at the University of Düsseldorf, Prof. Dr. Dr. h.c. Hans Schadewaldt, who devoted his life to the history of allergy as well as other textbooks of medical history [2–5].

We will proceed by considering different cultural regions. In the following we briefly want to show which symptoms or diseases regarding allergy have been described in antiquity, which therapeutic regimens were used and, finally, whether there have been historically identified individuals who were affected by allergic diseases.

Mesopotamia

According to many authors the cradle of culture – at least of Western culture – was in the area between the rivers Euphrates and Tigris when the Sumer people formed cities. Health and disease in antiquity were often related to religion – physicians were often priests and disease was commonly regarded as a consequence of sin.

In Mesopotamia, three means of disease development were known:

- the direct influence of gods,
- the withdrawal of divine protection, and
- the effect of black magic.

Breathing also had a very special importance. On old cuneiform script tablets therapeutic recommendations against cough and dyspnea can be found. An example is given here:

> When the patient suffers from cough, he should drink a mixture of *Lolium* and rose powder dissolved in oil and honey. Afterwards he should eat a broth of pork meat. When he has to defecate, a fire should be lighted where he should direct his anus. Then he will be cured. [2, vol. 1, p. 96]

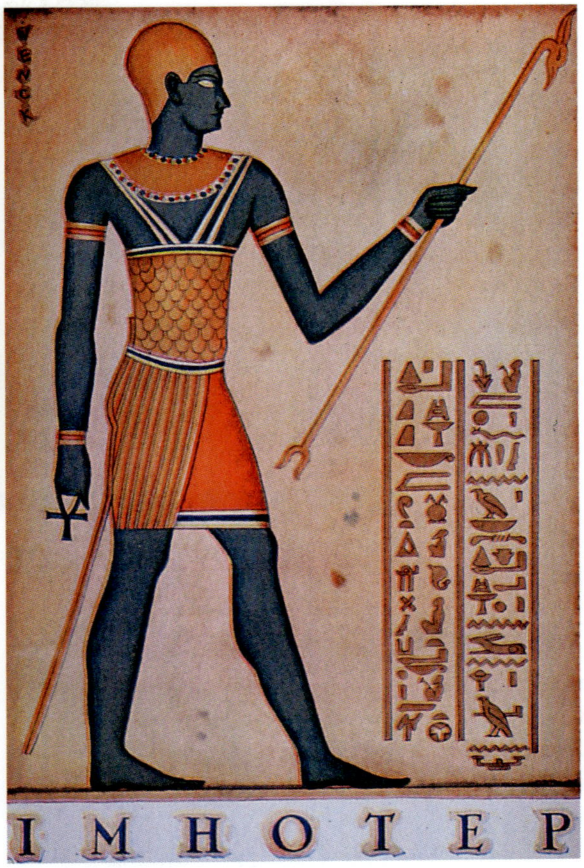

Fig. 1. Imhotep, deified priest from Old Egypt.

Egypt

Similar to Mesopotamia, physicians and priests in Egypt were often the same. Medical knowledge was supposed to originate from the god Thoth and was collected for history by Imhotep around 2700 BC in the third dynasty (fig. 1). Sir William Osler called Imhotep the 'first physician as a person which clearly appears in antiquity' [5, p. 40]. The Greeks identified Thoth with their god Hermes, whom they called three times great 'Trismegistos'. The books which contained his wisdom were known as the *Hermetic Collection.*

Although we do not know a lot about the teachings of Imhotep himself, he can be regarded as the first documented physician (fig. 1). Two or three centuries later we might have evidence for the first allergist, namely the Egyptian Sekhetnankh (Sekaetenanch) who was treating nasal disease as the personal physician of Pharaoh Sahura of the 5th dynasty. We find Sekhetnankh and his wife in stone at the tomb of the Pharaoh with the inscription 'he cured the noses of the kings' [6]. The pyramid of Pharaoh Sahura is located in Abusir, around 17 km to the south of Cairo [7].

People in Egypt estimated tradition very highly and accepted the high authority of existing texts. So, although some documents date from later times (from the new kingdom after 1650 BC), one can assume that they originated in much earlier times.

One of the most important documents of medical literature in old Egypt is the *Papyrus Ebers* (17th dynasty, 1650–1652 BC; fig. 2) which was bought by the German Egyptologist Georg Ebers for the museum of the city of Leipzig [8]. The *Papyrus Ebers* is more than 20 m long and contains 108 columns of text. A lot of therapeutic regimens are described which can also be used for the treatment of asthma. Therefore, many researchers believe that asthma was known in Egypt. The *Papyrus Ebers* was found in 1862 near Theben, between the legs of a well-preserved mummy. It was known in antiquity and quoted in the 2nd century AD by St. Clemens from Alexandria, who described it as a collection of the worldly wisdom of the god Thoth.

A total of 21 prescriptions against cough or dyspnea can be found, 12 of which name honey, dates, inhalation of myrrh and incense, as well as onions, ju-

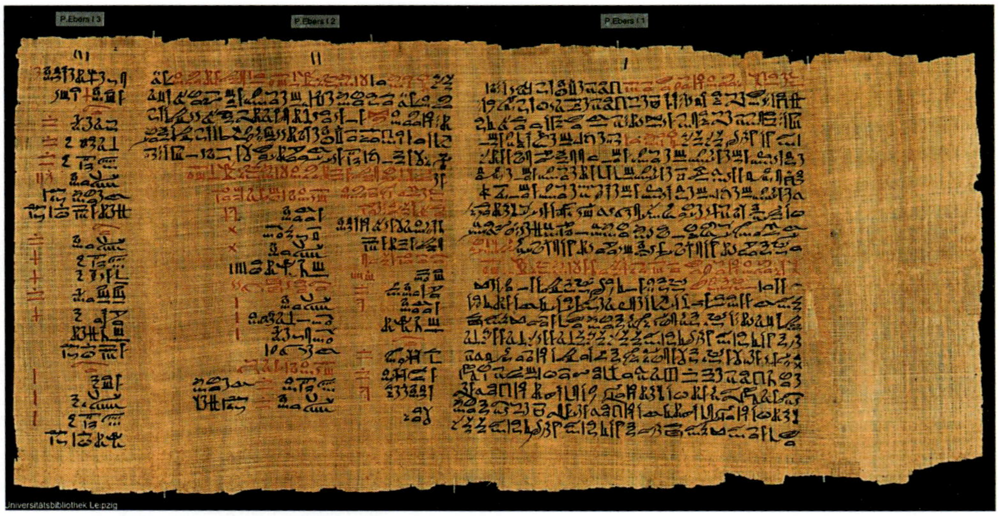

Fig. 2. Hieratic script from the *Papyrus Ebers*, in which remedies for asthma are described.

niper and beer. Against a 'running nose', lavations with palm wine were recommended, as well as topical application of smashed dates. Ebbell [8], who was a rather liberal translator, used 'asthma' for some not well-described diseases that were translated by Joachim [9] as 'major weakness'. Here is an original quotation:

> Thou shalt take seven stones and heat them by the fire, thou shalt take one of them and place a little of these remedies on it and cover it with a new vessel the bottom of which is perforated and place a stalk of reed in this hole; thou shalt put thy mouth to this stalk, so that thou inhalest the smoke of it. Likewise with all stones. [5, p. 43; 8]

In a prayer of Nefer-Abu, another source for the description of asthmatic dyspnea can be found:

> Day and night I was in her hand. I was sitting like a woman in labor on the birthing chair. I was gasping for air, it did not come to me. [10]

Indigenous Populations in America

Although there are few direct sources, we know of some remedies used by indigenous Indians from the reports of Spanish conquistadors and monks, and can draw conclusions with regard to several diseases. The so-called latex therapy was widely used where physicians used plasters of latex milk which then produced inflammation on the skin and thereby had effects upon internal organs. A curative root which the Spaniards and Portuguese found in South America was the dried root of the Brazilian *Ipecacuanha* (Cephaelis), which has strong expectorating properties that are used against cough to this day. In Mexico some other substances were used for inhalation:

> He who is troubled by a dripping nose or coryza is to sniff the herbs atochietl and tzompili-huizxihuitl and help thus against the coryza. [5, p. 58]

Another weed used against airway disease was tepopote, probably related to ephedra. The Indians also used dried leaves of *Erythroxylon coca*, which contains the alkaloid cocaine. Cocaine was used at the end of the 19th century with remarkable effects against rhinitic complaints.

A small figurine from Nayarit culture in the western part of Mexico dated to about 400 AD might represent a patient suffering from an asthma attack, with wide eyes and bent arms to support breathing. However, according to Prof. H. Krumbach from the Institute for American Ethnology, University of Düsseldorf, this is from a tomb and is not a didactic piece for physicians [7] (fig. 3).

China

According to the Chinese tradition, civilization was formed by ancient 'heroes', probably of legendary character. The three emperors, Fu Xi, Shen Nong and Huang Di, were regarded as fathers of traditional Chinese medicine.

In a dialogue of the Yellow Emperor (Huang Di) with his minister Qi Po in their *Su Wen* (meaning 'open questions'), there is an interesting part alluding to airway disease, possibly asthma, with even seasonal character:

> When the disease is located within the lungs, it should improve during winter. If it does not improve during winter, it will become more serious in summer. If death does not follow in summer, it can be warded off during the period of the long summer evenings, but the disease will again arise in fall. One should avoid eating and drinking cold things and one should not wear chilly clothing. [5, p. 36; 11]

It is of particular interest that in ancient Chinese medicine, 3,000 or 4,000 years ago, probably in the time of Emperor Shen Nong, the berries of the horse tail plant (ma huang), which were described corresponding to ephedra and are edible (*Ephedra distachya*; fig. 4), were used against a 'plant fever' which occurred predominantly in autumn and was characterized by increased nasal secretions. The drug's active substance ephedrine was isolated in 1878 by Nagai Nagayasi [5].

Other plants used for airway disease in ancient China comprise *Datura stramonium*, *Aconitum sinense* (from Ranuncula) and henbane *(Hyoscyamus)* against cough, and composite mixtures against harmful winds, parasites and diarrhea. Cannabis was used as a sedative. In Chinese medicine nervous disorders can manifest themselves as erythema of the face, red eyes and a running nose.

By feeling the pulse of Jen-Ying it can be measured whether the energy in the body is too superficial. When this is the case, muscle cramps, skin eruptions and tingling paresthesia can occur [2, vol. 1].

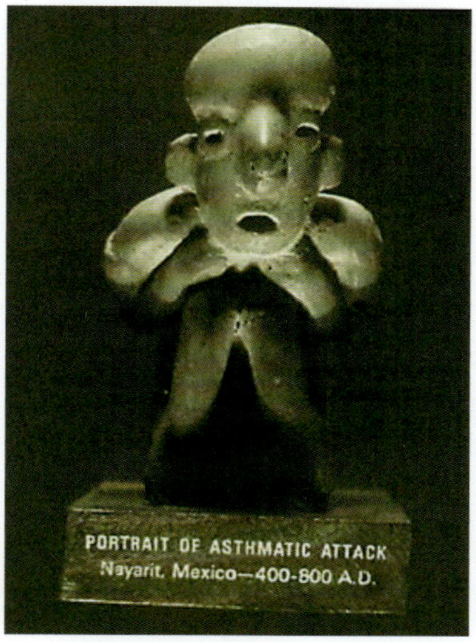

Fig. 3. Portrait of an asthmatic attack from ancient Mexico.

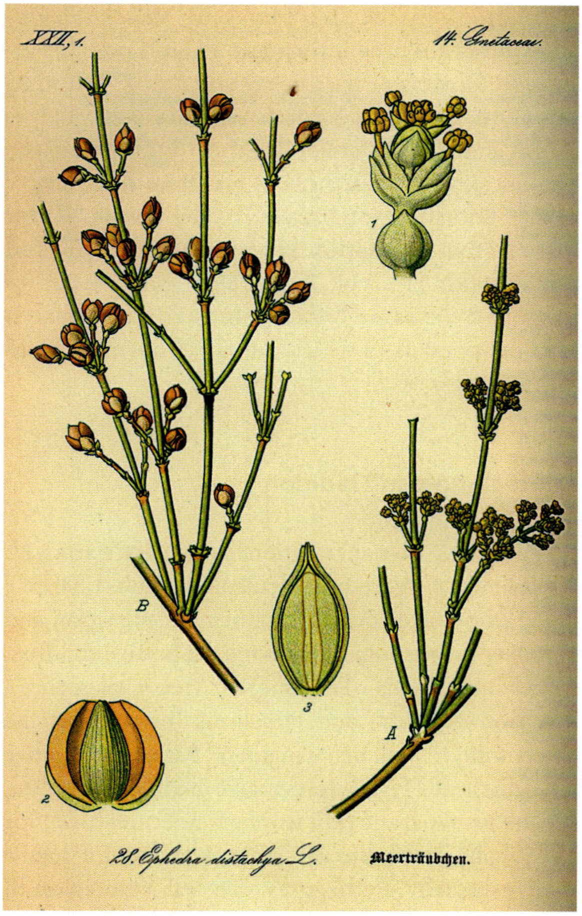

Fig. 4. *E. distachya.*

1

Ancient India

Medicine in ancient India gave special reference to different ways of breathing. The *Vedas* describe five winds: the Prana, Apana, Vyana, Samana and Udana.

All these words derive from the word 'breath'. Müller [12] found indications for heavy or powerful breathing in the *Bower Manuscript*, 350 AD, and in the collections named after the Indian physician Vagbhata, where it is described that patients with breathing difficulties should sit in an erect position in order to gain relief [13].

Allergy in the Bible

In spite of detailed dietary and hygienic recommendations in the five books of Moses *(Pentateuch)*, we find little information about possible allergies. However, in the second book (Exodus, chapter 6, verse 8) it is written that 'Moses told this to the children of Israel; but they didn't hear him because of their shortness of breath and the heavy work'. Shortness of breath in Hebrew is 'Kozer Ruach' (this translation is from Bergson [14] and Schadewaldt [15, vol. 2, p. 189]); Martin Luther translated the same words with 'sighs and fear'. It remains open as to which airway abnormality was meant in this text.

Greek-Roman Tradition

The Greek-Roman tradition in medicine starts with the legendary figure of Aesculapius (1200–1000 BC; fig. 5) who was deified as a charismatic physician and who gave his wisdom to mankind via his five children, namely the sons Telesphorus (reconvalescence), Machaon (surgery) and Podalirius (inventor of the phlebotomy), and his daughters Panacea (curative medicine) and Hygieia (preventive medicine) [2, 4, 16].

The pre-Socratic philosophers not only cared for philosophy and natural science, but also for medicine, especially Pythagoras. Several principles of medicine, which are still of interest today, are derived from this way of thinking, namely:

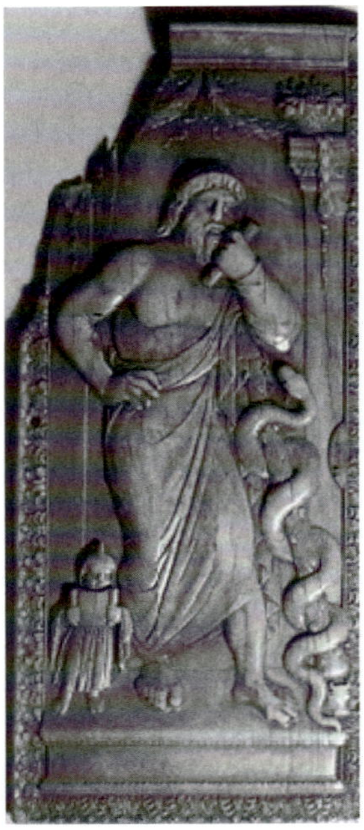

Fig. 5. Aesculapius: a diptych from around 400 AD.

- the so-called hylozoicism, describing common laws for living and dead material which today we would call physical laws;
- the concept of the four elements, fire, water, air and earth (derived from Empedocles) had direct influence upon the tradition of the four humors in the Hippocratic concept;
- that there is an interaction between the things which can be recognized as 'actio' and 'reactio';
- that there is a kind of evolution by which things develop from an origin; this thought is important with regard to the prognostic evaluation of diseases.

Hippocrates (circa 460–377 BC), who was born on the island of Kos, is generally regarded as the 'father of medicine' (fig. 6). He introduced the observation of the patient and the registration of symptoms into medicine. His work gave rise to various schools of medicine, the most important of which were the school of Knidos and the school of Kos, and is summarized in a collection of over 60 texts, the so-called *Corpus Hippocraticum*, translated by Littré [17] (see also Toellner [2, p. 303]).

The original parts, probably originating from himself, are the so-called *Aphorismata*, of which the most famous one is the following:

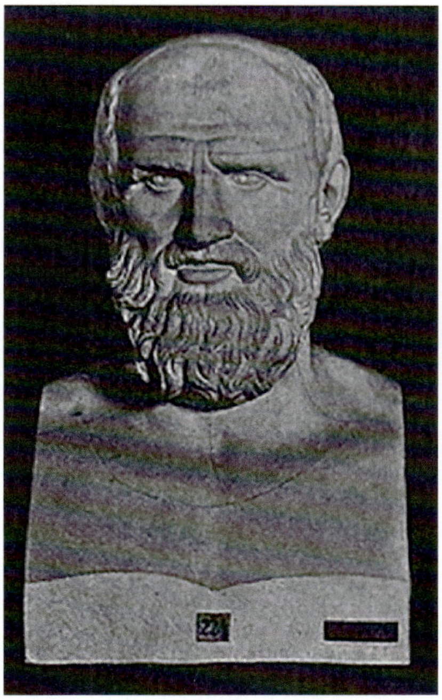

Fig. 6. Portrait of Hippocrates.

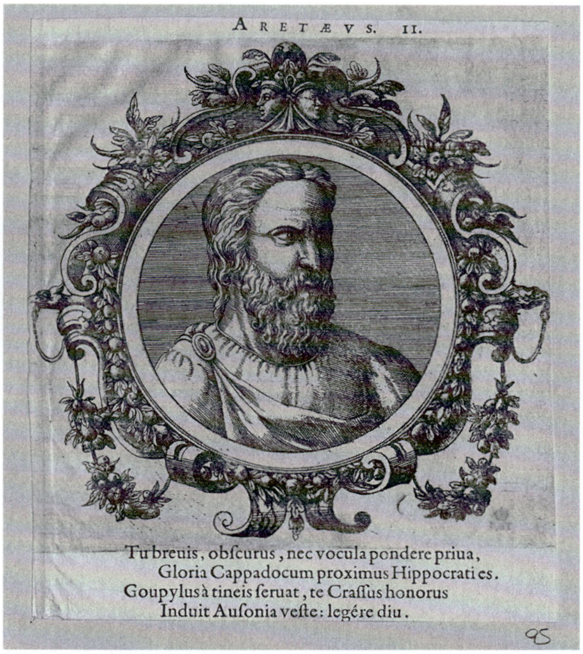
ARETÆVS. II.
Tu breuis, obſcurus, nec vocula pondere priua,
Gloria Cappadocum proximus Hippocrati es.
Goupylus à tineis ſeruat, te Craſſus honorus
Induit Auſonia veſte: legére diu.
95

Fig. 7. Aretaeus from Cappadocia.

> Time is short, art is long, occasions are vanishing and the decision is difficult.

The most famous work of Hippocrates is probably his oath which is, with minor modifications by the World Physicians Organization, still quoted by many medical students when they receive their certificates, for instance at the Medical Faculty of the Technical University of Munich.

The Hippocratic texts came via the city of Alexandria to Rome, where Greek physicians soon took over the healthcare. In Rome the names of Aulus Cornelius Celsus, who was actually an encyclopedist, as well as Aretaeus from Cappadocia (fig. 7) and finally Claudius Galenus (129–199 AD; fig. 8) have to be mentioned. The latter came from Pergamon via Corinth to Rome and became the physician of the Emperor Marcus Aurelius. But what can we find in these texts [18, 19] with regard to allergy or allergic disease?

Hay Fever/Rhinitis

There is no typical description of hay fever or seasonal rhinitis in these texts [17–19]. However, Hippocrates believed that conditions exist where the 'phlegm' which originates in the brain flows down via the nose to the lungs. The lungs would then be obstructed in the form of a strong 'catarrhus', which can be translated as 'flowing down' (similar to the term 'rheuma', which also means flowing movement).

Some others see an indication for the existence of hay fever in a text of Galen regarding the nose (peri osfresios organon) [15, 19]. However, it is most likely the effect of rose aroma and odor which may be able to cool the head when it is too hot in the sense of the principle 'contraria contrariis curantur'. The fact that a description of classical hay fever symptoms cannot be found in the entire *Corpus Hippocraticum* may either mean that they did not exist or that they were so transient that they were not a matter of importance to be mentioned to the physicians,

Fig. 8. Claudius Galenus.
Fig. 9. Aulus Cornelius Celsus.

8 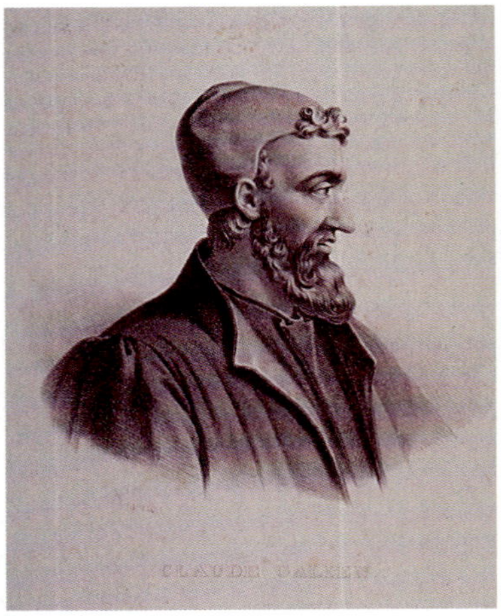

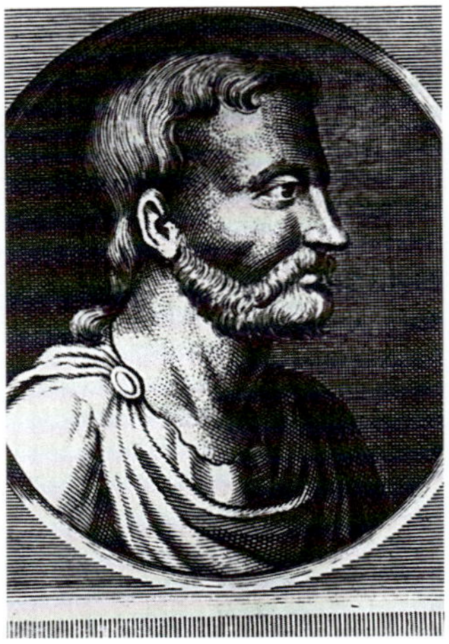 9

who rarely stayed at the same place over a longer period, but instead traveled from one place to another.

Herodotos

In the work of the father of history, Herodotus, one can find a single episode where he describes acute nasal problems in the Athenian traitor Hippias, who led the Persians to Marathon and, while he was directing the disembarkation of the Persian forces, was supposed to have suffered from an attack of nasal symptoms:

> While he was engaged in drawing the troops up in formation he had a fit of sneezing and coughing that was more intense than usual. Since he was of old age, most of his teeth were loose, and he lost one of them during his violent coughing; when he saw it falling into the sand he went to a great deal of trouble to find it again.

This text was discovered by Dr. Salazar Mallén and Dr. Cueva, who also speculated that pollen from *Helianthus annus* might be the cause of an attack of allergic rhinitis in the soldier Hippias in the year 490 BC [20, 21].

Plinius the Elder gives a report on the medical practice of the Greeks in his *Historia Naturalis*, where he writes that pollen, which he recognized as essential for the fertility of plants, may give rise to airway disturbance [5]. The reliability of this quotation, however, is questionable.

Marcus Terentius Varro

An interesting theory was brought forward by the Roman Scholar Marcus Terentius Varro, who lived at the time of Julius Caesar, when he wrote:

> In damp places grow very small animals, so tiny that they cannot be seen by the eye. Floating in the air that we breathe, they pass through the nose and the mouth into the body, where they give rise to serious diseases. [21, p. 31]

Asthma

The term 'asthma' can be found in Homer's *Iliad*, where he describes the loud noise of breathing during physical exercise in battle [15, 22]. There is also a note that asthma can be found in older children [23].

In the translation of the *Corpus Hippocraticum* by Littré [17], the term 'asthma' or 'asthmata' can be found ten times, sometimes in relation to diseases occurring in autumn or in the sense of increased respiratory frequency or 'panting'. On one occasion a breathing noise is described 'as if somebody was whistling through a pipe'. The patient 'is opening his nostril like a galloping horse, the tongue is hanging out like in a dog which suffers under the scorching heat of the air' [17].

Celsus (fig. 9) also gives a clear definition of asthma:

> Asthma is 'the inability to breath without making noise'. [18]

Aretaeus from Cappadocia

The first exact description of classical asthma comes from Aretaeus from Cappadocia, who practiced in Alexandria and Rome, and whose documents were rediscovered in 1954. He very exactly describes a disease which he calls 'asthma' or 'orthopnea'. Here is a part of his original description, from *Excerpts of Classics in Allergy* [24]:

> If from running, gymnastic exercises, or any other work, the breathing becomes difficult, it is called *Asthma*; and the disease *Orthopnoea* is also called *Asthma*, for in the paroxysms the patients also pant for breath. The disease is called *Orthopnoea*, because it is only when in an erect position that they breathe freely; for when reclined there is a sense of suffocation. From the confinement in the breathing, the name *Orthopnoea* is derived. For the patient sits erect on account of the breathing; and, if reclined, there is danger of being suffocated.
> The lungs suffer, and the parts which assist in respiration, namely the diaphragm and thorax, sympathize with them. But if the heart be affected, the patient could not stand out long, for in it is the origin of respiration and of life.
> The cause is a coldness and humidity of the spirit; but the *materiel* is a thick and viscid humor. Women are more subject to the disease than men, because they are humid and cold. Children recover more readily than these, for nature in the increase is very powerful to heat. Men, if they do not readily suffer from the disease, die of it more speedily. There is a postponement of death to those in whom the lungs are warmed and heated in the exercise of their trade, from being wrapped in wool, such as the workers in gypsum, or braziers, or blacksmiths, or the heaters of baths.
> The symptoms of its approach are heaviness of the chest; sluggishness to one's accustomed work, and to every other exertion; difficulty of breathing in running or on a steep road; they are hoarse and troubled with cough, flatulence and extraordinary evacuations in the hypochondriac region; restlessness; heat at night small and imperceptible; nose sharp and ready for respiration.
> But if the evil gradually get worse, the cheeks are ruddy; eyes protuberant, as if from strangulation a *râle* during waking state, but the evil much worse in sleep; voice liquid and without resonance; a desire of much and of cold air; they eagerly go into the open air since no house sufficeth for their respiration; they breathe standing, as if desiring to draw in all the air which they possibly can inhale; and, in their want of air, they also open the mouth as if thus to enjoy the more of it; pale in the countenance, except the cheeks, which are ruddy; sweat about the forehead and clavicles, cough incessant and laborious; expectoration small, thin, cold, resembling the efflorescence of foam; neck swells with the inflation of the breath; the praecordia retracted; pulse small, dense, compressed, legs slender: and if these symptoms increase, they sometimes produce suffocation, after the form of epilepsy. [25]

Galen's role with regard to asthma consists mainly in following the tradition of the Hippocratic concept with the flowing down of phlegm from the brain to the nose and lung leading to airway disturbance. The Roman physician Caelius Aurelianus (circa 400 AD) gave clear recommendations with regard to climatotherapy – he recommended stays at the seaside. He added to the symptomatology of asthma the presence of expiratory noises, thoracic pain and the feeling of anxiety [26].

Others who described asthmatic airway disturbances are Dioskurides and Oreibasios [3]. The following substances are mentioned among various therapeutics against breathing disturbance: 'purgatives, wine, incense, sulfur, ysop, mint, abrotanus, mustard, onions in honey, emetics, figs, starch, wax and honey'.

Urticaria

Urticaria can be recognized easily by the symptom of acute wheal formation and its similarity to contact with nettles. Early descriptions can be found in Hippocrates:

> The son of Euphranor suffered from skin rash similar to mosquito bites, but lasting shorter. [15]
> After exercise the pain occurs in one or another area on the chest or the back and the body will be covered with wheals like after contact with nettles. [15, p. 48]

Based on this description the disease got the corresponding Greek name derived from the plant 'he knide' and, over centuries, was called 'knidosis'. Aetius from Amida described the acute occurrence of skin lesions looking like the bites of bed bugs, but elicited by the juice of nettle weeds [15].

The famous myth of the death of Heracles (fig. 10) and its relation to the centaur Nessus should also be mentioned here. Nessus was supposed to carry Heracles' wife Deianeira over the river Euenos, but he molested her sexually during this journey. Heracles heard his wife crying out for help and shot the centaur with his arrow. The dying Nessus recommended Deianeira to collect his blood and soak a shirt belonging to her husband in it as a magic aphrodisiac for everlasting love. Maybe Deianeira suspected that this gift was a trick. Anyhow, some years later, when Heracles had an affair with the beautiful Iole, she sent the shirt to her husband in order to regain his love. After Heracles had put on the shirt during a sacrificial meal, he was hit by extreme pain which nothing could alleviate. After many days of raving he finally ordered his son Hyllos to take him home and burn him at the stake [15, vol. 3, p. 47]. It should be mentioned that there are other explanations for this myth and other possible diseases from which Heracles had suffered, such as scleroderma [27].

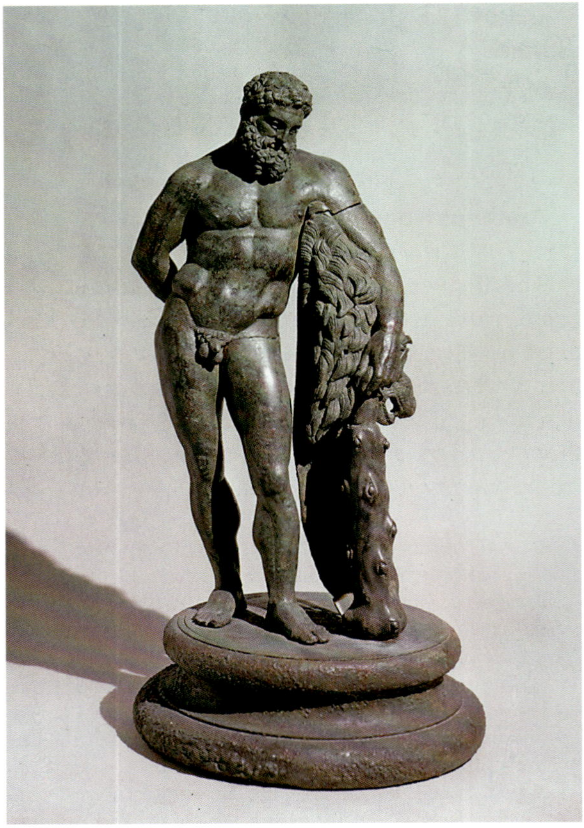

Fig. 10. Heracles.

Food Allergy

When untoward reactions to certain foods or drugs were described in Hippocratic medicine it was mentioned under the term 'idiosyncrasy' [see the chapter by Ring; this vol., pp. 46–52]. There was also an unusual ability to tolerate poisons in a few individuals, while others suffered with severe symptoms from only small doses. Here should be mentioned King Mithridates VI Eupator (132–63 BC; fig. 11), who was afraid of being poisoned and tried to adapt his organism by applying small doses of poison [15, vol. 4; 28]. He is also regarded as the inventor of the famous antidote, the 'Mithridate', which contained 54 different ingredients and was used over centuries.

When Mithridates finally lost the battle against Pompeius at the river Euphrates, he wanted to commit suicide. However, poison did not work and he had to ask his slave to kill him with a sword. Therefore, some authors regard Mithridates as an early precursor of the concept of 'hyposensitization' [29].

It was well known that individuals might become sick after eating normal food, as we learn from the poem 'De Natura Rerum' by Titus Lucretius Carus:

> Quod alii cibus est, aliis fuat acre venenum [What is normal food for some, can be deadly poison for others]. [30]

Eczema

Itchy skin conditions which are excoriated and bloody were also described in Hippocratic medicine. The term 'eczema' was first used by Aetius of Amida (circa 600 AD) and means the welling up of soup in a kettle ('ek' = out/up, 'zεo' = live/well).

Only modern pathophysiology and immunohistochemistry show how exact this name from 1,500 years ago describes a phenomenon of an inflammation arising in the dermis, leading to accumulation of fluid in the epidermis and spongiosis as the most characteristic sign of eczema [31].

Famous Allergic Individuals in Antiquity

Apart from the descriptions of disease conditions in medical literature, it is of special interest to know individuals who might have suffered from certain diseases, especially when they are famous in history. Here we want to briefly present 5 individuals:

- Pharao Menes from old Egypt
- Emperor Octavianus Augustus
- Emperor Claudius
- Britannicus
- Philosopher Seneca

It is clear that we do not have medical reports; medical secrecy existed in the Greek-Roman tradition of Hippocrates. It is general information gained from tombs, biographical notes or travel reports which lead us to the conclusion that these persons might have suffered from an allergic disease.

Pharaoh Menes from Egypt

In several allergy textbooks Pharaoh Menes is regarded as the first documented case of lethal anaphylaxis. He died in the year 2641 BC after the sting of a wasp, as can be concluded by the hieroglyphs from his tomb (fig. 12) [32–36].

This story has been critically commented on by several authors. It begins with the identity of the Pharaoh who, according to other sources, is regarded as founder of the first dynasty and unifier of lower and upper Egypt, and was also known by the name of 'Narner' or 'Aha'. This first dynasty reigned from 3100 to 2890 BC. However, there is a discrepancy as to the date of the tomb, which could be due to a later decoration.

Following the interpretation of Wadell [36], the Pharaoh died suddenly at the age of 63 years at the saltwater lake Birket el Karun near the earlier towns of Crocodilopolis and Arsinoe. His tomb was erected in the town of Saqqara, which was a little farther

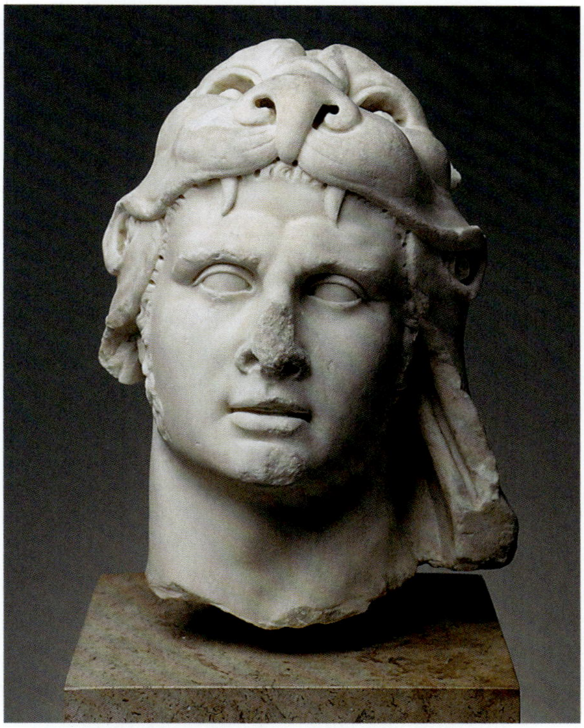

Fig. 11. Mithridates VI Eupator.

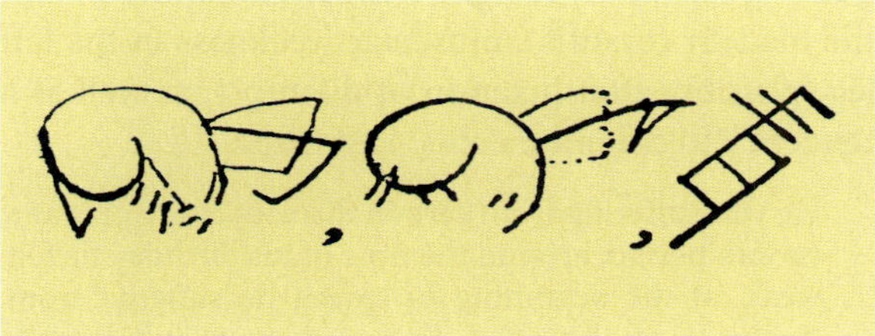

Fig. 12. Hieroglyphs from the tomb of Pharaoh Menes from Egypt (from Wadell [36]).

away. According to Wadell [36] and the corresponding allergological literature the symbols show that the pharaoh indeed died from the sting of a wasp. This does not necessarily mean that he was allergic – a sting into the larynx could also have been fatal. However, when a human being dies from the sting of an insect, it is most likely anaphylaxis.

Another critical question regards the meaning of the hieroglyphs. The symbols could not only mean 'wasp', but also 'hippopotamus'. It is interesting that the Egyptian town 'Hippo' shows a wasp in its emblem. Therefore, the interpretation of the hieroglyphs as an early indication for anaphylaxis can be viewed critically [37, 38].

Emperor Augustus, Emperor Claudius and Britannicus: The First Family History of Atopy in the Julio-Claudian Emperor Family

Octavianus Augustus

Emperor Augustus influenced the world and its history like few other people. After the confusion and the fighting following the death of Julius Caesar he created the Imperium Romanum, which lasted for another 500 years. He must have been extremely intelligent, which might be seen as being associated with atopy by some authors who, as should be mentioned, were mostly allergic themselves.

Suetonius [39] took biographical notes on the first Roman emperors in his book *De vita Caesarum*, and also gave a rather exact description of the physical appearance and the signs of the individuals. Besides the beauty and charismatic appearance of Emperor Augustus (fig. 13), Suetonius [39] mentioned a variety of signs which hint to possible diseases, as for example a large number of naevi, a disease of the liver, a strong sensitivity to light, frequent inflammation of the bladder (cystitis), muscular weakness in the left leg (possibly after luxation of the hip?), as well as a tendency to common colds. He writes:

> He was suffering from certain diseases every year at a certain period; around the time of his birthday he felt weak, at the beginning of spring he suffered from tightness of the chest ('precordiorum inflatione'), during the time of southern winds from catarrhus.

Furthermore, Suetonius [39] describes his skin:

> He also suffered from multiple lichenous skin lesions, which were characterized by extreme itch and had formed under continuous use of a scratching instrument.

Itch is the major symptom of atopic eczema. The seasonal occurrence of catarrhus can be a first indication for hay fever, and 'tightness of the chest' is interpretable as 'asthma'. We conclude that Emperor Augustus showed signs of all three atopic diseases. He also had a positive family history. Family relations in the Julio-Claudian emperor family are complex. It is rather difficult to follow genealogy; however, it is not impossible (fig. 14), and indeed we find two other members of the family with signs for atopy, namely Emperor Claudius and the young Britannicus.

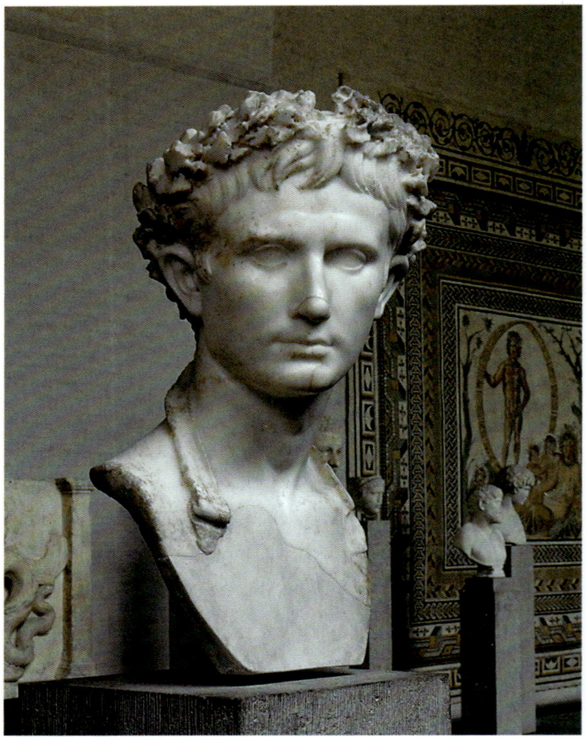

Fig. 13. Emperor Octavianus Augustus.

Emperor Claudius

Emperor Claudius was a great-nephew of Augustus and he is described as suffering from continuous runny nose and episodic acute redness of the eyes, which could be interpreted as perennial allergic rhinoconjunctivitis. Some authors describe him as being not so bright; however, this may be questioned with regard to his rather long life as emperor under the dangerous circumstances of the time, and he probably was, in fact, quite intelligent.

Britannicus

Britannicus was the son of Claudius and Messalina, and thus great-great-nephew of Emperor Augustus. He is supposed to have suffered from horse

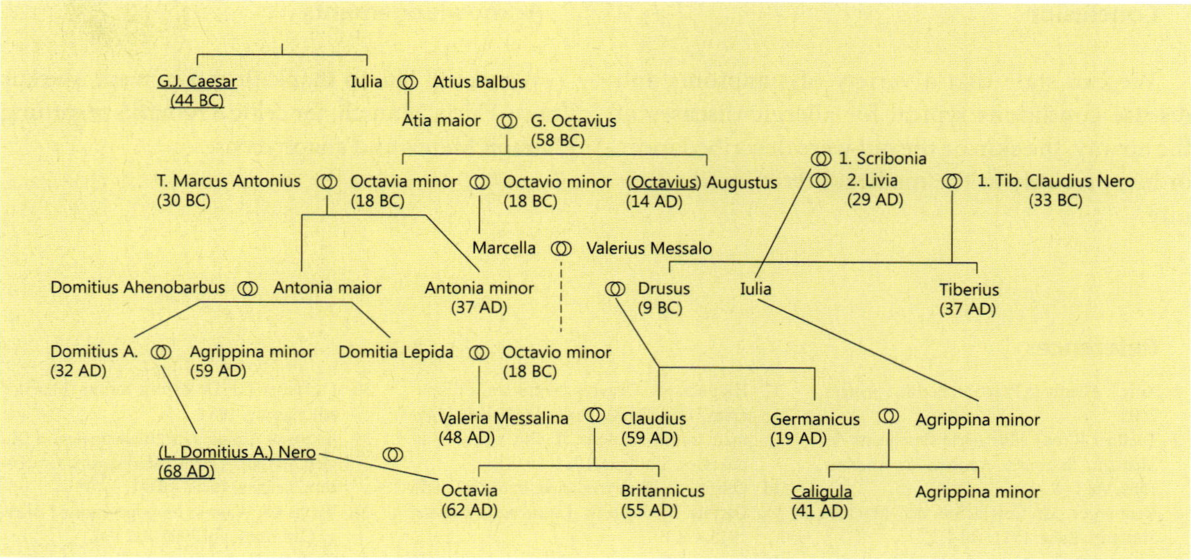

Fig. 14. Genealogy of the Julio-Claudian emperors' family.

allergy and, therefore, was not able to become a strong soldier. However, this information is derived from a historical novel by Mika Waltari who did not give exact references of antique literature [21, 40].

Positive family history is a cardinal criterion for atopic disease. Even if we apply the routine standards of today's genealogy, we can conclude that there was a positive family history for atopy in the Augustus family [41].

Seneca

In many books regarding the history of asthma, the philosopher Seneca (fig. 15) is named as the first asthmatic individual of history. This goes back to a note from Quecke [42] where he describes a disease condition which the philosopher himself describes in the *Moral Letters to Lucilius* [43].

However, it is possible that this condition was not asthma in sensu stricto. Seneca himself tries to find a name for the symptoms and does not use the then already well-known Greek term 'asthma', but rather the Latin word 'suspirium' ('uni tamen morbo quasi adsignatus sum, quem quare Graeci nomine appellem nescio, satis enim apte suspirium dici potest') [15, vol. 2; 43].

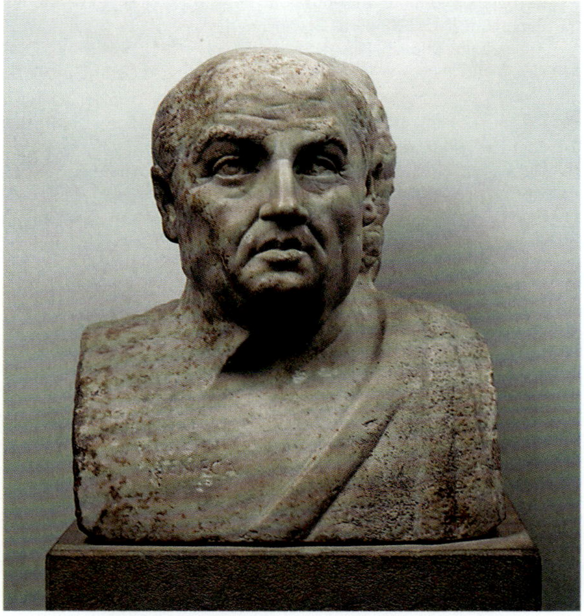

Fig. 15. Seneca.

Conclusion

We can state that a variety of symptoms and disease conditions typical for allergic diseases of the airway, the skin or the gut were described more or less precisely in the medical literature of antiquity.

Acknowledgements

We would like to thank Prof. Dr. med. Markus Braun-Falco, Munich, for critical remarks regarding Pharaoh Menes and anaphylaxis.

References

1 Ring J: Allergy in Practice. Berlin, Springer, 2005.
2 Toellner R (ed): Illustrierte Geschichte der Medizin. Salzburg, Andreas & Andreas, 1986, vol 1–6.
3 Neuburger M: Geschichte der Medizin. Stuttgart, Enke, 1911, vol 1, 2.
4 Diepgen P: Geschichte der Medizin. Berlin, Bergmann, 1949-1955, vol 1–4.
5 Simons E (ed): Ancestors of Allergy. New York, Global Medical Communications, 1994.
6 Stevenson RS, Guthrie Dl: A History of Otolaryngology. Edinburgh, Livingstone, 1949.
7 Bergmann K-C: Bebilderte Geschichte der Allergologie. Munich, Dustri, 2004.
8 Ebbell B: Papyrus Ebers. Copenhagen, 1937.
9 Joachim H: Papyros Ebers: Das älteste Buch über Heilkunde. Berlin, 1840.
10 Federn W: The oldest description of orthopnea. J Hist Med 1959;14:88.
11 Riedlin V: Observationum medicarum centuriae. Obs. 46. Augsburg, 1682.
12 Müller RFG: Kannten die altindischen Ärzte die Lunge? Dudhoffs Arch Gesch Med Naturw 1955;39:134.
13 Müller RFG: Über das indische 'Asthma'. Wiss Z Karl-Marx-Univ Leipzig Math-Naturw Reihe 1955/1956;5:105.
14 Bergson J: Das krankhafte Asthma der Erwachsenen. Nordhausen, 1850.
15 Schadewaldt H: Geschichte der Allergologie. Munich, Dustri, 1983, vol 1–4.
16 Buck AH: The Growth of Medicine from the Earliest Times to about 1800. New Haven, Yale University Press, 1917.
17 Hippocrates: Oeuvres complètes d'Hippocrate (Littré E ed, Paris, 1839–1861; German transl, Kapferer R: Die Werke Hippokrates. Stuttgart, 1934–1938).
18 Celsus AC: De re medicina; in Marx F (ed): Corpus Medicorum Latinorum, Leipzig, 1915, vol 1.
19 Galenos C: Opera (von Kühn CG ed). Leipzig, 1821–1833.
20 Salazar Mallén M, Cueva J: Allergy in the most ancient documents (in Spanish). Alergia 1965;13:1–5.
21 Avenberg KM, Harper DS, Larsson BL: Footnotes on Allergy. Uppsala, Pharmacia, 1986.
22 Homer: Ilias (Bolling GM ed, Lancaster and Oxford, 1950; German transl, Voss JH, ed von der Mühl P). Basel, Birkhäuser, 1953.
23 Fuchs L: Institutionum medicinae, sive methodi ad Hippocratis, Galeni, aliorumque veterum scripta libri quinque. Lyon, 1555.
24 Samter M (ed): Excerpts from Classics in Allergy. Columbus, Ross Laboratories, 1969.
25 Aretaeus: On the causes and symptoms of chronic diseases; in Adams F (ed): The Extant Works of Aretaeus the Capadocian. London, Sydenham Society, 1856.
26 Caelius Aurelianus: De morbis acutis et chronicis. Libri octo (Ammann JC ed). Amsterdam, 1722, vol 3, chapt 1, p 429.
27 Richter P: Geschichte der Dermatologie; in Jadassohn J (ed): Handbuch der Haut- und Geschlechtskrankheiten. Berlin, Springer, 1928, vol 14.
28 Letterer E: Allgemeine morphologische Immunologie. Stuttgart, Thieme, 1969.
29 Ring J, Gutermuth J: 100 years of hyposensitization: history of allergen-specific immunotherapy (ASIT). Allergy 2011;66:713–724.
30 Lucretius TC: De natura rerum (Martin J ed). Leipzig, 1934.
31 Aetius of Amida: Libri medicinales; in Olivieri A (ed): Corpus Medicorum Graecorum. Leipzig, 1935, vol 8.1.
32 Vetter RS: Wasp or hippopotamus? J Allergy Clin Immunol 2000;106:196.
33 Chaffee FH. Insect sting allergy. J Allergy 1969;43:309–310.
34 Cohen SG: The pharaoh and the wasp. Allergy Proc 1989;10:149–151.
35 Whiteley SM: The history of immediate hypersensitivity reactions. Anesthesiology 1995;82:316.
36 Wadell LA: Egyptian Civilization, Its Sumerian Origin and Real Chronology. London, Luzac, 1930, pp 60–63.
37 Krombach JW: Pharaoh Menes' death after an anaphylactic reaction – the end of a myth. Allergy Net 2004;59:1234–1240.
38 Kruszweski J: Up to allergy specialists' consideration: did Pharaoh Menes die of a wasp sting? (In Polish). Pol Merkur Lekarski 2003;14:708–710.
39 Suetonius: GT: De vita caesarum (Ihm M ed, editio minor). Stuttgart, Teubner, 1958, chapt 79–81.
40 Esser A: Caesar und die julisch-claudischen Kaiser im biologisch-ärztlichen Blickfeld. Leiden, 1958.
41 Ring J: Erstbeschreibung einer 'atopischen Familien-Anamnese' im Julisch-Claudischen Kaiserhaus: Augustus, Claudius, Britannicus. Hautarzt 1985;36:470–474.
42 Quecke K: An welcher Krankheit hat Seneca gelitten? Ärztl Praxis 1951;3:12.
43 Seneca MA: Epistulae Morales ad Lucilium. Ep 54 (Hänse O ed). Leipzig, 1898, vol 3, p 15.

Prof. Dr. med. Dr. phil. Johannes Ring
Department of Dermatology and Allergy Biederstein
Biedersteinerstrasse 29
DE–80802 München (Germany)
E-Mail johannes.ring@lrz.tu-muenchen.de

Bergmann K-C, Ring J (eds): History of Allergy. Chem Immunol Allergy. Basel, Karger, 2014, vol 100, pp 15–20
DOI: 10.1159/000358469

History of Allergy in the Middle Ages and Renaissance

Johannes Ring

Department of Dermatology and Allergy Biederstein, Christine Kuehne Center for Allergy Research and Education (CK-CARE), Technical University of Munich, Munich, Germany

Abstract

In the Middle Ages little innovative medical literature came from Western Europe. The Greek-Roman tradition with the scriptures of Hippocrates and Galenos was preserved in Byzantium and then in the Middle East by Arabic medicine; it then returned to Europe in Latin translations mostly made in Italy and Spain. There were innovative developments in Arabic medicine also with regard to the history of allergy, especially with the first description of 'rose fever', which is described as very similar in symptomatology to hay fever. Under Arabic influence, the first medical university in Salerno was famous for its well-known text *Tacuinum sanitatis* in which a description of asthma can be found. With the beginning of renaissance new developments were also registered in Europe, with new observations and a new way of thinking.

History of Medicine in the Middle Ages in the Middle East

When the power and influence of East Rome (Byzantium, Constantinople) decreased, the art of medicine also declined in the Imperium Romanum. At the same time a new power arose, namely the empire of the Caliphate, which soon was to expand all over North Africa, reaching Spain. In its wake a new period of active science and art developed. This period is often called 'Arabic' medicine; however, it should be mentioned that it was the mixture of many ethnicities which made this period so productive, most notably with influences from Persia, Syria and Egypt. The most famous Caliphs were Al-Mansur (750–775), Harun Al Rashid (786–809) and especially Kalif Al-Mamun (813–833) [1]. The most famous personalities of 'Arabic' medicine in the Middle Ages were Al Rhazes, Ibn Sina [2] and Moses Maimonides [3].

Al Rhazes

Born in Raj in Chorasan, Rhazes (865–932) came to Bagdad (fig. 1) where he worked in a hospital and became a famous teacher. He gave the first description of 'rose fever' in his treatise 'Dissertation regarding the course of Coryza occurring in spring, when the roses emit their odor' [4, p. 63; 5, vol. 2, p. 8; 6, 7]. Rhazes also wrote on asthma and gave practical therapeutic recommendations, for example:

> Two drachmae of dried and pulverized fox lung and fig extract mixed to a potion. [8]

Ibn Sina (Avicenna)

The second great personality in the Middle Ages was Ibn Sina (980–1037; fig. 2) who also came from

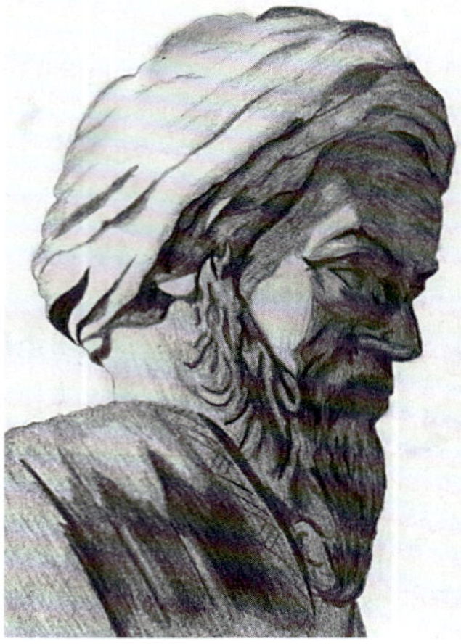

1

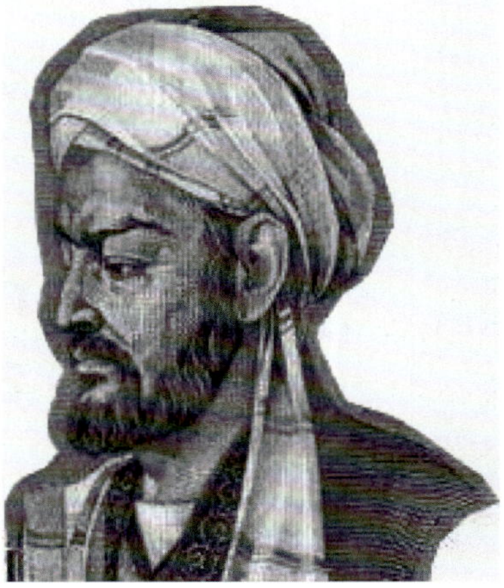

2

Fig. 1. Drawing of Muhammad Zakariya Razi.
Fig. 2. Ibn Sina (Avicenna).

Persia and became famous for his successful treatment of Prince Al-Mansur. Among others, Avicenna described a disease which was very similar to urticaria, namely itchy elevated lesions of the skin which in Arabic were called 'essera' (or 'sora', 'sera' or 'sare'), all derived from the same root 'As-Sarah' (meaning 'mountain' or 'elevation') [2, 5, vol. 3, p. 66]. Avicenna compared an asthma attack with epilepsy and used a word which was translated as 'caducus pulmonum', which fits well with the acute character of this condition.

Moses Maimonides

In the Almohade Caliphate, the Jewish physician Moses Maimon (fig. 3), also called Maimonides, grew up in Cordoba. He later went to Cairo via Morocco and became the personal physician to Sultan Saladin (1135–1204). He wrote a thesis on asthma and presented a concept for treatment which comprised relaxation, personal hygiene, avoidance of noxious environmental influences, avoidance of opium and intoxicating drugs, as well as 'equanimitas mentis', a relaxed state of mind. He recommended asthmatic patients to avoid the following foods: poultry, milk and nuts, whilst he allowed salad, cauliflower and eggplant [3, 4, p. 66; 5, vol. 2, p. 206; 7, 9, 10]. Here is one important passage on treating asthma:

> From what I have heard from others, and as is known to Your Highness, I conclude that this disorder starts with a common cold, especially in the rainy season, and the patient is forced to gasp for breath day and night, depending on the duration of the onset, until the phlegm is expelled, the flow completed and the lung well cleared. This is all I know about the prodromal phases of this illness. You have also told me you were in the habit of taking once or twice a year certain remedies to clear the nose and the lung and often, when resorted to during an attack, these tend to weaken you. I also know that you are about forty years of age, your body build moderate (neither fat nor lean), your bodily vigor about average, that you are rather hot-blooded and your head liable to become easily inflamed. You also remarked that strong winds tend to hurt you and sharp smells offend you much. Hair weighs on you heavily and repeated shaving of the head brings you some comfort. You wear no headdress and no turban, all of which goes to show that your head suffers from excessive heat. Your Highness has already confided in me that the air of Alexandria is harmful to you and whenever you fear an attack of the illness you prefer to move to Cairo where the air is much dryer and calmer, making the attack more tolerable for you. You also told me that many physicians prescribed for you remedies of all kinds, each one of them proclaiming his cure to be the best, but that none of them cured your disorder. …
>
> In all grave disorders marked by seizures, such as lumbago, inflammation of the joints, gravel (in the kidney), asthma (also called shortness of breath), migraine, – in all of them, provided the prescribed regimen is well kept and judiciously applied, the intervals between two onsets may be lengthened, the duration of the onset shortened and its intensity mitigated. However, should the rules of management go unheeded and one's desires and habits be followed indiscriminately, the gap between onset will grow shorter, and the duration and intensity gradually increase until a peak is reached which may well end in death. …

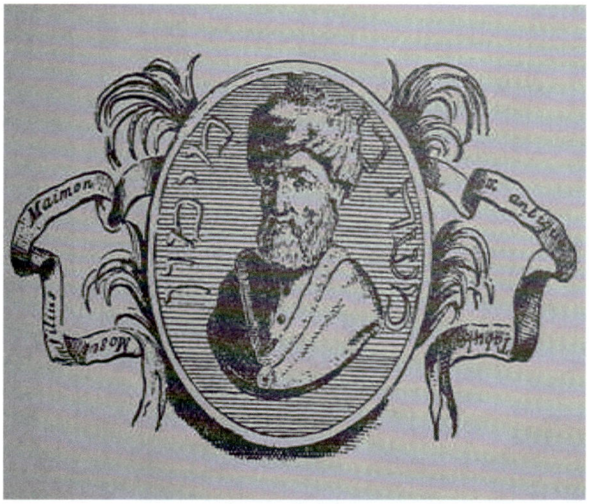

Fig. 3. The purported portrait of Moses Maimonides from which all modern portraits are derived.

> The six obligatory regulations are: (1) keeping clean the air which we breathe; (2) keeping an eating and drinking diet; (3) regulation of spiritual emotions; (4) regulation of bodily exercise, and lastly rest (5) sleep and waking up, (6) excretion, eventually keeping back of superfluous outflow. The seventh group is the one the body takes according to circumstances, such as bathing and massaging. [3]

The Period from 1300 to 1700 BC

One of the most colorful and famous figures from the end of the scholastic period when Arabic medical texts were translated into Latin, predominantly in Italy and Spain, is Arnaldus from Villanova (circa 1235–1311) who was active in Paris, Montpellier and Naples, and was the personal physician of several popes and kings. He wrote a remarkable number of books, among them a treatise *Reginem curativum* and *Praeservativum contra catarrheum* [1, vol. 1, p. 393].

In this period the constitution of a number of 'universities' was gradually improved at Bologna, Naples, Paris, Cambridge, Oxford and Coimbra, with medicine as the 4th faculty next to theology, philosophy and law.

While in Salerno anatomy was studied in pigs, autopsies were soon being performed more and more often in human bodies. The time of just rehearsing antique texts was about to end, and own observations led to an individual and new way of thinking.

In the following century, in England, we find Master John of Arderne (approximately 1306–1381), who worked as a pharmacist and surgeon and gave very detailed prescriptions for treatments, among them a 'sirup for the asthmatic' which contained:

> Root of Iris and hyssop, three handfuls of maidenhair, four seeds of the greater and lesser celandine, coriander seed, mallow seed, seed of the white poppy, cotton, fenugrek, bitter vetch, marmalade of licorice, marmalade of raisins, marmalade of pines and of almonds, and marmalade of husked barley, all which was to be boiled over a slow fire in sweet well water. Arderne claimed that it cleaned, purified, soothed nourished, healed and strenghtened, and drove out discharges. [11, p. 44]

Several books on therapy appeared in Germany in the 14th century, among them *Buch von den natürlichen Dingen* ('The Book of Natural Things') of the episcopal canonicus Konrad von Megenberg from Regensburg (1309–1378). This was like an encyclopedia and comparable to a bestseller towards the end of the Middle Ages. He described a disease called 'asthma' which can be treated with cress ('Nasturtium is nütz für das atem gepresten – der asma haizt') [12].

The 15th and 16th Centuries

Another famous figure of history who was supposedly allergic is King Richard III of England (1452–1485). According to a note by Sir Thomas More (1478–1535), who was the famous law expert of the English crown, Richard knew that he did not tolerate strawberries and reacted with a skin rash. So he uses this phenomenon in the council when he orders a bowl of strawberries and soon thereafter develops wheals on his forearms which he undoubtedly sees as result of an evil spell, and immediately he accuses Lord William Hastings, who is sentenced to death [12, 13].

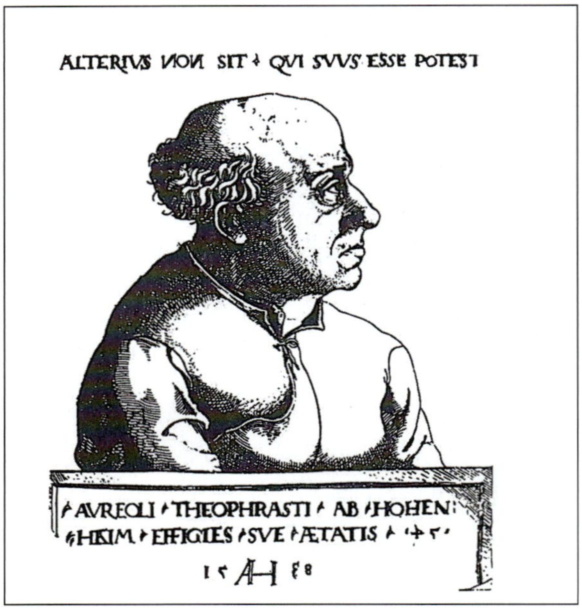
ALTERIVS NON SIT QVI SVVS ESSE POTEST
AVREOLI THEOPHRASTI AB HOHEN
HEIM EFFIGIES SVE ÆTATIS

Fig. 4. Paracelsus.

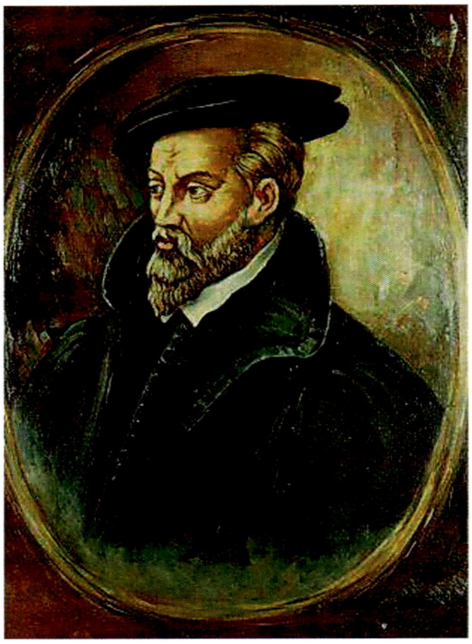

Fig. 5. Georgius Agricola.

A famous name at the beginning of this period is Theophrastus Bombastus von Hohenheim (called Paracelsus; 1493–1541) from Einsiedeln in Switzerland (fig. 4). He recognized that diseases were caused not only by dyscrasia or the wrong mixture of humors within the organism itself, but could also arise from outside. In a pathetic pose he burned the books of Galen and Avicenna. Once he briefly mentioned the noxious effect of rose odor, which he did not regard as a true poison, but as an 'alteration' of the organism [5, vol. 2, p. 12]:

> The roses can pass on their taste and thereby can elicit unconsciousness, while the body of the roses remains unchanged. Although the body of the venom is invisible, the evil is able to weaken the human being by causing serious sickness. [14]

For the skin disease causing wheals, which was known by the name of 'essera', he proposed the name 'Leusschiepen' [5, vol. 3, p. 73; 15]. The German physician Georg Bauer (also called 'Agricola'; 1494–1550; fig. 5) wrote on mining and mineralogy, and also a treatise on the art of mining in which he mentioned occupational airway diseases [4, p. 70].

Rose Fever

Following its first description by Rhazes, rose fever became an entity from the Middle Ages until modern times; in its symptomatology it was very similar to allergic rhinoconjunctivitis of our day. Many authors mention this 'condition' [5, vol. 2]. There are famous personalities, like Cardinal Carafi (who died in 1511), who sealed off his palazzo so that no roses could be brought inside [5, vol. 4, p. 14; 16]. Martin Cromer, who wrote down the history of Poland, mentioned that the archbishop of Wroclaw, Laurentius, died around 1230 after inhaling deadly rose odor [5, vol. 2, p. 16; 17, 18]. Similar descriptions were given by Botallo [19, 20] (fig. 6):

> Nosco sanae homines, qui prorsus rosae odorem, tamquam capitalem inimicum, odio habent eo quod capites dolorem iis faceat, vel sternutamenta moveat, vel navibus tam molestum pruritum inducat. [19]

An interesting episode can be found in the scriptures of Veit Riedlin (1656–1724), the physician of the city of Ulm. A merchant was described who suffered from a prickling sensation in the nose each year as soon as he noticed rose odor. He then suffered from catarrhus for several days which could only be prevented when he avoided contact with roses [5, vol. 2, p. 24; 21]. Riedlin was probably one of the first controlled provocation testers in this case, hiding a pouch of rose leaves in the coat of the patient without him knowing [22].

Rose fever also occurred in pharmacists when they prepared medications containing roses, as we learn from Ramazzini [23], the founder of occupational medicine [5, vol. 2, p. 28]. Amatus Lusitanus described the case of a woman with a very serious condition following a strong reaction to pharmacy containing the blossoms of lime trees, rose water and cinnamon [24].

Another well-known allergic patient was the Archbishop of St. Andrews in Edinburgh, Sir John Hamilton (1511–1571), who was the brother of James Hamilton, regent for the young and minor Queen Mary Stuart of Scotland. He suffered from airway disease at the time when it was considered 'catarrhus of the brain', with an accumulation of phlegm and mucus in the lung which was treated in the classical way. When the Italian physician Gerolamo Cardano (1501–1576) came from Milan his discomfort improved. Cardano documented his advice in a consilium of 20 pages. He removed the feather bed from the bedroom of the archbishop, probably in order to avoid too much heat at the spine. He also recommended dietary restrictions, more sleep and applications of cold water [5, vol. 2, p. 208; 25, 26].

In 1698 the English physician Sir John Floyer (1649–1734) published a book entitled *A Treatise of the Asthmas* in which he differentiated between a continuous and an episodic form of asthma [4, p. 73; 27]:

> I am certain no hot regimen can be proper for asthma, but the cold is very useful, viz. to drink water in the morning, to shave oft and wash the head every morning, and to cold bath in a month or fourteen days. [4, p. 71; 28]

His fellow countryman, Thomas Willis (1721–1675), wrote in his *Pharmaceuticae Rationalis* in extenso on asthma, and he observed that the nerves were also involved in the acute form of asthma:

> Among the diseases whereby the region of the breath is wont to be infested, if you regard their tyranny and cruelty, an asthma (which is sometimes by reason of a peculiar symptome denominated likewise an Orthopnea) doth not deserve the last place; for there is scarce anything more sharp and terrible than the fits thereof; the organs of breathing and the praecordia themselves, which are the foundations and Pillars of Life, are shaken by this disease as by an Earthquake, and so totter, that nothing less than the ruine of the whole animal Fabrick seems to be threatned; for breathing, whereby we chiefly live, is very much hindred by the assault of this disease, and is in danger, or runs the risque of being quite taken away. [4, p. 72]

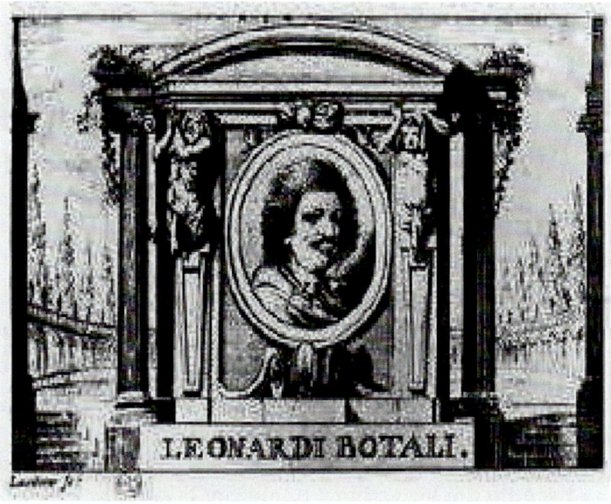

Fig. 6. Leonardo Botallo.

Amatus Lusitanus reported a case of heavy rhinorrhea with mostly aqueous secretion [5, vol. 3, p. 13; 24]. Cornelius Stalpaart van der Wiel (1620–1687) reported a case of 'an almost uncontrollable sneezing cramp (sternutatio) each time after the coitus with his wife' [29]. Giovanni Battista Morgagni (1682–1771) tells us about a patient who suffered from heavy aqueous nasal secretions over months [30].

The Italian physician Matteoli describes a patient in 1570 who was suffering from severe dyspnea due to a tomcat hidden in the same room. The patient developed anxiety, sweating and pallor together with airway symptoms, and he suspected the presence of the animal to be so noxious to him:

> Sed quamvis nec vi disset ille nec audisset catulum, cum pauco post tempore aerem felis alitum infectum inspirasset iritate statim eam temperamenti qualitate felium inimica, emissio, sudore, pallida ad modum facie omnibus sanae admirantibus cremebundus non clamare coepidi aliquo in angula latet felis. [31]

These are clear-cut descriptions of possible allergic reactions against indoor allergens such as feathers from a bed or pets.

The Belgian physician Jan Baptista van Helmont (1577–1644) reported a patient who was suffering from 'summer asthma' and at the same time from strongly itching whitish 'blisters' (probably wheals). It is interesting that van Helmont realized that not only the patient, but also his mother and sister were also suffering from the same symptoms [4]. Van Helmont saw similarities to epilepsy in the cramp-like acute attack, and he also differentiated between moist and dry asthma:

> Est ergo duplex asthma, humidum et seccum. [5, vol. 2, p. 226; 32]

There are more detailed descriptions of symptoms and signs of allergic airway and skin disease from this time which directly lead to the first classic description of allergic rhinitis in the 19th century.

Conclusion

Following the clear-cut descriptions of clinical symptoms very similar to hay fever under the name of 'rose fever' from Arabic medicine with Rhazes, and then over the whole period of the Middle Ages until modern times, more and more precise descriptions of similar disease entities can be found for acute seasonal rhinitis and perennial rhinitis by possible indoor allergens, as well as certain forms of asthma and urticaria.

References

1 Neuburger M: Geschichte der Medizin. Stuttgart, Enke, 1911, vol 1, 2.
2 Avicenna (Ibn Sina): Canon Medicinae (Plempius VF ed). Leuven, 1658.
3 Maimonides M: Treatise on asthma (Magali-vi-l-ra-bu). Historical document. Allergy 1956;14:382.
4 Simons E (ed): Ancestors of Allergy. New York, Global Medical Communications, 1994.
5 Schadewaldt H: Geschichte der Allergologie. Munich, Dustri, 1983, vol 1–4.
6 Elgood C: Persian science; in Arberry AJ (ed): The Legacy of Persica. Oxford, 1953, p 315.
7 Sarton G: Pollen allergy. Isis 1947;38:101.
8 Kamal H: Encyclopaedia of Islamic Medicine, with a Greco-Roman Background. Cairo, 1975.
9 Steinschneider M: Die Hebräischen Übersetzungen des Mittelalters und die Juden als Dolmetscher. Graz, 1956, p 767.
10 Muntner S: The Book on Asthma (Hebrew transl, Benveniste S). Jerusalem, 1940.
11 Avenberg KM, Harper DS, Larsson BL: Footnotes on Allergy. Uppsala, Pharmacia AB, 1980.
12 Bergmann KC, Bergman I, Schadewaldt H (eds): Bebilderte Geschichte der Allergologie. München, Dustri, 1980.
13 More T: The history of King Richard III; in Campbell WE (ed): The English Works of Sir Thomas More. London, Eyre and Spottiswoode, 1931, p 426.
14 Paracelsus von Hohenheim TB: De morbis metallicis; in Opera Omnia. Geneva, 1658, vol 1, chapt 2, p 711.
15 Paracelsus von Hohenheim TB: Von Apostemen, Geschwüren, offenen Schäden, Sironen und anderen Gewächsen, 1527; in von Sudhoff K (ed): Sämtliche Werke. Munich, vol 4, 1931, p 317.
16 Valerianus JP: Hieroglyphica, sive de sacris Aegyptiorum libris commentarii. Basel, 1556, vol 8, chapt 25, p 61.
17 Cromer M: De origine et rebus gestis Polonorum libri triginta. Basel, 1558, vol 8, p 207.
18 Sachs PJ: Gammarologia Curiosa. Frankfurt, 1665, vol 2, chapt 4, p 577.
19 Botallo L: Commentarioli due, alter de medici, alter de aegroti munere. Lyon, 1565, p 25.
20 Major RH: A History of Medicine, ed 1. Oxford, 1954, p 380.
21 Riedlin V Jr: Iter medicum sanitatis recuperandae causa non solum institutum, sed et feliciter finitum. Augsburg, 1702, p 25.
22 Riedlin V Sr: Observatorium medicarum centuriae tres (Riedlin V Jr ed). Augsburg, 1691.
23 Ramazzini B: De morbis artificum diatriba. Padua 1713 (Facsimile, Rome, 1953), Modena 1700.
24 Amatus Lusitanus (Rodriguez de Castello Branco J): Curationum medicinalium centuriae. Lyon, 1567 (first ed Venice, 1557).
25 Cardano G: De vita propria liber. Padua, 1575.
26 Cardano G: Consilia. No 52; in Opera Omnia. Leiden, 1663.
27 Floyer J: Treatise of the Asthma. London, 1698.
28 Floyer J: Essay to prove cold bathing safe and useful. 1706.
29 Stalpaart van der Weil O: Hondert seltsame aanmerkingen, so in de genees-als heelensuij-konst. Cent Post Obs 6. Amsterdam, 1682, p 45.
30 Morgagni GB: De sedibus et causis morborum per anatomen indagatis. Venice, 1761.
31 Mattioli PA: Commentarii in libris Dioscuridis; in Opera Quae Exstant Omnia. Frankfurt, 1598, vol 6, chapt 25, p 996.
32 van Helmont JB: Asthma et tussis; in Ortus Medicinae. Amsterdam, 1648, p 366.

Prof. Dr. med. Dr. phil. Johannes Ring
Department of Dermatology and Allergy Biederstein
Biedersteinerstrasse 29
DE–80802 München (Germany)
E-Mail johannes.ring@lrz.tu-muenchen.de

Bergmann K-C, Ring J (eds): History of Allergy. Chem Immunol Allergy. Basel, Karger, 2014, vol 100, pp 21–26
DOI: 10.1159/000358477

Landmarks in Allergy during the 19th Century

A. Barry Kay

Leukocyte Biology Section, National Heart and Lung Institute, Imperial College, London, UK

Abstract

There were remarkable achievements in the 19th century in our understanding of the cells of the allergic response, the clear descriptions of hay fever and asthma, as well as the role of pollen in seasonal rhinitis. Although allergy as a concept was not developed until well into the 20th century, the foundations of our present understanding of these diseases were laid in the 1800s. The outstanding physicians and scientists of this time included Paul Ehrlich (who described mast cells, eosinophils and basophils), John Bostock (who provided the first detailed account of hay fever), Charles Blackley (who showed that pollen was the cause of hay fever), Morrill Wyman (who demonstrated that autumnal catarrh was due to ragweed pollen), Henry Hide Salter (who made the first classic description of asthma) and Henri Laënnec (the inventor of the stethoscope).

Allergy as an immunological concept did not exist during the 19th century. The idea that antibodies may have a deleterious as well as a protective effect did not develop until well into the 1920s, and even then such ideas were greeted with scepticism. Great advances were made in the understanding of hay fever, asthma and anaphylaxis even though the cellular mechanisms involved were largely unappreciated. A pivotal landmark was the discovery of mast cells, basophils and eosinophils by Paul Ehrlich in the 1870s. Thus, the achievements made during the 19th century were largely those of description and causation, in particular the recognition of pollen as the cause of hay fever and identification of the major cells of allergic tissue reactions.

From about 1800 medical practice underwent fundamental changes in its perception of disease. The old ideas that every disease could exhibit every symptom and that each individual illness was a unique condition were being widely challenged. In 1800 the French surgeon, Xavier Bichat, recognised that disease was a specific phenomenon peculiar to certain tissue lesions. With the launch of systematic

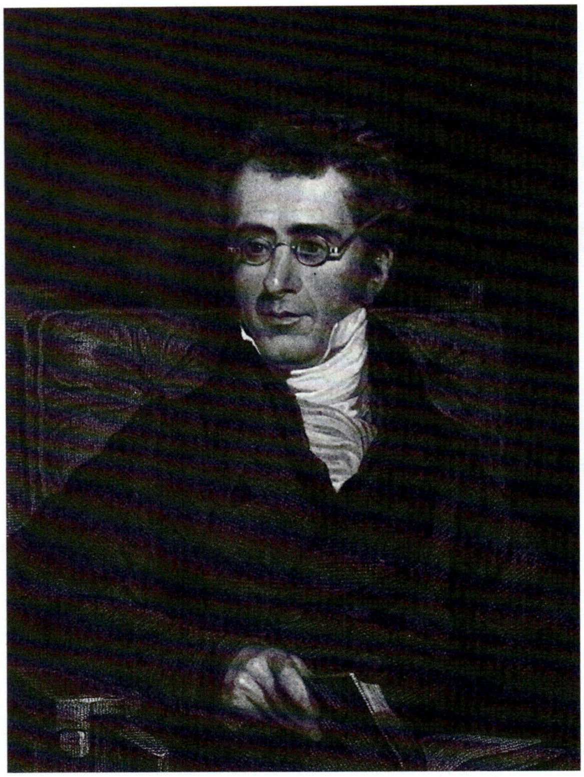

Fig. 1. John Bostock (1773–1846). Described 'catarrhus aestivus', later recognised as summer hay fever.

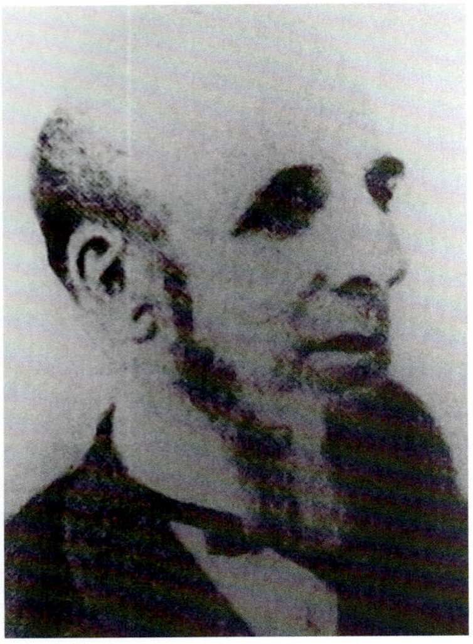

Fig. 2. Charles H. Blackley (1820–1900). Identified pollen as a cause of hay fever and devised methods for pollen counts and clinical challenge tests.

pathology, championed by the great Rudolf Virchow, came the realisation that diseases could be characterised by typical anatomic changes which, in turn, were related to clinical symptoms.

What, then, were the 19th century landmarks which increased our knowledge of hay fever, asthma and anaphylaxis, and what basic scientific advances occurred during this time which set the scene for a greater understanding of allergic diseases during the 20th and 21st centuries?

Hay Fever and Ragweed Pollinosis

Hay fever and ragweed pollinosis are good examples of clinical observation and experimentation leading to the recognition of a specific disease. Although William Heberden had described summer catarrh and asthma as early as 1802 [1], and differentiated it from the common cold, it was John Bostock (fig. 1) who gave the first detailed account of the disease to the Medical Society of London in 1819 [2]. He described the typical eye symptoms, profuse sneezing, itching and tightness of the chest of the hay fever sufferer during the summer months. His preferred name for the condition was 'estival catarrh' but the more popular term 'hay fever' persisted.

Unequivocal evidence that pollen was the cause of hay fever came from the meticulous experiments of Charles Blackley (fig. 2) in the 1870s [3]. A hay fever sufferer himself, he deliberately provoked symptoms by self-exposure to various pollens. He observed that dust stirred up by a passing carriage produced his symptoms and that samples of the dust contained grass pollen. Blackley applied pollen to his nose, eyes, tongue, lips and throat, and inhaled the pollens through his nose and mouth. The symptoms elicited were carefully documented. It became clear that, in general, it was grass pollen and not other pollens which caused hay fever-like symptoms. He went on to abrade his arms with grass pollen and observed lesions which we would now call immediate and late-phase allergic reactions. These skin tests were to form the basis of the standard diagnostic test used by all allergists to this day.

Blackley also invented devices for measuring pollens in the atmosphere and was able to study the effects of sunshine, rain, wind and humidity on the amount of pollen in the atmosphere. Using these instruments he related daily pollen counts to symptoms. Even more ingeniously, Blackley constructed devices for detecting and measuring pollen in the upper atmosphere using a box kite which in turn gave him an explanation as to why sufferers experienced symptoms while out at sea and in other localities free of grass.

The first epidemiological study of hay fever (1873) was performed by Dr. Philip Phoebus of Germany [4]. He distributed questionnaires concerning geographical distribution, gender, effect of social position, inheritance and time of occurrence, as they related to hay fever symptoms. Unfortunately his conclusions (that hay fever was due to 'the first heat of summer') were disappointing, but his methodology set the standards for subsequent field studies.

At more or less the same time as Charles Blackley was conducting his studies in England, Dr. Morrill Wyman, a professor of medicine at Harvard University, published his book on autumnal catarrh [5]. It was already appreciated by the 1850s that two distinct forms of hay fever existed in America, i.e. the early summer grass variety and the autumn, or ragweed, type. However, there was no firm proof that ragweed pollen caused symptoms. Accordingly, Dr. Wyman took some pollinating ragweed, wrapped securely, to the White Mountains where he was free of symptoms. After a few days he and his son, who was also a sufferer, sniffed the plant and both developed an attack of hay fever. The experiment was confirmed with other patients. Unfortunately some of his samples of pollinating ragweed were inactive and did not elicit symptoms in all patients, leading him to conclude that 'with our present knowledge Roman wormwood (ragweed) can be regarded as only a very active and general cause of paroxysms but not a cause of the whole disease'. Consequently his work was not fully appreciated. Nevertheless, by the end of the 19th century it was clearly established that pollen was the cause of seasonal catarrh, although it would be well into the 20th century before it was realised that the mechanism was immunological rather than 'toxic'.

Anaphylaxis

Although the discovery of experimental anaphylaxis in dogs was made early in the 20th century by Charles Richet and Paul Portier, there were a number of important observations prior to this. For example, Magendie [6] described in 1839 the sudden death of dogs following repeated injections with egg white and, in 1893, Von Behring noted that guinea pigs were frequently more sensitive to the second injection of toxin occurring some time after the first; he called it the 'paradoxical toxin reaction' [reviewed in 7]. In 1894, Samuel Flexner, working with rabbits, and Richet and Hericault, working with dogs, found that a second injection of a foreign serum led to a more or less violent reaction not seen with the reaction to the first injection [reviewed in 7]. However, these investigators focused largely on the concepts of toxins and toxic reactions. That these observations represented unique immunological reactions were not, at this time, seriously contemplated.

Asthma

Although asthma had been recognised since antiquity, and indeed Maimonides in the 13th century had written an insightful treatise on the subject, it was not until the 19th century that the first classical description of the condition appeared. We owe this largely to the work of the remarkable Dorset-born physician, Henry Hide Salter (fig. 3). His magnum opus *On Asthma: Its Pathology and Treatment*, published in 1860, was based on his experience of hundreds of cases and his own personal affliction from the disease [8]. Salter's definition of asthma was: 'paroxysmal dyspnoea of a peculiar character, generally periodic with intervals of healthy respiration between the attacks'. He believed that the disease was essentially a nervous disorder ('perverted nervous action') but also appreciated its hereditary nature and that there were many triggers (or 'idiosyncra-

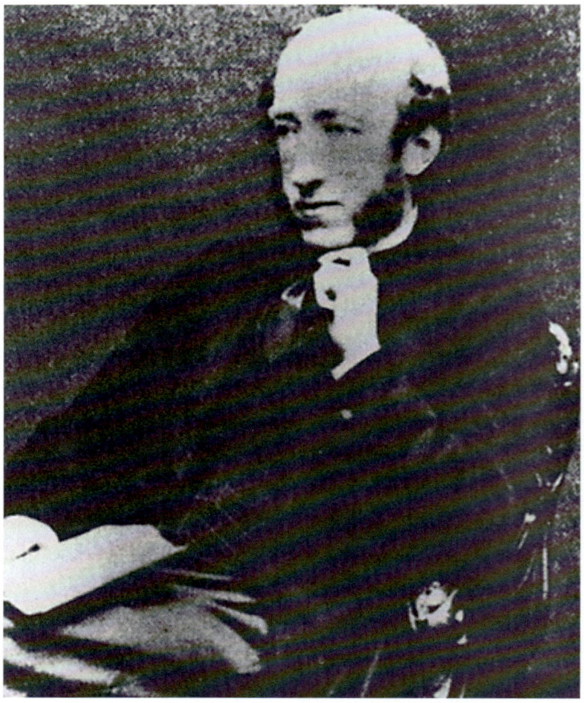

Fig. 3. Henry Hyde Salter (1823–1871). Description of the various causes of asthma and of cells (now known as eosinophils) in sputum.

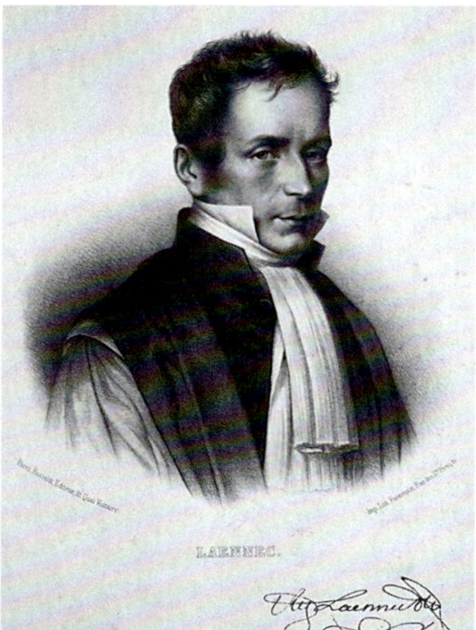

Fig. 4. René Laënnec (1781–1826). French physician who in 1816 invented the stethoscope.

sies') such as exposure to horses, cats and other animals. He recommended sleep and hot strong coffee and was opposed to the use of opiates.

The invention of the stethoscope in 1816 by René Laënnec (fig. 4) was also a monumental landmark for medicine in general, and chest diseases in particular [9]. Bronchospasm could now be readily identified by auscultation and shown to be an important component of asthma. It would not be until the early part of the 20th century that pathophysiological mechanisms were unravelled. However, important observations were made independently by Jean Martin Charcot (1853) [10] and Ernst van Leyden (1886; fig. 5) [11]. This was the discovery of characteristic crystals in the sputum of asthmatics. These are now known to be eosinophil derived; the role of the eosinophil in asthma fascinates investigators to this day.

Eosinophils and Mast Cells

The term eosinophil is derived from Paul Ehrlich's (fig. 6) discovery of blood cells with granules with an affinity for acid aniline dyes. His work was announced in a presentation to the Physiological Society of Berlin in 1879 [reviewed in 12]. However, more than 30 years previously, Thomas Wharton Jones (fig. 7), a technician working at St. Thomas's Hospital London, had described cells with retractile granules which were probably eosinophils, although his descriptions did not provide the methods for ready identification and quantification [13]. Ehrlich's early work on staining microscopic specimens arose from the expanding dye industry in Germany. He found that it was critical to use unfixed, thin, air-dried, heated specimens of blood for optimal staining. Using primitive optics he was able to describe the alpha granules of the eosinophils by their affinity for acid coal tar dyes. Ehrlich observed abundant eosinophils in the bone marrow and speculated that this was the site of their formation. He also proposed, with remarkable accuracy, that leucocyte granulations represented 'specific secretory cell activity', and that eosinophils and neutrophils had different chemotactic responses.

In Ehrlich's doctoral thesis submitted in 1878 he also described the mast cell ('maesten' in German,

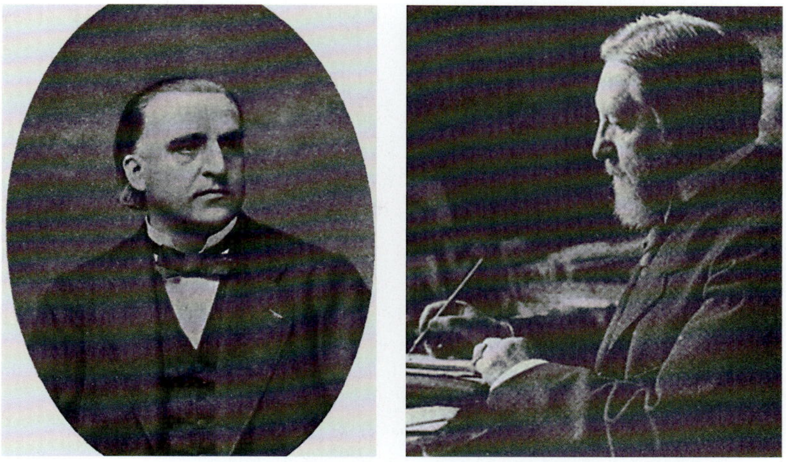

Fig. 5. Jean Martin Charcot (1825–1893; left) and Ernst V. von Leyden (1832–1910; right). The needle-like (eosinophil-derived) crystals characteristic of asthmatic sputum are named after Charcot and Leyden.

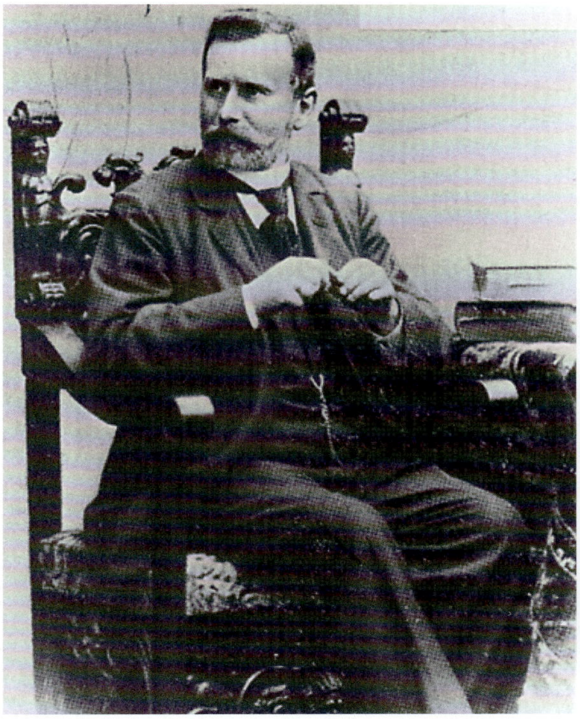

Fig. 6. Paul Ehrlich (1854–1915). An exceptionally creative bioscientist who, amongst many other accomplishments, described the side-chain theory of antibody formation and discovered the mast cell and the eosinophil.

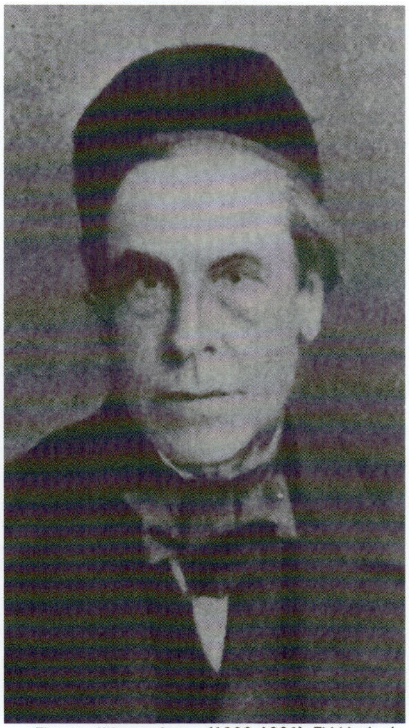

Thomas Warton Jones (1808-1891), TH Huxley's Physiology Tutor.

Fig. 7. Thomas Wharton Jones (1808–1891). Described course granular blood corpuscles which, 30 years later, Paul Ehrlich unequivocally identified and named 'eosinophils'.

meaning to stuff or force feed). He had found that mast cell granules stain with basic aniline dyes and speculated that the cell was associated with increased blood flow and nutrition as in, for example, chronic inflammation. Indeed, at this time Ehrlich was to go on to describe the basophil, neutrophil and lymphocyte, all on the basis of morphology and staining with dyes; techniques which have changed little even to this day.

References

1 Heberden W: Commentaries on the History and Cure of Diseases. Boston, Wells & Lilly, 1818, pp 108–111.
2 Bostock J: Case of a periodical affection of the eyes and chest. Med Chir Trans 1819;10:161.
3 Blackley CH: Experimental Researches on the Causes and Nature of Catarrhus Aestivus (Hayfever or Hay-Asthma). London, Dawson, 1959.
4 Waite KJ: Blackley and the development of hay fever as a disease of civilisation in the nineteenth century. Med Hist 1995;39:186–196.
5 Wyman M: Autumnal Catarrh. New York, Hurd & Houghton, 1872.
6 Magendie F: Lectures on the Blood. Philadelphia, Harrington, Barington & Hasswell, 1839.
7 Bulloch W: The History of Bacteriology. London, Oxford University Press, 1937.
8 Salter HH: On Asthma, Its Pathology and Treatment. London, Churchill, 1860.
9 Laennec RTH: De l'auscultation médiate ou Traité du diagnostic des maladies des poumons et du coeur. Paris, Brosson & Chaudé, 1819.
10 Charcot JM, Robin C: Observation de leucocythémie. CR Mem Soc Biol 1853;5:44.
11 Leyden E: Zur Kenntnis des Asthma bronchiale. Virchow Arch Pathol Anat 1872;54:324.
12 Hirsch JG, Hirsch BI: Paul Ehrlich and the discovery of the eosinophil; in Mahmoud AAF, Austen KF (eds): The Eosinophil in Health and Disease. New York, Grune & Stratton, 1980, pp 3–23.
13 Wharton Jones T: The blood corpuscle considered in its different phases of development in the animal series. Philos Trans R Soc Lond 1846;1:82.

Prof. em. A.B. Kay
Allergy and Clinical Immunology, Leukocyte Biology Section
National Heart and Lung Institute, South Kensington Campus
Imperial College, Sir Alexander Fleming Building
London, SW7 2AZ (UK)
E-Mail a.b.kay@imperial.ac.uk

Bergmann K-C, Ring J (eds): History of Allergy. Chem Immunol Allergy. Basel, Karger, 2014, vol 100, pp 27–45
DOI: 10.1159/000358478

Milestones in the 20th Century

Karl-Christian Bergmann

Allergy Centre Charité, Universitätsmedizin, Berlin, Germany

Abstract

From its very beginning, the 20th century represented the period of the main breakthrough for allergology as a clinical and scientific entity. The first years of this period were extraordinarily exciting because of the discovery of the anaphylactic reaction in 1902 and its clinical diagnosis as 'local anaphylaxis', 'serum sickness' (1903) or even as 'anaphylactic shock' (1907). The term 'allergy' was coined in 1906 and led to the recognition of allergic diseases as a pathogenetic entity. The first patient organization of hay fever sufferers was founded in Germany in 1900, the same year in which the very first report on immunotherapy was published in New York. In 1911 the era of actual immunotherapy started in London, becoming scientific with the first double-blind study in 1956, and still today being regarded as the backbone of allergology. In 1919 it was shown that allergy could be transferred by blood, in 1921 by serum (Prausnitz-Küstner test) and in 1966 the mystic 'reagins' were recognized as immunoglobulin (Ig) E. The development of the radioallergosorbent test for quantifying specific IgE antibody was a diagnostic landmark for allergists all over the world. The history of allergy diagnosis started with the introduction of a 'functional skin test', named the patch test in 1894. The scratch test was described in 1912 and the patch test in 1931. From 1908 the skin was tested by intracutaneous injections, and from 1930 by a 'puncture test' (a precursor of the prick test) which has been in worldwide use in modified variations since 1959. The rub test ('friction test') was added in 1961. Systematically applied provocation tests started with conjunctival provocation (1907), followed by nasal and bronchial provocation with allergens (1914 and 1925).

The 20th century is regarded as the era of modern times and was marked particularly by two world wars and the cold war arising from them. For medicine, the 20th century brought about huge progress in the diagnosis and therapy of many illnesses [1], promoted above all by the ever quicker and rapid developments in the natural sciences. This development had already started in the 19th century.

Table 1. Landmarks of medicine in the 20th century (from Halter [1])

1900	First 'X-ray congress' in Paris on the radiation discovered in 1895
1901	Karl Landsteiner describes the blood groups
1905	Fritz Schaudinn and Erich Hofmann discover the cause of syphilis, *Spirochaeta pallida*
1906	Alois Alzheimer describes the degeneration of the brain ('Morbus Alzheimer')
1910	Paul Ehrlich synthesizes the first chemotherapeutic drug against syphilis ('Salvarsan')
1921	Frederick Banting and Charles Best isolate insulin
1928	Alexander Fleming discovers *Penicillium notatum*, a mushroom which leads to the development of penicillin
1929	A 25-year-old assistant, Werner Forssmann, places the first heart catheter in a self-experiment
1948	The new antibiotic streptomycin is effective against tuberculosis and plague
1954	The first heart-lung machines are used for operations in the open heart at a standstill
1955	First polio vaccination
1958	In Sweden a heart pacemaker is implanted
1960	The anti-baby pill comes onto the market
1960	The development of the artificial kidney is finalized and the dialysis is applied clinically
1961	The first artificial heart flap is successfully implanted into a person
1964	First dilatation of narrowed heart coronary arteries
1967	Christiaan Barnard performs the world's first successful human-to-human heart transplant; the patient survives 18 days
1968	Bone marrow transplantation is applied successfully
1982	The HIV retrovirus causing deadly immune weakness – to be called Acquired Immunodeficiency Syndrome (AIDS) – is discovered by Luc Montagnier and Robert Gallo
1990	Microsurgical procedures ('key hole surgery') become established in all sections of medicine
1992	The microbe *Helicobacter pylori* is acknowledged, nearly one hundred years after its discovery, as a main cause of gastritis and ulcera
1995	Robots conduct millimeter-exact hip joint operations in California

Only in the 20th century, however, were drugs and methods developed, targeting illnesses efficiently and with lasting effect. Critics of medicine, but also some medicine historians, state that only from about 1900 did a doctor's visit really help the patient.

As a result, the population became increasingly aged in the industrialized countries of the world. In Germany, for example, life expectancy in this period increased by approximately 30 years.

The scale of progress made in medicine during the 20th century was huge. A small selection of especially important steps is shown in table 1.

Essential allergological landmarks began at the start of the 20th century, and were complemented during the following years in the area of diagnostics as well as therapy, in ever more rapid results. The author is completely aware that he cannot give an entire acknowledgment of all events and personalities involved in this progress. Besides, the article is written from a European-German view, influenced by personal allergological work since 1968. The author hereby gives his apologies should important developments not be appreciated extensively enough.

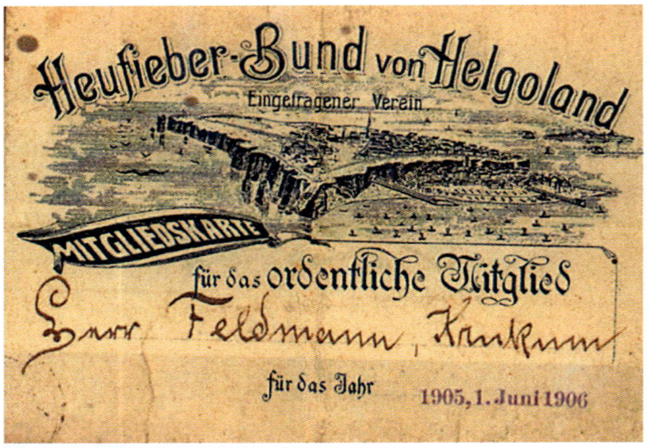

Fig. 1. Membership card of 1905/1906.

Patients First – The First Patient's Organization for Allergy Sufferers

In the first years of the 20th century, the very first patient organization ('Heufieber-Bund'; fig. 1) was founded in Germany for patients with hay fever. An association of hay fever sufferers was noted in the association register of the royal district court of Altona (Hamburg) on September 10, 1900. The patients had been meeting since 1897 on the island of Helgoland, where their hay fever did not occur as often as on the mainland.

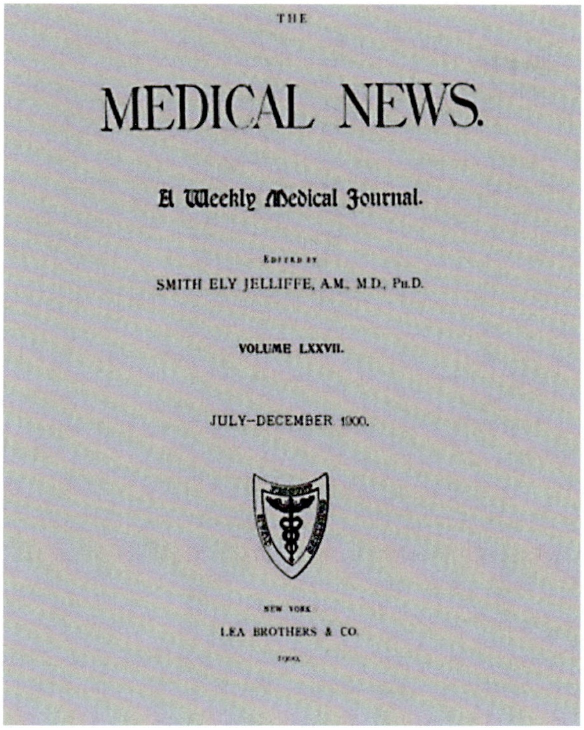

THE

MEDICAL NEWS.

A Weekly Medical Journal.

EDITED BY

SMITH ELY JELLIFFE, A.M., M.D., Ph.D.

VOLUME LXXVII.

JULY–DECEMBER 1900.

NEW YORK

LEA BROTHERS & CO.

1900.

Fig. 2. *The Medical News* dating from 1900 in New York, with one of the first reports on immunotherapy against ragweed allergy.

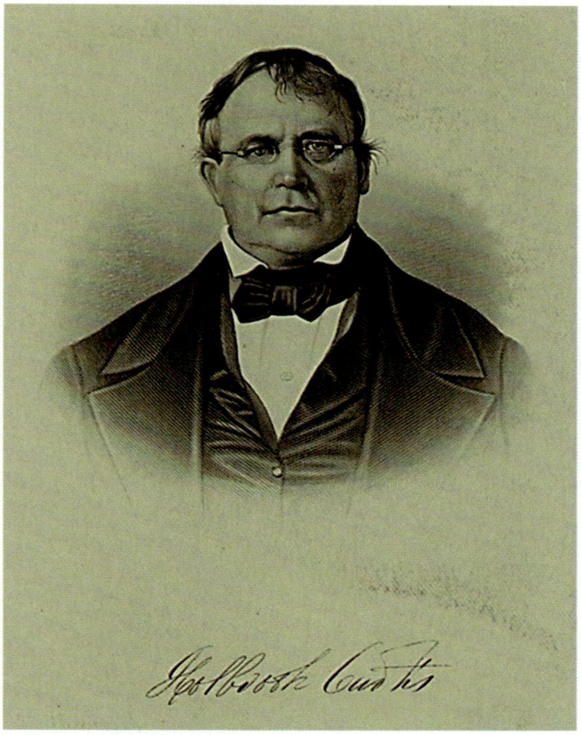

Fig. 3. H. Holbrook Curtis.

The number of members in the hay fever alliance rose rapidly from 157 in 1902 to 1,387 members only 6 years later. Among the members who joined during the first years were scientists, artists and members of the high-ranking nobility like 'Her Majesty Victoria Eugenia, Queen of Spain' (grandmother of the acting King of Spain, Juan Carlos).

The association had three aims:

(1) to give advice and information to patients with hay fever and their families;
(2) to collect money to allow the stay on the island of Helgoland to patients with less money during the pollen season;
(3) to provide sociable connections.

In 1929, the first 'advice center for allergic illnesses' was opened by the association, and after more than 100 years the association is still active today and is highly successful regarding the achievement of these aims. In many countries around the world, the value of patient organizations has been recognized where they contribute substantially to the understanding of the needs of allergy sufferers and cooperate with members to help themselves.

Today (summer 2013), the European Federation of Asthma and Allergy Associations (EFA; www.efanet.org) is an alliance of 41 organizations in 23 different countries across Europe. EFA's mission is to draw together a European community of patient organizations which share responsibility for substantially reducing the frequency and severity of allergies, asthma and COPD, minimizing their societal implications, improving health-related quality of life and ensuring full citizenship of people with these conditions, as well as pursuing equal health opportunities in the allergy and airways field in Europe.

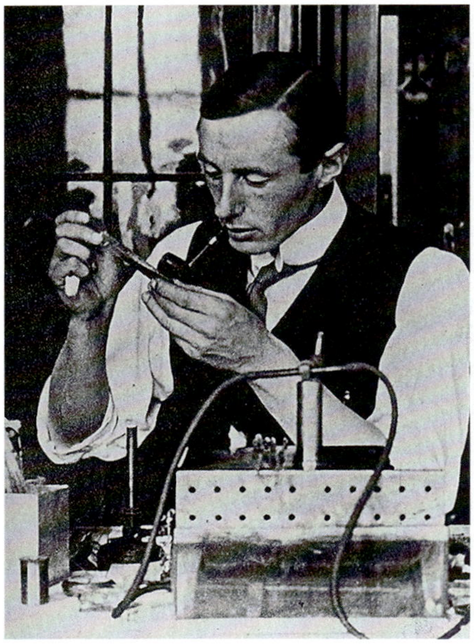

Fig. 4. Leonard Noon.

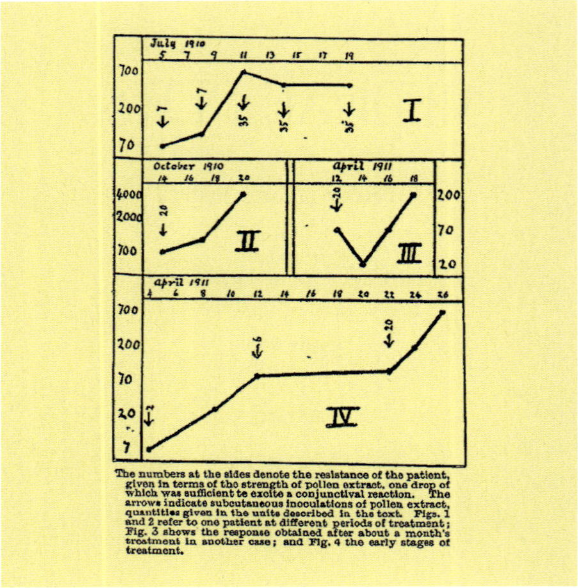

Fig. 5. Results of conjunctival tests done by Noon following subcutaneous injections of grass pollens given in threshold values of the extract to induce a conjunctival reaction.

Immunotherapy against Pollen and Other Allergens – The 'Backbone of Allergology'

In 1900, in *The Medical News* (fig. 2) from New York, one could read about one of the first reports on the use of watery pollen extracts with 'some eight or ten' patients with 'coryza' [2]. Henry Holbrook Curtis (1856–1920; fig. 3), the ENT physician, vocal therapist in the Metropolitan Opera and inventor of the tonograph, reported 'remarkable results' in these patients following the subcutaneous injection and oral application of pollen extracts from the 'old enemy rag-weed … the recognized king of pollens'. It seems that there were no other trials by him – but the idea was taken up successfully by Leonard Noon (1878–1913; fig. 4) in London.

Leonard Noon published in *The Lancet* in 1911 the first documentation of the effectiveness of subcutaneous immunotherapy (SCIT) in grass-allergic subjects with hay fever using conjunctival provocation testing [3]. Noon was working at St. Mary's Hospital in London when he began tests with injections of pollen extracts (fig. 5).

After Noon's early death, his friend John Freeman (1877–1962; fig. 6) continued this work and, only 3 months later, published a more detailed paper on the 'hypodermic inoculations of pollen toxin' in 20 patients [4]. In Freeman's opinion the results were 'disappointing', 'inconclusive' or a 'failure' in 3 cases, and 'moderately, fairly or eminently satisfactory' in 16 cases. He concluded:

> It is claimed that this increase in immunity produced by pollen vaccine is in itself the best proof of the soundness of this line of treatment, whether prophylactic or phylactic. It is true that one does not know if this increase is sufficient for all purposes, but the change is certainly in the right direction, and must be doing good.

Freeman and Noon administered increasing doses of crudely prepared whole allergen extracts to allergy patients until their symptoms were successfully lessened. These experiments represented the beginnings of the development of 'desensitizing immunotherapy'. Noon also made the first attempt at standardizing allergen doses and established the 'Noon unit' based on weight.

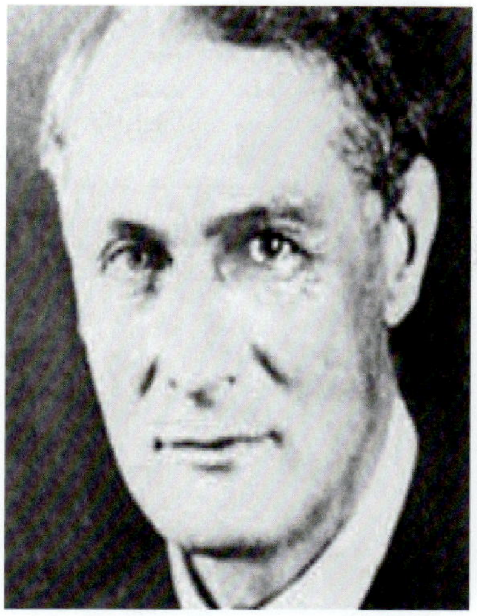

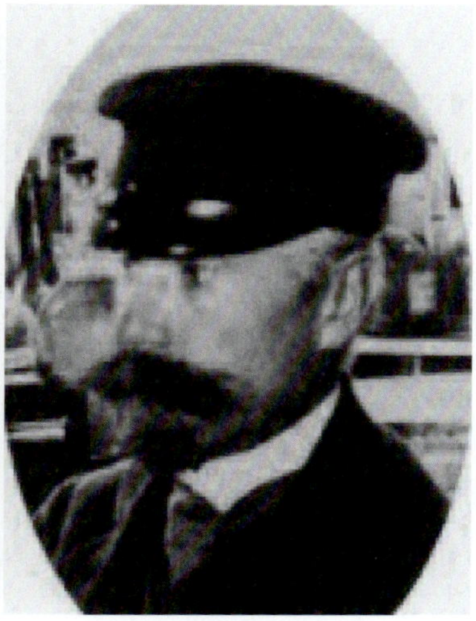

Fig. 6. John Freeman.
Fig. 7. Paul Portier.

For nearly 50 years following Noon's paper there have been only anecdotic reports on the efficacy of SCIT. The first study of SCIT purporting to be a controlled trial did not appear until 1950 [5], but the study did not seem to satisfy the criteria for experimental control.

In 1954, Frankland and Augustin [6] published the first double-blind placebo-controlled study of SCIT, followed by a DBPC study in the USA at the Harvard Medical School in 1965. In this study, 12 patients who were each suffering from allergic rhinitis due to ragweed pollen received verum or placebo injections. Medication and symptom score were significantly different in favor of the verum. Since then, many controlled clinical trials have confirmed the efficacy of SCIT and, although some concerns have arisen around safety, SCIT remains a valid option for treating allergic disease.

In the centenary year of 2011, data were presented by use of conjunctival provocation test and allergen-specific immunoglobulin (Ig) G that replicated this observation and additionally confirmed the allergen specificity of SCIT using a double-blind design employing either grass or mite SCIT in dual grass- and mite-allergic individuals [7]. A series of publications were issued in 2011 which summarized the development and success of immunotherapy [8].

The use of skin prick tests and new allergen extraction techniques accelerated the development of SCIT, which became a widespread practice. Recent developments include the introduction of sublingual immunotherapy, and clinical trials of recombinant and peptide vaccines.

Anaphylaxis – The Discovery of a New Field in 1902

In 1902, Paul Portier (1866–1962; fig. 7) and Charles Richet (1850–1935) [see fig. 1 in the chapter by Ring et al., this vol., p. 55] published a short, comprehensive publication, only a little more than two sides in length, after a talk before the Paris 'Société de Biologie' in which they first coined the term 'anaphylactic' reaction (anaphylaxis): 'Nous appelons anaphylactique (contraire de la phylaxie) la propriété dont est doué un venin de diminuer au lieu de renforcer l'immunité, lorsqu'il est injecté à doses non mortelles' [9] (fig. 8; online suppl. movie 1, see www.karger.com/chial100_movie1). OSM

Both authors meant to stimulate only one aspect in the field of serology and immunology, but they initiated a quite new working direction; in 1913 Richet received the Nobel Prize for this. Around the turn of the 19th century, the ideas of Robert Koch dominated the scene due to his new therapy for tuberculosis by means of tuberculin (from 1897). In 1897, Paul Ehrlich also coined the term

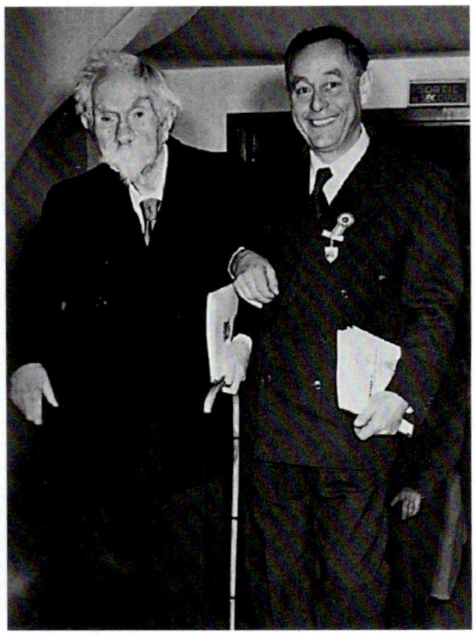

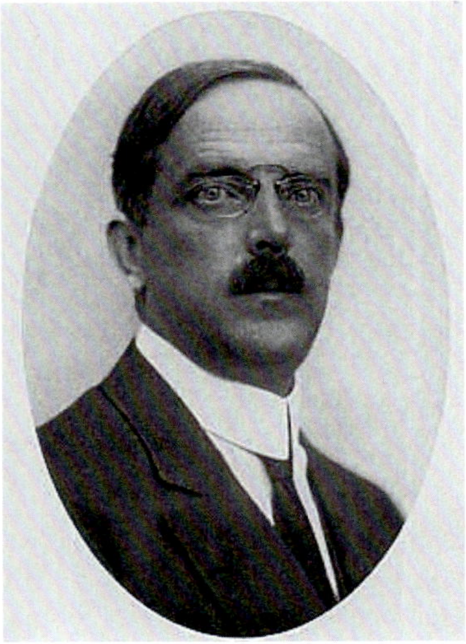

Fig. 8. Paul Portier enters the congressional hall in Paris on October 19, 1958, with Bernard Halpern, and reports on the experiments on anaphylaxis (see www.karger.com/chial100_movie1).
Fig. 9. Clemens von Pirquet (1906).

that was given to the side chain theory, and in 1892 Behring published his 'blood serum therapy' in Leipzig. The rapid rise of bacteriology and the possibilities of immunization against infectious diseases inspired the 'mainstream' of medicine during these years.

In 1901, using the lab on the yacht 'Princesse Alice II' [see fig. 3 and 5 in the chapter by Ring et al., this vol., p. 56 and p. 57] belonging to Albert I, Prince of Monaco, Charles Richet and Paul Portier studied the toxic qualities of certain kinds of jellyfish, with which contact led to urticarial reactions. Was it possible, by the repeated injection of toxins, to make animals insensitive, tolerant or even immune?

The answer was no; the opposite in fact occurred: with repeated injections after an incubation time, the slightest, subtle amount led to typical clinical reactions with tachycardia, blood pressure decrease, diarrhea, respiratory insufficiency and even death in the case of anaphylactic shock.

These phenomena deviated considerably from the picture of a primary poisoning, and therein quite a new form of hypersensitivity had been discovered. The term anaphylaxis should express a defenseless state with regard to the toxin; although philologically the word was criticized, it immediately found its entrance into medical language and substituted the oldest allergological name of 'idiosyncrasy'.

The phenomenon of anaphylaxis stimulated, in a broad sense, research on allergic reactions in humans and animals, leading to different 'forms of anaphylaxis'. The concept 'allergy' would follow that of 'anaphylaxis' 4 years later.

The Determining Word Is Born in 1906

On July 24, 1906, the word 'allergy' was first used in a publication by Clemens von Pirquet (fig. 9) in the Journal *Münchener Medizinische Wochenschrift*:

> We need a new ... word for the altered state which the organism finds out by the acquaintance with any organic, living or lifeless poison ... For this general concept of altered responsiveness, I suggest the term allergy. [10]

The meaning of the term has its origin in the Greek word 'allos' (other) and 'ergos' (activity). Within a few years the new expression had conquered the whole world and had edged out all older, varied names like idiosyncrasy, hypersensitivity, anaphylaxis and atopy, etc. The word 'allergy' represented a clinical concept which enabled one 'to understand' such clinical situations, the genesis of which were not yet understood.

What was the background for the new word? Pirquet was an eager doctor and researcher whose main interest was always the illness of children and who

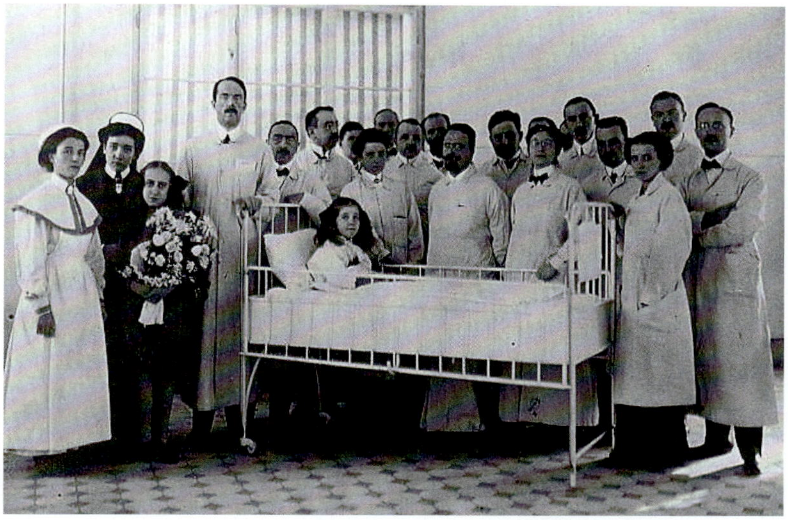

Fig. 10. Clemens von Pirquet in the Clinic for Pediatrics, Vienna, Austria.

constantly drew his conclusions from observations made at the sickbed. Around 1902, he first became aware of allergies when he observed that some children suffering from diphtheria developed non-disease-related and quite extreme side effects when treated with a horse serum antitoxin.

These observations and conclusions led to a new pathology; not only had the increase of the bacteria penetrating the body determined the course of the illness, but also the interaction between the organism and the bacteria. A repeated contact with the same material, which he called 'allergen', led to the reaction between the allergen (antigen) with the counter material, the antibody.

Pirquet was an all-round physician – he restructured the education of nurses and placed a high value on 'teamwork'. In addition, the nursing staff could introduce innovations in a patient's care and therapy. From 1924 onward, Pirquet also insisted that trainee doctors must finish a nursing training period to understand the problems in care better and to improve the cooperation between nurses and doctors. These were – at that time and still today – huge changes in the system of patient care (fig. 10).

He also became an excellent organizer in other areas: after the First World War he was able to activate a large-scale child relief operation in America through his good relations with American pediatricians, helping 400,000 malnourished children in Austria through the delivery of food.

Serum Sickness and the 'Case Langerhans'

The development and use of vaccines for the prophylaxis and therapy of infectious diseases, such as diphtheria and tetanus, led to an absolutely new clinical picture – that of serum sickness (or 'serum illness'). Firstly, only harmless side effects like urticaria and local exanthemas after injections were reported – then, however, a tragic event occurred.

On April 4, 1896, the well-known Berlin pathologist Robert Langerhans (1859–1904) injected 1.2 ml of diphtheria antitoxin ('Behring's antiserum') subcutaneously to his almost 2-year-old child for prophylactic reasons. Before his own eyes, his own child passed away 7 min later. Langerhans published a detailed report [11] and by 1910, 41 deaths had been described after injections of diphtheria vaccine [12].

The concept of 'serum sickness' as a result of anaphylactic reactions to foreign proteins was put forward by Clemens von Pirquet together with Béla Schick (1877–1967; fig. 11) in 1903 [13]. To avoid anaphylactic reactions Schick discovered a test for susceptibility to diphtheria (the Schick test), which

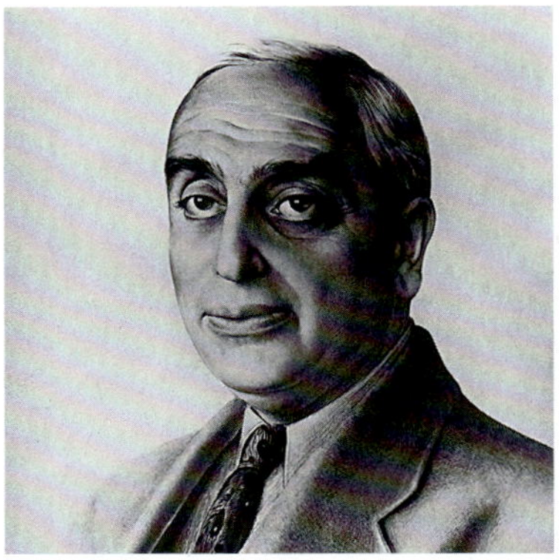

Fig. 11. Béla Schick.

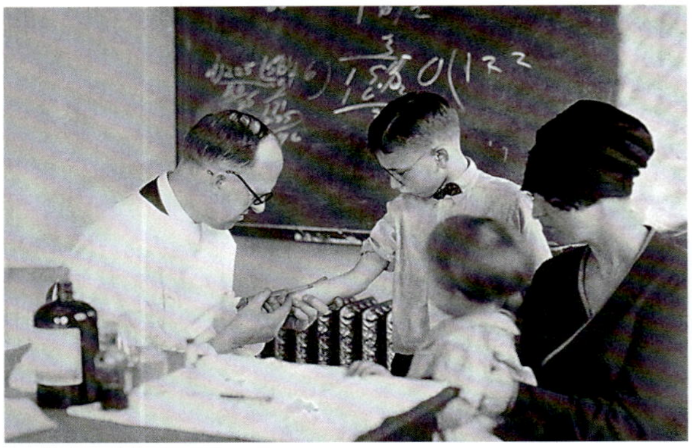

Fig. 12. Schick test, 1915.

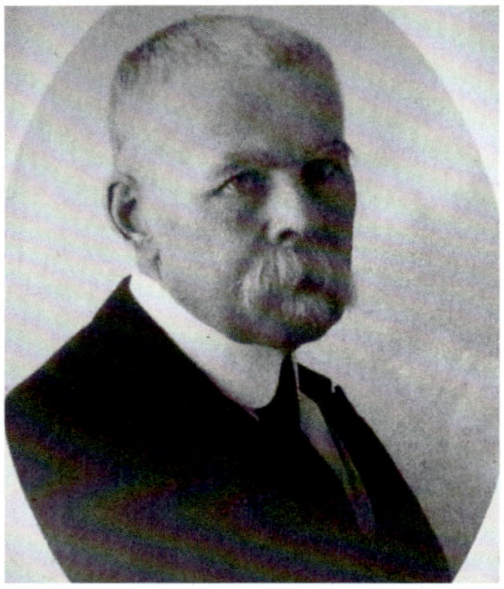

Fig. 13. Nicolas Maurice Arthus.

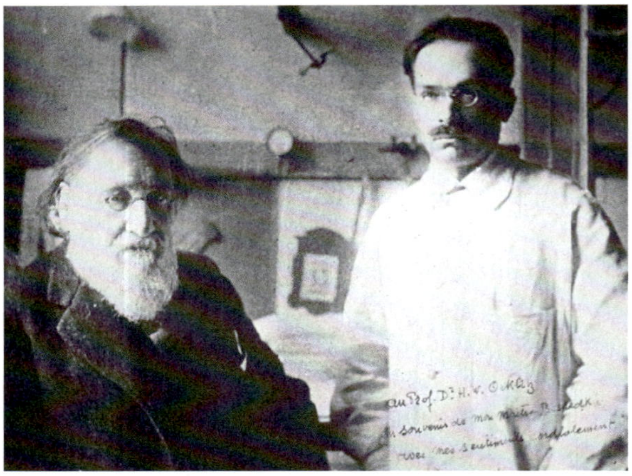

Fig. 14. Alexandre Besredka (right) beside Elias Metchnikoff (left) in the Institute Pasteur, Paris, France, 1914.

made him world famous (fig. 12). The test involved a small sample of toxin injected under the skin. If the subject did not have the necessary antibodies, a rash developed around the injection site, indicating a positive result, and a vaccine then could be administered. The test and vaccine eventually led to the eradication of the childhood disease that attacked 100,000 Americans in 1927, leading to about 10,000 deaths.

The observation of the 'serum illness' as a now and then fatal result of an injection of antiserum and its avoidance by way of the 'Schick test' shows the close connection of allergology and clinical immunology. This fruitful connection of both disciplines was particularly very clear at the beginning of 20th century.

The Idea of Anaphylaxis Received Growing Interest ...

Following the publication on anaphylaxis in 1902 [9], a number of allergologists around the world revealed more details on the phenomenon; hence, the 'local anaphylaxis'.

Local Anaphylaxis

Nicolas Maurice Arthus (1862–1945; fig. 13) postulated in 1903 the term 'local anaphylaxis', also known as 'Arthus reaction' [14]. Arthus had also observed that repeated injections of non-toxic materials (e.g. milk, horse serum) in the skin of rabbits led to stronger and stronger defensive reactions at the site of the injection. Inflammation and focal necro-

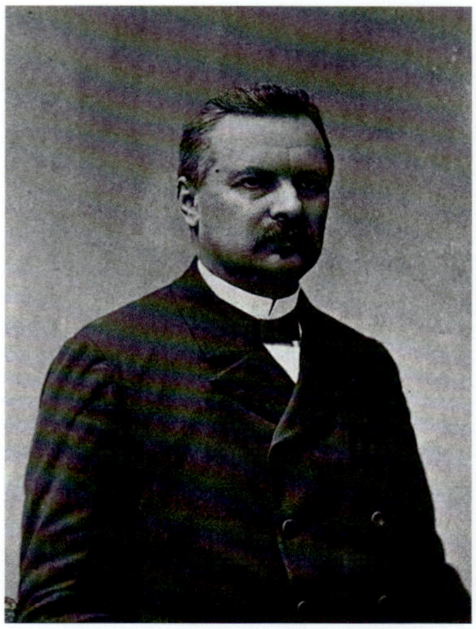

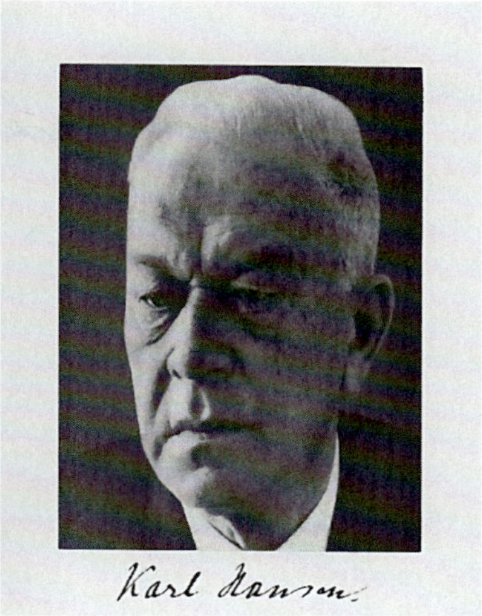

Fig. 15. Victor Henri Hutinel.
Fig. 16. Karl Hansen.

15 16

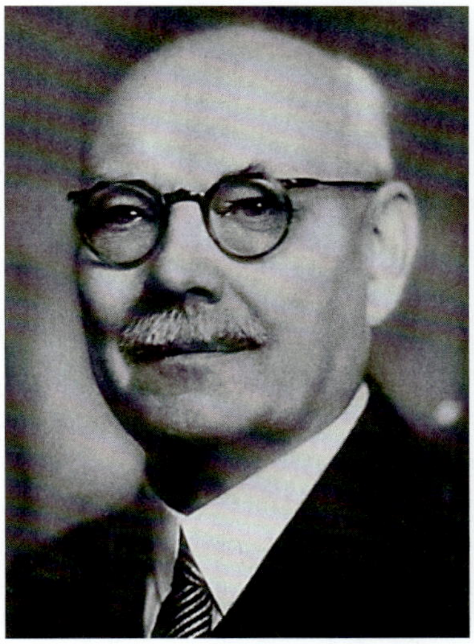

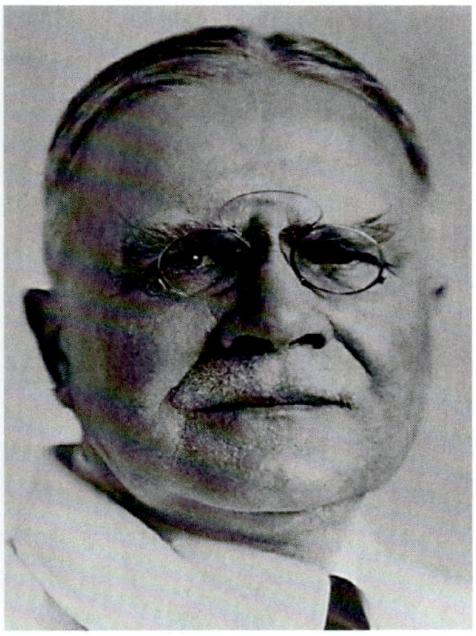

Fig. 17. Richard Otto.
Fig. 18. Paul Uhlenhuth.

17 18

sis of the skin appeared in increasing strength from injection to injection after approximately 6–8 h. Later the Arthus reaction was seen as a type of local type III hypersensitivity reaction (immune complex mediated), mainly as local vasculitis due to deposits of IgG-based immune complexes in dermal blood vessels.

Anaphylactic Shock and 'Local Immunity'

In 1907, Alexandre Besredka (1870–1940; fig. 14) published the term 'anaphylactic shock' [15]. At the Institute Pasteur in Paris, Besredka tried to inhibit the toxic (anaphylactic) effect from vaccines (foreign serums) by an 'anti-anaphylactic vaccination'. The attempts failed and the term anaphylactic shock has remained until this day.

In 1919, Besredka also published his ideas on 'local immunity'. This exists predominantly from secretory IgA, which works independently of the serum IgA. Therefore, he was later named as the father of 'mucosal immunity'.

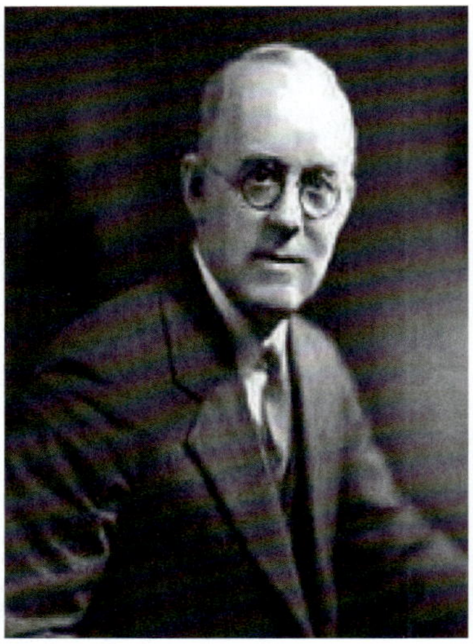

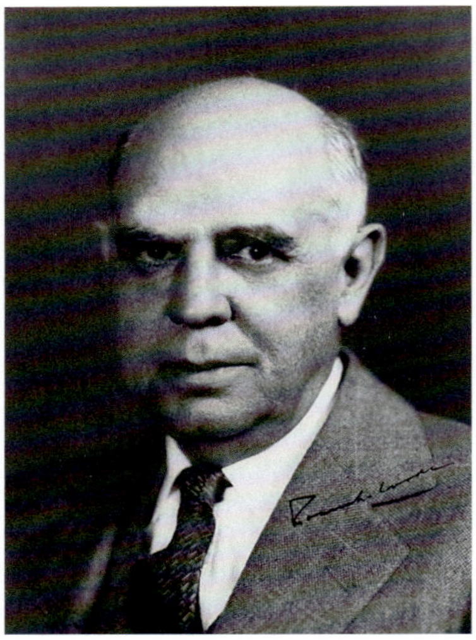

Fig. 19. Arthur Fernandez Coca.
Fig. 20. Robert Anderson Cooke.

19 20

Alimentary Anaphylaxis

In 1908 the French pediatrician Victor H. Hutinel (1849–1933; fig. 15) reported on cases of anaphylactic reactions induced by food – the 'alimentary anaphylaxis' [16].

Anaphylaxis in the Clinical Routine

Richet and Portiers' founding theory of anaphylaxis was first based only on findings from animal experiments and had great influence upon clinical allergy. Karl Hansen (fig. 16) later (1941) created the concept of the 'anaphylactic shock fragment' with asthma [17]. He wrote:

> However, in clinical reality with humans an universal shock mostly does not occur, rather only one or several symptoms of a shock are clearly apparent, which we want to call 'shock fragments'.

Richard Otto (1872–1952; fig. 17) worked at the Imperial Health Centre in Berlin and documented further important details of anaphylaxis: the incubation time is between 8–10 days, the reaction is specific and stops approximately 2–3 months later, the sensitization can be transferred passively by mothers to their newborns and a large number of antigens (animal, herbal, bacterial) are able to induce anaphylactic reactions, including non-toxic antigens [18]. That the anaphylactic reaction may also be used for the differentiation of proteins was shown by Paul Uhlenhuth (1870–1957; fig. 18), a hygienist and serologist in Freiburg, Germany [19].

The Word 'Atopy' Has Remained to This Day

Arthur Fernandez Coca (1875–1959; fig. 19) and Robert Anderson Cooke (1880–1960; fig. 20) first used the term 'atopy' at a congress in 1921 in Washington and published it in 1923 [20]. By the term 'atopy', Coca and Cooke understood the spontaneously (e.g. without former vaccination) appearing diseases hay fever and asthma, with a genetic disposition within families. The word 'atopy' was first used only in the USA, but later became global. Many physicians and scientists use the term for any IgE-mediated reaction (even those that are appropriate and proportional to the antigen), but many pediatricians reserve the word 'atopy' for a genetically mediated predisposition to an excessive IgE reaction. An exact definition is yet to be agreed.

In 1915 Coca founded the scientific journal, *Journal of Immunology*. As a young man, Cooke suffered from asthma which was particularly apparent when riding the horse-drawn ambulance as an intern. During his internship he was also exposed to diphtheria and suffered a nearly fatal reaction when given

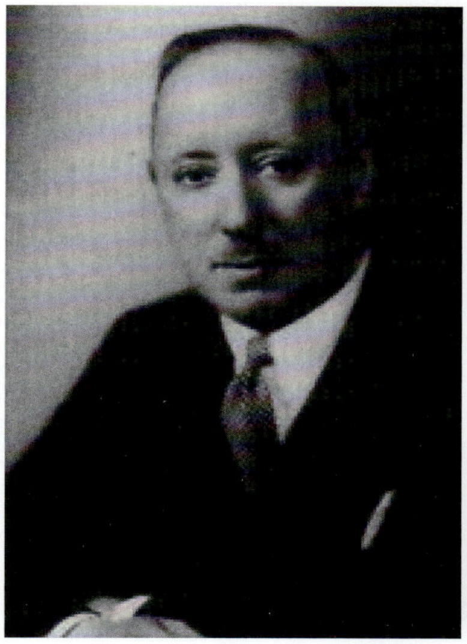

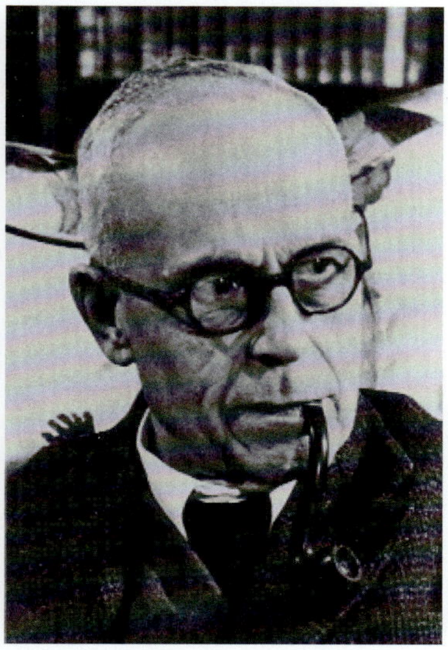

Fig. 21. Maximilian H. Ramirez.
Fig. 22. Karl Prausnitz.

21 22

a prophylactic injection of diphtheria antitoxin. These experiences certainly further stimulated his interest in allergy.

On February 19, 1919, at New York Hospital, he opened the first clinic devoted to allergy. This clinic served not only as an outpatient service for the treatment of allergic individuals, but also as a center for research and training in allergy. In 1932, the entire clinic was moved to Roosevelt Hospital, where Dr. Cooke was appointed Director of Allergy.

Cooke also helped establish the standardization of allergens by nitrogen content, as determined by the Kjeldahl method. He described 'blocking antibodies' and in doing so provided one of the earliest logical concepts for the clinical improvement of allergen immunotherapy.

The Transferability of an Allergy by Blood, or the Search for the 'Malefactor'

Following the observation and description of serum sickness as a result of treatment with foreign proteins by Pirquet [13] in 1903, the search for the trigger of these reactions in humans was intensified. The question arose as to whether these were cells, or if a protein in the serum triggered the reactions.

Among the first steps to clarification – with the final outcome being the discovery of IgE – an event in Central Park in New York has to be mentioned. A usually healthy 35-year-old waiter with negative family history underwent a blood transfusion (600 ml) for primary anemia. Two weeks later, and without recognizable reason, he suffered from an attack of asthma 5 min after entering a horse carriage in the park. He received epinephrine and when he entered the park again the next day another asthma attack occurred.

He was brought to the acute day ward by Dr. Ramirez (fig. 21), who tested the patient 'for a large number of food and bacterial proteins, pollens etc. with negative results, finally, however, obtaining a positive reaction to horse dandruff, measuring 1.5 cm in diameter and reacting as a 1:20,000 dilution'. The blood donor was a persistent asthmatic who was also positive to horse dandruff.

Dr. Ramirez rightly concluded that the allergy had been transferred along with the blood. He made the demand for future blood donors to be asked whether they were allergy sufferers, and concluded that 'the presence of these "anaphylactic bodies" in the donor's blood caused no untoward effects on the recipient during or immediately following the transfusion' in the absence of an allergen.

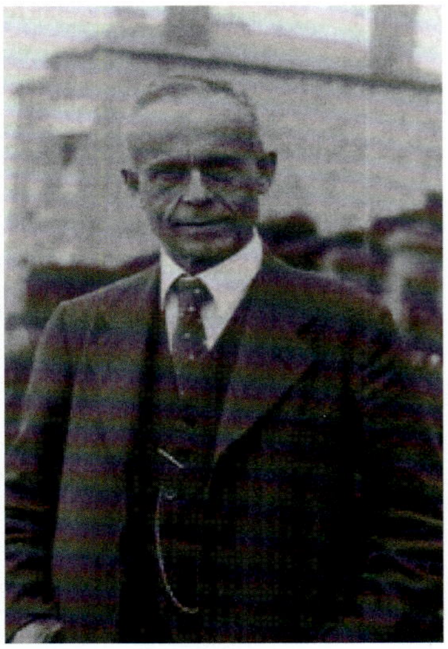

23

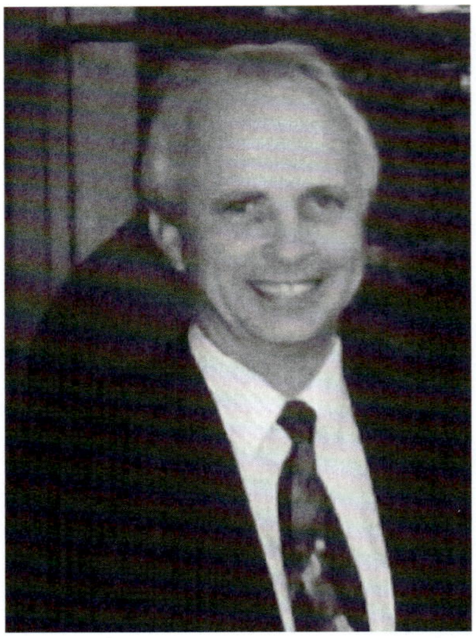

24

Fig. 23. Heinz Küstner.
Fig. 24. S.G.O. Johansson, June 1992.

This unusual case was published in 1919 [21]. The short case report shows exactly how history at this time was handled and from a single observation important conclusions could be gleaned.

Some years later, in 1922, Frugoni reported [22] a similar but experimentally induced case in which a rabbit allergy was transferred to a healthy 12-year-old girl. After playing with a rabbit she suffered from rabbit allergic rhinoconjunctivitis, urticaria and cough, which developed after she had received a blood transfusion from a donor with rabbit allergy.

The Transferability of an Allergy through Serum Is Proved

Only 3 years after Ramirez's observation, Karl Prausnitz (1876–1963; fig. 22) and his assistant Heinz Küstner (1897–1963; fig. 23) in distant Wroclaw (today in Poland) published their discovery that allergy can be transferred with serum, with cells playing no role [23]. Heinz Küstner worked at the Hygiene Institute in Wroclaw (1897–1963) as a junior scientist in Prausnitz's department. He was allergic to fish and provided an opportunity for Prausnitz to demonstrate the passive transfer of fish antibodies to somebody who was not allergic to fish, i.e. to himself. Prausnitz was allergic to pollen, but could eat fish without problems. Küstner's serum was injected in various dilutions into Prausnitz's skin. The next day he injected a fish extract near the injection sites of Küstner's serum as well as other areas. Only the areas where Küstner's serum had been injected reacted with an immediate wheal and flare.

With this experiment and publication in German (in 1921) [23] and English (in 1962), the earlier ideas of toxins and anti-toxins in allergic diseases were overcome. Sheldon Cohen (2004) summarized:

> Thus even though the allergic antibody had not yet been characterized, a scientific immunologic basis for investigating allergic phenomena had thereby been initiated. [24]

The Prausnitz-Küstner reaction remained the classical method for demonstrating and quantifying allergen-specific antibodies for many decades.

In 2005, Johansson (fig. 24) transfused defined amounts of IgE antibodies to an allergen and measured the degree and duration of IgE reactivity in the recipient by skin prick tests and basophil allergen threshold activation. It was concluded that after transfusion of plasma with >10 kU/l of IgE antibodies the recipient could have allergen-reactive basophiles for up to 7 weeks [25].

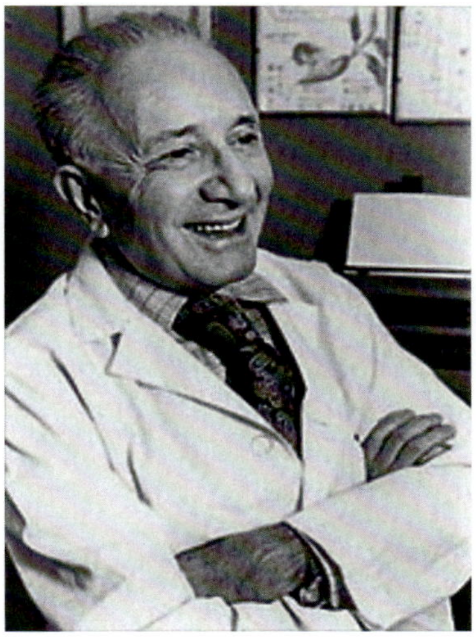

Fig. 25. Zoltan Ovary.

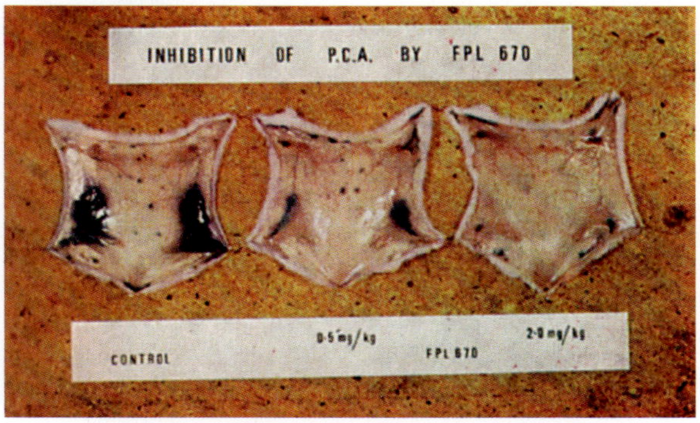

Fig. 26. Example of a passive cutaneous anaphylaxis reaction (Cox JSG, 5th March 1969).

Passive Cutaneous Anaphylaxis Test

In 1958, Zoltan Ovary (1907–2005; fig. 25) described the passive cutaneous anaphylaxis test (fig. 26). In this test an animal (usually a guinea pig) is injected intradermally with antibody (usually IgE) and subsequently challenged intravenously with a mixture of antigen and Evans blue dye 24–48 h later. A dark-blue area indicates a positive reaction due to the leakage of the dye at the site of antigen-antibody reactions. Ovary worked until his 98th year and summarized his fascinating life as an allergologist in his autobiography, entitled *Souveniers* [26]. The test was an advancement of the Prausnitz-Küstner tests for experimental purposes and was very important regarding the search for antibodies in small quantities.

Scientific Allergy Diagnostics

After earlier, predominantly casuistic observations about nasal, conjunctival and cutaneous reactions, mostly after accidental contact with allergens, diagnostic tests were scientifically founded by Charles Harrison Blackley. Before him the induction of allergic symptoms was generally only speculated about, and there were hardly any experiments. In 1873 he wrote:

> It is, however, much easier to try and theorise than to carry out experiments, and especially when these would have to be tried on the theoriser's own person. [27]

Scratch Test

The description of the scratch test on the skin by Blackley in 1873, involving pollen extracts scratched into his own skin, was a landmark in the development of allergy diagnostics. This 'scarification test' was described in more detail in 1912 by Oscar Menderson Schloss (1882–1952) [see fig. 2 in the chapter by Wüthrich, this vol., p. 111] as a 'scratch test' [28] and was made very popular by Isaac Walker as 'an asthma test' after 1917 [29].

According to Hans Schadewaldt this started 'the history of modern allergological skin tests ... after the introduction of the 'Läppchenprobe' (patch test), by the German dermatologist Josef Jadassohn (1863–1936; fig. 27) in the year 1894. In 1896 he named the simple application of test substances without injury a 'functional skin test' [30].

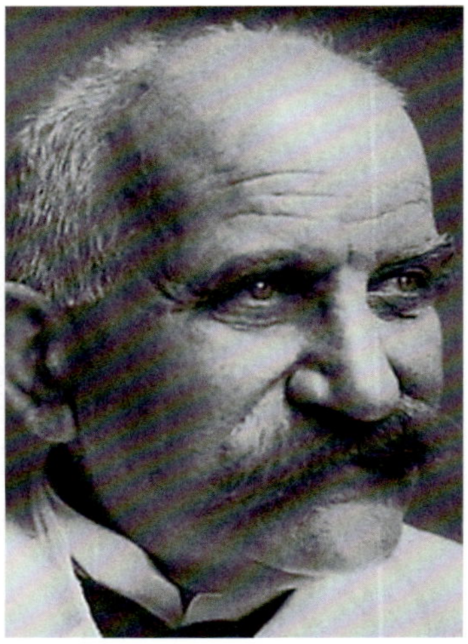

27

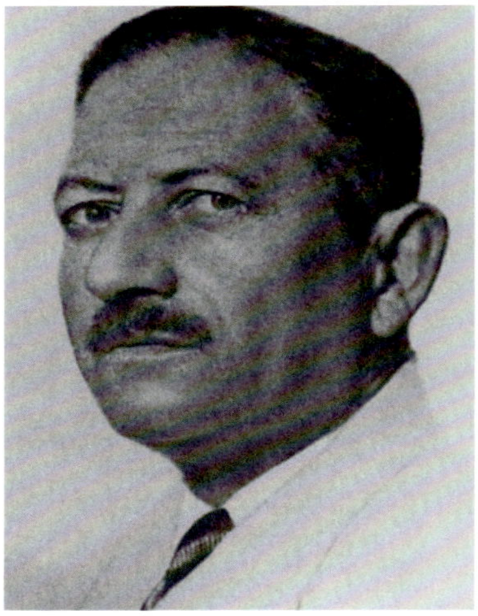

28

Fig. 27. Josef Jadassohn.
Fig. 28. Bruno Bloch.

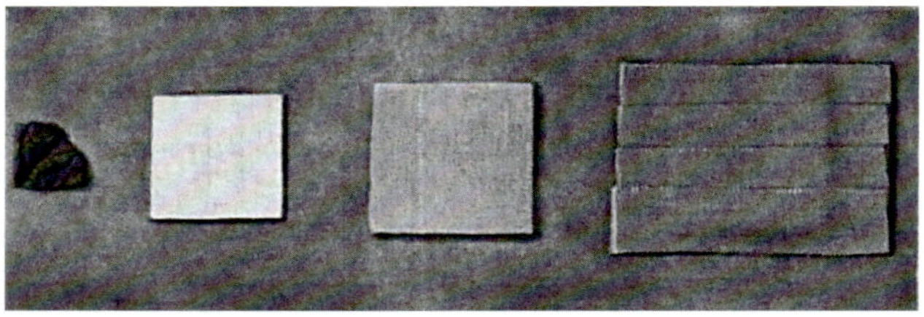

Fig. 29. Patch test with pieces of textiles.

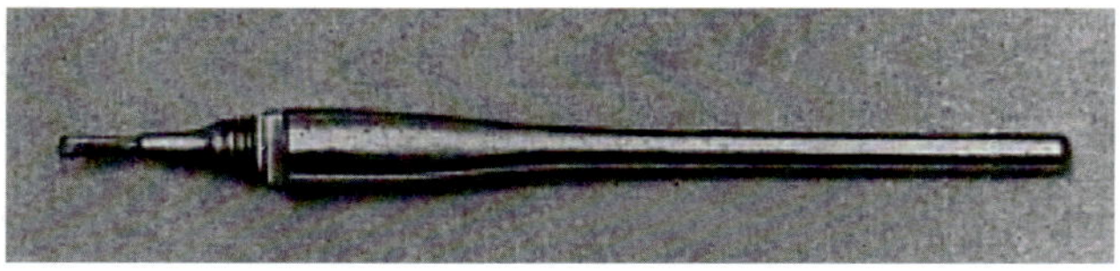

Fig. 30. Skin drill for prick test from Pirquet.

Around 1928, the patch test was popularized and developed further by Bruno Bloch (1878–1933; fig. 28), leading the test to general recognition as the 'Jadassohn-Bloch patch test' (fig. 29, from Berger and Hansen [31]). The generally accepted term 'patch test' was coined by Marion Baldur Sulzberger (1895–1983) [see fig. 6 in the chapter by Wallach and Taïeb, this vol., p. 88] in 1931, who, together with Fred Wise, popularized the test in the USA [32].

Precursor of the Prick Test

In 1890, Robert Koch presented his tuberculin at the 10th International Medical Congress in Berlin, and demonstrated a subcutaneous tuberculin test. Pirquet modified the tuberculin test by giving a drop of tuberculin on the skin of the forearm and then using a 'Pirquet-drill' (fig. 30) to scarify the skin under the tuberculin drop. This was the precursor of the skin prick test. Pirquet demonstrated his test for the first time in Vienna on June 6, 1907 [33].

The 'puncture method' was then further recommended by Freeman in 1930 for dermal testing and inoculation for vaccines [34]. This 'modified prick test', as it is used today, was developed by Mrs. Helmtraut Ebruster and was published in 1959 [35]. She worked for a short time at the University Clinic for Dermatology in Vienna. The test became the most commonly used allergy test worldwide; however, of H. Ebruster there are no known pictures and we know very little about her life.

Intracutaneous Test

On March 22, 1908, Felix Mendel (1862–1925), working in Essen, Germany, recommended the intracutaneous application of tuberculin, not as a diagnostic tool but as a way of vaccination [36]. His name is almost forgotten. Some months later, on August 10, 1908, Charles Mantoux (1877–1947) published the tuberculin test in the same way, known today as the Mendel-Mantoux test [37]. Béla Schick used the intracutaneous test (fig. 31) for the detection of immunity to diphtheria and Robert A. Cooke published the method in New York in 1915 [37].

In the early years there was considerable disagreement as to the relative advantages of the intracutaneous (or 'endermal') test in comparison to the scratch test, which was simpler and safer. The endermal test was more sensitive, but more dangerous when not properly used, and fatalities had been reported as a consequence [38]. So it was proposed by Vaughan [39]:

> The safe procedure is invariably to apply scratch tests before testing endermally with the same allergens.

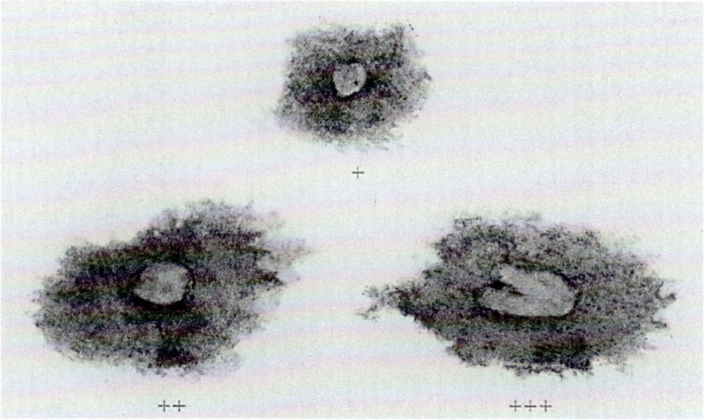

Fig. 31. Positive intracutaneous tests; from + to +++.

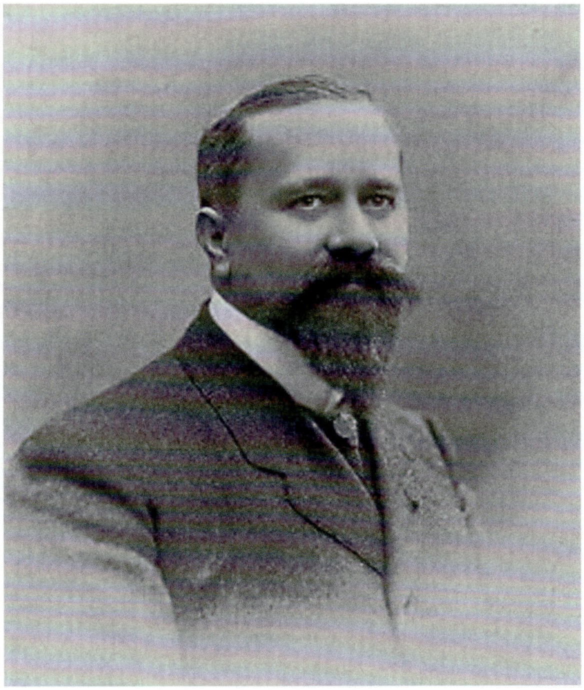

Fig. 32. Albert Calmette.

Rub Test

The technically easiest skin test for proving a sensitization was first described in 1961 as a 'rub test' by Albert Oehling [40]. He demonstrated the test in a carpenter with an allergy to obeche wood using the native wood. The 'rub test' has proven to be a very reliable, easily demonstrable and extremely simple method for detection of IgE-mediated allergy, inducing an immediate reaction with various inhalative and ingestive allergens.

Conjunctival Provocation

The 'ophthalmo reaction' was used by Blackley in 1873 for the diagnosis of hay fever, but the method fell into oblivion. In 1907, Léon Charles Albert Calmette (1863–1933; fig. 32) and Alfred Wolff-Eisner (1877–1948) published the usefulness of the conjunctival test for the diagnosis of tuberculosis [41, 42]. Therefore, for some years the test was named the Calmette and Wolff-Eisner ophthalmo reaction. Noon and Freeman used the test successfully in 1911 for measuring the effectiveness of immunotherapy (fig. 33, from Urbach [43]).

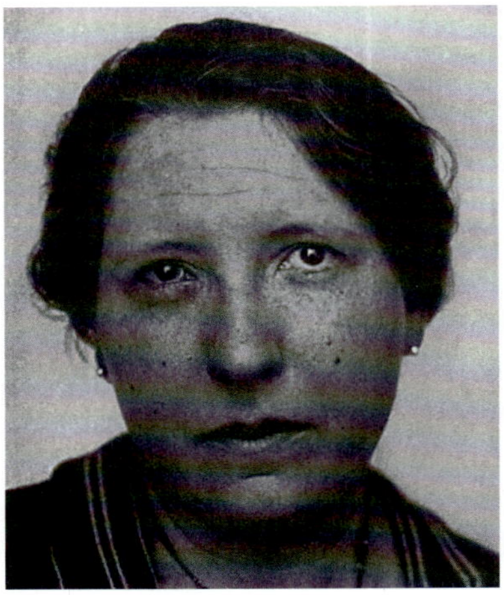

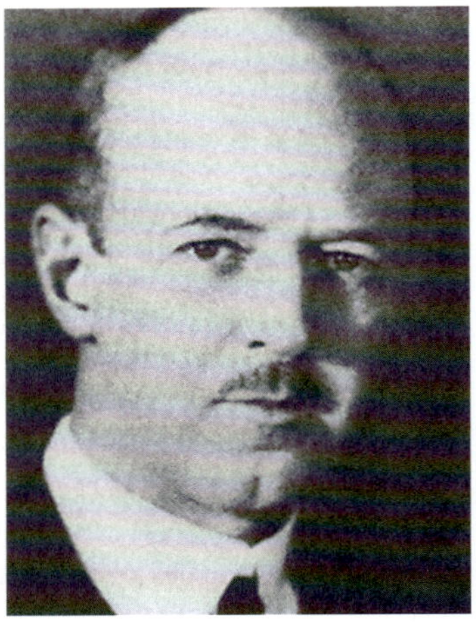

Fig. 33. Positive conjunctival test.
Fig. 34. William Duke.

Nasal Provocation Test

The development of the nasal provocation test started with the publication of a case report by the British physician William P. Kirkman (1827–1852), who reported in a local medical journal in 1852 [44]. In 1851 at around Christmas time, Kirkman, who suffered from hay fever, had a flowering grass in his greenhouse 'loaded well with pollen'. He took some pollen in his hand and inhaled them through his nose. He sneezed immediately and developed all the symptoms of hay fever over the next hour. In this way, the deliberate nasal application of pollen had led to hay fever symptoms outside of the pollen season in an experiment.

The Boston laryngologist Joseph Lincoln Goodale (1868–1957) systematically studied the nasal allergen provocation in the diagnosis of allergic rhinitis and, in 1914, published the test in detail for the diagnosis of horse asthma [45]. Between 1914 and 1916 he tested more than 400 patients suffering from rhinitis due to animal dander, food and pollen on the nasal mucosa.

In 1925, William W. Duke (1883–1946; fig. 34) suggested the test as a routine procedure [46]. He made modifications in an effort to avoid overly intense reactions by spraying dilutions of 1:1,000 pollen extract into the nose.

In 1930, outside of the pollen season, Efron and Penfound blew a small amount of dried pollen into one side of the nose [47]. When the patient was allergic to pollen hay fever, symptoms of varying severity ensued; it was reported that some patients had severe nasal and conjunctival symptoms.

In 1933, Erich Urbach (1893–1946) developed and proposed the 'cotton applicator method' (Stieltupfermethode; fig. 35) to allow provocation with allergen extracts [48]. From 1935 the allergens were given as powder into the nose, termed the powder puff test [49].

Inhalation Tests

In 1925, the brothers Simon S. (1892–1957) and Charles S. Leopold (1896–1960) developed and published an inhalation technique for allergens, primarily for experimental tests and not for routine diagnostics [50]. It seems that the test was not popular.

Later, in 1952, Schiller and Lowell used aerosolized allergens for inhalation with special emphasis on house dust, but also with extracts of pollen and *Alternaria*. Following the inhalation, vital capacity and expiratory rates were measured at intervals of 1 min. A reduction of 10% in vital capacity was considered as evidence of sensitivity. The incidence of skin reactions was much higher than of pulmonary reactions, and there were no pulmonary reactions with allergens which did not result in skin reactions [51].

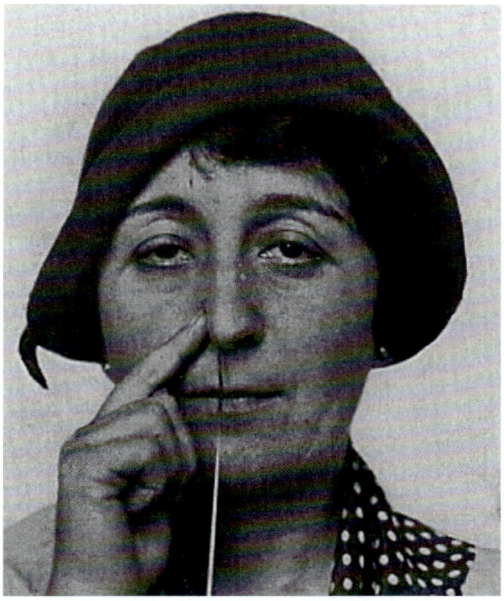

Fig. 35. The cotton applicator method according to Urbach.

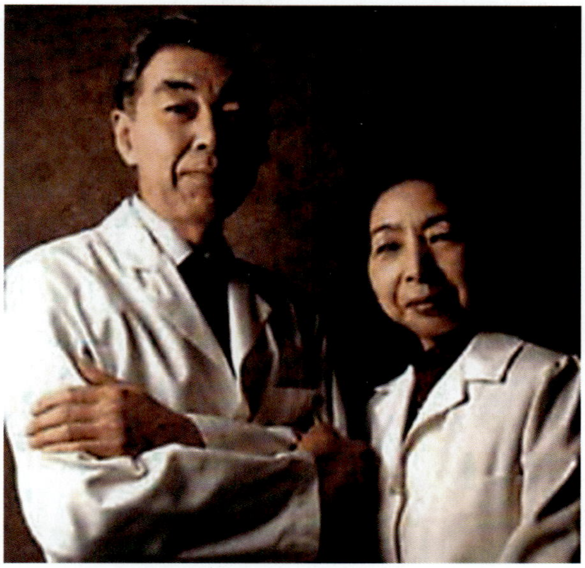

Fig. 36. Teruko and Kimishige Ishizaka.

In 1956, Wilhelm Gronemeyer (1912–1990) and Erich Fuchs (1921–2008) published the 'inhalation pneumometry test' as a routine method in Germany which was especially designed for the diagnosis of occupational asthma. A positive inhalation test was seen as the ultimate proof of a clinically relevant sensitization [52].

Discovery of IgE and Slow Reacting Substances

Kimishige Ishizaka (born in 1925) and Teruko Ishizaka (born in 1926; fig. 36) isolated IgE from the serum of sufferers of hay fever caused by ragweed, immunized rabbits and absorbed the antiserum with IgG, IgA, IgM and IgD. Using the supernatant after the absorptions, a Prausnitz-Küstner reaction was induced, and a new Ig class, named gamma E (erythema), had been detected [53].

The time had come for the discovery of IgE. S.G.O. Johansson and H. Bennich had at the same time identified a previously unknown Ig in a patient with a myeloma, which they named after his initials, IgND [54]. It turned out that this IgND was identical to IgE, and the long search for the 'reagins' was over!

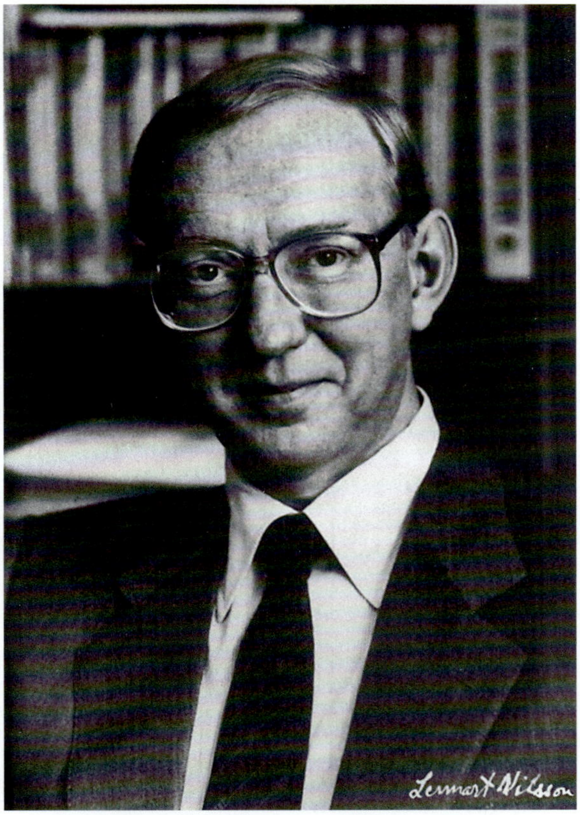

Fig. 37. Bengt Ingemar Samuelsson.

Allergological research was inspired by the discovery of IgE. Its quantitative determination in serum for diagnostic purposes was groundbreaking. In the blood of healthy individuals only small quantities of IgE could be found, while patients with type 1 allergies had elevated amounts – just as in an IgE-induced allergy. The quickly following development of the radioallergosorbent test and its wide use was another diagnostic landmark for the work of allergists all over the world.

Discovery of Leukotrienes

In 1982, Bengt Ingemar Samuelsson (born in 1934; fig. 37) received the Nobel Prize in Medicine/Physiology for identifying leukotrienes as the little-understood 'slow reacting substance of anaphylaxis', which had been found in allergic inflammation many years earlier. Samuelsson's work greatly advanced the understanding of the biological role of leukotrienes as mediators in asthma, allergy and inflammation.

References

1 Halter H: Traum vom ewigen Leben. Spiegel 1999;14:131–138.
2 Curtis HH: The immunizing cure of hay-fever. Med News 1900;77:16–18.
3 Noon L: Prophylactic inoculation against hay fever. Lancet 1911;i:1572–1573.
4 Freeman J: Further observations on the treatment of hay fever by hypodermic inoculations of pollen vaccine. Lancet 1911;ii: 814–817.
5 Bruun E: Le traitement des états allergiques par désensibilisation spécifique. Acta Allerg 1950;3(suppl 1):239.
6 Frankland AW, Augustin R: Prophylaxis of summer hay-fever and asthma: a controlled trial comparing crude grass-pollen extracts with the isolated main protein component. Lancet 1954;1055–1057.
7 Dreborg S, Lee TH, Kay AB, Durham SR: Immunotherapy is allergen-specific: a double-blind trial of mite or timothy extract in mite and grass dualallergic patients. Int Arch Allergy Immunol 2012;158:63–70.
8 Ring J, Gutermuth J: 100 years of hyposensitization: history of allergen-specific immunotherapy (ASIT). Allergy 2011;66:713–724.
9 Portier P, Richet C: De l'action anaphylactique de certain nénins. CR Soc Biol 1902; 54:170.
10 Pirquet C: Allergie. Münch Med Wochenschr 1906;53:1457.
11 Langerhans R: Tod durch Heilserum! Berl Klin Wochenschr 1896;33:602.
12 Lamson RW: Sudden death associated with the injection of foreign substances. J Am Med Assoc 1924;82:109.
13 Pirquet C, Schick B: Zur Theorie der Inkubationszeit. Wien Klin Wochenschr 1903; 16:758.
14 Arthus M: Injections répétées de sérum de cheval chez le lapin. CR Soc Biol 1903;55: 817–820.
15 Besredka A, Steinhardt E: De l'anaphylaxie et de l'antianaphylaxie vis-a-vis du serum de cheval. Ann Inst Pasteur 1907;21:117.
16 Hutinel VH: Intolérance pour le lait et anaphylaxie chez les nourrissons. Clin Paris 1908;3:227.
17 Hansen K: Asthma als Schockfragment. Wien Klin Wochenschr 1941;54:175.
18 Otto R: Zur Frage der Serumüberempfindlichkeit. Münch Med Wochenschr 1907;54: 1665.
19 Uhlenhuth P, Haendel L: Untersuchungen über die praktische Verwertbarkeit der Anaphylaxie zur Erkennung und Unterscheidung verschiedener Eiweissarten. Z Immun Forsch 1909/1910;4:761.
20 Coca AF, Cooke RA: On the classification of the phenomenon of hypersensitiveness. J Immunol 1923;8:163.
21 Ramirez MH: Horse asthma following blood transfusion: report of case. J Am Med Assoc 1919;73:984–985
22 Frugoni C: Studi sull'astma bronchiale cum particolare riguardo all'asma anafilattico. Policlinico Med 1922;29:179.
23 Prausnitz K, Küstner H: Studien über die Überempfindlichkeit. Zbl Bakt 1921;86: 160–169.
24 Frankland AW: Carl Prausnitz: a personal memoir. J Allergy Clin Immunol 2004;114: 700–705.
25 Johansson SG, Nopp A, van Hage M, Olofsson N, Lundahl J, Wehlin L, Söderström L, Stiller V, Oman H: Passive IgE-sensitization by blood transfusion. Allergy 2005;60: 1192–1199.
26 Ovary Z: Souveniers: Around the World in Ninety Years. New York, India Ink Press, 1999.
27 Blackley CH: Experimental Researches on the Causes and Nature of Catarrhus Aestivus (Hay-Fever or Hay-Asthma). London, Bailliere, Tindeall & Cox, 1873, p 73.
28 Schloss OM: A case of allergy to common food. Am J Dis Child 1912;3:341.
29 Walker I: Studies in the sensitisation of patients with bronchial asthma to bacterial proteins. J Med Res 1917;37:487.
30 Jadassohn J: Zur Kenntnis der medikamentösen Dermatosen. Verh Dtsch Derm Ges 1986;5:103.
31 Berger W, Hansen K: Allergie. Leipzig, Thieme, 1940.
32 Sulzberger MB, Wise F: The contact or patch-test in dermatology. Arch Dermatol Syph 1931;23:519.
33 von Pirquet C: Tuberkulindiagnose durch cutane Impfung. Berlin Klin Wochenschr 1907;1907:644.
34 Freeman J: Rush inoculation. Lancet 1930;i: 744.
35 Ebruster H: Der Pricktest, eine neuere Cutanprobe zur Diagnose allergischer Erkrankungen. Wien Klin Wochenschr 1959; 71:551–554.
36 Mendel F: Die von Pirquetsche Hautreaktion und die intrakutane Tuberkulinbehandlung. Med Klin 1908;4:402.
37 Cooke RA: The treatment of hay fever by active immunization. Laryngoscope 1915;25: 108.
38 Harris LH, Shure N: Sudden death due to allergy tests. J Allergy 1950;21:208.
39 Vaughan WT, Black JH: Practice of Allergy, ed 3. St Louis, Mosby, 1984, p 168.
40 Oehling A, Gronemeyer W: The use of rub test in wood allergy. Abstract 143 of the 4th International Congress. International Congress Series No 42. New York, Allergology, 1961.
41 Calmette LCA: Sur un nouveau procédé de diagnostic de la tuberculose chez l'homme par l'ophthalmo-réaction à la tuberculine. CR Acad Sci 1907;144:1324–1326.

42 Wolff-Eisner A: Die kutane und konjunktivale Tuberkulinreaktion, ihre Bedeutung für Diagnostik und Prognose der Tuberkulose. Z Tuberk 1907;12:21–25.
43 Urbach E: Klinik und Therapie der allergischen Krankheiten. Vienna, Maudrich, 1935.
44 Kirkman W: Case of hay fever. Prov Med Surg J 1852;12:360.
45 Goodale JL: Studies regarding anaphylactic reactions occurring in horse asthma and allied conditions. Ann Ot 1914;23:273.
46 Duke WW: Allergy, Asthma, Hay Fever, Urticaria and Other Manifestation of Reaction. St Louis, Mosby, 1925.
47 Efron BG, Penfound WT: A nasal test with dry pollens in the diagnosis of seasonal hay fever. J Allergy 1930;2:43.
48 Urbach E: Methodik des Allergennachweises. Münch Med Wochenschr 1933;80:134.
49 Urbach E: Fortschritte in der Testung und Behandlung allergischer Kranker. Wien Klin Wochenschr 1935;48:251.
50 Leopold SS, Leopold CS: Bronchial asthma and allied allergic disorders. J Am Med Assoc 1925;84:731.
51 Schiller IW, Lowell FC: The inhalation test as a diagnostic procedure with special emphasis on the house dust allergen. J Allergy 1952;23:234.
52 Fuchs E, Gronemeyer W, Iwanoff I: Der inhalative Antigen-Pneumometrie-Test zur Ermittlung des aktuellen Allergens bei berufsbedingtem Asthma bronchiale. Dtsch Med Wochenschr 1956;81:339.
53 Ishizaka K, Ishizaka T, Hornbrook MM: Physicochemical properties of reaginic antibody. 5. Correlation of reaginic activity with γE-globulin antibody. J Immunol 1966;97:840–853.
54 Johansson SG: Raised levels of a new immunoglobulin class (IgND) in asthma. Lancet 1967;ii:951–953.

Prof. Dr. med. Karl-Christian Bergmann
Allergie-Centrum-Charité, Charité – Universitätsmedizin
Luisenstrasse 2
DE–10117 Berlin (Germany)
E-Mail karlchristianbergmann@googlemail.com

Bergmann K-C, Ring J (eds): History of Allergy. Chem Immunol Allergy. Basel, Karger, 2014, vol 100, pp 46–52
DOI: 10.1159/000358500

Terminology of Allergic Phenomena

Johannes Ring

Department of Dermatology and Allergy Biederstein, Christine Kuehne Center for Allergy Research and Education (CK-CARE), Technical University of Munich, Munich, Germany

Abstract

Over the last 2,000 years a variety of terms have been used for the description of phenomena possibly related to allergy. Many have been forgotten, while some of them have remained. In Greco-Roman literature the term 'idiosyncrasy' was used to describe an individual characterization of a health condition, possibly comparable to 'constitution'. The same term was also used to describe individual reaction patterns, and the term 'antipathy' was used in a similar sense. 'Hypersensitivity' originated from the German word 'Überempfindlichkeit' and was first used in a medical sense by Emil von Behring when he described untoward reactions to his antitoxin containing serum therapy. 'Anaphylaxis' was coined by Richet and Portier to describe the new phenomenon of a life-threatening general pathogenic reaction after repeated injection of antigen. In 1906, Clemens von Pirquet introduced the term 'allergy' in order to bring more clarity to the confusing debate regarding protective and harmful immunity. In order to characterize the familial occurrence of hypersensitivity reactions such as asthma, hay fever and others, the American allergists A.F. Coca and R.A. Cooke introduced the term 'atopy'. Contrary to anaphylaxis, which was experimentally induced, this type of 'hypersensitiveness' occurred spontaneously. The nature of the pathogenic factor was called the 'atopic reagin' and was found to be transferable with serum by Prausnitz and Küstner. After the detection of immunoglobulin (Ig) E as the carrier of this type of hypersensitivity, the term 'atopy' gained a new sense, since IgE is a characteristic – yet not exclusive – parameter of the so-called atopic diseases. Clinically similar diseases such as asthma, rhinoconjunctivitis or eczema can be found in the absence of IgE, and are then called 'intrinsic' variants of the same disease.

It is impossible to write a history of allergy without discussing terminology. This is because many and contrasting terms were and are used for the description of a variety of clinical conditions. Over the centuries or millennia it was not the development of new diseases – as shown in the opening two chapters of this volume – and neither was it the occurrence of new elicitors (pollen or indoor allergens), but rather a new understanding of a pathophysiologic mechanism on the basis of an altered and thereby pathogenic immune response which was new. That was the intention of Clemens von Pirquet when he created the term 'allergy' in his short essay in the *Münchner Medizinische Wochenschrift* of 24 July 1906 [1]. This term itself is neither the beginning nor the end of the history of allergy terminology, it has itself changed in meaning over the decades, including in the 20th century.

In the following we want to briefly discuss some of the most important terms used in the description of allergic phenomena in the past. From time to time regional and international organizations have tried to standardize terminology and give clear-cut definitions [2–4]. Not all these endeavors were successful. With increasing knowledge new concepts arose and new interpretations and names developed.

Idiosyncrasy

The earliest term we can find in the context of descriptions of possible allergic phenomena in medical history might be the term 'idiosyncrasy', which was used in Hippocratic medicine and was better described probably, for the first time, by Ptolemaios (885–960 AD) [5, vol. 1, p. 8; 6, 7]. This term described the uniqueness or individuality of a single human being and was based on the Hippocratic concept of the four humors, which have to be in the correct mixture within the individual. Earlier sources possibly described the term 'symmixis', which was used by the philosopher Anaxagoras [8]. Today, the term 'idiosyncrasy' could probably be best translated as 'constitution'. The word is derived from the Greek 'synkerannimi', meaning 'mix', and 'idios', meaning 'own' or 'itself'. Occasionally the expression also describes the specific reaction patterns of an individual.

In some sources, besides or instead of idiosyncrasy, the terms 'idiosystasy', 'idiaesthesy' or 'idiosynkrisy' are found [5, vol. 1, p. 12]:

> Quite often (susceptible) people are suffering with regard to their body from idiosynkrasy, e.g. certain foods or drinks as for example after heavy intake of wine. [9]

Galen uses the term in a pharmacological sense when he describes unexpected drug effects which cannot be explained by the effect of the substance, but rather by the property of a certain patient [5, vol. 1, p. 13]:

> And someone who did not know this drug, prepared it in a weaker form and in a finer powder, and thus it did not have any effect with regard to the stool but a rather stronger effect with regard to the urine. He reported this observation because he was surprised and he wanted to find the true cause. He himself thought that a certain idiosyncrasy of the respective patient was the cause of the phenomenon and he called it like that. [10]

In a variety of texts of antiquity, idiosyncrasy is used to explain various phenotypes or differences between races and skin colors, as well as different tolerability of foods or luxury foods [8]. The same author used this term in the description of a special tolerance regarding poisons, in cases where certain persons were tolerating otherwise fatal or lethal poisons without any adverse reactions, or when it described different degrees of susceptibility to pain in different individuals or population groups.

Later, the term was used for psychological phenomena or philosophical conditions. For example, Immanuel Kant [11] (1724–1804) spoke about this in the sense of 'hobby' or 'crank':

> Idiosyncrasy ... wanted to be popular term which does not find acceptance with wise people ... but rather behaves like a cricket in the head and is chirping without to be heard by anybody else.

In a letter from November 24, 1812, to a lady serving the Empress of Austria, Johann Wolfgang von Goethe (1749–1832) used the word 'idiosyncrasy' to describe his distaste of writing letters [5, vol. 1, p. 21; 12, vol. 9, p. 677]. The same Goethe also used the term in a medical sense when he described a strange disease with complaints in the throat and the esophagus which could not be explained by the physicians and which he suspected to be caused by his activity in etching and erasing copperplates [5, vol. 1, p. 28].

> I felt quite well in this time after my work, although during these days I was attacked by an evil which I had never known before. The throat was quite sore and especially the part which is called uvula was inflamed.

I could only swallow with great pain and the doctors did not know what to do. They tortured me with gargling and brushing yet without relieving me from this pain. Finally I realized intuitively that when I was etching not carefully and especially when I did it more often and with passion, I acquired this evil and it came back repeatedly. Now the doctors agreed and saw the plausibility and finally when I stopped the etching and erasing – especially because my experiments were not at all good – ... I found the easier consolation the sooner I was liberated from this unpleasant evil. [12, vol. 10, p. 382]

Other authors used the term 'idiosyncrasy' in order to describe compulsory neurotic conditions, like an acute desire to urinate when listening to lute music or singultus after coitus [5, vol. 1, p. 27; 13]. By such widely differing meanings the term became more and more diluted, leading Wolf Eissner [14] (1877–1848) to feel it should be preserved for allergic reactions:

A large number of idiosyncrasies can now be explained as hypersensitivity against the application of foreign protein, especially occurring after previous injections of the respective protein when a hypersensitivity against this substance has developed.

In modern allergology the term was used to distinguish certain genetically defined non-allergic hypersensitivity reactions, for instance together with enzyme defects like the favism or lathyrism, when intoxication symptoms occur after the application of chickpeas. Today, idiosyncrasy is used in Anglo-Saxon literature in order to describe non-immunologic hypersensitivity reactions, the symptoms of which differ in quality from the pharmacological effect of the substance, e.g. aspirin idiosyncrasy [15, 16].

Antipathy

Over the centuries another term – today mostly used in a psychological context – was 'antipathy', which also described incompatibility symptoms against certain substances or against colors. Occasionally classic allergic conditions were also described as sequels of antipathy, such as by Johann Samuel Eggers from Halle in the year 1730, who classified cases of rose fever under 'antipathy' [5, vol. 1, p. 41; 17].

In the sense of 'constitution', the term idiosyncrasy was also sometimes replaced by the following other terms: 'idiopathy' (Galenos), 'diathesis' (in Latin 'dispositio'), 'schisis' (posture of body and appearance; in Latin 'habitus'), and 'physis' (in Latin 'natura'). The term 'diathesis' will be discussed together with 'atopy', below.

Hypersensitivity

It is surprising that the term 'hypersensitivity', which today is the main term for the various immunologically or non-immunologically mediated reactions against environmental substances, was only discovered in the 19th century for medical use. It was Emil von Behring (1854–1917) who used it in the year 1893 in order to describe untoward reactions to his serum therapy [5, vol. 1, p. 45; 18, 19]:

Let us understand the result of the milk and serum tests: so maybe at a first glance it looks paradoxical that an animal which in its blood and also in the secretions contains considerable amounts of tetanus antitoxin should develop less resistance against the tetanus poison than it had at a time, when it had not developed antitoxin in its organism. [20]

Von Behring and his co-worker Wladimiroff used the term 'paradoxical reaction' for a phenomenon when organisms, which should actually be protected by immunization, reacted pathogenically. The phenomenon itself was not new; Robert Koch had already noted – and von Behring [21] also mentioned this – that stronger skin reactions could be observed after repeated injections of tuberculin.

Clemens von Pirquet and Béla Schick also used the term in the sense of the later introduced term 'allergy' when they wrote an article entitled 'Überempfindlichkeit und beschleunigte Reaktionen' ('Hypersensitivity and accelerated reactions') [22]. There they described increased second-set reactions by an increased reaction of the organism to a second injection of antigen in the form of hypersensitivity.

Coca and Cooke used the German term as 'hypersensitiveness' in English, and later as 'hypersensitivity' when they described a special form of this hypersensitiveness as 'atopy' [23]. Today, hypersensitivity is used in order to describe a 'reaction exceeding the normal'.

This does not necessarily have immunological implications [4, 16]; the term can also be used for psychological phenomena or increased pain sensitivity.

Anaphylaxis

The birth of the term 'anaphylaxis' has been described and commented on often in allergy history, and rightly so: it shows the importance of giving names to a newly discovered phenomenon. This will be discussed in detail in the chapter by Ring et al. [this vol., pp. 54–61]. Here we only reflect the terms used in context with the discovery of Richet and Portier [24, 25] in the 20th century and beyond.

Richet used the term to describe potentially life-threatening generalized reactions after repeated injection of protein. As an adjective, 'anaphylactic' was very well accepted. Von Behring, who had seen such reactions and called them 'paradoxical' or 'hypersensitivity', now called reactions without preceding antigen injections which showed a clinically similar symptomatology 'anaphylactoid':

> These processes which are symptomatic for anaphylactic (anatoxic) poisoning, in their origin yet markedly differ and occur not in an organism which is hypersensitive or sensitized, I want to call 'anapyhlactoid'. [21]

Later, several authors tried to differentiate non-immunologic reactions with the symptoms of anaphylaxis by calling them 'anaphylactoid' [26]; other terms used include 'allergoid', 'allergy-like' or 'pseudo-allergic' [27]. The new definition of the World Allergy Organization (WAO) is based on the clinical symptomatology and defines anaphylaxis as 'acute generalized potentially life-threatening reaction with varying symptomatology' [4].

It is independent from the pathomechanism; there is an immunologic (allergic) anaphylaxis and a non-immunologic anaphylaxis. With this all other terms, such as anaphylactoid, are superfluous [28].

Several authors tried to improve the etymologically incorrect term 'anaphylaxis' by calling it 'paraphylaxis' [29–31] or 'aristophylaxy' (Karl Momsen) when there is natural sensitization [32]. However, these ideas were not acknowledged by the public.

After a large dose of antigen a phase of tolerance was sometimes observed and was called 'sceptophylaxis' ('sceptos' means 'acute thunderstorm'). Alexandre Besredka used the term 'antianaphylaxis' for a state of tolerance after desensitization [33].

In modern pharmacology, the term 'tachyphylaxis' is still used to describe a phenomenon where the effect of a substance is weakened after its repeated application [34]. Elicitors of these reactions were called 'anaphylactogen' or 'anaphylactin'.

In the decades after the term was born, 'anaphylaxis' conquered the world; many authors used it equally with allergy or to describe all kinds of hypersensitivity. The term became so popular that some authors felt they should warn of the 'myth of anaphylaxis' or the danger of an 'anaphylactomania' [35]. Today, 'anaphylaxis' is a clearly defined term which describes a subgroup of hypersensitivity reactions which may be allergic but also non-immunologic in nature.

Allergy

When in 1906 Clemens von Pirquet wrote his famous essay of one and a half pages, he used an artificial new creation which he justifies as follows:

> We need a new general not-prejudicing word for the change in condition which exists in an organism after knowing some organic living or dead poison … For this general condition of altered reactivity I propose the term 'allergy'. 'Allos' means the deviation of an original condition, of a behavior of normality, like allorhythmy, allotropy, … The new names do not alter the existing special nomenclature. The well-defined terms like antitoxins, cytolysins, hemolysins, precipitins, agglutinins, coagulins are not affected. Hypersensitivity is a new field in which only recently the formation of terms takes place under painful adaptation to old names. From this feeling and in order to bring clarity in this formation of terms I propose the new terms and hope that by making the external forms more simple, the investigation of the interesting processes in this field will be facilitated for the co-workers. [1]

This proposal was based on the clinical situation which he had observed in his studies on serum sickness together with Béla Schick. The term did not contain bacteriological or immunological mechanisms [22]. From the philological viewpoint, the word is not strictly correct since the melting of 'o' (omicron) and 'ε' (epsilon) in Greek would lead to 'ου'.

In his meaning, von Pirquet's altered reactivity also included deviations from the norm to the lesser, i.e. weakened reactions. This has been lost over time. After many discussions in international nomenclature committees, the following was decided at the 3rd International Congress for Allergology in 1958 in Paris:

> Allergy is an acquired qualitatively altered capacity of living tissue to react induced by a specific allergen. [2]

Besides this term others were developed, such as 'parallergy' or 'metallergy', which aimed to describe that during the development of hypersensitivity against one antigen, increased reactions to another non-related antigen can be observed [36, 37]. The inherent dilemma of one common definition for clinical symptoms and basic pathomechanisms at the same time continues. Often the fact that these are different categories which are not necessarily connected is not considered.

Four aspects remain until today:
(1) altered reactivity (mostly increased);
(2) specificity;
(3) involvement of the immune system, and
(4) a pathogenic effect.
Therefore, in agreement with most authors, 'allergy' can today be defined as follows:

> Allergy is a specific alteration of the immune response leading to a pathogenic hypersensitivity. [16]

The nomenclature task force of the WAO made the following definition:

> Allergy is an immunologically mediated specific hypersensitivity. [4]

Terms like 'neuroallergy', 'psychoallergy' or 'panallergy' should be mentioned, although they did not become established [5]. Other authors tried to describe the phenomenon as 'pathobiosis' [38] and 'allobiosis', or, in the example of the surgeon August Bier, 'metakinesis' [5, vol. 1, p. 91; 39, p. 11].

In the description of allergy-related diseases various names were created, like the term 'allergoses', further divided into 'rhinallergoses', 'ophthallergoses', 'bronchiallergoses', 'enterallergoses', 'dermallergoses', etc. Erich Hoffmann subsumed allergic occupational diseases in the term 'ergasidermatoses' (in Greek 'ergasia', meaning 'occupation') [40]. The tendency of an individual to develop allergic reactions was called allergic diathesis by Kämmerer [41]. This leads us directly to the term 'atopy'.

Atopy

While the immense progress of early allergology was mainly due to experimental investigations (e.g. anaphylaxis) or immunological studies following active of passive vaccinations, the mere clinical observation was not so important. It was well known that diseases like hay fever and asthma, and also the skin disease called 'neurodermite' by Brocq and Jacquet [42], often occurred in one and the same patient, but even more often in various family members. This familial disposition – in contrast to the artificially induced situation of anaphylaxis – was adopted by the American allergists Arthur Fernandez Coca (1875–1955) and Robert Anderson Cooke (1880–1960), and was newly defined. They were modest with regard to their linguistic etymologic competence and consulted the Graeco-philologist Edward Perry (1856–1938) from the Columbia University of New York. Perry proposed the term 'atopy', which he created from the Greek word 'atopos' (meaning 'unusual, strange, not in the right place').

Coca and Cooke [23] proposed this term in an article in 1923 in a series on 'Phenomena of hypersensitiveness', and intended to describe patients who suffered either from seasonal allergic rhinitis, bronchial asthma or other allergic phenomena:

> The individuals as a group possess a peculiar capacity to become sensitive to certain proteins to which the environment and habits of life frequently expose them. [43, p. 122]

Since there were no precipitating antibodies in hay fever patients, which were well-known from serum sickness, other relevant agents were suspected which were named 'atopic reagins' and were transferrable by serum, as shown by Prausnitz and Küstner [44] in 1921.

For certain forms of food hypersensitivity where Coca could not see positive skin tests, as well as certain forms of drug hypersensitivity, he proposed the term 'idioblapsis' ('idios' meaning 'own, itself' and 'blaptein' meaning 'damage'), equally following the advice of the Graeco-philologist Kurt von Fritz [5, vol. 1, p. 101]. This term did not succeed, whereas 'atopy' was well accepted and gained increasing importance, especially after the detection of the nature of reaginic antibodies such as immunoglobulin (Ig) E [see the chapter by Johansson, this vol., pp.150–154). Yet also here, as was the case with the term 'allergy', the discussion between immunological-experimental investigators and clinicians continued, meaning there are at least two similar but not identical definitions for 'atopy', one originating from the tendency to form IgE, the other from the clinical situation (WAO definition):

> Atopy is the tendency to produce immunoglobulin E antibodies against environmental substances leading to clinical symptoms. [4]

The other definition from the *Handbook of Atopic Eczema* is:

> Atopy is the familial tendency to develop certain diseases (asthma, rhinoconjunctivitis, eczema) on the basis of a hypersensitivity of skin and mucus membranes against environmental substances associated with increased IgE production and/or altered non-specific reactivity. [45]

This latter definition originates from the clinical symptom observed by the physician, before he or she is able to measure IgE in the serum. Today one might connect this altered reactivity probably to epithelial barrier dysfunction.

Both definitions differ essentially insofar as in the first (WAO), increased IgE levels must be present per definition in order to call a disease 'atopic'. However, it is a general clinical experience that exactly the same clinical diseases, namely rhinoconjunctivitis, bronchial asthma and eczema, can occur with and without elevated IgE levels.

This may be due to a lack of methodology for measuring IgE antibodies against specific allergens not yet known. However, it is more likely that the disease itself can exist as hypersensitivity of the skin and mucus membranes without a necessary involvement of IgE antibodies. Therefore, the concept for asthma with an 'intrinsic' versus 'extrinsic' form is also valid for rhinoconjunctivitis where the non-IgE-associated form is often called 'vasomotor'. Wüthrich [46] transferred this concept to atopic eczema and postulated an extrinsic and intrinsic variant of atopic eczema.

The problem of the term 'intrinsic' is its negative nature – it can only be diagnosed by exclusion of detectable immune reactions. This weakens the defining potency. As soon as there was a positive marker of the intrinsic variant, this dilemma would be solved.

For allergy practice it is important to measure IgE antibodies. Only when they are detectable should specific therapeutic regimens, such as avoidance recommendation or allergen-specific immunotherapy, be commenced.

Conclusion

The knowledge and the discussion of terminology is no child's play, nor is it for sophisticated self-purpose [47, 48]. Underlying each term there is a more or less well thought out concept regarding the understanding of a disease or a pathomechanism, and their practical consequences for diagnosis and therapy. Therefore, it is important to clearly define what one is talking about!

References

1 von Pirquet C: Allergie. Münch Med Wochenschr 1906;53:1457.

2 International Association of Allergology and Clinical Immunology (IAACI): Definitions of 'allergy' and 'allergen'. Ann Allergy 1958;16:680.

3 Johansson SG, Hourihane JO, Bousquet J, Bruijnzeel-Koomen C, Dreborg S, Haahtela T, Kowalski ML, Mygind N, Ring J, van Cauwenberge P, van Hage-Hamsten M, Wuthrich B; EAACI (the European Academy of Allergology and Clinical Immunology) Nomenclature Task Force: A revised nomenclature for allergy. An EAACI position statement from the EAACI nomenclature task force. Allergy 2001:56:813-824.

4 Johansson SG, Bieber T, Dahl R, Friedmann PS, Lanier BQ, Lockey RF, Motala C, Ortega Martell JA, Platts-Mills TA, Rng J, Thien F, Van Cauwenberge P, Williams HC: Revised nomenclauture for allergy for global use: report of the Nomenclauture Review Committee of the World Allergy Organization, October 2003. J Allergy Clin Immunol 2004;113:832–836.
5 Schadewaldt H: Geschichte der Allergie. Munich, Dustri, 1979/1980, vol 1.
6 Nielsen CB: History and present status of tissue anaphylaxis. Stanf Med Bull 1961;19: 120.
7 Ptolemaios: Tetrabiblos; in Doll F, Boer AE (eds): Opera quae exstant omnia. Leipzig, 1957, vol 3.1.
8 Sextus Empiricus: Pyrrhoniarum hypotyposeon; in Bury RG (ed): Opera Graece et Latine (first ed Leipzig 1718: Opera). London, Loeb Classical Library 1, 1933, vol 1.
9 Dioskorides: Pedanii Dioscorides Anazerbei libri; in Kühn CG (ed): Medicorum Graecorum Opera. Leipzig, 1829, vol 25-1, p 184/ Leipzig, 1830, vol 26-2, p 4.
10 Galenos: Opera (Kühn CG ed). Leipzig, 1821–1833. Corpus Medicorum Graecorum. (Mewaldt J et al/Koch UK et al eds). Leipzig, 1914/1923, vol 5.4.2/5.9.1. Oeuvres anatomiques, physiologiques et médicales (von Daremberg C ed). Paris, 1854, vol 1, p 549.
11 Kant I: Anthropologie in pragmatischer Hinsicht; in Schbert F (ed): Sämtliche Werke. Leipzig, vol 7.2.
12 von Goethe JW: Gesammelte Werke Artemis Ausgabe. Zürich, 1949, vol 9, p 677/vol 10, p 382.
13 Baumgarten-Crusius M: Periodologie oder die Lehre von den periodischen Veränderungen im Leben des gesunden und kranken Menschen (Gruber JGG ed). Halle, 1831, vol 344, p 296 ff.
14 Woff-Eisner A: Das Heufieber, sein Wesen und seine Behandlung. Munich, 1906.
15 Middleton H, Ellis F, Reed C (eds): Allergy: Principles and Practice. St Louis, Mosby, 2008.
16 Ring J: Allergy in Practice. Berlin, Springer, 2005.
17 Eggers HS (Präses: M. Alberti): De sensibilitate personali. Med Inaug Diss, Halle-Magdeburg, 1730, p 23.
18 von Behring E: Über Idiosynkrasie, Anaphylaxie, Toxin-Überempfindlichkeit, Disposition und Diathese. Schmidts Jb Ges Med 1914;319:113.
19 von Behring E: Experimentelle Analyse und Theorie der anaphylaktischen und apotoxischen Vergiftung. Dtsch Med Wochenschr 1914;40:1749.
20 Wladimiroff A: Über die antitoxinerzeugende und immunisierende Wirkung des Tetanusgiftes bei Thieren. Hyg Infekt Kr 1893;15:405.
21 von Behring E: Über Idiosynkrasie, Anaphylaxie, Toxin-Überempfindlichkeit, Disposition and Diathese. Schmidts Jb Ges Med 1914; 319: 113/Gesammelte Abhandlungen, NF No 23. Bonn, 1915, p 175 ff.
22 von Pirquet C, Schick B: Überempfindlichkeit und beschleunigte Reaktion. Münch Med Wochenschr 1906;53:66.
23 Coca AF, Cooke RA: On the classification of the phenomena of hypersensitiveness. J Immunol 1923;8:163.
24 Richet C: De l'anaphylaxie ou sensibilité croissante des organismes à des doses successives de poison. Arch Fisiol 1903/1904;1: 129.
25 Portier P, Richet C: De l'action anaphylactique de certains vénins. CR Soc Biol 1902; 54:170–172/Trav Labor Physiol 1902;5:506.
26 Hanzlik PJ, Karsner HT: Anaphylactoid phenomena from the intravenous administration of various colloids, arsenicals and other agents. J Pharmacol Exp Ther 1920; 14:379.
27 Kallos P, Schlumberger HD: Allergie und allergische Krankheiten. Cologne, 1978, p 28 ff.
28 Ring J: Anaphylaktoische Reaktionen nach Infusion kolloidaler Volumenersatzmittel. Berlin, Springer, 1978.
29 Danielopolu D: Paraphylaxie et choc paraphylactique. Paris, 1943.
30 Danielopolu D: Rôle réspectif de l'acétylcholine et de l'histamine dans le choc paraphylactique (anaphylactique). Schweiz Med Wochenschr 1948;78:567.
31 Danielopolu D: Nouvelles preuves de la nature acétylcholinique du choc paraphylactique (anaphylactique). Recherches sur l'organe isolé. Acta Med Scand 1947;126: 589.
32 Momsen K: Allgemeine Bemerkungen zum Thema Allergie, speziell der pathologischen Physiologie; in Holler G, et al (eds): Das akute allergische Phänomen. Wien, 1958, p 7.
33 Besredka A, Steinhardt E: Du mécanisme de l'antianaphylaxie. Ann Inst Pasteur 1907; 21:384.
34 Champy C, Gley E: Sur la toxicité des extraits de corps jaune. Immunisation rapide consécutive à l'injection de petites doses de ces extraits (tachyphylaxie). CR Soc Biol 1911;63:159.
35 Jousset A: The myth of anaphylaxis. Med Press 1919;108:250.
36 Schadewaldt H: Premières mentions historiques des affections allergiques. Acta Allerg 1959;13:223.
37 Moro E, Keller W: Über die Parallergie. Klin Wochenschr 1935;14.
38 Heubner W: Über Pathobiose. Nachr Ges Wiss Göttingen (Math Phys Klasse) 1929; 96.
39 Abderhalden R: Grundriss der Allergie. Basel, Schwabe, 1950.
40 Rössle R: Geschichte der Allergieforschung; in Hansen K (ed): Allergie, ed 3. Stuttgart, Thieme, 1957.
41 Kämmerer H: Allergische Diathese und allergische Erkrankungen. Munich, Bergmann, 1926.
42 Brocq L: L'eczéma considéré comme une réaction cutaneé. Ann Dermatol Syph 1903;4:172.
43 Simons E (ed): Ancestors of Allergy. New York, Global Medical Communications, 1994.
44 Prausitz K, Küstner H: Studien über die Überempfindlichkeit. Zbl Bakt (Orig) 1921; 86:160.
45 Ring J, Ruzicka T, Przybilla B (eds): Handbook of Atopic Eczema, ed 2. Berlin, Springer, 2006.
46 Wüthrich B: Neurodermitis atopica sive constitutionalis. Ein pathogenetisches Modell aus der Sicht des Allergologen. Aktuel Dermatol 1983;9:1–7.
47 Otto R: Zur Frage der Serumüberempfindlichkeit. Münch Med Wochenschr 1907;54: 1665.
48 Rackemann FM: Professor Willem Storm van Leeuwen and the asthma problem. Acta Allerg 1958;12:407.

Prof. Dr. med. Dr. phil. Johannes Ring
Department of Dermatology and Allergy Biederstein
Biedersteinerstrasse 29
DE–80802 München (Germany)
E-Mail johannes.ring@lrz.tu-muenchen.de

2 Most Common Allergic Diseases: Historical Reflections in Understanding

Bergmann K-C, Ring J (eds): History of Allergy. Chem Immunol Allergy. Basel, Karger, 2014, vol 100, pp 54–61
DOI: 10.1159/000358503

Anaphylaxis

Johannes Ring[a] · Martine Grosber[a] · Knut Brockow[a] · Karl-Christian Bergmann[b]

[a]Department of Dermatology and Allergy Biederstein, Christine Kuehne Center for Allergy Research and Education (CK-CARE), Technical University of Munich, Munich, and [b]Allergy Centre Charité, Universitätsmedizin, Berlin, Germany

Abstract

The term anaphylaxis was coined by Charles Richet and Paul Portier when they tried to immunize dogs with actinia extracts, but after a repeated injection of a small amount of the toxin the dog died within 25 min. The new term rapidly spread all over the world. The discovery of the phenomenon of anaphylaxis showed that by immunization not only protection but also harmful events could be induced. For this discovery Richet received the Nobel Prize in 1913, but he still believed the condition of anaphylaxis was a lack of protection to the poisonous effect of the substance. Already earlier similar clinical phenomena had been observed but not well described. A major breakthrough in understanding the pathophysiology came through the experiments of Dale and Laidlaw who showed that the newly discovered histamine was able to induce quite similar symptoms to anaphylaxis. For decades reactions mimicking anaphylaxis but without involvement of the immune systems were called 'anaphylactoid', 'allergy-like' or 'pseudo-allergic'. Since the new definition of the World Allergy Organization (WAO) anaphylaxis is defined on the basis of clinical symptoms independent of pathomechanisms involved: one distinguishes between allergic and non-immune anaphylaxis. Epinephrine (Adrenalin) was soon recognized as treatment of choice of this dramatic condition.

Although the term 'allergy' was coined in 1906 by Clemens von Pirquet [1], it was the short lecture given by Paul Portier and Charles Richet [2] on February 15, 1902, at the Societé de Biologie in Paris that is regarded by many authors as representing the birth of modern allergology with the discovery of the phenomenon of anaphylaxis. The phenomenon itself was not totally new. We find descriptions of similar and sometimes dramatic and untoward reactions in ancient history [see the opening two chapters by Ring, this vol., pp. 2–20], especially with regard to the famous Pharaoh Menes, who supposedly died in 2641 BC after being stung by a wasp, hornet or honey bee [3, 4; see the chapter by Ring, this vol., pp. 2–14].

The first detailed description of an unusual reaction to the sting of a honey bee was found by Ulrich Müller [5] in an article written in Latin ('De curiosis post apium ictus symptomatibus') by Udalricus

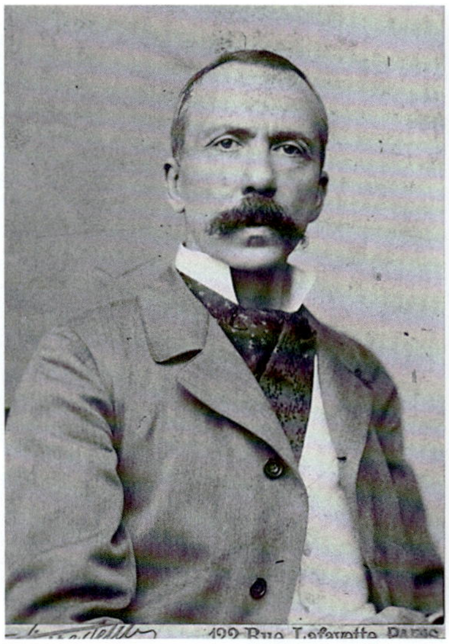

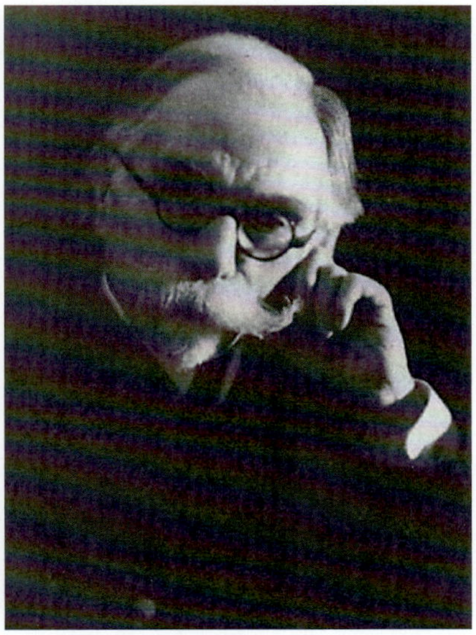

Fig. 1. Charles Richet.
Fig. 2. Paul Portier.

Staudigelius (Ulrich Staudigl), who was a monk at the Benedictine monastery of Andechs in Bavaria, situated south-west of Munich. In France in 1765, Dr. Desbrest described a 30-year-old man who was stung on his eyelid by a honey bee while he was working in the garden; a short time later he collapsed and died. Similar case reports from the 19th century of fatal insect stings have been reported in Europe and the USA [6]. A first experimental description of this phenomenon goes back to experiments done on rabbits with injections of ovalbumin by François Magendie, who noted that some rabbits died after the second or third injection [7]. These reactions were generally attributed to some poisonous substances or toxin given to the animals.

The Voyage on the Yacht Princesse Alice II

The French physiologist Charles Richet (1850–1935; fig. 1), son of Alfred Richet, professor of clinical surgery in Paris, became interested in the toxic effects of *Physalia* (Portuguese man o' war). He had studied medicine in Paris and received his doctoral degree in 1869 and his doctor in science in 1878. From 1887 he worked as a professor of physiology at the faculty of medicine in Paris and published a variety of papers on physiology, thermoregulation, serotherapy of tuberculosis and the effect of injections of proteins on the chemical constitution of bodily fluids as well as electrolytes.

Together with Héricourt he described possible protective effects of the blood of animals infected with staphylococci [8]. This was 2 years before the finding made by Emil von Behring who, together with Shibasaburo Kitasato (1852–1931), observed this type of immunity with diphtheria toxin and the production of toxin-neutralizing 'antitoxin' in animals [9].

In 1898, Héricourt and Richet [10] studied the effect of eel serum in dogs, observing that a second or third injection made the dogs sicker, sometimes severely so. However, Richet later stated that he did not really recognize this phenomenon worthy of deeper investigation.

Paul Portier (1866–1962; fig. 2) was born in Bar-sur-Seine in France and began his career as a clerk in a country registry [11]. Through his interest in entomology and general natural science, he came to the faculty of science and medicine in Paris in 1889. In 1920, he was appointed professor of comparative physiology at the Sorbonne. Portier was a personal friend of Prince Albert I of Monaco, who was an enthusiastic oceanographer; thus, he was regularly invited to participate on cruises organized by the prince aboard the yacht 'Princesse

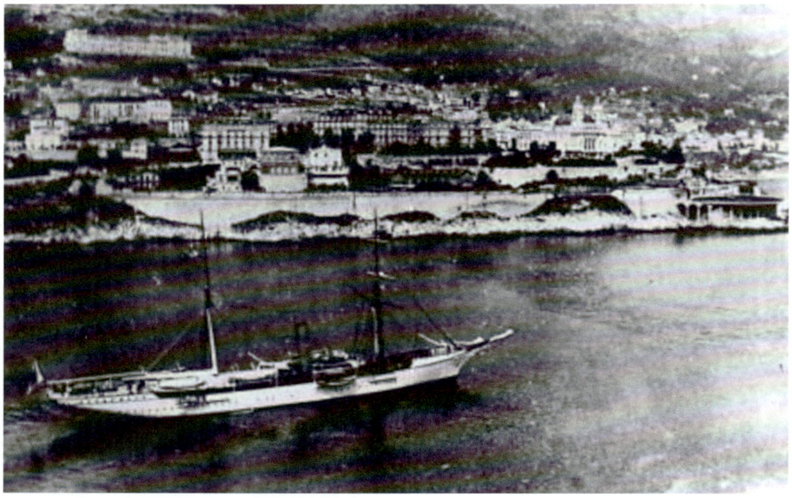

Fig. 3. The yacht 'Princesse Alice II' in front of Monaco.

Alice II' (fig. 3). Charles Richet was also invited on one of these cruises, and they travelled via the Mediterranean Sea to the Canary Islands, Madeira and Cape Verde Islands (fig. 4). Due to his interest in oceanographic studies, Prince Albert founded the Oceanographic Institute in Monaco, which today hosts a multitude of objects attractive to visitors.

During this particular cruise the prince and G. Richard suggested to Charles Richet and Paul Portier that they study the toxic properties of certain *Physalia* species found in the South Seas, using a special laboratory on the boat (fig. 5, 6) [12]. Richet and Portier later decided to continue their studies in Paris, but could not obtain any *Physalia*. Thus, they continued with extracts of another species of *Actinia:*

> On board the prince's yacht experiments were carried out proving that an aqueous glycerin extract of the filaments of *Physalia* is extremely toxic to ducks and rabbits. On returning to France I could not obtain any *Physalia* and decided to study comparatively the tentacles of actinaria, which resemble *Physalia* in certain respects and are easily procurable. Owing to the kindness of Y. Delage I was able to obtain a large quantity; the tentacles, cut close to the body, were placed in glycerin and thus we had in Paris several liters of an intensely toxic fluid, the glycerin dissolving and extracting the active principle. [13]

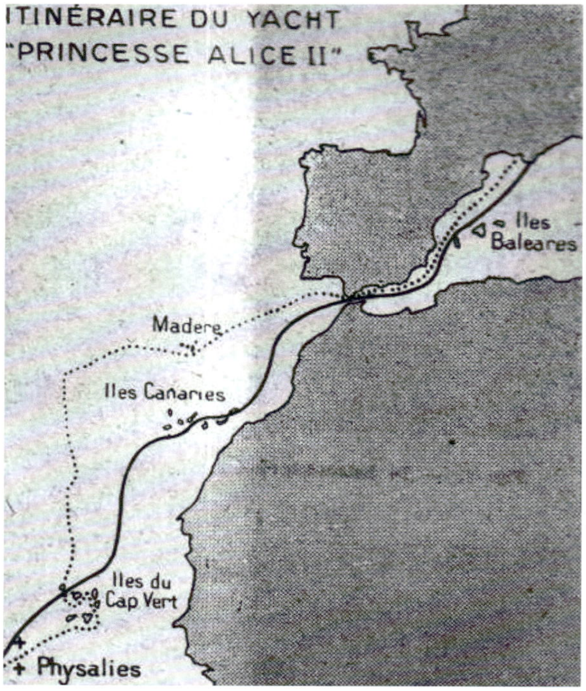

Fig. 4. Travel route of the 'Princesse Alice II' via the Mediterranean Sea to the Canary Islands, Madeira and Cape Verde Islands [12].

One fraction of these *Physalia* extracts contained a substance which was called 'hypnotoxin', which induced very painful urticarial reactions after contact with the skin, coupled with a drop in body tempera-

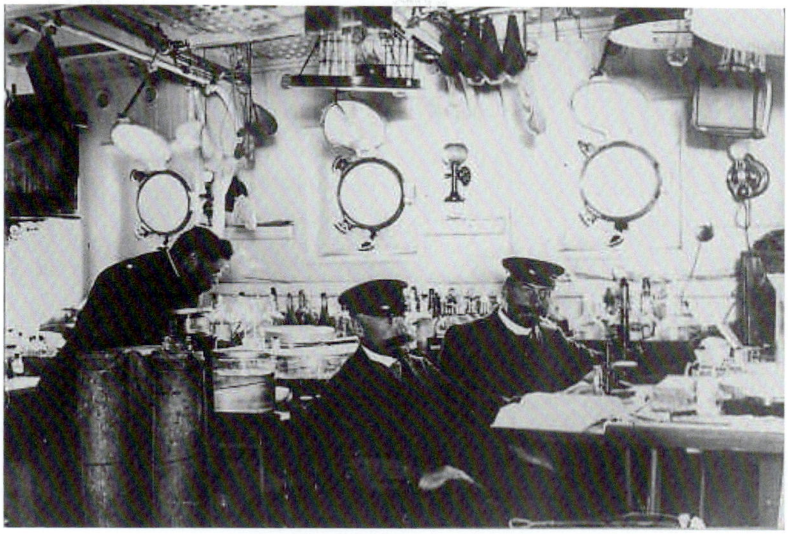

Fig. 5. The laboratory on board the yacht 'Princesse Alice II' of Prince Albert I of Monaco (1848–1922). Paul Portier is to the left side of the table, on his right is Dr. Richard [12].

ture and somnolence. The *Actinia* species was *Anemonia sulcata*. Richet described the toxic properties of his extract:

> One dog (Amphitryon) of 31 kg received 1.6 cc on 8 March 1902 of this liquid (corresponding to 0.8 cc of tentacles) and he died on the third day. If one admits that only 10% of the extract of the tentacles corresponds to solid material, 0.08 g are sufficient to poison the dog weighing 31 kg; therefore the minimal quantity per kg dog to produce fatal effects are 0.0025 g out of the total of extractable substances of the tentacle. [14]

Richet described the toxic effects of these extracts very precisely in several dog experiments and concluded that there were two different toxins, one which he called 'thalassine', which induced violent pruritus and urticaria but was not fatal. The other one he called 'congestine', which led to an intestinal and cardiovascular congestion with finally lethal outcome.

The aim of the studies was to immunize the dogs against the toxin. However, the opposite in fact occurred. They noted that dogs, having previously received small amounts earlier, reacted with more symptoms at the second or third injection. The critical illustrative experiment was performed on a dog called Neptune which Richet [15] described in his article from 1904:

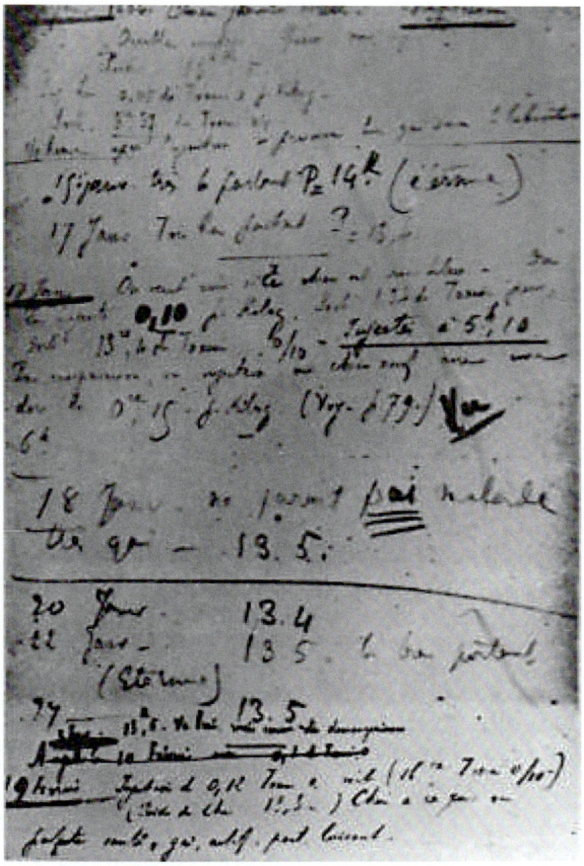

Fig. 6. Handwritten notes from the protocol book used by Charles Richet and Paul Portier regarding the first experiments from January 15–19, 1902 [12].

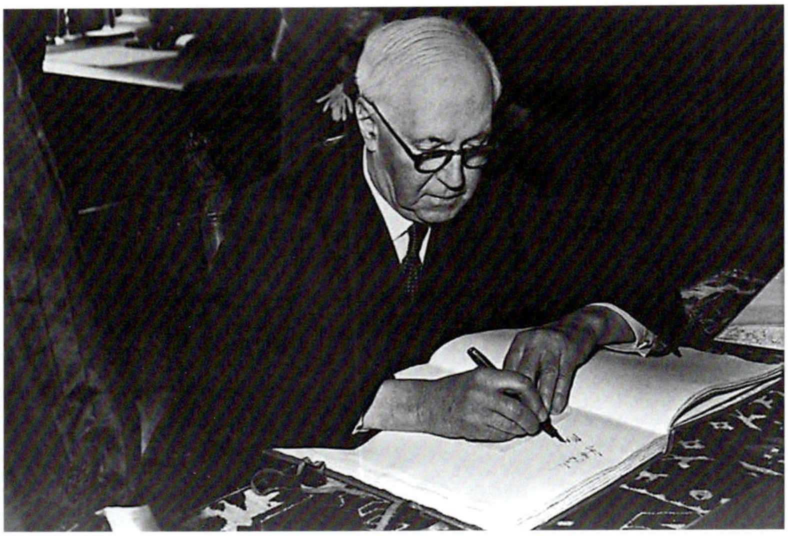

Fig. 7. Sir Henry Hallett Dale. Photo taken at the Honorary Doctor Award in Graz, Austria, 1954.

> Je prendrai notamment pour exemple le chien *Neptune*, gros matin á poil ras, très vigoureux, qui, après avoir reçu, 22 jours auparavant la dose de 0,10 qui ne l'avait presque pas rendu malade, reçoit du même liquide la même dose de 0,10. Alors aussitôt quelques secondes après que l'injection a été terminée, il est extrêmement malade: la respiration devient angoissée, haletante. Il peut à peine se trainer; se couche sur le flanc, est pris de diarrhée et de vomissements sanguinolants. La sensibilité est aboulie, et il meurt en vingt-cinq minutes.
> Or, chez des chiens non injectés antérieurement, des doses dix fois plus fortes, 1 cc par kilogramme, ne tuent pas les animaux avec cette même rapidité. [15]

Portier wrote about the experiment in the dog Neptune in which the phenomenon later called 'anaphylaxis' was first seen. This strong and healthy animal had received a low dose of actinium toxin on January 14 and 17, 1902 [16–18], which was tolerated with 'almost no reaction'. After 22 days, on February 10, he received the same dose when in excellent general condition. However, some seconds after the injections the dog began to gasp and to wheeze, the animal was agonized, was not able to stand and lay on his side, developed bloody vomiting and died within 25 min.

When notified by Portier, Richet recognized immediately that this surprising phenomenon was new ('C'est un phénomène nouveau, il faut le baptiser!'). In trying to find a name he wanted to express 'lack of protection' and should have used the word 'aphylaxis' (from the privative alpha in Ancient Greek grammar, meaning 'negation'). However, for euphonic and rhythmic reasons he preferred 'anaphylaxis' [15], and this term rapidly spread all over the world.

In the reminiscences of Paul Portier and Charles Richet there is a slight discrepancy with regard to the number and timely sequence of injections the dog Neptune actually received. According to Richet there were two injections within an interval of 22 days. However, Portier states that the dog received the first injection on January 14 followed 3 days later by another low dose, which was tolerated well, and only then, 22 days later on February 10 – on which there is total agreement – the dramatic reaction occurred.

The researchers had a similar experience with another dog called Galathee, who received 0.05 ml of the actinotoxin on January 14, and 0.1 ml on January 22, which was tolerated with 'almost no reaction'. He was in perfect health on February 10 when he received an injection of 0.12 ml/kg of actinotoxin and 'immediately produced vomiting of mucus and blood, some bloody defecation and very marked stupor'. These symptoms became worse in the following hours and he died in the night.

The small discrepancies concerning the details of the first experiment are obviously of no importance with regard to the discovery of the new phenomenon. The term anaphylaxis was – as always in medicine – only accepted with some criticism. Especially Emil von Behring remarked in 1914 (note that it was the beginning of World War I) that Richet's report described nothing else than what he had previously called 'hypersensitivity' [19].

Untoward reactions to foreign, heterologous serum injection had been observed earlier. The most tragic event was probably published by Robert Langerhans (1859–1904), a pathologist in Berlin, who injected 1.2 ml of Behring's 'Heilserum' subcutaneously into his almost 2-year-old child on April 7, 1896. The child died within 7 min in the presence of the helpless father [20]. By 1910, 41 fatalities after injection of diphtheria serum had been described [21].

Regarding pathophysiology, Richet still believed that the dramatic symptoms elicited by the second or third injections represented an increased toxic effect. Interestingly, he obviously did not notice a difference in the quality of symptoms between the injection of a high dose of the toxin and the symptoms of 'anaphylaxis' after repeated low doses. This was correctly commented on by Paul Kallós and Kallós-Defner [22] in 1937.

In 1913, Richet was awarded the Nobel Prize. In his address on receiving the award, he humbly stated:

> The discovery of anaphylaxis is not at all the result of thinking, but of simple observation, almost accidental. It had no other merit than that of not refusing to see the facts which presented themselves before me completely evident. [13, 23]

There is a movie clip of a very emotional address given by the aged Paul Portier at the World Congress in Paris on October 19, 1958 (online suppl. movie 1, see www.karger.com/chial100_movie1).

The story of the discovery of anaphylaxis also illustrates the importance of terminology. It remains an object of speculation whether the findings of Richet and Portier would have gained such rapid interest in the scientific community without the new name.

In the following decades anaphylaxis was regarded as an experimental phenomenon after the 'artificial' injection of proteins. The similarity to human disease was only slowly recognized. When they coined the term 'atopy', Coca and Cooke clearly distinguished this 'natural' occurring hypersensitivity from the 'artificial' symptoms of anaphylaxis in animal experiments.

In his Nobel address, Richet clearly stated:

> These two factors – (a) increased sensitivity to a poison after previous injection of the same poison and (b) an incubation period necessary for this state of increased sensitivity to develop – constitute the two essential and sufficient conditions for anaphylaxis. [13]

Earlier on, through the works of Louis Pasteur, Robert Koch, Emil von Behring and others, immunization was only connected with a positive and desired effect of protection against pathogenic organisms. The discovery of the phenomenon of anaphylaxis showed that by immunization harmful events and severe disease could also be induced. Similar observations regarding the example of serum sickness then led Clemens von Pirquet to coin the term 'allergy' in order to bring some clarity to these seemingly contradictive phenomena [1].

Pathophysiology

During the search for an active substance to induce the symptoms of anaphylaxis it soon became clear that it was not the effect of the toxin itself, but rather some principle in the organism. The credit for the elucidation goes to Sir Henry Dale (1875–1968; fig. 7), born in London, who studied at Trinity College in Cambridge and began his career in neuroanatomy together with J.N. Langley. He had been working since 1903 in the laboratory with E.H. Starling at the University College in London, from where he visited Paul Ehrlich in his laboratory in Germany. In 1904, he became director of the Wellcome Physiological Research Laboratories. His studies covered many fields of pharmacology, physiology and biochemistry. In 1910, he studied the physiological action of histamine together with his coworker, P.P. Laidlaw, and developed the concept of histamine shock as a basis of anaphylaxis [24]. They clearly described the effect upon the smooth muscle of different organs, as well as an effect (mildly stimulating) on cardiac muscle, but the absence of an effect on skeletal muscle. They noted the similarity to the effect of Witte's peptone after several injections:

> This symptom complex has recently acquired interest in another direction. Biedl and Kraus drew attention to the identity of the symptoms of anaphylactic shock with those produced by intravenous injection of 'peptone' which, as we have seen, are again very largely identical with those of β-iminazolylethylamine. The correspondence cannot yet be regarded as sufficient for theoretical speculations, and we content ourselves with recording, as a point of interest and possible significance, the fact that the immediate symptoms with which an animal responds to an injection of a normally inert protein, to which it has been sensitized, are to a large extent those of poisoning by β-iminazolylethylamine. [24]

In later works Dale also noticed that anaphylactic antibodies had to attach themselves to cells before reacting with antigen. This was more clearly established by Prausnitz and Küstner [25] in 1921 when they were able to transfer individual hypersensitivity to fish via serum from one allergic individual to another non-allergic individual.

The French physiologist Nicolas-Maurice Arthus (1862–1945) reported that after repeated injection of sterile horse serum into the skin increased inflammatory reactions with redness, edema, bleeding and necrosis could be observed. He called this 'local anaphylaxis' and it later became known as 'Arthus phenomenon' [26].

In the USA, M.J. Rosenau (1869–1946) and John F. Anderson (1873–1958) established animal experiments, particularly in the guinea pig [27]. Laboratory notes of the American pathologist Theobald Smith (1859–1934) were given to Paul Ehrlich (1854–1915) when he was visiting America. Recognizing the value of these experiments, Ehrlich gave the notebooks to Richard Ernst Wilhelm Otto (1872–1950) and asked him to continue the experimental work. Otto finally published his and Theobald Smith's results and coined the term' 'Theobald Smith's phenomenon' for anaphylactic shock in guinea pigs [28].

In the years following the discovery of anaphylaxis some researchers noticed that similar symptoms can also be elicited in animals that had not been previously immunized, as well as through the direct injection of histamine. The term 'anaphylactoid reaction' was used for this non-immunological type of induction of symptoms [29–31; see also the chapter by Ring, this vol., pp. 46–52]. A direct histamine release evoked by several substances (e.g. codeine, dextran) in certain rat strains or gelatin blood substitutes led to the development of the concept of pseudo-allergic reactions by Paul Kallós [22, 32, 33].

Only at the beginning of the 21st century did the nomenclature task forces of both the European Academy of Allergy and Clinical Immunology (EAACI) and the World Allergy Organization (WAO) come to a new terminology and define 'anaphylaxis' on the basis of clinical symptoms independent of the pathomechanism evolved in elicitation [34]. Thus, one now distinguishes between an allergic and a non-immune anaphylaxis, formerly called a 'pseudo-allergic reaction'.

Today, anaphylaxis seems to be increasing in prevalence all over the world, maybe due to the pollen-associated food allergies which follow the rising prevalence of atopic diseases. Since anaphylaxis describes a syndrome of clinical symptoms involving several organ systems with varying intensity, attempts have been made to classify the severity of this reaction using so-called severity scales, as proposed by Mueller [35] or Ring and Messmer [36], which are the most commonly used.

While we know a lot about the events in IgE-induced sensitization and IgE-induced mast cell activation and degranulation, there is still only limited knowledge on the final pathophysiological events at the smooth muscle and microcirculatory level which finally lead to the fatal symptoms.

Epinephrine (Adrenalin) as a treatment of choice has been known for more than a hundred years. There is no new therapeutic substance on the horizon with a less dangerous or narrow therapeutic profile between beneficial effect and pharmacological side reaction [28, 37; see also the chapter by Starke, this vol., pp. 288–301].

Guidelines for acute treatment of anaphylaxis have been developed at the national [38] and international level [39]. The complex interactions between elicitors, pathophysiology, pharmacotherapy and general measures have to be explained to the patient together with prescribing emergency medication, including the epinephrine autoinjector. It has been shown that educational programs ('anaphylaxis school') may be helpful in this context [40].

References

1 von Pirquet C: Allergie. Münch Med Wochenschr 1906;53:1457–1458.
2 Portier P, Richet C: De l'action anaphylactique de certains vénins. CR Soc Biol 1902; 54:170–172/Trav Labor Physiol 1902;5:506.
3 Waddell L: Egyptian Civilization. London, Luzac, 1930.
4 Avenberg KM, Harper DS, Larsson BL: Footnotes on Allergy. Uppsala, Pharmacia, 1980.
5 Müller U: Geschichte der Insektenstichallergie. Allergo J 2009;18:342–352.
6 Galli S (ed): Anaphylaxis. Novartis Foundation Symposium 157. Chichester, Wiley, 2004.
7 Magendie F: Lectures on the Blood and on the Changes It Undergoes during Disease. Philadelphia, Harrington Barungton & Haswell, 1939.
8 Héricourt J, Richet C: Sur un microbe pyrogène et septique *(Staphylococcus pyosepticus)* et sur le vaccination contre ses effets. CR Acad Sci 1888;107:690.
9 von Behring E, Kitasato S: Über das Zustandekommen der Diphterie-Immunität und der Tetanus-Immunität bei Thieren. Dtsch Med Wochenschr 1890;16: 1113/1145.
10 Héricourt J, Richet C: Effets lointains des injections de serum d'anguille. CR Soc Biol 1989;50:137.
11 Samter M: Excerpts from Classics in Allergy. Columbus, Ross Laboratories, 1969.
12 Schadewaldt H: Die Lehre von der Allergie und den allergischen Krankheiten in ihrer historischen Entwicklung; Habilitation Diss, Medizingeschichtliches Institut der Albert-Ludwigs-Universität Freiburg im Breisgau, 1960.
13 Richet C: Anaphylaxies. Liverpool, University Press, 1913.
14 Richet C: De l'anaphylaxie après injection de congestine chez le chien. CR Soc Biol 1905;57:112.
15 Richet C: Des effets prophylactiques de la thalassine et anaphylactiques de la congestine dans le virus des actiniés. CR Soc Biol 1904;56:302.
16 Richet C: Des poisons contenus dans les tentacules des actiniés (Congestine et Thalassine). CR Soc Biol 1903;55:246.
17 Richet C: De l'anaphylaxie au sensibilité croissant des organismes à des doses successives de poison. Arch Fisiol 1903/1904;1: 129.
18 Richet C: De l'action de la congestine (virus des actinides) sur les lapins et de ses effets anaphylactiques. CR Soc Biol 1905;57:109.
19 von Behring E: Über Idiosynkrasie, Anaphylaxie, Toxin-Überempfindlichkeit, Disposition and Diathese. Schmidts Jb Ges Med 1914;319:113/Gesammelte Abhandlungen, NF No 23. Bonn, 1915, p 175 ff.
20 Langerhans R: Tod durch Heilserum! Berl Wochenschr 1896;33:602.
21 Lamson RW: Sudden death associated with the injection of foreign substances. JAMA 1924;82:1091–1098.
22 Kallós P, Kallós-Defner L: Die experimentellen Grundlagen der Erkennung und Behandlung der allergischen Krankheiten. Ergebn Hyg 1937;19:178.
23 Richet C: De l'anaphylaxie ou sensibilité croissante des organsimes à des doses successives de poison. Arch Fisiol 1904;1:129.
24 Dale HH, Laidlaw PP: The physiological action of beta-imidazolethylamine. J Physiol 1910;41:318–344.
25 Prausnitz C, Küster H: Studien über die Überempfindlichkeit. Zbl Bakt Abt 1 Orig 1921;86:160.
26 Arthus N-M: La séro-anaphylaxie du lapin. Arch Int Physiol 1909;7:471.
27 Rosenau MJ, Anderson JF: Hypersusceptibility. JAMA 1906;47:1007.
28 Simons FER (ed): Ancestors of Allergy. New York, Global Medical Communications, 1994.
29 von Behring E: Experimentelle Analyse und Theorie der anaphylaktischen und apotorischen Vergiftung. Dtsch Med Wsch 1914;40:1857.
30 Hanzlik PJ, Karsner HT: Anaphylactoid phenomena from the intravenous administration of various colloids, arsenicals and other agents. J Pharmacol Exp Ther 1920; 14:379.
31 Lorenz W, Doenicke A, Dittmann I, Hug P, Schwarz B: Anaphylaktoide Reaktionen nach Applikation von Blutersatzmitteln beim Menschen. Verhinderung dieser Nebenwirkung von Haemaccel durch Praemedikation mit H_1 und H_2-Antagonisten. Anaesthesist 1977;26:644.
32 Dukor P, Kallos P, Schlumberger HD, West GB (eds): Pseudo-Allergic Reactions. Basel, Karger, 1980, vol 1–3.
33 West G: 5-Hydroxytryptamine, tissue mast cells and skin oedema. Int Arch Allergy Appl Immunol 1957;10:257–275.
34 Johansson SGO, Bieber T, Dahl R, Friedmann PS, Lanier BQ, Lockey RF, Motala C, Martell JAO, Platts-Mills TAE, Ring J, Thien F, Cauwenberge PV, Williams HC: Revised nomenclature for allergy for global use: report of the nomenclature review committee of the World Allergy Organization. J Allergy Clin Immunol 2004;113:832–836.
35 Mueller HL: Diagnosis and treatment of insect sensitivity. J Asthma Res 1966;3:331–333.
36 Ring J, Messmer K: Incidence and severity of anaphylactoid reactions to colloid volume substitutes. Lancet 1977;i:466–469.
37 Ring J: Anaphylaktoide Reaktionen. Berlin, Springer, 1978.
38 Ring J, et al: Leitlinie Akuttherapie der Anaphylaxie. Allergo J, in press.
39 Simons FE, Ardusso LR, Bilò MB, El-Gamal YM, Ledford DK, Ring J, Sanchez-Borges M, Senna GE, Sheikh A, Thong BY, et al: World Allergy Organization anaphylaxis guidelines: summary. J Allergy Clin Immunol 2011;127:587–593.
40 Ring J, Beyer K, Dorsch A, Biedermann T, Fischer J, Friedrichs F, Gebert N, Gieler U, Grosber M, Jakob T, Klimek L, Kugler C, Lange L, Pfaar O, Przybilla B, Reese I, Rietschel E, Schallmayer S, Schnadt S, Szczepanski R, Worm M, Brockow K (für AGATE): Anaphylaxieschulung – ein neues Behandlungsprogramm zur tertiären Krankheitsprävention nach Anaphylaxie. Allergo J 2012;21:96–102.

Prof. Dr. med. Dr. phil. Johannes Ring
Department of Dermatology and Allergy Biederstein
Biedersteinerstrasse 29
DE–80802 München (Germany)
E-Mail johannes.ring@lrz.tu-muenchen.de

Bergmann K-C, Ring J (eds): History of Allergy. Chem Immunol Allergy. Basel, Karger, 2014, vol 100, pp 62–68
DOI: 10.1159/000358505

Allergic Rhinitis

Niels Mygind

Otopathological Laboratory, ENT Department, Rigshospitalet, Copenhagen, Denmark

Abstract

Allergic rhinitis is a very frequent disease with a prevalence of 15–20%. Symptoms are most pronounced in young people while, for some unknown reason, the elderly become clinically hyposensitized. Pollen is the cause of seasonal allergic rhinitis, and house dust mite and animals are the main causes of perennial allergic rhinitis. Histamine is the main cause of sneezing and hypersecretion, while other mediators probably also play a role in nasal blockage. In polyposis, a local denervation is an important cause of vascular leakage, edema and polyp formation. Antihistamines have a positive effect on sneezing and hypersecretion, but not on blockage. As they have a quick onset of action they are useful in patients with mild and occasional symptoms. A nasal steroid is preferable in patients with persistent symptoms, since it is more effective on all nasal symptoms. Short-term use of a systemic steroid can be a valuable adjunct to topical treatment, especially in nasal polyposis, when there is a temporary failure of topical treatment in a blocked nose. A nasal vasoconstrictor can be added for short-term treatment, and an ipratropium spray can be beneficial in perennial non-allergic rhinitis, when watery secretion is the dominant symptom. Immunotherapy can be added in allergic rhinitis, when pharmacotherapy is insufficient. This chapter is based on the author's personal experience with allergic rhinitis, as a patient, a doctor and a researcher. Therefore, it is not a balanced review and the references will be highly selected as they largely consist of the author's own publications. As the text is mainly based on personal research, steroids are described in detail, while, with regard to immunotherapy, the reader is referred to another chapter. In addition to allergic rhinitis, nasal polyposis will be described. It was formerly believed to be an allergic disease, but we now know that it is not. However, with regard to histopathology and drug responsiveness this disease is very similar to allergic rhinitis.

An Allergy Giant in 1873

In 1873, Charles Blackley wrote a book on 'catarrhus æstivus' (hay-fever or hay-asthma) [1]. At that time the cause of the disease was largely unknown, although it was suspected to be produced by 'the effluvium from new hay'.

As a patient himself, Blackley sampled pollen and rubbed them into a scratch on his arm, which caused a reaction measuring 2.5 inches. He also provoked conjunctivitis, rhinitis and asthma, and even made single-blind provocations. He counted pollen in the air, and showed a correlation between the count and his symptoms. Finally, he sampled pollen by attaching sticky glass slides to the strings of kites and found a high count 100 m above ground level. This discovery explained to him why he suffered from hay fever even in a large city. He produced nice figures of daily pollen counts during the season and showed how they correlated with his symptoms.

Blackley also noted that 'the presence of cats, rabbits, or guinea pigs will in some cases cause a form of asthma which cannot be distinguished from hay-asthma'. However, he stated that 'the fur of the animals may be simply a carrier of the granular matter and of the pollen. I have never met with a case in which the attacks could be shown to be due entirely to the odour given off by animals'. Not so good Blackley!

Overall, it was indeed a very impressive body of work that Charles Blackley presented more than 100 years ago.

Terminology and Definition

The term 'allergy' is based on the Greek words 'allos', meaning 'different' or 'changed', and 'ergos', meaning 'work' or 'action'. 'Rhinitis' means 'inflammation in the nose'. However, an inflammatory reaction is not essential for the disease and symptoms can be produced by allergen provocation in a non-inflammatory nose. Thus, 'rhinopathy' is a more correct term, but it is not used.

Hippocrates, in 400 BC, described nasal polyps and named them 'polypous' ('poly' means 'many'; 'pous' means 'foot' or 'feet'). However, a polyp has only one stalk or food. Therefore, the more correct word is a 'monop'; but I believe that it is too late to change Hippocrates' diagnosis of this disease to 'monoposis'.

In clinical practice the diagnosis of rhinitis is based on the occurrence of the symptoms of sneezing, nose blowing and nasal blockage. As all people occasionally have these symptoms it can be difficult to make a clear distinction between a normal state and a disease.

In a consensus report on rhinitis, the disease was defined as 2 or more symptoms lasting for more than 1 h on most days [2]. The clinician can be guided by asking the patient how many hours a day he or she has symptoms and how many times he or she sneezes and blows the nose.

2

Epidemiology and Natural History

During his career Charles Blackley was only able to find a few patients with hay fever. A series of studies have now shown a 15–20% cumulative prevalence figure for allergic rhinitis in the general population [3, 4], and it is the most common immunologic disease.

National population surveys in Switzerland identified a change in prevalence of hay fever from 0.3% in 1926 to 5% in 1958, 10% in 1985 and 14% in 1995 [5]. Thus, there is no doubt that the prevalence of allergic rhinitis has increased considerably since the days of Blackley, and the cause is unknown.

Blackley wrote that 'the predisposition to hay-fever is more common among the educated than it is among the illiterate'. In addition, 'Hay-fever is said to be an aristocratic disease. I have myself never seen a case among the working part of the population and if they occur at all, they do so very seldom' [1].

That later studies have found a higher prevalence rate of positive skin tests and of clinical allergic rhinitis in university students than in the population as a whole gives some support to Blackley's observations. In addition, a correlation between a positive skin test and the level of education and income has been described [3].

Blackley commented: 'There is the curious phenomenon that hay fever is apparently less common in rural than in urban areas.' One would believe that children living in the country more frequently develop hay fever than children in cities, but this does not seem to be the case, and the reason is unknown.

The symptoms of hay fever are worse in the age range of 15–20 years, and old people never suffer from severe symptoms, although they are still sensitized [4]. We do not know the cause of this spontaneous cure of the disease but not the allergic sensitization. A detailed study is deserving of the underlying immunological and inflammatory mechanisms.

Allergens

The nose acts as a filter for inhaled particles. Filtration is very effective for large particles (>10 μm), which are retained in the nose, but less so for smaller particles which can reach the lower airways. This explains the difference in rhinitis and asthma symptoms related to the particle size of the allergen.

Pollen grains, as relatively large particles (20–30 μm), impinge against the eye and are trapped in the nasal filter. Although they do not reach the lower airways in any significant number, pollen asthma can be induced by allergen-containing dust.

Grass is of considerable importance worldwide. Birch is an important cause of allergy in Scandinavia and Japanese cedar is the most important cause in Japan. Ragweed holds a leading position in North America.

Only 50 years ago extracts of house dust and of bird feathers were used for skin testing and also for treatment. However, considerable progress was made in the Netherlands in 1964 when Voorhorst et al. [6] showed that the mite *Dermatophagoides pteronyssinus* is the chief cause of 'house dust allergy'. 'Feather allergy' is also largely accounted for by contamination with this mite, which in Greek means 'the skin-eating feather mite'. Predominantly, the fecal pellets, which have the same size as pollen, are the cause of the airway symptoms.

Cats deposit allergen in saliva on their pelt by licking themselves. This allergen is continuously airborne in the home as small particles. Allergy to mold spores, with a size of 3–10 μm, is a well-known cause of rhinitis in asthmatic children, while its role in non-asthmatic patients is probably insignificant. As a general rule, food allergy and intolerance will seldom cause isolated rhinitis. However, food, and alcoholic beverages in particular, frequently precipitate nasal symptoms by non-allergic mechanisms.

Histopathology and Pathogenesis

The Epithelial Lining

Findings and opinions about epithelial changes in allergic rhinitis are somewhat contradictory. In studies of sensitized animals it has been described that pollen grains can destruct and penetrate the epithelial lining in the nose [quoted in 7]. However, we have not been able to confirm this after pollen provocation of allergic patients [7].

In allergic rhinitis patients, experienced researchers using transmission electron microscopy have found a loss of epithelial junctions, dilated intercellular spaces and extrusion of epithelial cells into the nasal lumen [quoted in 8]. Using scanning electron microscopy, we have found only minor changes in the surface epithelium [8]. However, we found that scraping of the nasal mucosa detached more epithelial cells in patients with perennial rhinitis than in normal controls [9]. Thus, allergic rhinitis patients may have slight intercellular edema which reduces cohesion between the cells, but there is no marked pathology of the epithelial lining in allergic rhinitis.

The Mast Cell

The mast cell ('the well-fed cell') was first described in 1879 by Paul Ehrlich. This cell has a unique role to play in the pathogenesis of allergic rhinitis since it expresses high-affinity receptors for immunoglobulin E and, together with the basophil leukocyte, is the only cell that synthesizes and releases histamine. During the early-phase response to allergen challenge there are morphological and biochemical signs of mast cell degranulation, and in allergic rhinitis there is an increased number of mast cells in the surface epithelium [9].

Histamine

In contrast to bronchi, histamine is definitely the most important mediator of allergy in the nose. The good effect of antihistamines clearly demonstrates that histamine accounts for the great majority of sneezing and associated watery hypersecretion. This is due to an effect on H_1 receptors on sensory nerves, causing sneezing, and hypersecretion by stimulation of the submucosal glands. Histamine also induces nasal blockage, but H_1 antihistamines have a poor effect on this symptom. This may in part be due to the significance of H_2 histamine receptors in blood vessels. In a study of nasal histamine provocation we found an equal effect on nasal blockage by pretreatment with an H_1 and an H_2 antihistamine [10]. The insignificant effect of H_1 antihistamines on nasal blockage in allergic rhinitis also indicates that other mediators are important in causing this symptom.

The Eosinophil

In 1879, Paul Ehrlich described the eosinophil leukocyte, which he named after 'Eos', the Greek goddess of dawn. The simple counting of eosinophils in nasal secretion/smear, which was introduced in 1922, is still the best morphological sign of allergic inflammation in the nose. The role of the eosinophil in the pathogenesis of allergic rhinitis, however, is not clear. It is possible that eosinophils may contribute to nasal hyperreactivity, as it is shown that molecules from eosinophils can have an effect on airway epithelial cells [11]. However, as stated above, there does not seem to be any marked morphological changes in the surface epithelium in an allergic nose. In addition, the nasal response to a provocation with histamine and with allergen is only increased by a factor of three during the pollen seasons [12]. Thus, although hyperreactivity occurs in allergic rhinitis, it is far less pronounced than in asthma.

Nasal Polyps

Nasal polyposis was earlier believed to be an allergic disease, but it is now clear that such patients do not have a positive skin test to allergen more frequently than the general population. Thus, the etiology of nasal polyps is unknown.

In nasal polyposis mast cell degranulation is present to a considerably higher degree than in an allergic nasal mucous membrane, and the histamine level in the edema fluid in a polyp is much higher than in allergic nasal tissue. In addition, there is pronounced eosinophilia [13].

Polyps largely consist of edema fluid, which is formed because the blood vessels have wide open cell junctions due to a total lack of nerves in the polyps. These structures are merely formed in a few square centimeters of the nose, i.e. in the middle meatus, where the nasal mucosa joins that of the paranasal sinuses. This marginal zone contains thin nerve fascicles which may have an increased sensitivity to damage from, for example, eosinophil-derived proteins [13].

Symptoms

Itchy eyes are a considerable nuisance, as is itching or tickling in the nose, because the allergen-exposed patient is constantly aware of the eyes and the nose. An itchy nose will also result in serial sneezing (25 sneezes is my personal record) and in watery rhinorrhea, which necessitates frequent use of a handkerchief.

In perennial rhinitis, and especially in nasal polyposis, a blocked nose, resulting in mouth breathing and a nasal voice, is very unpleasant. In nasal polyposis an abolished sense of smell, and with that 'taste', considerably reduces the quality of life.

Treatment

Antihistamines

The first antihistamine, Antergan, was introduced in 1942. In the early 1980s, a second generation of non-sedating antihistamines was introduced, which marked important progress in the management of allergic rhinoconjunctivitis.

Antihistamines have an established and valued place in the treatment of pollen allergy because they have a positive effect on itching in the eyes, sneezing and hypersecretion in the nose. In addition, they have a quick onset of action and can therefore be used on an as-needed basis.

When we gave the non-sedating antihistamine astemizole to patients with perennial rhinitis, it reduced sneezing to 41%, nose blowing to 55% and nasal blockage insignificantly, as compared to placebo. When a steroid spray was added the corresponding figures were 24, 37 and 64%. The effect of the antihistamine was equal in allergic and in nonallergic perennial rhinitis [14].

When antihistamine treatment is insufficient in hay fever, it should be replaced by a nasal steroid spray, which is definitely more effective on nasal symptoms, especially on blockage. Combined therapy with oral antihistamine and a topical steroid is often used, although a series of studies have shown that combined therapy is not more effective on nasal symptoms than a steroid spray alone [15]. Oral antihistamine tablets are often used in small children, who prefer oral and not intranasal therapy.

In summary, the place for oral antihistamines in allergic rhinitis is mainly for patients with occasional symptoms and in those who, in addition to the nasal symptoms, suffer from severe eye symptoms. Antihistamine eyedrops are very useful as they work instantaneously. They are a very good supplement to a nasal steroid spray.

Cromoglycate

Intranasal cromoglycate, introduced in 1967 by Roger Altonyan, has a prophylactic effect in allergic rhinitis, probably by stabilizing mast cells. The effect on sneezing and nasal discharge is mild-to-moderate, while the effect on blockage is weak. Cromoglycate, used four times daily, is considerably less effective than a nasal steroid spray, used once daily. Therefore, according to a consensus statement on the treatment of allergic rhinitis, 'cromoglycate cannot be considered a major therapeutic option in the treatment of allergic rhinitis' [16]. Cromoglycate may be more useful in the eyes than in the nose.

Topical Steroids

The drug company Allen and Hanburys (later Glaxo) wanted to test a newly developed asthma aerosol with the corticosteroid beclomethasone dipropionate. Dr. Harry Morrow Brown from Derby, UK, quickly showed that inhalation of this drug (later called Becotide) had a remarkable effect in asthma [17].

A representative from the drug company showed this spray to me and explained the remarkable results in asthma. Therefore, I performed a trial in hay fever with the beclomethasone dipropionate asthma aerosol equipped with a homemade nasal adapter. The effect on nasal symptoms was pronounced [18]. Measurement of urine cortisol concentration and a lack of effect on eye symptoms clearly showed that the spray had a local mode of action. In children the effect was even more pronounced [19].

In perennial rhinitis, we also found a pronounced effect on all nasal symptoms [20]. For the first time, however, it was noted that the steroid spray could result in hemorrhagic nasal secretion, and it raised the question of whether there was a risk of development of atrophic rhinitis, similar to skin atrophy from steroid ointment. Fortunately, later studies clearly showed that the observed side effect was not an increasing problem, and a biopsy study after long-term treatment showed no signs of the development of atrophic rhinitis [21].

In hay fever, symptom relief can be achieved within 12 h, reaching a maximum after 2–4 days. Topical treatment of nasal symptoms necessitates a prescription of antihistamine eyedrops. In a study of nasal polyposis this spray significantly reduced sneezing, hypersecretion and nasal blockage [22].

In a consensus report on the diagnosis and management of rhinitis, intranasal steroid was described as a first-line therapy in moderate and severe cases of hay fever, perennial allergic and non-allergic rhinitis [2]. There do not seem to be any significant differences between the steroid molecules on the market with regard to efficacy and side effect profile.

Systemic Steroids

Systemic steroids, synthesized in the 1950s, are effective in rhinitis and in nasal polyposis, but their use is restricted by their well-known side effects. However, the risk is very small when treatment is confined to a few weeks. Physicians agree that systemic steroids should not be used for rhinitis in children, during pregnancy and when there are contraindications. Otherwise opinions vary considerably. In contrast to antihistamines, systemic steroids have a pronounced effect on nasal blockage but a poor effect on sneezing and rhinorrhea [23].

Allergic Rhinitis. When a steroid spray is insufficient in hay fever, a short course of systemic steroids is often added. However, although an added efficacy seems likely, it has not been proven in controlled studies. A short course of systemic steroids can probably play a role when there are breakthrough symptoms in a blocked nose in perennial rhinitis, in spite of treatment with a nasal steroid. Clinical experience speaks in favor of this, but it has not been proven in controlled trials. In summary, systemic steroid is not used as the first-line treatment in rhinitis. While it may have a place as an additional treatment in chronic perennial rhinitis, its place in seasonal allergic rhinitis is less certain.

Nasal Polyposis. In this disease, however, the treatment can be of considerable value by opening up a blocked nose before topical therapy and when there is a temporary failure of this treatment, for example after a common cold. Preoperative treatment with systemic steroid can also make surgery easier. An effect on all parts of the nasal mucosa is important, including the ostiomeatal area, where the polyps are formed, and also on the paranasal sinuses. It is of particular importance that only systemic steroids can improve the sense of smell [24]. In summary, there is no doubt that systemic steroids have a place in nasal polyposis. Personally, I find that short-term treatment, given not more frequently than every 3 months, can be of considerable value in this disease.

Oral Treatment or a Depot Injection. Systemic steroid can be given as prednisolone tablets or as a depot injection (corresponding to 100 mg of prednisolone). There have been no placebo-controlled studies of oral prednisolone in rhinitis, but a few exist in nasal polyposis [25]. As there are no dose-response studies, the choice of dosage is uncertain. There is a definite effect of 30 mg of prednisolone daily, while 7.5 mg seems to have merely a marginal effect. There have been a few placebo-controlled studies of a depot injection. The effect on the hypothalamic-pituitary-adrenal axis lasts for 3 weeks and the clinical effect for 4–5 weeks [26]. Generally, oral treatment is recommended by almost all authors [2, 16] due to a fear of side effects from a depot injection. However, when all side effects of this treatment reported to the Danish Register for Side Effects were requested over a 10-year period, we found only one side effect reported per 11,785 injections [26]. However, there is no doubt that this is a considerable underrepresentation of subcutaneous atrophy with a depression over the injection site, which can occasionally occur after a depot injection, especially when it is given subcutaneously instead of intramuscularly.

Vasoconstrictors

Ephedrine is an active constituent of ma huang, a Chinese herbal medicine, which has been used for more than 5,000 years. This compound was introduced for clinical use in 1927 [27].

An intranasal vasoconstrictor has a pronounced effect on nasal blockage, starting after a few minutes and lasting for 10 h. There is no risk of systemic side effects, but, as was shown by Hüberman in 1942, prolonged use of this medication can result in the development of rhinitis medicamentosa. Therefore, a nasal vasoconstrictor is only recommended for short-term use (10 days).

It seems logical to add an oral vasoconstrictor to an antihistamine as they have supplementary effects. However, it is not elegant pharmacotherapy to constrict every blood vessel in the body in order to give a slight effect on nasal blockage. In addition, the dosage used can have systemic side effects, and there are a number of contraindications [27].

Ipratropium Bromide

A nasal spray with this drug has a moderate effect on watery rhinorrhea and it can be used when this is the dominant symptom in patients with perennial non-allergic rhinitis [28]. It also reduces rhinorrhea induced by cold weather and the common cold [29].

Immunotherapy

Specific immunotherapy, which was introduced by Noon and Freeman in 1911, is described in the chapter by Raulf [this vol., pp. 248–255]. It has a place in the management of allergic rhinitis when pharmacotherapy is insufficient, especially when systemic steroids are necessary.

References

1 Blackley CH: Experimental Research on the Causes and Nature of Catarrhus Æstivas (Hay-Fever or Hay-Asthma). Oxford, Oxford Historical Books, 1988.

2 Lund VJ, Aaronson D, Bousquet T, et al: International consensus report on the diagnosis and management of rhinitis. Allergy 1994;49(suppl 19):1–34.

3 Hagy GW, Settipane GA: Bronchial asthma, allergic rhinitis and allergy skin tests among college students. J Allergy 1969;45:323–332.

2

4 Mygind N, Dahl R: Epidemiology of allergic rhinitis. Pediatr Allergy Immunol 1996; 7(suppl 9):57–62.
5 Wüthrich B, Schindler C, Leuenberger P: Prevalence of atopy and pollinosis in the adult population in Switzerland. Int Arch Allergy Appl Immunol 1995;106:149–156.
6 Voorhorst V, Spieksema-Boezaman MIA, Spieksma FTM: Is a mite (*Dermatophagoides* sp) the producer of the house-dust allergen? Allerg Asthma 1964;10:329–336.
7 Wihl J-Å, Mygind N: Studies of the allergen-challenged human nasal mucosa. Acta Otolaryngol 1977;84:281–286.
8 Mygind N: Scanning electron microscopy of the human nasal mucosa. Rhinology 1975; 13:57–75.
9 Mygind N, Thomsen J: Cytology of the nasal mucosa: a comparative study between a replica-method and a smear-method. Arch Klin Exp Ohren Nasen Kehlkopfheilkd 1973;204:123–129.
10 Secher C, Kirkegaard J, Borum P, Maansson A, Osterhammel P, Mygind N: Significance of H_1 and H_2 receptors in the human nose: rationale for topical use of combined antihistamine preparations. J Allergy Clin Immunol 1982;70:211–218.
11 Ohashi Y, Motojima S, Fukuda T, Makino S: Airway hyperresponsiveness, increased intercellular spaces of bronchial epithelium, and increased infiltration of eosinophils and lymphocytes in bronchial mucosa in asthma. Am Rev Respir Dis 1992;145:1469–1476.
12 Borum P, Grønborg H, Brofeldt S, Mygind N: Nasal reactivity in rhinitis. Eur J Respir Dis 1983;64(suppl 128):65–71.
13 Mygind N, Dahl R, Bachert C: Nasal polyposis, eosinophil dominated inflammation, and allergy. Thorax 2000;55(suppl 2):S79–S83.
14 Wihl J-Å, Petersen BN, Gundersen G, Bresson K, Mygind N: Effect of the nonsedative H_1-receptor antagonist astemizole in perennial allergic and nonallergic rhinitis. J Allergy Clin Immunol 1985;75:720–727.
15 Navarro A, Valero A, Rosales MJ, Mullol J: Clinical use of oral antihistamines and intranasal corticosteroids in patients with allergic rhinitis. J Investig Allergol Clin Immunol 2011;21:363–369.
16 van Cauwenberge P, Bachert C, Passalacqua G, et al: Consensus statement on the treatment of allergic rhinitis. Allergy 2000;55: 116–134.
17 Brown HM, Storey G, George WHS: Beclomethasone dipropionate: a new steroid aerosol for the treatment of allergic asthma. Br Med J 1972;1:585–590.
18 Mygind N: Local effect of intranasal beclomethasone dipropionate in hay fever. Br Med J 1973;4:464–466.
19 Prahl P, Wilken-Jensen K, Mygind N: Beclomethasone dipropionate aerosol in treatment of hay fever in children. Arch Dis Child 1975;50:875–878.
20 Hansen I, Mygind N: Local effect of beclomethasone dipropionate aerosol in perennial rhinitis. Acta Allergol 1974:29:281–287.
21 Mygind N, Sørensen H, Pedersen CB: The nasal mucosa during long-term treatment with beclomethasone dipropionate aerosol: a light and scanning electron microscopic study of nasal polyps. Acta Otolaryngol 1978;85:437–443.
22 Mygind N, Pedersen CB, Prytz S, Sørensen H: Treatment of nasal polyps with beclomethasone dipropionate aerosol. Clin Allergy 1975;5:159–164.
23 Borum P, Grønborg H, Brofeldt S, Mygind N: Seasonal allergic rhinitis and depot injection of a corticosteroid. Allergy 1987;42: 26–32.
24 Mygind N, Lildholdt T: Nasal polyps treatment: medical management. Allergy Asthma Proc 1997;17:275–282.
25 Martinez-Devesa P, Patiar S: Oral steroids for nasal polyps. Cochrane Database Syst Rev 2011:CD005232.
26 Mygind N, Lund V: Intranasal corticosteroids for nasal polyposis: biological rationale, efficacy, and safety. Treat Respir Med 2006;5:93–102.
27 Malm L, Änggård A: Vasoconstrictors; in Mygind N, Naclerio RM (eds): Allergic Rhinitis: Clinical Aspects. Copenhagen, Munksgaard, 1993, pp 95–100.
28 Borum P, Mygind N, Larsen FS: Intranasal ipratropium: a new treatment for perennial rhinitis. Clin Otolaryngol 1979;4:407–411.
29 Østberg B, Winther B, Borum P, Mygind N: Common cold and high-dose ipratropium bromide: use of anticholinergic medication as an indicator of reflex-mediated hypersecretion. Rhinology 1997;35:58–62.

Prof. Niels Mygind
Kildegaarden 9
DK–8000 Aarhus (Denmark)
E-Mail niels.mygind@dadlnet.dk

Bergmann K-C, Ring J (eds): History of Allergy. Chem Immunol Allergy. Basel, Karger, 2014, vol 100, pp 69–80
DOI: 10.1159/000358575

Asthma

Karl-Christian Bergmann

Allergy Centre Charité, Universitätsmedizin, Berlin, Germany

Abstract

'Asthma' is derived from the Greek root ασθμαινω, meaning 'gasp for breath'. The term originally did not define a disease, but was employed to describe respiratory symptoms of a variety of pulmonary conditions. Over the centuries, several models have been proposed to understand the pathophysiologic abnormalities of asthma. By the beginning of the 20th century, asthma was seen to be a unique illness characterized by 'spasmodic afflictions of the bronchial tubes'. Consistent with the nature of asthma as a complex disease, the models for asthma pathogenesis have become increasingly complex. Research has moved from antiquated ideas to a descriptive functional approach to one that relies on pathophysiology in cellular and molecular biology, immunology, microbiology and genetics/genomics. As more advanced technologies for measuring lung function were developed, the features of asthma were steadily unraveled and its pathophysiology clarified. Asthma was shown to be associated with transient increases in airway resistance, reductions in forced expiratory volumes and flows, hyperinflation of the lungs and increased work of breathing, as well as abnormalities in the distribution of ventilation, perfusion and arterial blood gases. Today, asthma is seen as a chronic inflammatory disease which is not yet fully understood in its pathophysiology; therefore, therapy is still on the path to becoming optimal.

> Asthma is doubly capricious; the disease in general is capricious, and each case is capricious in itself.
> *Henry Hyde Salter*

Asthma is a Greek word that means panting or difficulty in breathing. It was used for the first time by Homer, one of the epic poets of ancient Greece, in the *Iliad*, which narrates the last year of the legendary war between the Greeks and the inhabitants of the city of Troy. The term was also quoted by the ancient Greek lyric poet from Thebes, Píndar (522–443 BC), by the Greek writer Aeschylus (525–456 BC) and the Greek philosopher Plato (427–347 BC).

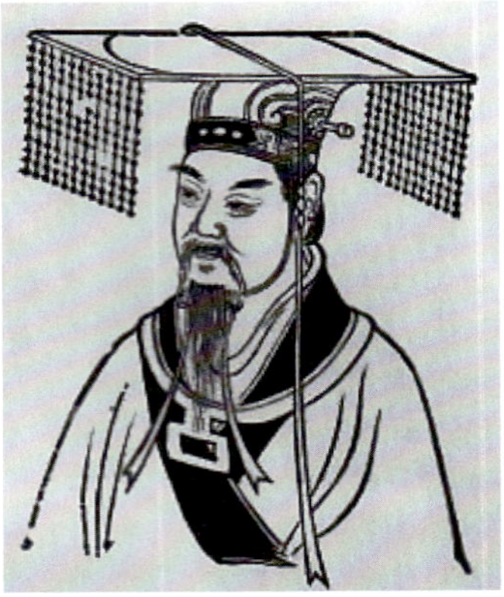

1

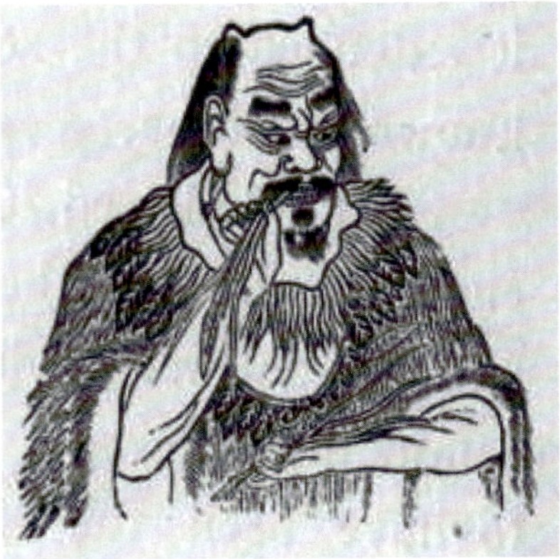

2

Fig. 1. Huangdi. The Yellow Emperor.
Fig. 2. Shen-Nung, the Farmer God, tasting herbs to discover their qualities.

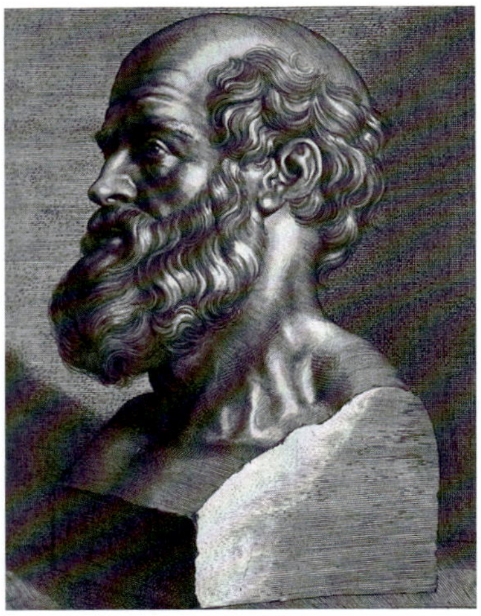

Fig. 3. Hippocrates. Engraving by Peter Paul Rubens, 1638.

The Beginning in the East

Asthma was described in 2600 BC in the medical book *Huangdi Neijing*, also known as *The Inner Canon of Huangdi* or *Yellow Emperor's Inner Canon.* This is an ancient Chinese medical text that has been treated as the fundamental doctrinal source for Chinese medicine for more than 2 millennia. It is comparable in importance to the *Hippocratic Corpus* in Greek medicine or the works of Galen in Islamic and medieval European medicine.

This source seems to be the most ancient book of internal medicine, written by the mythical Huangdi (Yellow Emperor or, more correctly, Yellow Thearch; fig. 1) who practiced medicine during the third millennium BC. Written in the form of a dialogue between the emperor and six of his equally legendary ministers, the emperor discusses the causes of noisy, troubled breathing.

Shen-Nung (fig. 2) is said to have compiled the first Chinese pharmacopoeia *(Pen Tsao)* written under the form of a dialogue between the emperor and his doctor. One of the included plants is quoted as 'ma huang', *Ephedra.* Drinks prepared from this native plant of Asia and America, of which the ephedrine began to be extracted at the beginning of 20th century, were prescribed by physicians for a variety of respiratory conditions, including cough. About 350 remedial plants are named in the book *Shen Nung Pen Tsao Ching.*

The Beginning in the West

Hippocrates of Kos (fig. 3), the ancient Greek physician of the Age of Pericles (Classical Greece), used the term asthma, 'I gasp for breath', to signify 'hurried breathing' [1]. He is considered one of the most outstanding figures in the history of medicine and referred to as the father of Western medicine in recognition of his lasting contributions to the field as the founder of the Hippocratic School of Medicine. This intellectual school revolutionized medicine in ancient Greece, establishing it as a discipline distinct from other fields that it had traditionally been associated with philosophically, thus establishing medicine as a profession.

Asthma was described by Hippocrates as a paroxysmal attack, more severe than simple dyspnea. The spasmodic condition of the asthma was compared to an epileptic convulsion, which was regarded as a divine punishment.

Aulus Cornelius Celsus (circa 25 BC to 25 AC) [see fig. 9 in the chapter by Ring, this vol., pp. 2–14] was a Roman encyclopedist, known for his extensive medical work, *De Medicina*. He was familiar with the loud breathing noise with complicated expiration of the asthmatic, and suggested the cause to be a narrowing of the respiratory tract. He classified the difficulties in breathing into three degrees:

(1) dyspnea – quickened breathing, especially after running or physical exercise;
(2) asthma – breathing disturbance without exercise;
(3) orthopnea – disease of the heaviest degree for which the patient must sit upright to get enough air.

This classification of asthma made by Celsus was recognized until the 18th century. One of his proposals for treatment was:

> Sit down in a half straight position, apply warm wraps around the breast and drink a little bit of sulphurized wine to which the powdered liver and lung of a fox is added. [2]

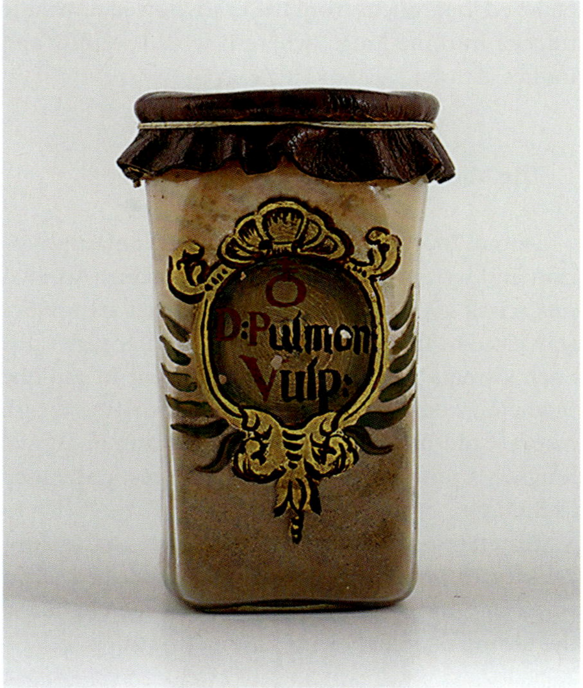

Fig. 4. The vessel 'Pulmon Vulpis' from the medicine cabinet of the monastery of the Unbeschuhten Karmeliten in Schongau, 18th century.

In the collection of the German Pharmacy Museum in Heidelberg, a vessel for the powdered lung of a fox is part of the exhibition (fig. 4).

Aretaeus (circa 80 AD to circa 130 AD) [see fig. 7 in the chapter by Ring, this vol., pp. 2–14], generally known as 'the Cappadocian', is one of the most celebrated of the ancient Greek physicians. He first described the asthmatic paroxysm, calling attention to this very characteristic feature of the disease [3]. According to Hans Schadewaldt [4], Aretaeus made the first and also the best description of asthma in antiquity.

His definition of asthma still comprises all the difficulties in breathing. His subtle clinical description enclosed remarks on bronchial hyperreactivity. He described the life-threatening danger of the status asthmaticus and he localized the disease in the lung.

Aelius Galenus or Claudius Galenus (129 AD to about 200 or 216 AD) [see fig. 8 in the chapter by Ring, this vol., pp. 2–14], better known as Galen of Pergamon, did not include this concept in his records. Galen was the most famous physician of his time in Rome and the personal physician of Emperor Marcus Aurelius. His apprenticeship and writings dominated European medicine until the Middle Ages.

In his writings he defined every quickened respiration as asthma [5]. With this he was less exact than his predecessor, Aretaeus. Galen tried to generate breath disturbances experimentally. He wrote:

> If you cut the spinal cord in the area of the 3rd or 4th vertebra, the animal experiences immediately a heavy breath disturbance. [6]

Galen had raised the teaching of the four juices for more than 1,000 years to the medical dogma of his time and, hence, was persuaded that asthma would originate from a 'dyskrasia' of the juices. He believed that mucus from the brain flowed down the trachea into the lungs, where it would solidify and induce asthma [7].

The Middle Ages

About 200 years after Galen, the Roman physician and writer on medical topics, Caelius Aurelianus (circa 400 AD), recommended that asthmatics stay close to the seashore and near water generally. Such climate therapy was not unusual in antique medicine, representing the predecessor of a health resort. Cold baths, diet and the drinking of animal lungs as a powder in wine were also recommended as therapy.

Aurelianus still added some nuances to the clinical description of Aretaeus. He described clear wheezing during expiration, pain in the chest and the feeling of anxiety with asthma [8].

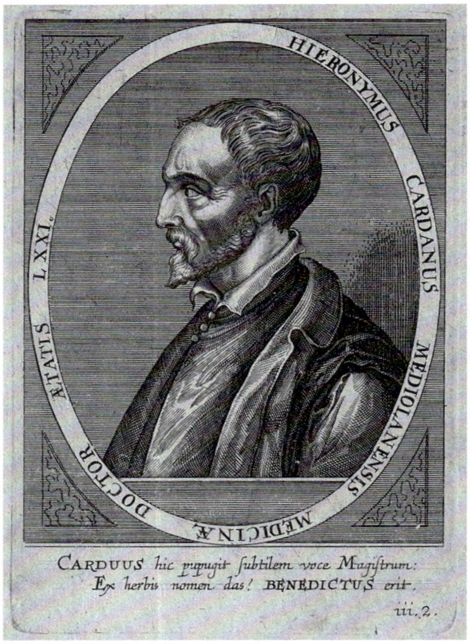
HIERONYMUS CARDANUS MEDIOLANENSIS
MEDICINÆ DOCTOR
ÆTATIS LXXI.
CARDUUS hic pupugit subtilem voce Magistrum:
Ex herbis nomen das! BENEDICTUS erit.
iii.2.

Fig. 5. Girolamo Cardano. Line engraving by C. Ammon the younger, 1652.

Modern Times

The superiority of Italian medicine was also demonstrated at the beginning of the 16th century by the physician and mathematician Girolamo Cardano (1511–1571; fig. 5). He was able to 'cure' John Hamilton (1511–1571), the Roman Catholic archbishop of St. Andrews in Scotland, who suffered from an increasingly severe asthma characterized by cough, expectoration and shortness of breath. Cardano was invited by Hamilton's physician, Dr. Cassanate, to treat Hamilton. He accepted and observed carefully the nocturnal difficulty in breathing of the bishop for more than 40 days. He then decided that his pillows and bedding filled with feathers had to be substituted with a silk cover and a pillow filled with straw. Also, he recommended that the bishop should receive less food, more sleep, and showers with cold water [9].

The therapy was very successful. The asthma attacks, possibly induced by an allergy to bed feathers (or perhaps to mites in the bed feathers), disappeared. This was clearly a great success for Cardano, who received a luxuriant wage of 1,800 crowns in gold and a golden necklace. Cardano was also an astrologer, interpreter of dreams and a mathematician.

Although Cardano's treatment of asthma was very successful in his famous patient, the ancient understanding of asthma in terms of accumulation of cold, moist humors persisted and remained the main explanation of asthma during the 16th and 17th centuries. According to Jackson [10], Cardano's rejection of feather mattresses cannot be taken as a precursor of later allergic theories on asthma, as some allergy-interested historians have suggested.

With the renaissance of medicine, Jan Baptist van Helmont (1577–1644; fig. 6), a Flemish chemist, physiologist and physician who was himself asthmatic, first called attention to the spastic (bronchial obstruction) element of sudden attacks amidst intervals with freedom to breath. Van Helmont was critical to Galenic medicine and kept a distance from Hippocratic notions of phlegm descending from the brain to the lungs. He insisted that the disease originated in the lungs, not the head. Van Helmont worked during the years just after Paracelsus and is sometimes considered to be 'the founder of pneumatic chemistry'.

In his major medical work [11] he included a chapter on 'The asthma or arrest of breathing, and cough'. Van Helmont described two separate clinical phenotypes of the disease, one a 'moist' asthma with expectoration or 'spitting' of phlegm (it is possible that he meant bronchitis), the other a 'dry' asthma. However, he recognized that in some patients a mixture of both could occur. Therefore, van Helmont provided a constructive framework for subsequent discussions about the causes and manifestations of asthma.

Van Helmont described the heredity of asthma with the example of the mother and sister of an asthmatic monk. Amongst his other achievements he also discovered carbon dioxide and he coined the word 'gas'.

Thomas Willis (1621–1675; fig. 7) recognized the peculiar episodes of shortness of breath and the absence of evidence of bronchial or pulmonary disease at autopsy. He described two types of asthma, the 'pneumonic' and the 'convulsive' asthma, which may be recognized as chronic, persistent or acute episodic. In 'pneumonic asthma' the bronchi were obstructed or not sufficiently open as the result of 'thick humours and viscious, or purulent matter or blood extravasated' into the bronchi. In contrast, the 'convulsive form' of asthma resulted from a 'morbific cause or matter', adversely affecting the muscular fibers, nerves or the brain. He asserted that some patients may have a mixed clinical picture, especially if the asthma had become habitual [12].

Sir John Floyer (1649–1734; fig. 8) stated in his book, *A Treatise of the Asthma* (fig. 9), that he himself 'had suffered under the tyranny of the disease for at least thirty years' [13]. He was an excellent observer and gave vivid descriptions of the asthmatic episodes and the many causes of the acute attacks he or his patients had experienced. Floyer attributed the disease to 'straightness or constriction of the bronchi' and argued that the immediate triggers of asthma included any agent that encouraged 'a slow effervescence, or ebullition of our blood'. Examples were great heat or cold, any excess in eating and drinking, changes in the weather to rain or snow, or from frost to thaw.

Floyer's monograph, *A Treatise of the Asthma*, was translated into French and German and went

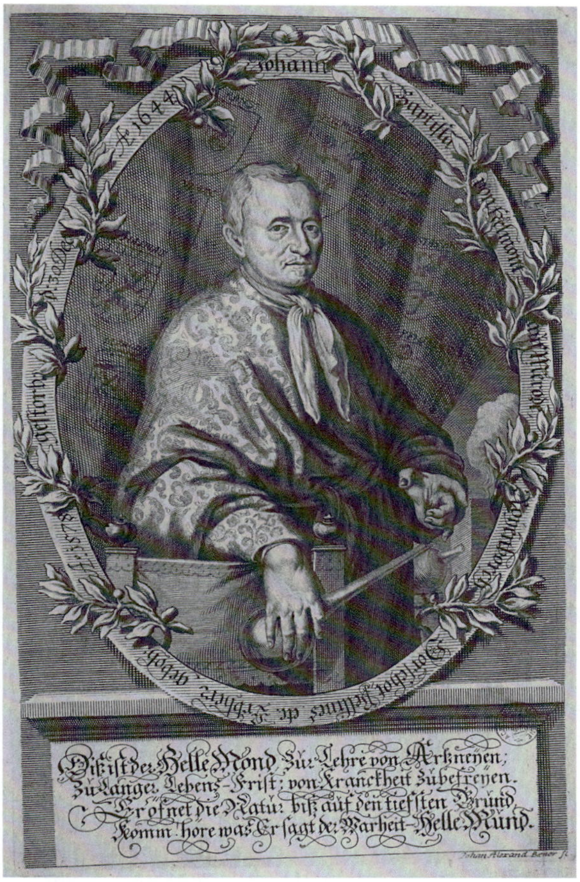

Fig. 6. Jan Baptist van Helmont.

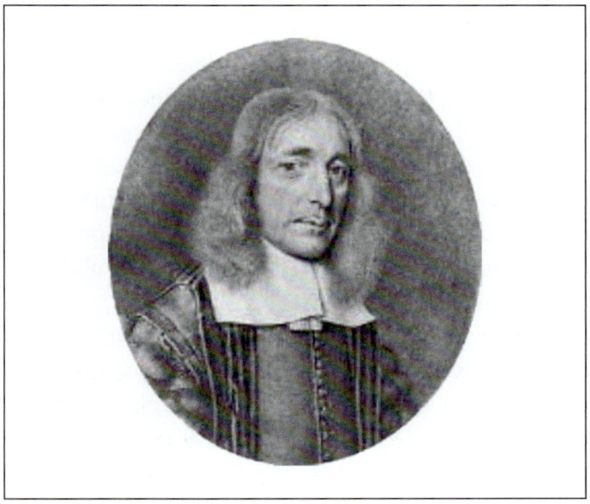

Fig. 7. Thomas Willis.

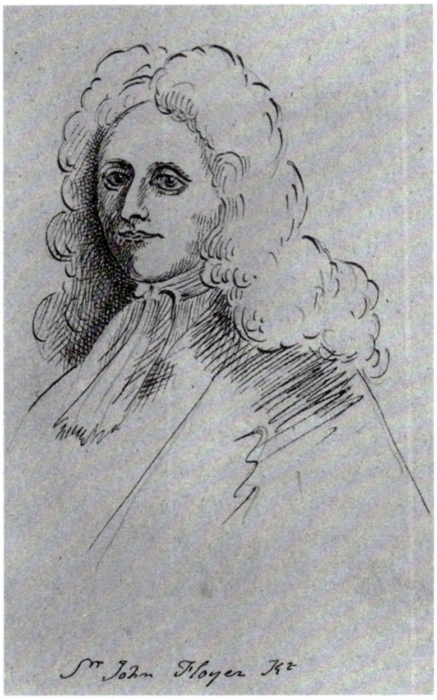

8

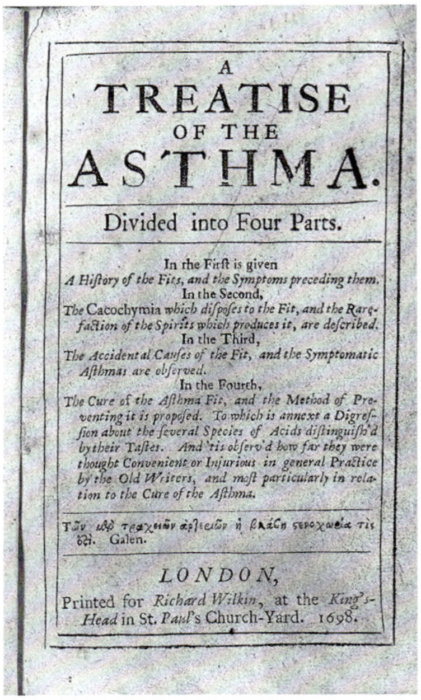
A
TREATISE
OF THE
ASTHMA.

Divided into Four Parts.

In the First is given
A History of the Fits, and the Symptoms preceding them.
In the Second,
The Cacochymia *which disposes to the Fit, and the Rarefaction of the Spirits which produces it, are described.*
In the Third,
The Accidental Causes of the Fit, and the Symptomatic Asthmas are observed.
In the Fourth,
The Cure of the Asthma Fit, and the Method of Preventing it is proposed. To which is annext a Digression about the several Species of Acids distinguish'd by their Tastes. And 'tis observ'd how far they were thought Convenient or Injurious in general Practice by the Old Writers, and most particularly in relation to the Cure of the Asthma.

Galen.

LONDON,
Printed for *Richard Wilkin*, at the *King's-Head* in St. *Paul's* Church-Yard. 1698.

9

Fig. 8. John Floyer.
Fig. 9. Title page of *A Treatise of the Asthma* (1698) by John Floyer.

through several popular and influential English editions. It is regarded as a pivotal moment in the history of asthma 'comprising an extensive overview of the causes, diagnosis, pathology and treatment of the condition, was often cited and quoted by subsequent authors, becoming a standard, if sometimes contested, reference point for all modern Western discussions of the disease' [10, p. 66]. Floyer returned to his own experiences of asthma at key moments in his text, using personal insight to explain the symptoms, periodicity and prognosis of the disease.

Following the epochal work of Willis and Floyer, which received acceptance over some time, a tendency developed to revert to the concept of the ancient times, calling all manner of difficult breathing asthma, usually with the addition of descriptive adjectives such as nervous, arthritic, cardiac, abdominal, plethoric or dry asthma, and so on.

Bernardino Ramazzini (1633–1714; fig. 10) was the first to systematically describe occupational diseases, among them the asthma of bakers, in his book on the subject, *De Morbis Artificum Diatriba* ('Diseases of Workers') [14]. He thought that baker's asthma was the result of a blockage of the respiratory tract caused by flour, forming a paste. At the beginning of the 18th century, the anatomy of bronchi and the lungs was described more precisely and aided the understanding of the pathophysiology of asthma.

One of the best anatomists of his time was Frederik Ruysch (1638–1731), who is remembered for his improvements to anatomical preservation. He assembled one of Europe's most famous anatomical collections, which he sold 1717 to Peter the Great for 30,000 guilders. In his *Opera Omnia* from 1721 [15], he published pictures of diffuse bullous emphysema from an asthmatic who had died during an acute asthma attack (fig. 11). He diagnosed the emphysema before the methods of percussion and auscultation were used (fig. 12).

William Cullen (1710–1790; fig. 13), a Scottish physician, chemist and agriculturalist, recognized again the spastic character of asthma ('asthma convulsive') as an entity. He described the hereditary tendency in the onset of asthma, the nocturnal symptoms and the effect of weather on the outbreak of the disease. He believed that the disease affected more men than women and usually appeared first at, or after, puberty. For Cullen, asthma constituted a form of dyspnea or breathing difficulty caused primarily by 'an affection of the nervous system' rather than by the accumulation of mucus. He stated that the term asthma should be confined to cases as 'spasmodic asthma' or 'asthma convulsivum'. For treatment he recommended identifying and avoiding any occasional or exciting causes, including tea and coffee [16].

The charm of 'spasmodic asthma' was that it explained not only the symptoms of asthma, but also the inefficacy of old and newer treatments that did not include anti-spasmodic agents. There were disputes over the use of mucus-expectorating treatments versus the use of spasmolytics.

The idea of spastic asthma was underlined by the diagnostic studies and observations of René Théophile Hyacinthe Laënnec (1781–1826; fig. 14). He invented the stethoscope in 1816 (fig. 15) and pioneered its use in diagnosing various chest conditions. In 1819, he published the results of his research on the auscultation in patients with chest diseases [17]. He showed that many cases of supposed asthma were actually due to cardiac (referred to by subsequent authors as 'cardiac asthma') and pulmonary lesions, discoverable during life and demonstrable after death. Shortness of breath is recognized as a symptom which may be due to many causes. Among the causes he distinguished affection, characterized by paroxysmal dyspnea without demonstrable associated lesions, in which no evidence of the disease could be found on auscultation during the free interval. He also realized that patients with both dry and humid asthma exhibited identical wheezing during inspiration and expiration. Therefore, the respiratory distress in asthmatics was not caused by mucus, but rather by spasms of the bronchi. He concluded that the cause of asthma must be a spasm of the muscle of the bronchi and believed that asthma was primarily a neurosis [18].

During the 19th century, Laennec's idea of the spasmodic theory of asthma was supported by various studies in experimental pathology. The concept of neurosis influenced the history of asthma. Longet (1842) showed that stimulation of the distal end of the vagus would produce bronchial construction [19]. A number of scientists contributed to the idea of a nervous etiology of asthma. Among them were Bergson, Ramagde, Andral, Salter and the great French physician Armand Trousseau (1801–1867).

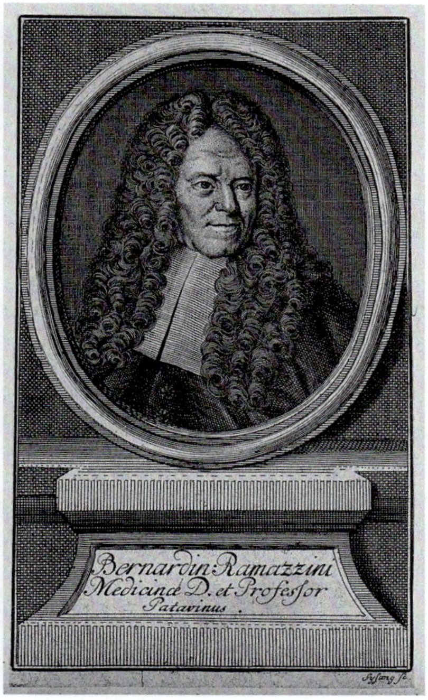

Fig. 10. Bernardino Ramazzini. Engraving by J.C. Sysang.

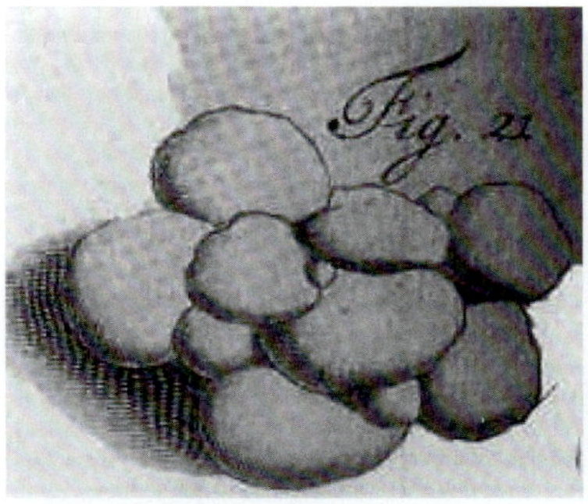

Fig. 11. The first picture of emphysema bullae in the lung of an asthmatic.

He regarded asthma as a dietetic neurosis dependent upon spastic obstruction of the bronchi that was interchangeable with eczema, rheumatic infection and periodic headaches.

In the second half of the 19th century, three principle theories dominated and overcame the 'neurotic theory' of asthma. These were bronchial spasm,

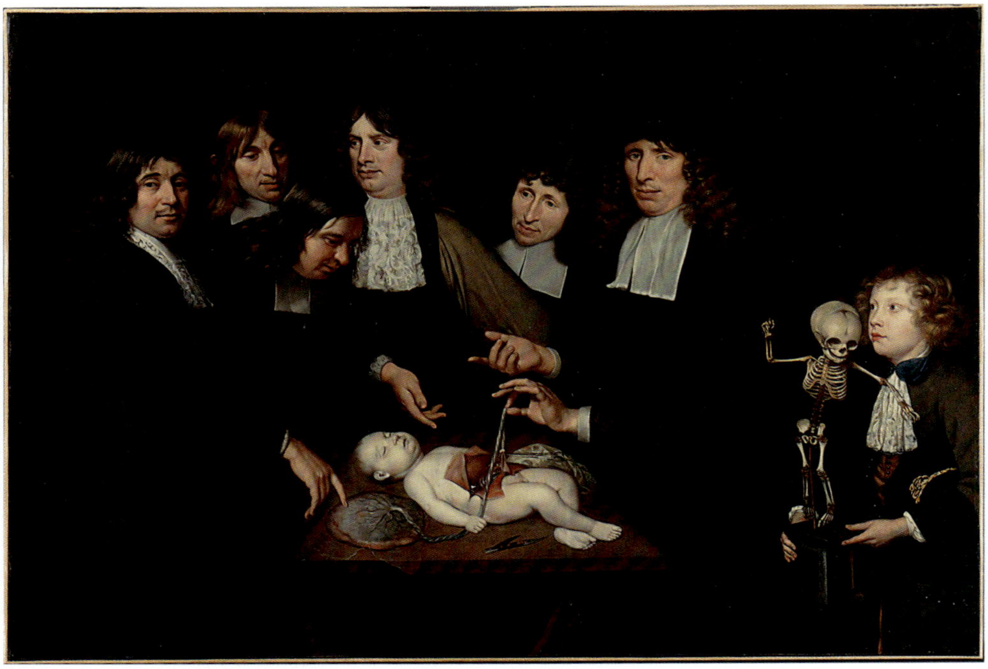

Fig. 12. Anatomy lesson of Dr. Frederik Ruysch, by Jan van Neck (1683).

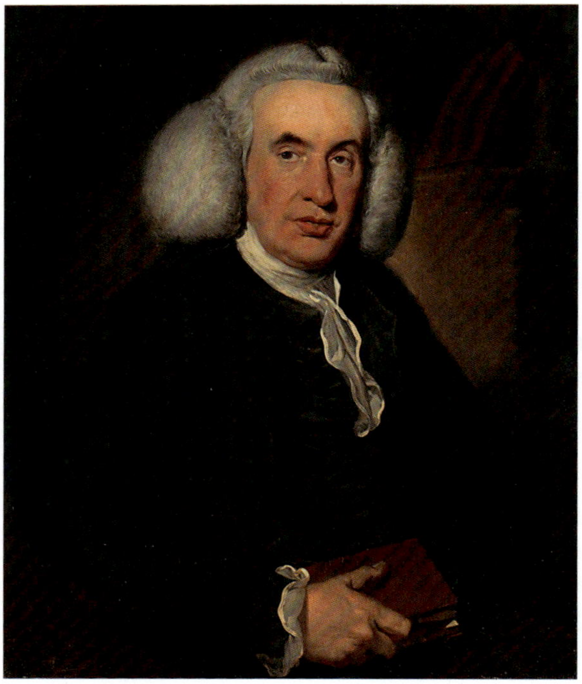

Fig. 13. William Cullen.

spastic contraction of the diaphragm and sudden turgescence of the bronchial mucosa [10].

The English physician Henry Hyde Salter (1823–1871) was an asthmatic himself and published his treatise of asthma in London in 1860 [20]. He suggested that bronchial obstruction was the product of 'excite-motory or reflex action' initiated by 'deleterious material' in the bronchi. He accepted that asthma attacks may be induced by a variety of factors, which had been familiar since Hippocrates, including fatigue or emotions, but he also indicated the greater pressures of modern civilization:

> The rich might be really more liable to asthma than the poor, from a more irritable nervous organization engendered by the state of hyper-civilization in which we live. [21, cited by 10]

Salter's concept was similar to that of Sir William Osler [22] (1849–1919; fig. 16). He taught that both direct and psychogenic stimulation of the nervous system could produce asthma exacerbations. Because of his prestige in the medical world, his writ-

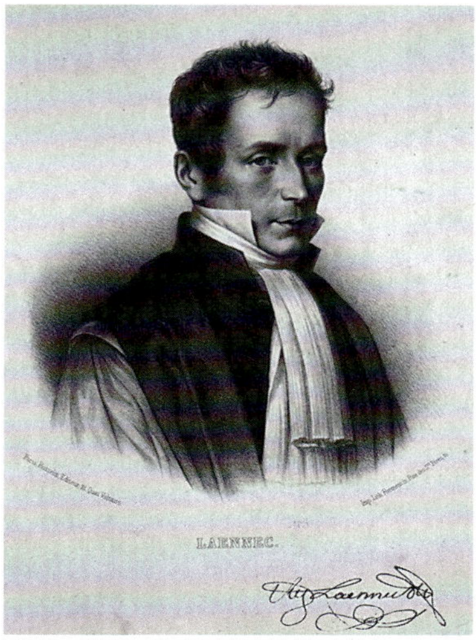

Fig. 14. Lithograph of René Théophile Hyacinthe Laënnec.

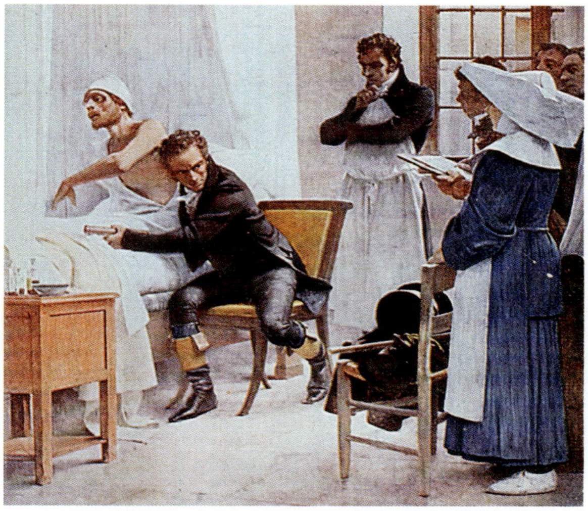

Fig. 15. 'Laënnec examines a consumptive patient with a stethoscope in front of his students at the Hospital Necker in Paris'. Painting by Théobald Chartran.

ings ultimately led to asthma becoming synonymous with a psychoneurosis.

Beside the development of a lung function diagnostic, new tools for asthma diagnosis were developed; mechanical irritants in the bronchi such as Charcot-Leyden crystals (fig. 17), Curschmann's spirals and eosinophils were regarded as asthma triggers. Jean-Martin Charcot (1825–1893; fig. 18) described special crystals in the sputum of a woman who suffered from bronchitis [23]. They aroused the interest of other colleagues in the following years. Ernst Viktor von Leyden (1832–1910; fig. 19) examined these colorless crystals closer and found them in the sputum of asthma patients; he thought that they were the cause of the asthma [24]. The Charcot-Leyden crystals became famous and were valid for decades as an important diagnostic parameter of asthma, especially following an asthmatic attack.

Heinrich Curschmann (1846–1910; fig. 20), a German internist, completed the sputum diagnosis in 1882 with his description of spirals as coiled mucous fibrils sometimes found in the sputum of bronchial asthma sufferers ('Curschmann's spirals') [25]. The crystals were recognized as crystallized eosinophil-cationic protein.

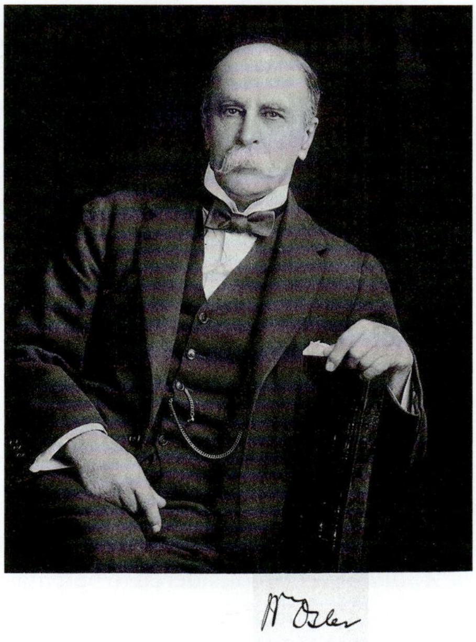

Fig. 16. Sir William Osler, at the age of 70.

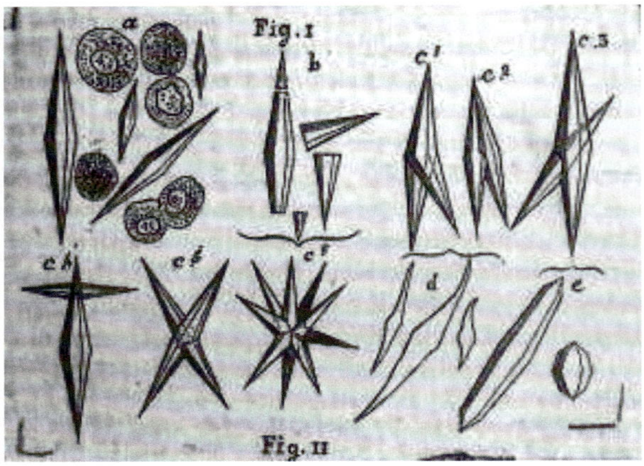

Fig. 17. Charcot-Leyden crystals (Charcot, 1860).

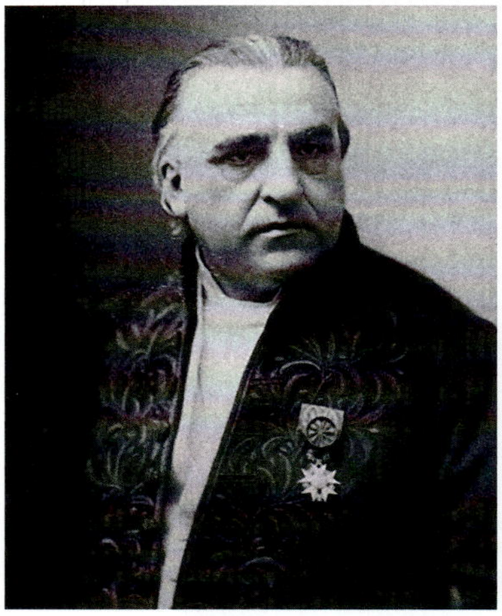

Fig. 18. Portrait of Jean-Martin Charcot.

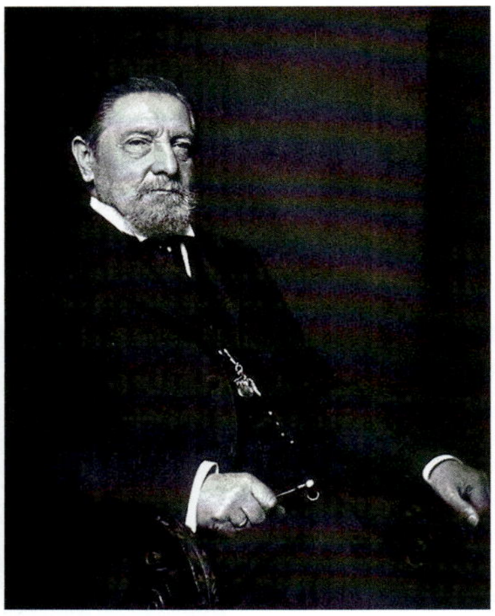

Fig. 19. Ernst Viktor von Leyden.

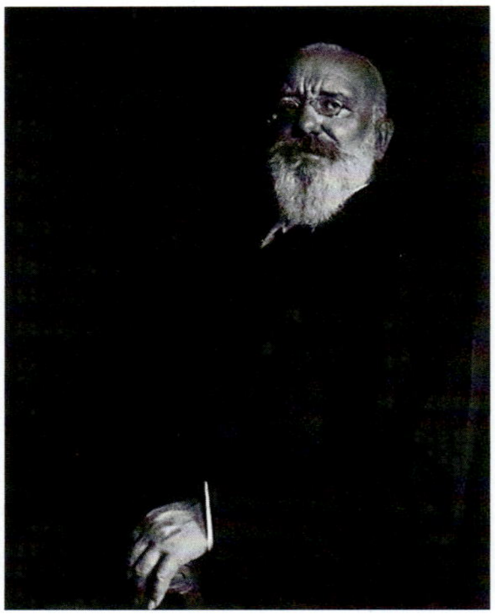

Fig. 20. Heinrich Curschmann.

Curschmann is remembered for the 1894 publication of *Klinische Abbildungen* ('clinical illustrations'), a collection of photos, involving changes in the outer human appearance caused by internal disease. *Klinische Abbildungen* is considered to be a major pioneering work in medical photography [26].

At the beginning of the 20th century, asthma was quite generally considered to be a neurosis, as recorded in the famous *Osler's Modern Medicine* from 1907 [27]. However, even though the nervous factor was emphasized, the importance of extrinsic excitants in the precipitation of asthma attacks was increasingly recognized. Such etiologic agents were seen in pollen, through the handling of fresh coffee beans, oak wood, mattress dust, in the odor of a cat, house dust, the ingestion of certain foods and climatic changes. However, the potential pathogenesis of asthma was about to take a new form.

In 1873, Charles Blackley [28] demonstrated that pollen was the cause of hay fever and 'hay asthma'. In 1910, Meltzer theorized that asthma in humans and anaphylaxis in guinea pigs were equivalent phenomena because they both involved the airways, and thus a new school of thought was created. Asthma was no longer just a 'neurosis'. Since asthma and hay fever were often associated, and because pollen produced hay fever, it followed that the sensitizing proteins in pollen and plant material in general also produced asthma. The role of sensitizing allergens became understood in greater depth and dermal tests became popular in diagnosing asthma. However, some asthmatics had negative skin tests; they were categorized as 'intrinsic' in contrary to the 'extrinsic' or allergic asthmatics. It was also theorized that some asthmatics might be sensitive to the bacteria resident in places such as the nose, sinuses and tonsils. These groupings also had therapeutic implications: allergen avoidance and immunotherapy was advised for the allergic group, while antibiotics or specific vaccines were prescribed for the 'intrinsic' patients [29].

Bronchoscopy had been performed in asthmatics since at least 1914, but the histologic features of biopsies were not reported until 1985. It was established that chronic inflammation was a feature of asthma in all of its stages. On this basis, anti-inflammatory therapies were introduced to limit the inflammatory cascades which led to airway remodeling with permanent functional impairments. Glucocorticoids offered the first hope in this area. They were applied in acute asthma in 1956 [30], and then in chronic disease.

The bronchial hyperresponsiveness characteristic of asthma was described in 1946 by Curry [31], who examined the effects of graded doses of histamine in individuals with and without asthma. In the 1960s and 1970s, peak flow meters were introduced to assess airway obstruction at home and at the working place.

With the systematic research on mast cells, basophils and eosinophils, knowledge about the biology of asthma grew exponentially. New tools emerged in immunology, allergology, genetics and virology, leading to an increasingly better understanding of the inflammatory processes in the lung, including intercellular and intracellular pathways in the disease process [32]. Measuring quality of life in asthmatics became a new branch in research on the disease in the 1970s using genetic or disease-specific questionnaires. Later, the measurement of disease control using asthma control tests which try to quantify the stability of asthma was a new aspect. Finally, in 1991, the first international consensus was reached on the diagnosis and management of asthma [33] – a big step forward in the worldwide control of the disease.

2

Acknowledgments

This article could not have been written without knowledge of the excellent book *Asthma: A Biography* by Mark Jackson. Also indispensable were the articles by McFadden on the history of asthma, and the *Geschichte der Allergie* by Hans Schadewaldt, the nestor of the history of allergy.

References

1 Hippocrates: On the nature of bones, 13.19, cited in Marketos SG, Ballas CN: Bronchial asthma in the medical literature of antiquity. J Asthma 1982;19:263–269.
2 Celsus AC: De re medicina; in Marx F (ed): Corpus Medicorum Graecorum. Leipzig, 1915, vol 1.
3 Aretaeus of Cappadocia; in Hude K (ed): Corpus medicorum Graecorum, ed 2. Berlin, Akademie, 1958.
4 Schadewaldt H: Geschichte der Allergologie. Munich, Dustri, 1983, vol 1–4.
5 Galen; in Kühn CG (ed): Opera. Leipzig, 1821–1833.
6 Galen; in Mewaldt J (ed): Corpus medicorum graecorum. Leipzig, 1914, vol 17, p 633.
7 Galen; in Mewaldt J (ed): Corpus medicorum graecorum. Leipzig,1914, vol 7, p 957.
8 Aurelianus: De Morbus acutis et chronicis. Libri octo (ed JC Ammann). Amsterdam, 1722, Lib 3, Cap 1.
9 Dana CL: The story of a great consultation. Jerome Cardan goes to Edingburgh. Ann Med Hist 1921;3:122.
10 Jackson M: Asthma: The Biography. Oxford, Oxford University Press, 2009.
11 van Helmont JB: Asthma et Tussis; in van Helmont (ed): Ortus medicinae. Amsterdam, 1648.
12 Willis T: Pharmaceutice rationalis: Or, the Operations of Medicines in Human Bodies, Part II. London, Dring, Harper & Leigh, 1679.
13 Floyer J: A Treatise of the Asthma. London, 1698.
14 Ramazzini B: De morbis artificum diatriba. Modena, 1700 (Facsimile Rome, 1953).
15 Ruysch F: Opera Omnia. Anatomica-medico-chiurgia. Amsterdam, 1721.
16 Cullen W: Lectures of the Materia medica. London, 1773.
17 Laennec RHT: De l'auscultation médiate. Paris, 1819.
18 Laennec RHT: Traité de l'auscultation médiate et des maladies des poumons et du coeur. Paris, 1826.
19 Longet FA. Anatomie et physiologie du système nerveux de l'homme et des animaux vertèbres. Paris, 1842, vol 2.

20 Salter H: On Asthma: Its Pathology and Treatment. London, Churchill, 1860.
21 Salter H: Spasmodic asthma. Lancet 1869; 75:152–153.
22 Osler W: Diseases of the respiratory system: bronchial asthma; in Osler W (ed): The Principles and Practice of Medicine, ed 4. New York, Appleton, 1901, pp 628–632.
23 Charcot JM, Robin CP: Observation de leucodythemie. C R Soc Biol 1853;5:44.
24 Leyden EV: Zur Kenntnis des Bronchialasthmas. Arch Pathol Anat 1872;54:324.
25 Curschmann H: Über Bronchiolitis exsudativa und ihr Verhältnis zum Asthma nervosum. Dtsch Arch Klin Med 1882;32:1.
26 Curschmann H: Klinische Abbildungen. Berlin, Julius Springer, 1894.
27 Osler W: Modern Medicine. Philadelphia, Lea Brothers, 1907.
28 Blackley CH: Experimental Researches on the Causes and Nature of Catarrhus Aestivus (Hay Fever or Hay-Asthma). London, Ballière, Tindall & Cox, 1873.
29 McFadden ER Jr, Steven JB: History of asthma; in Middleton E, Reed C, Ellis E (eds): Allergy: Principles and Practice, ed 2. St Louis, Mosby, 1983, pp 805–809.
30 Brown HM, Storey G, George WH: Beclomethasone dipropionate: a new steroid aerosol for the treatment of allergic asthma. Br Med J 1972;1:585–590.
31 Curry JJ: The action of histamine on the respiratory tract in normal and asthmatic subjects. J Clin Invest 1946;25:785–791.
32 McFadden ER Jr: A century of asthma. Am J Respir Crit Care Med 2004;170:215–221.
33 National Heart, Lung and Blood Institute, National Asthma Education and Prevention Program: Expert panel report: guidelines for the diagnosis and management of asthma, executive summary. NHLBI NAEPP Publication No 92–3091. Washington, US Government Printing Office, 1991.

Prof. Dr. med. Karl-Christian Bergmann
Allergie-Centrum-Charité
Charité – Universitätsmedizin, Luisenstrasse 2
DE–10117 Berlin (Germany)
E-Mail karlchristianbergmann@googlemail.com

Bergmann K-C, Ring J (eds): History of Allergy. Chem Immunol Allergy. Basel, Karger, 2014, vol 100, pp 81–96
DOI: 10.1159/000358606

Atopic Dermatitis/Atopic Eczema

Daniel Wallach[a] · Alain Taïeb[b]

[a]Department of Dermatology, Hôpital Tarnier-Cochin, Paris, and [b]Department of Dermatology and Pediatric Dermatology, National Reference Centre for Rare Skin Disorders, Hôpital St. André, Bordeaux, France

Abstract

Atopic dermatitis was described in 1933 but exists since antiquity. We review descriptions of a childhood skin disease compatible with our modern diagnosis of atopic dermatitis, in ancient medicine and in nineteenth century dermatology texts. We identify Hebra's prurigo and Besnier's diathetic prurigo as forerunners of atopic dermatitis, the latter being a synthesis of infantile eczema and prurigo. The pathogenic theories which link atopic dermatitis to humoralistic medicine, to digestive diseases, to allergy may have had consequences on today's reluctance to consider atopic dermatitis as a skin disorder, the treatment of which relies mainly on topicals.

Atopic dermatitis is one of the most prevalent skin disorders. It is estimated that approximately 10% of young children receive a diagnosis of atopic dermatitis [1], and in some individuals the disease persists into adulthood. Severe atopic dermatitis is a burdensome disease, with painful repercussions on the daily life of the patient and his or her family, and significant economic consequences [2].

Atopic dermatitis is relatively easy to diagnose and is well known by dermatologists, as well as general practitioners and pediatricians. Even the lay public is aware of the main clinical features of atopic dermatitis as an eczema involving infants.

In spite of its prevalence, ease of diagnosis and the availability of efficient treatments, atopic dermatitis still remains a mysterious disease, and many aspects of atopic dermatitis knowledge are controversial. A huge amount of literature is available, reflecting diverse, if not contradictory opinions, which may be confusing. Recently, two comprehensive textbooks have gathered and attempted to synthesize recent publications [3, 4]; one of these textbooks contains a historical text by ourselves [5]. The goal of this chapter is to review the historical aspects of atopic dermatitis in order to understand not only the ancient descriptions and conceptions of the disease, but also to find explanations for our current difficulties with the understanding and management of atopic dermatitis.

When looking at the historical aspects of the disease that we today call atopic dermatitis or atopic eczema, the question of semantics is unavoidable. One can identify three levels of complexity in analyzing the meaning of the terms we use: (1) the significance of ancient medical terms, which have long been vague and indefinite; (2) translation problems, from Greek and Latin into current languages, and between current vernacular languages, and (3) current controversies about the meaning of medical terms.

In order to avoid too many citations, we will only indicate briefly how the three terms – 'atopic', 'dermatitis' and 'eczema' – can be considered as specifically controversial.

Atopic derives from the Greek 'a-topos', and means a strange disease without a precise place, a disease with no known place in the medical nosology. This word was coined in 1923 to designate a special state of immunologic hypersensitivity; it is self-mysterious.

Dermatitis is an inflammation of the skin. Many diseases can be included under this heading, such as urticaria, lichen planus, psoriasis, pemphigoid and eczema. Some authors use dermatitis as a synonym for eczema, as indicated in the title of this chapter. For other authors, dermatitis indicates an inflammation of the dermis, separate from eczema, which is primarily an inflammation of the epidermis.

Eczema was defined by Bateman in 1813 and has a rather precise meaning for the majority of dermatologists (clinical vesicles, microscopic spongiosis). The word eczema is often used as a synonym for dermatitis and would probably be a well-accepted denomination since the general public has always considered the disease called atopic dermatitis to be an eczema, as it is identical to infantile eczema. However, eczema is also a controversial term and it is possible to find in the literature such contradictory statements about eczema that some authors wish to see this term disappear from the dermatologic nomenclature [6].

Therefore, we are left with a 'strange' inflammation of controversial denomination. To add disturbing arguments to this brief review into the uncertainties of medical semantics would render the place of atopic dermatitis in allergic diseases (and with it the justification of this chapter of the book) very questionable. Atopic dermatitis indeed is not an allergic disease in the sense that the clinical manifestations are usually not directly induced by contact with an allergen [7]; the place of allergic factors in atopic dermatitis will be one of the controversies we will examine. To add to the confusion, even the atopic nature – in the sense of associated immunoglobulin (Ig) E sensitization – of atopic dermatitis is questioned [8].

For these and many more reasons, atopic dermatitis is a fascinating disease, and hundreds of papers are written every year on this topic. In 2004, we edited a book, in French, on the history of atopic dermatitis [9]. This book, which contains hundreds of references, forms the basis of this chapter, enriched with additional reflections.

Chronological Agenda

Atopic dermatitis has existed since antiquity, but was only described in 1933. For didactic purposes, we will divide the history of atopic dermatitis (an anachronism when it refers to pre-1933) into four periods:

- ancient medicine, from antiquity to 1800: descriptions compatible with atopic dermatitis can be found in ancient texts;
- clinical dermatology, from 1800 to 1933: dermatologists describe diseases which resemble atopic dermatitis, under different denominations, including eczemas and prurigos; infantile eczema and Besnier's prurigo appear as the most faithful forereunners of atopic dermatitis;
- immunologic medicine, from 1933 to 2006: discoveries in immunology and allergology allow the definition of atopic dermatitis as a special form of hypersensitivity;
- cutaneous medicine, since 2006: progress in genetics focuses on the importance of the epidermis in the pathophysiology of atopic dermatitis.

In spite of all these achievements, in 2011, our understanding of atopic dermatitis is far from complete.

Atopic Dermatitis before 1800

Atopic dermatitis was described and named in 1933 by Fred Wise and Marion Sulzberger [10]. Before 1933, however, the dermatological literature contained many clinical descriptions compatible with the modern diagnosis of atopic dermatitis.

Atopic dermatitis has probably existed since antiquity. Mier [11] attracted attention to a text by Suetonius, clearly describing cutaneous and respiratory atopic symptoms in Emperor Augustus.

From antiquity to 1800, skin disorders were not particularly looked at because the skin was considered one of the emunctories of the human body. Skin eruptions, especially oozing ones, were viewed as a salutary way of elimination of noxious or vitiated humors. With this conception, the individuality of skin diseases was not important, and it was dangerous to try and heal them.

This Hippocratic humoralist conception of skin diseases was prevalent until at least the 19th century and is still present in today's popular culture, as well as some alternative medicines. A few authors, however, paid special attention to the skin and its disorders. The first book committed to skin diseases was published in 1572 in Venice. It reported the oral lessons of Girolamo Mercuriali (1530–1606) and was recently translated into English [12] and French [13]. For the purpose of this chapter, we have selected Mercuriali's book as a good example of the ancient conceptions of skin diseases. Following Galen, Mercuriali classified skin disorders into two groups: the ones involving the head (hair and scalp, and less importantly the face), and the ones involving the remainder of the body. The ninth chapter of the cephalic dermatoses is called 'achores and favus'. Achores, a term close to tinea or to head ulcerations, designates oozing cephalic dermatoses, which are particularly frequent in children. This is attributed to the need to eliminate humors accumulated during intrauterine life. Mercuriali here describes an itchy cephalic dermatosis in infants, where one can recognize atopic dermatitis.

Similar precise descriptions of pruriginous dermatoses in infants, starting or predominating on the head, can be found in all the books of authors of this 'pre-Willanist' era, including Turner, Astruc and Alibert.

In *A Treatise of Diseases Incident to the Skin*, written in English and published in 1714, Daniel Turner (approx. 1667–1741) mentions crusts and scabies (pruritus) in infants. He indicates that it is one of the most prevalent of infantile diseases, that these lesions are a way of evacuating sick humors, and that it is wiser not to treat them in order to avoid more severe, even lethal, diseases. One can, however, try and modify the wet nurse's diet, or ask for another wet nurse.

In his *Traité des tumeurs et des ulcères* (1759), Jean Astruc (1684–1766) describes in detail infantile milky crusts, secondary to the milk and its influence on the sebaceous glands. He differentiates stick crusts with little pruritus, probably infantile seborrheic dermatitis, from wet crusts with violent pruritus, probably atopic dermatitis.

Jean-Louis Alibert (1768–1837), the founder of French dermatology, described tinea mucosa (teigne muqueuse) as an oozing and violent disease not to be mistaken for the trivial milky crusts. In his *Description des maladies de la peau observées à l'hôpital Saint-Louis et exposition des meilleures méthodes suivies pour leur traitement*, published in 1806, he gave detailed reports of 4 infants with tinea mucosa. One of these patients (Joseph Buisseret, aged 20 months) became ill after his wet nurse's husband was taken to jail. In spite of these precise and lively clinical descriptions, it is difficult to find forerunners of atopic dermatitis in Alibert's classifications of diseases. In his 1829 classification, very famous for its illustration of the 'tree of the dermatoses', the mucous tinea became the mucous achore, which belongs to the branch of tinea, the third group of dermatoses. The fourth group, the 'dartres', includes herpes (in the old sense), and one of these herpes, 'herpes squamosus madidans', is considered to be an eczema. Alibert indicated that this kind of 'dartre' alternates with dyspnea and asthma, which is a clue for diagnosing atopic dermatitis. However, the corresponding illustration was not convincing. Prurigos, which belong to another group, may also have included cases of atopic dermatitis. Therefore, we can say that Alibert observed genuine cases of atopic dermatitis, described them and mentioned their relation with asthma, but his nosological conceptions and personal vocabulary innovations prevented him from a logical classification.

To summarize, dermatologists prior to the scientific era had precisely described cases which fit well into the modern criteria for atopic dermatitis that we will detail below: a frequent, cephalic oozing (ulcerated) skin condition of infants, with violent pruritus.

Atopic Dermatitis in Willanist Dermatology

Robert Willan (1757–1812) and his talented pupil Thomas Bateman (1778–1821) created clinical dermatology by giving precise descriptions of elementary lesions, a concept created in 1776 by Jacob Plenck (1735–1807), and classifying skin diseases according to these elementary lesions. In this truly revolutionary approach, skin diseases were defined by their primary lesion. For example, psoriasis is scaly and pemphigus is bullous. But what is atopic dermatitis?

In Willan and Bateman's [14] classification, eczema is precisely described in the order of vesicles. Thomas Bateman is credited with the first definition of eczemas:

> The eczema is characterized by an eruption of small vesicules, on various parts of the skin, usually set close or crowded together, with little or no inflammation round their bases, and unattended by fever. It is not contagious. This eruption is generally the effect of irritation, whether internally or externally applied, and is occasionally produced by a great variety of irritants, in persons whose skin is constitutionally very irritable.

Considering the fact that almost 200 years later there is still controversy concerning the definition of eczema, it is interesting to point out that Bateman clearly indicated that eczemas may have external and internal causes, and occur in predisposed individuals. However, the eczemas described by Bateman are eczema solare (sunburn), eczema impetiginodes (close to impetigo) and eczema rubrum (probably mercurial dermatitis and other drug reactions). All are of external origin and none of Bateman's eczemas resemble atopic dermatitis. In the writings of Willan and Bateman, there is nothing like a chronic, infantile eczema. The reason they did not describe atopic dermatitis can be found in their epistemological way of thinking. For them, one disease must have one elementary lesion, and atopic dermatitis has many lesions: vesicles, papules, scales, pustules and erythema. Therefore, it cannot be found under only one heading in Willan's and Bateman's works.

A careful reading of Willan's and Bateman's writings, innovatively illustrated by engravings [15], shows that diseases compatible with the modern diagnosis of atopic dermatitis can be found in four different chapters: 'Strophulus', 'Lichens' and 'Prurigos' contain three varieties of the papules (order I), and 'Porrigo' contains one of the pustular dermatoses (order V). Porrigo larvalis (fig. 1) is considered by many as one of the best forerunners of atopic dermatitis. The Latin word porrigo is very close to the ancient vague terms 'tinea', 'favus' and 'achores', and designates an oozing and crusty scalp eruption. Larvalis means 'similar to the mask of a ghost', or 'frightening'. Porrigo larvalis is similar to the milky crusts (or milky tinea) of many ancient authors.

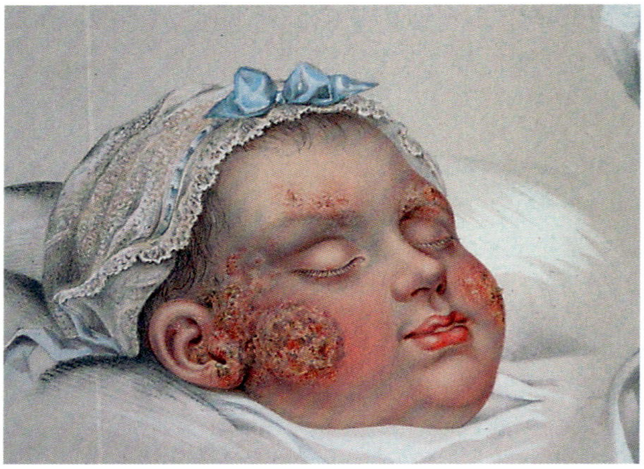

Fig. 1. Porrigo larvalis Willan has been identified as one of the earliest faithful descriptions and representations of atopic dermatitis [16]. Instead of the well-known initial picture, we chose to show this plate to pay tribute to the most beautiful dermatological atlas ever published. The illustrators, Anton Elfinger (1821–1864) and Carl Heitzmann (1836–1896), were gifted painters and physicians. Hebra describes chronic eczemas according to their localization. In scalp eczema, he alludes to the old porrigos and achores, for which he proposes the synonyms eczema impetiginosum and porrigo larvalis Willan. As seen here, the term 'head and scalp' clearly includes the face.

Ancient terminology is a difficult problem, and the majority of the terms used before Willan to describe dermatoses are impossible to understand or to translate into modern dermatological descriptions. Fortunately, starting with Willan, dermatological books included atlases with drawings, engravings and paintings of the diseases described in words. Even though modern dermatologists may be unable to understand ancient words, they are able to look at ancient images and to make diagnoses. The position of a modern dermatologist looking at an ancient picture is very similar to his or her position as a teleder-

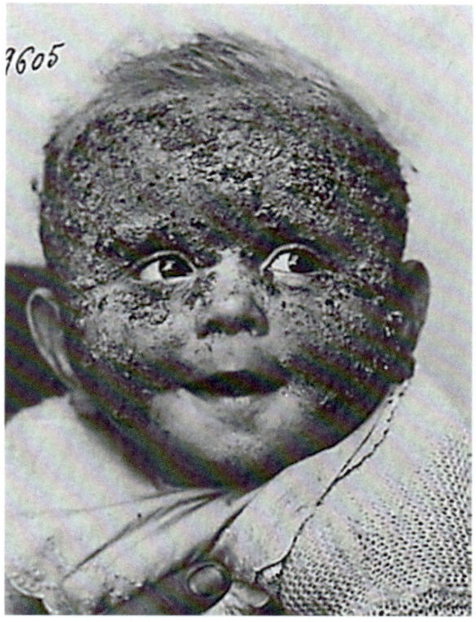

Fig. 2. Infantile eczema is a rather stereotyped condition. In the majority of cases, the general health and the moral and intellectual qualities are unaffected, as illustrated by this photograph of Maurice, a 10-month-old patient of Prof. Degos.

matologist, or as an expert indicating, with his or her own undetailed criteria, whether a given patient has atopic dermatitis or not. Accordingly, we recently asked 31 experts in pediatric dermatology to examine selected ancient pictures in order to identify the first images of atopic dermatitis in the dermatological literature. Consensus could be reached to indicate that the first three iconographic representations of atopic dermatitis are strophulus confertus (Willan, 1796), lichen agrius (Willan, 1796) and porrigo larvalis (included in Willan's works, but formally described by Bateman in 1816) [16]. Hidden among papular and pustular diseases, absent from eczema descriptions, atopic dermatitis was present, but was not identified as a single skin disease by dermatology pioneers.

The method used by Willan and Bateman for diagnosing skin diseases and for classifying them was soon adopted by the majority of dermatologists [17]. Rayer (1793–1867), in the first edition of his influential *Treatise* [18], proposed to distinguish acute and chronic eczemas. Chronic eczemas are clearly different from the three categories of Bateman's eczemas, but Rayer does not insist on any infantile form. In the second edition of *Treatise* [19], however, Rayer gives a detailed description of scalp eczema, a synonym for mucous tinea Alibert and porrigo larvalis Willan. The onset of this chronic eczema is between 3 and 8 months of age and it is violently pruriginous.

One of the best descriptions of infantile eczema must be credited to Erasmus Wilson (1809–1884), delivered at the 1856 Meeting of the British Medical Association. His lecture and the subsequent publication in the *British Medical Journal* were so successful that he wrote the same description again many times, including in his 1870 lectures on eczema [20]. He asserted that infantile eczema (synonyms: crusta lactea, tinea lactea, porrigo larvalis, tinea mucosa, tinea granulata) commences at 4–6 weeks of age and its cause resides in the mother's milk. To support this assumption, Wilson reported the case of a mother who, distressed by the death of her husband, transmitted eczema to her child. In this case, which is similar to the one described by Alibert and cited above, one can see that at this time not only nutriments, bacteria and allergens, but also emotions, were considered to be transmitted by the milk.

Wilson indicated that many different types of lesions can be seen in infantile eczema, which was not limited to a vesicular disease. These included 'erythema, lichen, strophulus, eczema, impetigo, pityriasis, psoriasis', all of them 'on the same skin and in gross defiance of the order, genera and species of the Plenckio-Willanean method of classification' [20]. Figure 2 shows the well-known typical aspect of infantile eczema.

Atopic Dermatitis as a Diathetic Prurigo

According to Willan and Bateman's classification, prurigos are one of the three varieties of papules, but no prurigo is predominantly a pediatric disease. The infantile papules are included in the strophulus. The nosological status of prurigos changed when Ferdinand von Hebra (1816–1880), head of Viennese dermatology and considered to be the leader of European (world) dermatology during the second half of the 19th century, described prurigo not only as a lesion, but also as a disease [21]. Hebra's prurigo ('prurigo mihi') is essentially a papular disease. These papules are severely pruriginous. Hebra's prurigo is a lifelong disease, which follows the patient 'to his

2

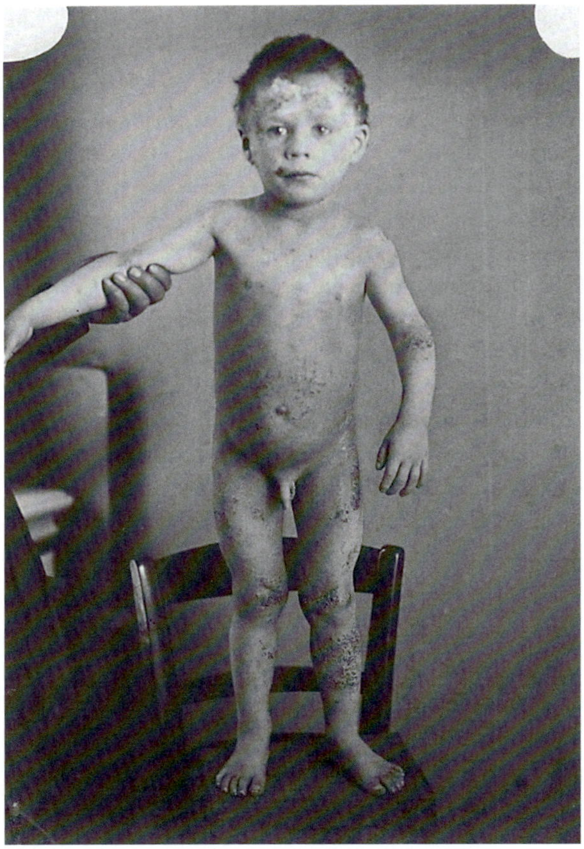

Fig. 3. Hebra's prurigo in a 4-year-old (French variety). French dermatologists were never comfortable with the diagnosis of Hebra's prurigo and thought that this typical and precisely described form was very rare. They invented the term 'French variety' for these atypical cases, probably identical to Besnier's prurigo. The photograph was taken on March 12, 1902, Hôpital Broca, Dr. Brocq's department.

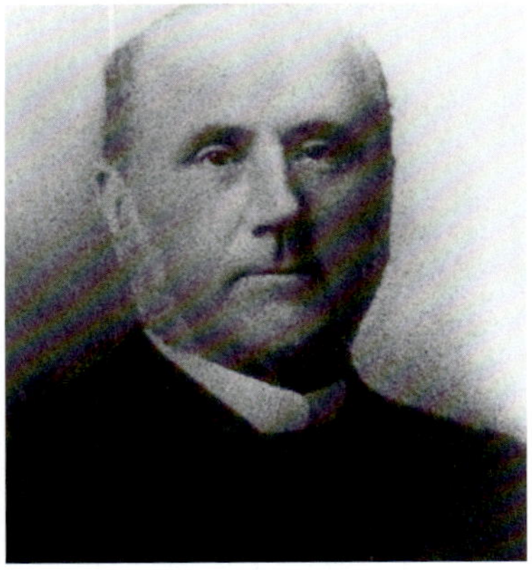

Fig. 4. Ernest Besnier (1831–1909) was the leader of French dermatology between 1890 and 1900. He was the first editor of *La pratique dermatologique*, the first French multi-author textbook, published in 1900. Diathetic prurigo, described by Besnier in 1892, is identical to atopic dermatitis.

grave' and there is no mention of infantile forms or of a pediatric predominance. The distribution of lesions is characteristic and Hebra insisted on the involvement of the extensor parts of the limbs. The folds, including the elbows, are 'almost always unaffected'. Hebra's prurigo has always been considered as a severe, rare disease, and French and British dermatologists, although acknowledging the talent and authority of the Viennese master, often indicated that they saw very few genuine cases [22] (fig. 3).

Another disease named prurigo was described in 1892 by Besnier (1831–1909; fig. 4), under the name diathetic prurigo [23]; more precisely, 'paroxystic and chronic polymorphous and pruriginous dermatoses, Hebra's prurigo type'. In this communication to the French Society of Dermatology, Besnier, helped by his resident Sabouraud, described a disease in three young men which began in early infancy and was mainly a pruritus. Pruritus came first and lesions followed. Besnier's prurigo was, so to say, a 'pruritic diathesis, a diathetic prurigo'. This denomination is very significant because Besnier, like the majority of dermatologists of his time (in opposition to Hardy and Bazin) did not think that diatheses really exist. At an early age, the lesions which follow pruritus in Besnier's prurigo are non-specific. It may be 'infantile erythema, urticaria, pseudo-lichen, or one of the eczematisations or lichenisations…'. Besnier did not relate his prurigo to infantile eczema, but he related it to asthma and hay fever, and differentiated it from the narrow description of Hebra's prurigo.

The French dermatologists of these times, including Besnier, Brocq and Vidal, wrote many pages about eczemas, prurigos, lichens and pruriginous dermatoses. However, since a picture is worth a thousand words, it is appropriate to examine figure 5, which represents the nebula of cutaneous reactions according to Louis Brocq (1856–1928), one of the smartest of the dermatology clinicians. Accord-

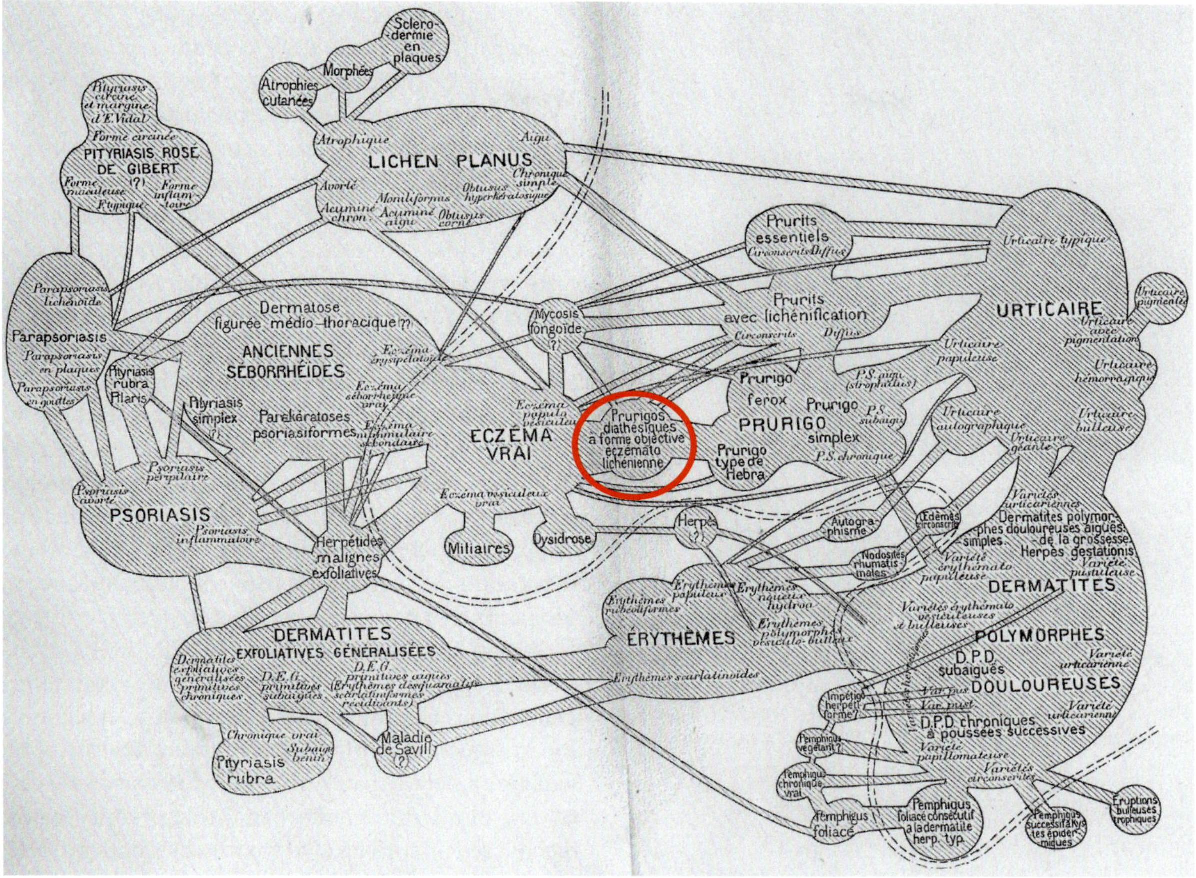

Fig. 5. The turning point in the history of atopic dermatitis was the discovery that infantile eczema and some prurigos are in fact the same disease. This discovery was anticipated by some clinicians at the end of the 19th century and is well illustrated in this graphic representation of Brocq's conception of cutaneous reactions. The pruritic reactions are situated to the right of the double dotted line. Brocq's main idea was that clinical entities are linked with one another by 'faits de passage' (transitions) which are represented by 'corridors'. The width of the corridors represents the frequency of these transitions and their length represents the closeness between the entities. We have added a circle to point out the nosological position of Besnier's prurigo, the forerunner of atopic dermatitis. It is rightly positioned between eczemas and prurigos, especially the severe prurigo Hebra, synonym of prurigo ferox. Short, wide corridors indicate the closeness of these entities. By contrast, the corridor between Besnier's prurigo and mycosis fungoides is both long and narrow, indicating that these entities are rather distant, although some relationship may exist.

ing to Brocq, skin diseases are not separated, but linked by many 'faits de passage' (transitions), represented by the corridors between the circles. As clearly indicated on the figure, diathetic prurigo (Besnier's prurigo) is situated between eczemas (true eczemas) and prurigos, rather close to Hebra's prurigo, the most severe form of prurigos. Indeed, it was necessary to link infantile eczema and chronic prurigo to conceive such a disease as atopic dermatitis. A few years earlier, J. Hutchinson had suggested such a link when indicating that severe cases of infantile eczema, persisting into adulthood, are similar to Hebra's prurigo [24].

Birth of Atopic Dermatitis

Before the years of *Index Medicus* and Medline, *The Year Book of Dermatology* was a publication most awaited for. Once a year, experts analyzed the

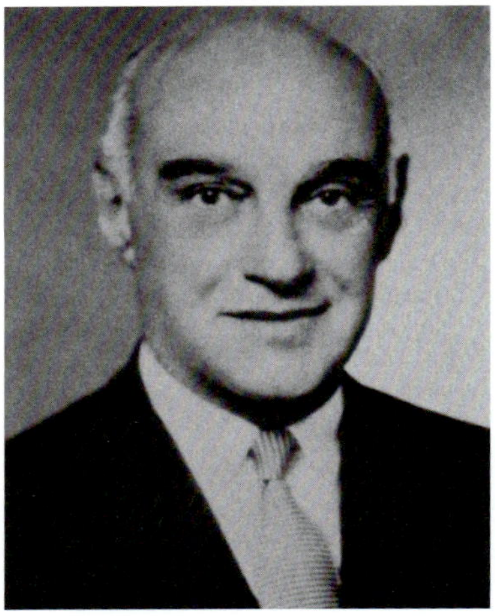

Fig. 6. Marion Baldur Sulzberger (1895–1983) was born in New York and studied in Geneva and in Zurich with Bruno Bloch, a pioneer in cutaneous allergy. Back in the USA, he was associated with Fred Wise, his mentor and friend. Sulzberger was professor of dermatology in New York from 1949 to 1961, and in San Francisco from 1964 to 1970. He was one of the most brilliant and influential of American dermatologists. His contribution to the history of atopic dermatitis is unique – he denominated and described the disease, and indicated the main criteria and the clinical course. Twenty years later, he discovered the efficacy of topical corticosteroids.

international literature. In the 1933 edition, Fred Wise and Marion Sulzberger (fig. 6) tried to simplify the problem of eczemas [7]. They commented on Rost's early and late 'exudative eczematoids' and their link to allergy, and on Ormsby's discussion of neurodermatitis (Brocq) and lichenification, similar to Vidal's lichen simplex chronicus. In an illuminating footnote, Wise and Sulzberger indicated that from this confused and confusing group of diseases, 'at least one is now emerging as a fairly distinct and clear-cut entity. This is probably best called atopic dermatitis.' As soon as they denominated atopic dermatitis, Wise and Sulzberger indicated the nine qualities, or criteria, of this condition:

(1) atopic family history;
(2) antecedent infantile eczema;
(3) localizations: creases of elbows and knees, neck, chest, face and mainly eyelids;
(4) a grayish/brownish coloration of the skin;
(5) the absence of true vesicles, both clinically and histologically;
(6) vasomotor instability or irritability;
(7) negativity of patch tests to contact irritants;
(8) many positive reactions of immediate wheal type to scratch or intradermal testing;
(9) presence of many reagins in the blood serum.

Immediate allergy, or atopic hypersensitivity, was therefore the main argument for isolating atopic dermatitis from other chronic eczemas, and skin tests were considered as a valuable scientific diagnostic test for this condition. An earlier attempt to link skin manifestations to constitutional disturbances, including food reactions and respiratory disorders, had been proposed by Czerny with the concept of 'exsudative diathesis' (1905), but it lacked the biological support that skin and blood tests brought to establish the allergic nature of atopic dermatitis [25]. Consequently, the logical treatment of atopic dermatitis was the elimination of all foods and all inhalants that gave positive reactions.

Atopy had been defined in 1923 as a type of inherited hypersensitivity to environmental allergens, different from anaphylaxis and hypersensitivity to infection [26]. Other chapters in this book will give a detailed account of the history of the discovery of allergic phenomena. Richet and Portier discovered anaphylaxis to toxic substances in 1902, von Pirquet described allergy to infectious antigens in 1906. In 1909, Smith described positive tests in a patient allergic to buckwheat, and in 1912 Schloss described hypersensitivity to egg in a child with urticaria. In 1916, Blackfan [27] published the first article on skin tests in children with eczema. Considering the fact that many patients with asthma had infantile eczema, he thought it would be 'of interest to determine the frequency of proteins reactions in eczema, to see if a relation existed between the disease and protein sensitization…'. Indeed, in a group of 27 patients with eczema, including 18 infants, he found a majority of positive tests: 21 to egg white, 17 to cow's milk, 10 to human milk, 7 to horse serum and 6 to meat extract. In a control group, no test was positive.

In older children and adults, the removal of the food that gave positive tests improved some patients. However, this was not the case in infants exposed to the dangers of unnecessary avoidance diets. So, the discrepancy between the positivity of skin tests and the consequences of food intake or food exclusion was noted as soon as tests were performed. This remark is of paramount importance.

In 1921, Prausnitz and Küstner demonstrated that allergy can be transferred by serum and so, when Wise and Sulzberger described atopic dermatitis in 1933, they could consider skin and blood tests as reliable criteria for this new condition, the main criteria to differentiate atopic dermatitis from other eczematoid dermatoses.

Soon afterwards, Hill and Sulzberger [28] gave a precise description of the evolution of atopic dermatitis, indicating clearly that the hypersensitivity to proteins was the link unifying different clinical aspects: eczema in infants, neurodermatitis in children, and the numerous denominations of what is now called atopic dermatitis in adults (prurigos, among others).

The denomination of atopic dermatitis was rapidly adopted by American and British dermatologists. In France, it was long considered to be an Anglicism, and Degos, leader of French dermatology until the 1970s, always spoke of constitutional eczema. In Germany, the term 'neurodermitis' was long favored. When Nexmand [29], in 1948, wrote a thesis on this disease in Copenhagen, he preferred to call it Besnier's prurigo, explaining that it was not an eczema, not always atopic (although he favored an allergic pathogenesis) and always pruriginous.

Criteria and Scores in the Contemporary Era

Neither the skin or blood tests which helped the individualization of atopic dermatitis nor the discovery of an increase of circulating IgE in the 1960s [30] proved to be pathognomonic, or even very helpful for the diagnosis of atopic dermatitis. Although the majority of physicians had no major problem in diagnosing atopic dermatitis, precise clinical criteria were felt necessary for epidemiological and clinical research, as well as for communication between dermatologists, immunologists, allergists and pediatricians from different countries, who were still using different denominations. Jon Hanifin (USA) and Georg Rajka (Norway), who had worked independently on this topic, organized an international symposium in Oslo in June, 1979. In a short article, one of the most frequently cited of the dermatological literature, they proposed clinical criteria for atopic dermatitis [31]. Although Hanifin and Rajka's criteria are based on personal experience and informal discussions, and have never been formally validated, they have been widely accepted and used in the majority of the works published in the last 30 years.

According to Hanifin and Rajka, a diagnosis of atopic dermatitis is certain if a patient has 3 or more of 4 major features, and 3 or more of 21 minor features.

The major criteria are (abridged text):

- pruritus
- typical eczema, according to age (flexural in adults...)
- chronicity
- personal or family history of atopy

The minor criteria are:

- xerosis
- ichthyosis/keratosis pilaris
- immediate skin reactivity
- elevated serum IgE
- early age of onset
- tendency toward cutaneous infections (*Staphylococcus aureus* and Herpes simplex)
- non-specific hand and foot dermatitis
- nipple eczema
- cheilitis
- conjunctivitis
- Dennie-Morgan fold
- keratoconus
- cataracts
- orbital darkening
- facial pallor/facial erythema
- pityriasis alba
- anterior neck folds
- itch when sweating
- intolerance to wool and lipid solvents
- perifollicular accentuation
- food intolerance
- influence of environmental/emotional factors
- white dermographism

Hanifin and Rajka's criteria were found to be relevant for clinical research, but they required derma-

2

tological skills. They were considered later to be too complicated to be used in a primary care setting, and in 1994 a British Working Group headed by Hywel Williams elaborated the criteria using an epidemiological methodology. Thirty-two physicians examining 224 patients established and validated diagnostic criteria for atopic dermatitis based on the presence and frequency of 13 symptoms and 18 signs. The main conclusion of this impressive work [32] was that the diagnosis of atopic dermatitis requires pruritus, or 'an itchy skin condition'; no atopic dermatitis can exist without pruritus. In addition to this compulsory criterion, the patient must have 3 or more of the following criteria: (1) history of flexural involvement, (2) visible flexural dermatitis, (3) history of a generalized dry skin, (4) history of asthma or hay fever and (5) onset of rash before the age of 2 years.

There is a historical sense in comparing these three sets of criteria for atopic dermatitis. Wise and Sulzberger's 1933 criteria can be considered allergists' criteria, in which one third of the criteria relate to skin or blood tests. Hanifin and Rajka's 1979 criteria are those of dermatologists – none of the major criteria and only 2 of the 21 minor criteria are related to immunological data. Williams' 1994 criteria are those of epidemiologists – immunological skin and blood tests have disappeared and the diagnosis requires no dermatological skills; all the criteria can be obtained by interview or questionnaire, except one (visible flexural dermatitis), which can be established by a non-physician health professional or a caring mother.

Atopic dermatitis is a polymorphous disease and, in addition to ascertaining the diagnosis, it is helpful for clinical research as well as everyday practice to gather some information on the severity of the disease. In 1990, Alain Taïeb and Jean-François Stalder co-ordinated 29 specialists from 9 European countries in a European Task Force on Atopic Dermatitis [33]. Through expert discussions on clinical photographs, consensus meetings and statistician expertise, this group was able to set up a score called SCORAD (scoring atopic dermatitis) following a suggestion by A. Oranje. The SCORAD index takes into account the intensity of the lesions and the extent of the disease, as well as pruritus and sleep disturbance. The SCORAD index has been widely accepted and used, although other indexes are also used (e.g. EASI), resulting in somewhat disturbing confusion [34].

Will Semantic Discussions End?

The progressive abandonment of immunological criteria in the diagnosis of atopic dermatitis paralleled the observation that many patients did not have atopic biologic criteria, i.e. positive immediate skin tests and elevated circulating IgE. Many authors questioned the adequacy of the terms 'atopic' and 'dermatitis'. They proposed separating atopic dermatitis into an extrinsic and an intrinsic form, the latter lacking atopic stigmata. Others, skeptical of an atopic disease without atopy, preferred to speak of an atopiform dermatitis. The Task Force for Nomenclature of the European Academy of Allergology and Clinical Immunology proposed in 2001 to replace atopic dermatitis with 'atopic eczema/dermatitis syndrome' (AEDS), which could be allergic or non-allergic. Allergic AEDS is further divided into IgE-associated and non-IgE-associated forms [35]. The World Allergy Organization made a somewhat different proposal 3 years later, in which eczema is considered to be one of the dermatitis, and divided into atopic eczema and non-atopic eczema [36]. No doubt the discussions will continue, and no doubt there is also a clear advantage, at least from the bibliographic point of view, to consider that atopic dermatitis is a pragmatically useful, if not very precise, denomination.

Pathogenic Theories and Their Therapeutic Consequences

Atopic dermatitis is a complicated disease. In the chapter on atopic dermatitis of the first edition of *Dermatology in General Medicine*, issued in 1971, Sulzberger [37] represents a multifactorial chain of causation which does not prioritize any of the 10 factors cited (fig. 7). However, the majority of authors tend to favor an etiological hypothesis and to recommend therapy according to their preferred hypothesis.

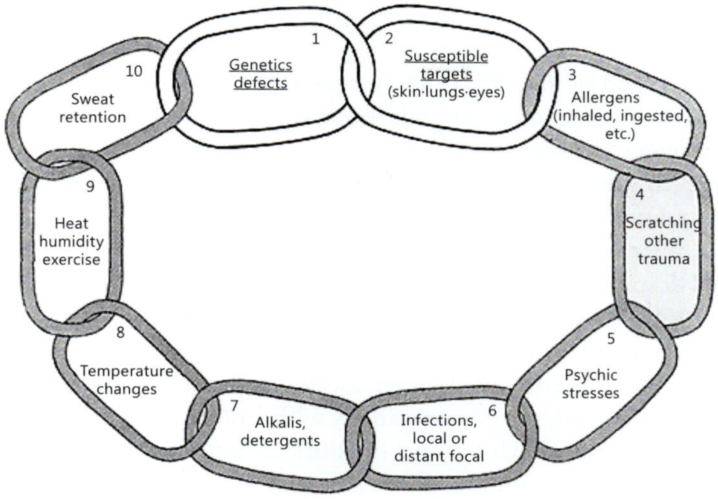

Fig. 7. In the first edition of Fitzpatrick's famous textbook, *Dermatology in General Medicine*, published in 1971, Marion B. Sulzberger [37] represents the etiology of atopic dermatitis as a chain of 10 elements, without hierarchy between them.

Humoralistic Theories and Reluctance to Treat

The Hippocratic conception of a beneficial oozing, allowing the elimination of vitiated humors, was the main cause of contemplative medicine or a refusal to try and heal eczematous eruptions [38]. This was the attitude of the majority of French dermatologists until the middle of the 20th century, in contrast with the position of Viennese dermatologists who favored a local cause and a local therapy. Not only did French dermatologists advise to respect the eruptions, but they also invented ways to increase them. The so-called serous bloodletting was used for this purpose from 1870 until at least 1924 [39]. We hypothesize that modern controversies about the use of water [40], topical corticosteroids [41] and topical immunomodulators [42] are due in part to the persistence of such a Hippocratic thinking in the lay public and some alternative practitioners, as well as in some mainstream physicians.

Digestive Theories and Diet

Atopic dermatitis begins a few weeks after birth and in the majority of patients stops before the age of 2 years. This special timing, which seems incompatible with a genetic disease or an infectious disease, suggested to many physicians that it could be due to milk, the only food taken at this age. This belief led to much contradictory therapeutic advice. The psychological stress and the physical health of the wet nurse was implicated. Human and animal milk were compared and their supposed influence on the health of children was questioned. Marfan, a leading French pediatrician, taught that infantile eczema is linked to digestive disturbances [43]. The nervous component of eczema was also attributed to dyspepsia. When biochemistry developed, the content of the milk in fat, sugar and proteins was studied, and many attempts were made to modify the milk. The pediatric and the dermatologic literature contain hundreds of dietetic advices, none of which have ever proved useful.

The positivity of skin tests to food (milk and mainly egg) in children with atopic dermatitis but no digestive symptom has never been clearly understood. Some authors considered they had no causal relationship, others advised the suppression from the diet of foods which were tested positive. However, the advantage of food avoidance has never been clearly established [44, 45], and some cases of severe malnutrition resulted from unwise food evictions [46].

Parasitic/Bacteriological Dimension of Eczema

At the end of the 19th century, medicine could rely not only on clinical grounds, but also on modern biologic discoveries. The discovery of microscopic parasites, including bacteria, by Pasteur and other researchers led to the belief that all diseases had a microbial cause. Paul Gerson Unna (1850–1929) described seborrheic eczema and was a talented advocate of the microbial (parasitic) cause of all eczemas [47]. This theory was much discussed at the 1900 Paris International Congress, and the complexity of eczemas, the non-specificity of the morococcus described by Unna, and the difficult interpretations of inoculation experiments led the majority of dermatologists to reject the microbial theory of eczemas.

The skin of patients with atopic dermatitis is almost constantly colonized by *S. aureus* [48], but the meaning of this colonization is not fully understood. Staphylococci are rarely the cause of clinical superinfection. They are believed to trigger eczema flare-ups, possibly by a superantigenic mechanism [49]. The interest of anti-infectious treatments for the management of atopic dermatitis, however, remains controversial [50].

The severe varicelliform eruption identified by Kaposi and Juliusberg in the 19th century is a specific consequence of vaccinia or herpes inoculation on the skin of atopic individuals [51]. It is currently believed that the reason for atopic individuals' cutaneous susceptibility to staphylococcal and herpetic infections lies in a defect of innate immunity, one of the constituents of the barrier function of the epidermis [52].

The relationship between micro-organisms and atopy is even more complex. The hygiene hypothesis proposed by Strachan [53] in 1989 postulates that a lack of contacts with bacteria in early childhood could favor an orientation of the immune system towards Th2-related responses, including allergy and auto-immunity. This hypothesis could theoretically explain the apparent recent increase in prevalence of atopic diseases in westernized countries. One of the aspects of the complex interaction between micro-organisms and allergy is the influence of the gut microflora on the development of digestive and systemic immunity, and the tendency to Th2-oriented, allergic-type responses. A much-publicized clinical trial indicated that probiotics could prevent allergy in newborns at risk [54]. Such favorable results, however, could not be reproduced and this topic remains controversial.

Allergological Theories, Hyposensitization and Allergen Eviction

In non-atopic allergic diseases, for example in allergic contact dermatitis, the introduction of the allergen induces the lesions. Its responsibility can be further proved by skin tests which reproduce the lesions, and its eviction eradicates the symptoms.

In atopic dermatitis, there are many positive skin tests and elevated circulating IgE against many substances. However, the significance of these allergological data is not clear. They do not point to an external causation (allergens), but rather to an internal condition (atopy, also called the atopic diathesis). The true nature of the interaction between internal (genetic) and external (environmental) factors has never been understood in atopic dermatitis, leaving all physicians and patients experimenting with their own belief of these mysterious relationships.

The discovery of elevated IgE blood levels in atopic dermatitis [30] stimulated the hope that this could represent a faithful biologic diagnostic test. IgE is indeed important in the pathophysiology of atopy, and its presence on Langerhans cells of atopic individuals is also an important discovery [55], but these are non-specific findings which cannot be used as diagnostic tests.

Elevated IgE against dietary allergens, skin tests, scratch tests, prick tests, intradermal tests and the more recent atopy epidermal patch tests were never considered a convincing proof of the allergens' responsibility. Double-blind placebo-controlled oral food challenges have been advocated as the gold standard for food allergy in conditions such as atopic dermatitis [56], yet are seldom performed. Children with atopic dermatitis and digestive symptoms could possibly benefit from a digestive investigation. However, for the majority of children with atopic dermatitis there is usually no digestive clinical disease and investigation of sensitization to food is left to severe cases. Hyposensitizations are similarly useless, with the occasional exception of food allergy symptoms, and are rarely employed for eczema itself.

Fear of Treatment Side Effects

At the beginning of the 20th century, infantile eczema was known among pediatric diseases for a lethal threat through the rapid death of eczematous children when they were hospitalized. Eczema has been long considered a contra-indication to hospital admission because of the frequency of a syndrome consisting of apparent improvement of the skin condition coupled with pallor, high fever and death. Some authors thought that the cause of death was the rapidity with which eczema had improved, and many theories were discussed. The infectious nature of this syndrome was claimed by Hutinel and Rivet [57] and became evident after the use of antibiotics in the 1950s.

Since the report by Sulzberger and Witten [58] in 1952, it has become well established that topical corticosteroids are highly efficient in the treatment of atopic dermatitis. In acute, early eczema, daily applications stop the oozing and bring an almost complete resolution in a few days. Maintenance treatment (currently called proactive therapy) prevents relapses in the majority of cases. Safety is excellent with careful use of topical corticosteroids. In spite of this truly revolutionary progress, many children are not adequately treated and this is probably the cause of many chronic evolutions and complications. The reason for this underutilization of an efficient treatment has been identified as a corticophobia, or topical corticophobia. It is mainly due to an overestimation of the side effects of corticosteroids and confusion between the safety of oral and topical corticosteroids. Corticophobia [41] is a widespread problem that should be solved by a more careful attention to patients' beliefs and wishes in order to increase their confidence in physicians and scientific medicine. Atopy schools and workshops for therapeutic education are the modern answer to this sequel of the humoralistic way of thinking [59].

Topical immunomodulators were recently developed as a new class of anti-inflammatory topical drugs [60]. They were widely accepted, partly due to the reluctance to use topical corticosteroids in the long term, particularly in children and on the face or areas of thin skin, such as the eyelids. In February 2005, the Food and Drug Administration recommended 'black box' warnings for these drugs because of concern of potential increased risk of skin cancer and lymphoma. This issue is still controversial [61]. This warning and the following controversy can be viewed by clinicians and patients as an additional argument for fearing efficient treatments.

Neuropsychological Considerations

Psychological factors have long been recognized as important triggers of atopic dermatitis flares. The wet nurses' or nursing mothers' stresses were considered to be the cause of milk modifications, inducing eruptions. The link between psychologic or psychiatric events, however, is difficult to rationalize and little attention has been paid to a psychiatric approach in the dermatological literature.

Brocq, who created the term 'neurodermitis/névrodermite', and his contemporary dermatologists discussed the importance of the nervous system in pruritus, prurigos and lichenifications. Some even advocated the removal of cerebrospinal fluid by spinal tap for the treatment of prurigos [62], although this produced irregular results. Psychology-based treatments are less aggressive, if not easier to evaluate.

The attention to the psychological and sociological consequences of chronic diseases has recently led to the concept of quality of life scores. Atopic dermatitis is a condition which severely impairs quality of life. Some quality of life scales are valid for all diseases, some are specific for skin diseases in general, some are specific for atopic dermatitis [63], and some also evaluate the consequences of atopic dermatitis on the quality of life of family members. The neurological pathogenesis of pruritus is another component of the link between atopic dermatitis and the central nervous system [64].

Other Hypotheses

Szentivanyi [65] proposed that a relative blockade in β-adrenergic responses could explain immediate respiratory and cutaneous allergy. Abnormalities in the functions of many immunological cells, such as T cell subpopulations, B cells, antigen-presenting cells, eosinophils and basophils, have been described in atopic dermatitis. One unifying explanation has been proposed: the increase in phosphodiesterase activity [66].

Dermatological Approach and Topical Therapy

It is clear from the above considerations that until recently the skin itself played a small role, if any, in the attempts to understand the pathophysiology of atopic dermatitis. Humoralist physicians believing in the importance of humors, pediatricians believing in the importance of diet and immunologists believing in the importance of circulating IgE had little consideration for the skin itself, not to speak of the stratum corneum, the outer layer of the epidermis, commonly considered as being made of 'dead' cells. Things began to change in the 1990s with hypotheses speculating on the importance of the epidermal barrier in epicutaneous allergenic sensitization and possibly other aspects of atopic dermatitis [67, 68]. Dryness of the skin is one of the most important minor criteria of atopic dermatitis. Epidermal abnormalities had been described which could explain this dryness, such as a decreased level of ceramides [69] or an abnormality in the metabolism of essential fatty acids [70]. These biochemical discoveries led to numerous trials of topical or oral interventions on the metabolism of epidermal lipids, with conflicting results.

We have not reported the numerous genetic studies which have led to the identification of many loci and candidate genes linked and associated with atopic dermatitis. Some of them code for molecules of acquired immunity, including interleukins 4 and 5, their receptors, and chains of IgE receptors. The most significant genetic discovery, however, was made in 2006 when an Irish-Scottish team headed by I. McLean discovered that mutations in the filaggrin gene are a major predisposing factor for atopic dermatitis [71]. It was later demonstrated that filaggrin mutations are correlated with the severity of atopic dermatitis and, more importantly, with respiratory atopy, including asthma [72]. A new paradigm thus emerged, which gives priority to the epidermis in the pathophysiology of cutaneous and respiratory atopy. Recent experimental work has shown that skin barrier defects such as filaggrin deficiency or proteases hyperactivity can induce the epidermal production of TSLP (thymic stromal lymphopoietin), a cytokine inducing an asthmatic phenotype [73]. This is a contemporary area of research which is not yet part of history. We wish to underline, however, that this epidermal pathogenesis of atopy already has therapeutic implications [74], including the important role of emollient therapy to maintain the epidermal homeostasis, prevent allergenic transepidermal penetration and the subsequent induction of inflammation.

Conclusion

Atopic dermatitis is a complex disease. Many of the theoretical and practical unsolved questions are enlightened by a consideration of the medical doctrines that have been prevalent in Western medicine since antiquity. The humoralist doctrine led to the belief that skin eruptions should not be treated. The allergological doctrine implies that hypersensitivity is the cause of the eczematous eruptions. A more dermatological approach leads to a pragmatic synthesis of epidermal defects, including the permeability barrier and innate immunity, atopic hypersensitivity, and the interaction between the nervous system and the skin.

References

1 Shaw TE, Currie GP, Koudelka CW, Simpson EL: Eczema prevalence in the United States: data from the 2003 National Survey of Children's Health. J Invest Dermatol 2011;131:67–73.

2 Mancini AJ, Kaulback K, Chamlin SL: The socioeconomic impact of atopic dermatitis in the United States: a systematic review. Pediatr Dermatol 2008;25:1–6.

3 Ring J, Przybilla B, Ruzicka TR (eds): Handbook of Atopic Eczema, ed 2. Berlin, Springer, 2006.

4 Bieber T, Leung DYM (eds): Atopic Dermatitis, ed 2. New York, Informa Healthcare, 2009.

5 Taïeb A, Wallach D, Tilles G: The history of atopic eczema/dermatitis; in Ring J, Przybilla B, Ruzicka TR (eds): Handbook of Atopic Eczema. New York, Springer, pp 10–20.

6 Ackerman AB, Ragaz A: A plea to expunge the word 'eczema' from the lexicon of dermatology and dermatopathology. Am J Dermatopathol 1982;4:315–326.

7 Halbert AR, Weston WL, Morelli JG: Atopic dermatitis: is it an allergic disease? J Am Acad Dermatol 1995;33:1008–1018.

8 Flohr C, Johansson SG, Wahlgren CF, Williams H: How atopic is atopic dermatitis? J Allergy Clin Immunol 2004;114:150–158.

9 Wallach D, Taïeb A, Tilles, G: Histoire de la dermatite atopique. Paris, Masson, 2004.

10 Wise F, Sulzberger MB: 1933 Year Book of Dermatology and Syphilology. Chicago, Year Book Medical, 1933, pp 38–39.

11 Mier PD: Earliest description of the atopic syndrome? Br J Dermatol 1975;92:359.

12 Sutton RL Jr: Sixteenth Century Physician and His Methods. Mercurialis on Diseases of the Skin. Kansas, Lowell, 1986.

13 Mercuriali G: Traité des maladies de la peau (transl Gombert P and Chevallier J). Lyon, Bioderma, 2008.

14 Bateman T: A Practical Synopsis of Cutaneous Diseases, ed 4. London, Longman, 1817, p 250.

15 Bateman T: Delineations of Cutaneous Diseases. London, Longman, 1817.

16 Wallach D, Coste J, Tilles G, Taïeb A: The first images of atopic dermatitis: an attempt at retrospective diagnosis in dermatology. J Am Acad Dermatol 2005;53:684–689.

17 Tilles G, Wallach D: Robert Willan and the French Willanists. Br J Dermatol 1999;140: 1122–1126.

18 Rayer P: Traité théorique et pratique des maladies de la peau. Paris, Baillière, 1826.

19 Rayer P: Traité théorique et pratique des maladies de la peau, ed 2. Paris, Baillière, 1835.

20 Wilson E: Lectures on Ekzema and Ekzematous Affections. London, Churchill, 1870.

21 Hebra F: On Diseases of the Skin. London, New Sydenham Society, 1868.

22 Civatte A: Formes cliniques et pathogénie des prurigos. IVe congrès des dermatologistes et syphiligraphes de langue française. Paris, Masson, 1929, pp 243–308.

23 Besnier E: Première note et observations préliminaires pour servir d'introduction à l'étude des prurigos diathésiques (dermatites multiformes prurigineuses chroniques exacerbantes et paroxystiques, du type du prurigo de Hebra). Ann Dermatol Syphil 1892;3:634–648.

24 Hutchinson J: On incurred infantile eczema and its occasional persistence through life: remarks on the relation of such cases to Hebra's prurigo. Arch Surg 1889–1890;1:365–367.

25 Faber HK, Roberts DB: Serum proteins and lipoids in the eczema of infants and children. J Pediatr 1933;3:78–83.

26 Coca AF, Cooke RA: On the classification of the phenomena of hypersensitiveness. J Immunol 1923;8:163–182.

27 Blackfan KD: Cutaneous reactions from proteins in eczema. Am J Dis Child 1916;11: 441–454.

28 Hill LW, Sulzberger MB: Evolution of atopic dermatitis. Arch Derm Syph 1935;32: 451–463.

29 Nexmand PH: Clinical Studies of Besnier's Prurigo. Copenhagen, Rosenkilde, 1948.

30 Juhlin L, Johansson GO, Bennich H, Högman C, Thyresson N: Immunoglobulin E in dermatoses: levels in atopic dermatitis and urticaria. Arch Dermatol 1969;100:12–16.

31 Hanifin JM, Rajka G: Diagnostic features of atopic dermatitis. Acta Derm Venereol (Stockh) 1980;92(suppl):44–47.

32 Williams HC, Burney PG, Pembroke AC, Hay RJ: The UK Working Party's Diagnostic Criteria for Atopic Dermatitis. 3. Independent hospital validation. Br J Dermatol 1994;131:406–416.

33 European Task Force on Atopic Dermatitis: Severity scoring of atopic dermatitis: the SCORAD index. Dermatology 1993;186: 23–31.

34 Schmitt J, Langan S, Williams HC, European Dermato-Epidemiology Network: What are the best outcome measurements for atopic eczema? A systematic review. J Allergy Clin Immunol 2007;120:1389–1398.

35 Johansson SG, Hourihane JO, Bousquet J, Bruijnzeel-Koomen C, Dreborg S, Haahtela T, Kowalski ML, Mygind N, Ring J, van Cauwenberge P, van Hage-Hamsten M, Wuthrich B, EAACI (the European Academy of Allergology and Cinical Immunology) Nomenclature Task Force: A revised nomenclature for allergy: an EAACI position statement from the EAACI nomenclature task force. Allergy 2001;56:813–824.

36 Johansson SG, Bieber T, Dahl R, Friedmann PS, Lanier BQ, Lockey RF, Motala C, Ortega Martell JA, Platts-Mills TA, Ring J, Thien F, van Cauwenberge P, Williams HC: Revised nomenclature for allergy for global use: report of the Nomenclature Review Committee of the World Allergy Organization, October 2003. J Allergy Clin Immunol 2004; 113:832–836.

37 Sulzberger MB: Atopic dermatitis; in Fitzpatrick TB, Arndt KA, Clark WH Jr, Eisen AZ, Van Scott EJ, Vaughan JH (eds): Dermatology in General Medicine. New York, McGraw Hill, 1971, pp 680–684, pp 687–697.

38 Tilles G, Wallach D, Taïeb A: Topical therapy of atopic dermatitis: controversies from Hippocrates to topical immunomodulators. J Am Acad Dermatol 2007;56:295–301.

39 Lortat-Jacob L: Traitement des eczémas suintants par l'enveloppement caoutchouté. Médecine 1924;6:118–123.

40 Scholtz JR: Management of atopic dermatitis. Calif Med 1965;102:210–216.

41 Charman CR, Morris AD, Williams HC: Topical corticosteroid phobia in patients with atopic eczema. Br J Dermatol 2000; 142:931–936.

42 Berger TG, Duvic M, van Voorhees AS, VanBeek MJ, Frieden IJ, American Academy of Dermatology Association Task Force: The use of topical calcineurin inhibitors in dermatology: safety concerns: report of the American Academy of Dermatology Association Task Force. J Am Acad Dermatol 2006;54:818–823.

43 Marfan A: Les eczémas des nourrissons: leurs rapports avec les vices de l'alimentation et les troubles digestifs. Semaine Méd 1894;14:138–140.

44 Bath-Hextall F, Delamere FM, Williams HC: Dietary exclusions for established atopic eczema. Cochrane Database Syst Rev 2008;1:CD005203.

45 Sinagra JL, Bordignon V, Ferraro C, Cristaudo A, Di Rocco M, Amorosi B, Capitanio B: Unnecessary milk elimination diets in children with atopic dermatitis. Pediatr Dermatol 2007;24:1–6.

46 Ladoyanni E, Cheung ST, North J, Tan CY: Pellagra occurring in a patient with atopic dermatitis and food allergy. J Eur Acad Dermatol Venereol 2007;21:394–396.

47 Unna PG: On the nature and treatment of eczema. Br J Dermatol 1890;2:231–245.

48 Leyden JJ, Marples RR, Kligman AM: *Staphylococcus aureus* in the lesions of atopic dermatitis. Br J Dermatol 1974;90: 525–530.

49 Taskapan MO, Kumar P: Role of staphylococcal superantigens in atopic dermatitis: from colonization to inflammation. Ann Allergy Asthma Immunol 2000;84:3–10.

50 Huang JT, Abrams M, Tlougan B, Rademaker A, Paller AS: Treatment of *Staphylococcus aureus* colonization in atopic dermatitis decreases disease severity. Pediatrics 2009;123:e808–e814.
51 Barton RL, Brunsting LA: Kaposi's varicelliform eruption. Arch Derm Syph 1944;50: 99–104.
52 Hata TR, Gallo RL: Innate immunity in atopic dermatitis; in Bieber T, Leung DYM (eds): Atopic Dermatitis, ed 2. New York, Informa Healthcare, 2009, pp 101–119.
53 Strachan DP: Hay fever, hygiene, and household size. BMJ 1989;299:1259–1260.
54 Kalliomäki M, Salminen S, Arvilommi H, Kero P, Koskinen P, Isolauri E: Probiotics in primary prevention of atopic disease: a randomised placebo-controlled trial. Lancet 2001;357:1076–1079.
55 Bruynzeel-Koomen C, van Wichen DF, Toonstra J, Berrens L, Bruynzeel PL: The presence of IgE molecules on epidermal Langerhans cells in patients with atopic dermatitis. Arch Dermatol Res 1986;278: 199–205.
56 Sampson HA, McCaskill CC: Food hypersensitivity and atopic dermatitis: evaluation of 113 patients. J Pediatr 1985;107:669–675.
57 Hutinel V, Rivet L: Septicémies graves au cours des affections cutanées des jeunes enfants. Arch Méd Enfants 1909;12:1–20.
58 Sulzberger MB, Witten VH: The effect of topically applied compound F in selected dermatoses. J Invest Dermatol 1952;19: 101–102.
59 Staab D, Diepgen TL, Fartasch M, Kupfer J, Lob-Corzilius T, Ring J, Scheewe S, Scheidt R, Schmid-Ott G, Schnopp C, Szczepanski R, Werfel T, Wittenmeier M, Wahn U, Gieler U: Age related, structured educational programmes for the management of atopic dermatitis in children and adolescents: multicentre, randomised controlled trial. BMJ 2006;332:933–938.
60 Ruzicka T, Bieber T, Schöpf E, Rubins A, Dobozy A, Bos JD, Jablonska S, Ahmed I, Thestrup-Pedersen K, Daniel F, Finzi A, Reitamo S: A short-term trial of tacrolimus ointment for atopic dermatitis. N Engl J Med 1997;337:816–821.
61 Ring J, Möhrenschlager M, Henkel V: The US FDA 'black box' warning for topical calcineurin inhibitors: an ongoing controversy. Drug Saf 2008;31:185–198.
62 Thibierge G: Ponction lombaire dans les dermatoses prurigineuses. CR du Xe congrès français de médecine. Paris, Masson, 1910.
63 Whalley D, McKenna SP, Dewar AL, Erdman RA, Kohlmann T, Niero M, Cook SA, Crickx B, Herdman MJ, Frech F, Van Assche D: A new instrument for assessing quality of life in atopic dermatitis: international development of the Quality of Life Index for Atopic Dermatitis (QoLIAD). Br J Dermatol 2004;150:274–283.
64 Tominaga M, Ogawa H, Takamori K: Possible roles of epidermal opioid systems in pruritus of atopic dermatitis. J Invest Dermatol 2007;127:2228–2235.
65 Szentivanyi A: The beta-adrenergic theory of the atopic abnormality in bronchial asthma. J Allergy 1968;42:203–232.
66 Hanifin JM, Chan SC: Monocyte phosphodiesterase abnormalities and dysregulation of lymphocyte function in atopic dermatitis. J Invest Dermatol 1995;105(suppl 1):84S–88S.
67 Ogawa H, Yoshiike T: A speculative view of atopic dermatitis: barrier dysfunction in pathogenesis. J Dermatol Sci 1993;5:197–204.
68 Taieb A: Hypothesis: from epidermal barrier dysfunction to atopic disorders. Contact Dermatitis 1999;41:177–180.
69 Imokawa G, Abe A, Jin K, Higaki Y, Kawashima M, Hidano: Decreased level of ceramides in stratum corneum of atopic dermatitis: an etiologic factor in atopic dry skin? J Invest Dermatol 1991;96:523–526.
70 Melnik BC, Plewig G: Is the origin of atopy linked to deficient conversion of omega-6-fatty acids to prostaglandin E1? J Am Acad Dermatol 1989;21:557–563.
71 Palmer CN, Irvine AD, Terron-Kwiatkowski A, Zhao Y, Liao H, Lee SP, Goudie DR, Sandilands A, Campbell LE, Smith FJ, O'Regan GM, Watson RM, Cecil JE, Bale SJ, Compton JG, DiGiovanna JJ, Fleckman P, Lewis-Jones S, Arseculeratne G, Sergeant A, Munro CS, El Houate B, McElreavey K, Halkjaer LB, Bisgaard H, Mukhopadhyay S, McLean WH: Common loss-of-function variants of the epidermal barrier protein filaggrin are a major predisposing factor for atopic dermatitis. Nat Genet 2006;38:441–446.
72 Weidinger S, O'Sullivan M, Illig T, Baurecht H, Depner M, Rodriguez E, Ruether A, Klopp N, Vogelberg C, Weiland SK, McLean WH, von Mutius E, Irvine AD, Kabesch M: Filaggrin mutations, atopic eczema, hay fever, and asthma in children. J Allergy Clin Immunol 2008;121:1203–1209.
73 Demehri S, Morimoto M, Holtzman MJ, Kopan R: Skin-derived TSLP triggers progression from epidermal-barrier defects to asthma. PLoS Biol 2009;7:e1000067.
74 Elias PM: Therapeutic implications of a barrier-based pathogenesis of atopic dermatitis. Ann Dermatol 2010;22:245–254.

Dr. Daniel Wallach
Department of Dermatology
Hôpital Tarnier-Cochin
89, rue d'Assas
FR–75006 Paris (France)
E-Mail dwallach@noos.fr

Bergmann K-C, Ring J (eds): History of Allergy. Chem Immunol Allergy. Basel, Karger, 2014, vol 100, pp 97–100
DOI: 10.1159/000358608

Allergic Contact Dermatitis

Ali Alikhan[a] · Howard I. Maibach[b]

[a]Department of Dermatology, Mayo Clinic, Rochester, Minn., and [b]Department of Dermatology, University of California at San Francisco School of Medicine, San Francisco, Calif., USA

Abstract

Allergic contact dermatitis is one of the most important dermatologic disorders worldwide – it can cause significant morbidity and decreased quality of life, as well as having major economic implications and loss of vocational productivity. Patch testing is the most important discovery in allergic contact dermatitis and the best diagnostic modality to date; the thin-layer rapid-use epicutaneous (TRUE) test is a more recent patch test development which has improved the convenience and feasibility of the test. The future of allergic contact dermatitis is bright as we continue to learn more about the science of the disorder, as well as ways to improve diagnosis and patient care. Furthermore, it is important to remember, in this global age, that cooperation between health care providers worldwide is essential.

Awareness of contact dermatitis has been present since ancient Greek and ancient Egyptian times, as evidenced by the writings of Hippocrates and Pliny the Younger [1, 2]. Knowledge of the disorder grew rapidly during the 19th century, with Ferdinand von Hebra demonstrating that croton oil could provoke eczematous dermatitis on normal human skin [1].

Patch Testing – Jadassohn and Bloch

The standard diagnostic test in allergic contact dermatitis is the patch test, the discovery of which is credited to Josef Jadassohn. Jadassohn was the first dermatologist 'to apply objective experimental methods to the study of cutaneous immunology' [3]. In 1895, while professor of dermatology at Breslau University, he developed the contact test ('funktionelle Hautprüfung') in order to objectively diagnose a patient who had developed an eczematous reaction to mercury plasters, which had been prescribed for pediculi pubis [2, 4]. In doing so, he recognized the potential for certain chemicals (when placed on the skin) to cause eczematous reactions in sensitized individuals. Bruno Bloch, a student of Jadassohn and a professor at Basel and Zurich Universities, expanded the work of Jadassohn, increasing the knowledge base of contact dermatitis immunology [3, 4]. He further described the patch test methodology and grading of skin reactions, postulated the idea of cross-reactivity, described the first cases of systemic contact dermatitis and, with Paul Karrer, synthesized primin [2], the specific chemical in *Primula obconica* that is responsible for allergic contact dermatitis [5]. Perhaps most importantly, he developed and promoted a primitive standard series for patch testing [5]. Among his influential disciples are Marion Sulzberger, who brought patch testing to America, and Paul Bonnevie.

Between 1895 and the 1960s, patch testing was used in certain European clinics, but ignored by others [4]. No consensus was reached regarding material, allergen concentrations, reading times or reading scores. Additionally, differentiating between allergic and irritant dermatitis, as well as understanding the significance of a positive patch test, was unclear.

Important Early Basic Science Discoveries

Important discoveries in basic immunology as it relates to allergic contact dermatitis have been reviewed extensively by Krueger and Stingl [6]. Some of these scientists and their discoveries include:

(1) Landsteiner and Jacobs – their experiments underlined the relationships between chemical structure and allergenicity [7, 8];
(2) Sulzberger and Baer – demonstrated in man a relationship between the in vitro reactivity of a chemical and its ability to produce allergic contact dermatitis [9];
(3) Landsteiner and Chase – using guinea pig modeling, they found that allergic contact hypersensitivity could be transferred to naïve recipients by live lymphoid cells from affected donors [10].

Standard Series – Bonnevie

Understanding that most clinical cases of allergic contact dermatitis are caused by a relatively small number of chemicals, Paul Bonnevie, a student of Bruno Bloch and professor of occupational medicine in Copenhagen, expanded Bloch's limited standard allergen series and published it in his famous textbook of environmental medicine [4, 5]. Bonnevie's [11] twenty-one allergen series is considered the predecessor to the current standard series utilized by various countries and continents. It was employed for several decades in Copenhagen, allowing Marcussen [12] to publish a large epidemiological survey on contact allergies in 1962. Later, it was modified and updated by the fledgling International Contact Dermatitis Research Group (ICDRG).

Contact Dermatitis and Public Health – Ramazzini and Prosser White

The fields of contact dermatitis and public health are inextricably linked. Bernardo Ramazzini (1633–1714), the author of *A Treatise of the Disease of Tradesmen*, is considered the father of occupational medicine – he 'emphasized the connection of many diseases with the occupations of patients and urged that medical students study ways to protect workers' [2]. He described hand dermatitis in laundry women and soapworkers, attributing their condition to direct contact with substances.

Two-hundred years later, Robert Prosser White would expand the field of occupational dermatology. Prosser White saw and diagnosed thousands of work-related skin disorders in Wigan, UK, a large industrial town in the heart of Lancashire [1, 13]. He published and lectured extensively on occupational dermatoses, holding various international positions and receiving numerous honors. His textbook *Occupational Affections of the Skin* was considered the definitive reference for occupational skin disease [1, 13].

Contact Dermatitis Societies

The first contact dermatitis society, the Scandinavian Committee for Standardization of Routine Patch Testing, was created in 1962. In 1967, this committee enlarged and joined with various national or European groups interested in contact dermatitis to form the ICDRG, whose tasks were to standardize (at an international level) the patch testing procedure (e.g. allergen vehicles, allergen concentrations, etc.), encourage cooperative research among different countries, and promote interest by dermatologists in allergic and environmental skin disorders [1, 5]. Founding members included H.J. Bandmann, C.D. Calnan, E. Cronin, S. Fregert, N. Hjorth, B. Magnusson, H.I. Maibach, K.E. Malten, C. Meneghini, V. Pirilä, and D.S. Wilkinson. The first international standard series was published in 1997 by the ICDRG [14], with an updated revision in 2011 [14].

Niels Hjorth was the first chairman of the ICDRG and organized the first international symposium on contact dermatitis in 1974. This symposium was followed by many others, which elevated the stature of contact dermatitis throughout the world and resulted in the establishment of numerous national and continental contact dermatitis groups [5, 15]. Among these groups are the European Environmental and Contact Dermatitis Research Group (EECDRG), the European Society of Contact Dermatitis (ESCD), which is responsible for the journal *Contact Dermatitis*, the North American Contact Dermatitis Group (NACDG), and the American Contact Dermatitis Society (ACDS), which is responsible for the journal *Dermatitis* [1]. Many of these groups have their own standard allergen series, allergen concentrations, and patch testing methodology and techniques (e.g. when to read the tests, use of Finn chambers, etc.) [16].

Improving Convenience – The TRUE Test

The thin-layer rapid-use epicutaneous (TRUE) test was developed by Fischer and Maibach in 1985 [17]. It is a standardized, ready-to-apply patch test system requiring no pre-mixing or preparation time, and contains 29 common allergens. The allergens are incorporated in hydrophilic gels, coated on a water-impermeable sheet of polyester, and dried to a thin film. The coated polyester sheet is cut into squared patches that are mounted on non-woven cellulose tape with acrylic adhesive, covered with siliconized plastic (a protect sheet), and packed in an airtight and light-impermeable envelope [18]. When the test strip is taped on the skin, perspiration hydrates the film and transforms it to a gel, causing the allergen to be released. The TRUE test has been demonstrated to be accurate and safe, and allows for greater consistency in terms of allergen distribution, quantity, stability and location. Unfortunately, development costs and regulatory hurdles have limited its expansion to the much larger baseline series of today.

Moving into the Computer Age – The CARD Database

First developed at the Mayo Clinic in 1998, the Contact Allergen Replacement Database (CARD) is an internet database which enables clinicians to find suitable skin care products for their patients with contact allergies; it contains over 8,100 known ingredients catalogued in over 5,500 commercially available skin care products [19]. By entering allergens that the patient should avoid (based on patch test positivity and clinical relevance), the program creates a list of safe products for the patient to use. This innovative use of technology has enhanced patient care as allergen avoidance education can be quite overwhelming given complexly named allergens as well as avoidance of allergen cross-reactors. The Contact Allergen Management Program (CAMP), which is similar to the CARD, has been developed by the ACDS.

The Future of Allergic Contact Dermatitis

While the study of allergic contact dermatitis has blossomed since Jadassohn developed the patch test over 100 years ago, further improvements will significantly strengthen the field. Alikhan and Maibach [20] suggest various strategies to enhance our understanding of allergic contact dermatitis and our practice of patch testing. Categories for improvement include: understanding allergen stability, identifying true allergens, expanding and refining the TRUE test, separating irritant reactions from allergic reactions, investigating patch wearing and application periods, developing patch test banks, approaching false-negative patch test results, re-examining the utility of intradermal testing, understanding the significance of positive patch testing, developing contact allergy certifications and fellowships, increasing discussion of chemical identification of allergens in publications, improving international collaboration between worldwide contact dermatitis groups, and improving technology (e.g. utilization and refinement of skin bioengineering tools, in vitro diagnostic methods and use of a patient's genetic code).

Conclusion

This brief overview omits many important contributors and contributions. Lachapelle's [21] *Giant Steps in Patch Testing: A Historical Memoir* provides extensive detail and is highly recommended.

References

1 Smith DR: The continuing rise of contact dermatitis. 1. The academic discipline. Contact Dermatitis 2009;61:189–193.
2 Wright RC, Goldman L: Contact dermatitis: a historical perspective. Int J Dermatol 1979;18:665–668.
3 Crissey JT, Parish LC, Holubar K: Historical Atlas of Dermatology and Dermatologists. Boca Raton, Parthenon, 2002.
4 Lachapelle J-M, Maibach HI: Patch Testing and Prick Testing: A Practical Guide – Official Publication of the ICDRG. Berlin, Springer, 2009.
5 Rycroft RJG: Textbook of Contact Dermatitis. Berlin, Springer, 2001.
6 Krueger GG, Stingl G: Immunology/inflammation of the skin – a 50-year perspective. J Invest Dermatol 1989;92:32S–51S.
7 Landsteiner K, Jacobs J: Studies on the sensitization of animals with simple chemical compounds. J Exp Med 1935;61:643–656.
8 Landsteiner K, Jacobs J: Studies on the sensitization of animals with simple chemical compounds. II. J Exp Med 1936;64:625–639.
9 Sulzberger MB, Baer RL: Sensitization to simple chemicals. 3. Relationship between chemical structure and porperties, and sensitizing capacities in the production of eczematous sensitivity in man. J Invest Dermatol 1938;1:45–58.
10 Landsteiner K, Chase MW: Experiments on transfer of cutaneous sensitivity to simple chemical compounds. Proc Soc Exp Biol Med 1942;49:688–690.
11 Bonnevie P: Aetiologie und Pathogenese der Ekzemkrankheiten. Klinische Studien über die Ursachen der Ekzeme unter besonderer Berücksichtigung des diagnostischen Wertes der Ekzemproben. Copenhagen, Busch, 1939.
12 Marcussen PV: Variations in the incidence of contact hypersensitivities. Trans St Johns Hosp Dermatol Soc 1962;48:40–48.
13 Ashworth J: Robert Prosser White (1855–1934). Clin Exp Dermatol 1994;19:186–187.
14 Lachapelle JM, Ale SI, Freeman S, Frosch PJ, Goh CL, Hannuksela M, et al: Proposal for a revised international standard series of patch tests. Contact Dermatitis 1997;36:121–123.
15 Cheng LS, Alikhan A, Maibach HI: Compilation of international standards for patch testing methodology and allergens. Dermatitis 2009;20:257–260.
16 Cheng LS, Alikhan A, Maibach HI: Creating an electronic collaboration between international contact dermatitis groups. Contact Dermatitis 2009;61:59–60.
17 Fischer TI, Maibach HI: The thin layer rapid use epicutaneous test (TRUE-test), a new patch test method with high accuracy. Br J Dermatol 1985;112:63–68.
18 Fischer T, Maibach HI: Easier patch testing with TRUE Test. J Am Acad Dermatol 1989;20:447–453.
19 Yiannias JA, Miller R, Kist JM: Creation, history, and future of the Contact Allergen Replacement Database (CARD). Dermatitis 2009;20:322–326.
20 Alikhan A, Maibach HI: Allergic contact dermatitis: the future. Dermatitis 2009;20:327–333.
21 Lachapelle JM: Giant Steps in Patch Testing: A Historical Memoir. Phoenix, SmartPractice, 2010.

Dr. Ali Alikhan
Department of Dermatology, Mayo Clinic
200 First Street SW
Rochester, MN 55905 (USA)
E-Mail alikhan.mirza@mayo.edu

Bergmann K-C, Ring J (eds): History of Allergy. Chem Immunol Allergy. Basel, Karger, 2014, vol 100, pp 101–104
DOI: 10.1159/000358614

Urticaria and Angioedema

Marcus Maurer

Department of Dermatology and Allergy, Charité-Universitätsmedizin Berlin, Germany

Abstract

Urticaria and angioedema are ancient diseases. Many different names have been used to describe them, and many different theories have been postulated to explain their origin and pathogenesis. The current classification and nomenclature of urticaria and angioedema have evolved over several millennia, with many detours and problems, some of which still remain to be solved. This chapter describes the history of urticaria and angioedema. The evolution of selected aspects of today's understanding of both conditions is also traced, based on the review of original sources and previously published research on this topic.

Urticaria

Urticaria is a group of diseases characterized by the occurrence of itchy wheals (urticae), angioedema or both. Research on the history of this common skin condition is complicated by several independent problems. Firstly, wheals and/or angioedema occur in diseases other than urticaria, many of which have only been recognized as separate entities within the last centuries (e.g. hereditary angioedema; HAE) or even decades (e.g. Schnitzler syndrome, urticarial vasculitis). Secondly, the name 'urticaria' is fairly new, being less than 250 years old [1]. Many different names had been used before then, including knidosis, uredo, Nesselsucht and Nesselfieber, urticatio and randados, among others (see below). This happened, in part, because of changes in the understanding of the pathogenesis and the underlying causes of this condition. Thirdly, urticaria is a heterogeneous group of conditions, and subgroups differ substantially in their clinical course and features, their underlying causes and the relevance and nature of eliciting triggers. Nevertheless, the history of urticaria and angioedema is well researched and understood, which is mainly due to the work of Schadewaldt [1], who published detailed descriptions of the history of both conditions.

Urticaria and angioedema are ancient conditions. Both are believed to have troubled even our earliest ancestors since they are also found in other animals such as horses and dogs. Also, mast cells, the key effector cells of all urticarias and most angioedemas, have been found in the skin of all mammals investigated so far. One of the earliest descriptions of urticaria comes from China, and is more than 2,000 years old. In the *Huangdi Neijing* [2], written before and during the early Han period around 200 BC, urticaria is referred to as Feng Yin Zheng ('wind type concealed rash'), very similar to one of today's traditional Chinese medicine (TCM) terms for urticaria, Feng Sao Yin Zhen ('wind itch concealed rash'). In TCM, wind is held to be the major pathogen in urticaria, therefore other names for urticaria are wind rash (Feng Zhen) and wind rash lumps (Feng Zhen Kuai).

The 'father of Western medicine', Hippocrates (460–377 BC), used the term 'knidosis' to describe elevated itching lesions caused by nettles (knido in Greek), which would appear to be the first reference to what today is called contact urticaria. Hippocrates is also believed to have first described gastrointestinal disorders as a cause of urticaria. Urticaria, in the ancient Latin medical literature, was called 'uredo' (urere means 'to burn'), and 'essera' (meaning 'elevation') in the old Persian medical texts. Paracelsus (1493–1541) introduced the first German name, Leusschieppen, but this was neither useful nor used for long. The term 'urticaria', derived from *Urtica urens* (stinging nettle), was first introduced by William Cullen in the 18th century [3].

Today, urticaria is understood to be a group of diseases, most commonly classified as either acute or chronic, and spontaneous or induced by specific eliciting triggers. The underlying causes of spontaneous urticaria are still under investigation and discussion. Autoreactivity, intolerance to food components and/or bacterial infections are held to be relevant by most, but not all, contemporary authors. Even in some of the oldest reports known, urticaria is postulated to be due to food intolerance or food poisoning. Interestingly, the first case report on death from urticaria also involves hives that developed in response to food consumption [4]. In his book, *The History of King Richard III*, Sir Thomas More (1478–1535) tells the following story: King Richard, who apparently knew that strawberries would make him break out in hives, convened the lords of the privy council and demanded to be served strawberries, which he ate in their presence. He then left and returned after several hours to show them the urticarial rash that had developed on his arm in the meantime. King Richard blamed this on one of the lords, who he disliked. He accused the lord of witchcraft and had him killed, claiming that the lord had poisoned him [1].

Over the years, many other conditions and factors have been claimed to be responsible for the onset of urticaria. The wide array of theories on the etiology of urticaria, which includes but is not limited to the idiosyncratic theory, the humoral theory, the toxin theory, the nervous theory, the microthrombosis theory, the menstrual theory, the angioneurotic theory, the theory of inflammation, and even the meteorological theory, have previously been reviewed in detail by Czarnetzki [5].

The group of induced (or inducible) urticarias includes contact urticaria (first described by Hippocrates, see above), which occurs at skin sites exposed to contact with urticariogenic substances, as well as cholinergic urticaria and the physical urticarias. The latter are characterized by wheals and/or angioedema that occur in response to skin exposure to a physical trigger, e.g. cold (cold urticaria), pressure (delayed pressure urticaria) or friction (symptomatic dermographism). Symptomatic dermographism is believed to be the first physical urticaria to be described in the literature, in 1767 by Heberden [6]. Today, symptomatic dermographism is used synonymously with urticaria factitia, derived from the term 'factitious urticaria' coined by Gull in 1859 [7]. In the Middle Ages, patients with urticaria factitia/symptomatic dermographism were beheaded or burnt alive because they were assumed to be related to the devil [8]. Solar urticaria was also first described in the 18th century and later, in 1887, identified as being sunlight dependent [9, 10]. Cold urticaria is held to have been first described in 1792 by Frank [11], cholinergic urticaria in 1924 by Duke [12], pressure urticaria in 1929 by Urbach and Fasal [13], and aquagenic urticaria in 1964 by Shelley and Rawnsley [14].

Angioedema

Angioedema is a common symptom in patients with wheals, either during anaphylactic reactions or in patients with chronic urticaria. The coexistence of both wheals and angioedema was recognized early on, primarily in patients with hypersensitivity reactions to food. In 1586, Marcello Donati [15] described lip swelling in a young male patient in response to the ingestion of eggs. Later reports from the mid-1600s described similar cases of angioedema in response to honey or mussels [1]. Until the late 1800s, angioedema was seen exclusively as a sign of, and linked to, urticaria, even though some cases of isolated angioedema, i.e. without wheals, were reported as early as the mid-1800s. Diez or Graves, for example, noted the danger of laryngeal edema and speculated that similar swellings may involve the mucosa of the gastrointestinal tract [1].

In 1882, it was Eugen Dinkelacker and his teacher Heinrich Irenäus Quincke [16] (1842–1922), a German internist and surgeon in Kiel, who first described HAE. Dinkelacker's doctoral thesis (fig. 1) documented 14 cases of angioedema, some with and some without wheals. In retrospect, at least 2 of the patients described had HAE: a 22-year-old male patient with chronic recurrent facial, laryngeal and abdominal angioedema attacks of up to 3 days duration since early childhood, and his infant son. Both patients apparently used to develop prodromal symptoms, including erythema marginatum.

Quincke and Dinkelacker used the term 'acute circumscript angioedema' for the condition they described, which soon became known as Quincke's edema. At the time, urticaria was held to be of 'angioneurotic' origin, i.e. caused by an increased permeability of capillaries due to a spasm in response to neurogenic influences. It is, therefore, not surprising that Quincke and Dinkelacker both suggested that the cases of angioedema they had observed were also due to 'angioneurosis'. In fact, the term 'angioneurotic edema' had been used by other authors earlier, for example by Bannister in 1880 in his description of suddenly appearing and inflammatory swellings [17]. Although Quincke, who is also known for introducing lumbar puncture as a procedure for diagnostic and therapeutic purposes, postulated that pa-

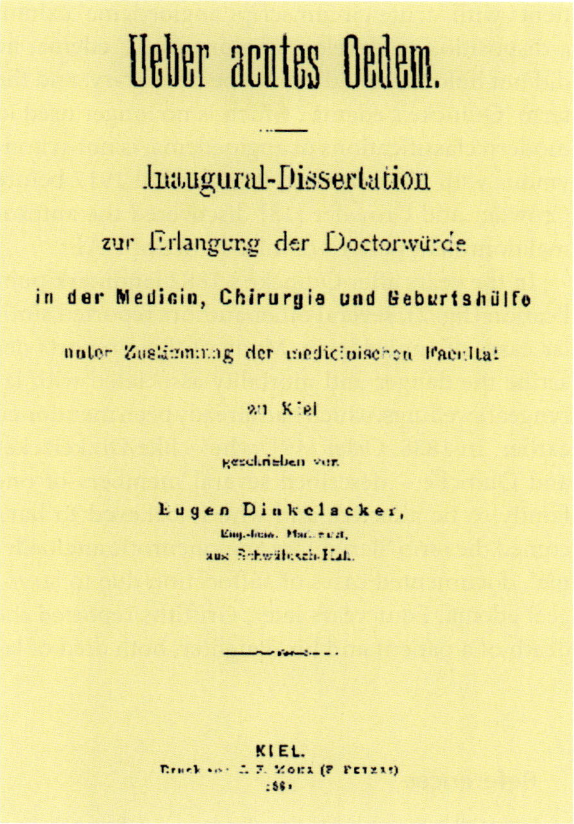
Ueber acutes Oedem.

Inaugural-Dissertation

zur Erlangung der Doctorwürde

in der Medicin, Chirurgie und Geburtshülfe

unter Zustimmung der medicinischen Facultat

zu Kiel

geschrieben von

Eugen Dinkelacker,

aus Schwäbisch-Hall.

KIEL.

Fig. 1. Title page of Eugen Dinkelacker's doctoral thesis on 'acute circumscript angioedema' in which he describes the first cases of what is today designated HAE type I/II.

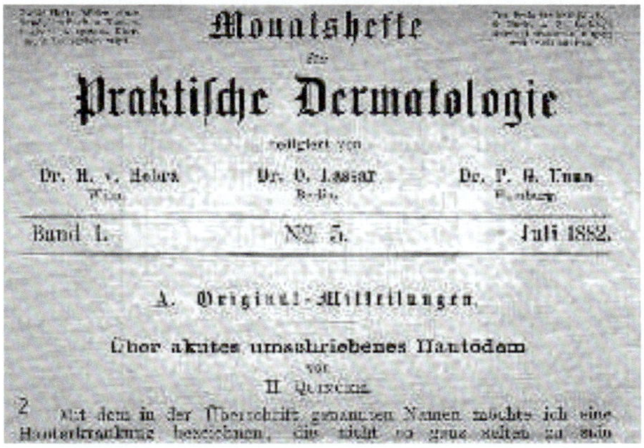
Monatshefte für Praktische Dermatologie

redigiert von

Dr. H. v. Hebra, Wien | Dr. O. Lassar, Berlin | Dr. P. G. Unna, Hamburg

Band I. | Nº 5. | Juli 1882.

A. Original-Mittheilungen.

Über akutes umschriebenes Hautödem

von

H. Quincke.

Mit dem in der Überschrift genannten Namen möchte ich eine Hauterkrankung bezeichnen, die nicht so ganz selten zu sein

Fig. 2. Title page of Quincke's landmark paper on angioedema, which linked his name to the condition for more than 200 years.

tients with 'acute circumscript angioedema' exhibit a disposition to develop 'angioneurotic' edema, he did not hold this condition to be hereditary, and the term 'Quincke's edema', which is no longer used in modern classifications of angioedema, is not synonymous with HAE. In fact, it took until 1917 before Crowder and Crowder [18] discovered the autosomal dominant pattern of inheritance of HAE.

In the years after Quincke's 1882 landmark publication (fig. 2), several other authors reported similar cases of angioedema. Many of these reports describe the danger and mortality associated with laryngeal swellings, which had already been mentioned earlier. In 1888, Osler [19], who – like Dinkelacker and Quincke – described several members of one family to be affected, and who is believed to have coined the term 'hereditary angioneurotic angioedema', documented cases of suffocation due to laryngeal edema. Four years later, Griffiths reported the death of a patient and his daughter, both died of laryngeal edema [1]. Within the following 5 years, two large families, with 33 and 110 affected members and 12 and 30 fatalities from laryngeal edema, respectively, were published [1].

Today, we know that recurrent angioedema is either inherited or acquired, and that HAE is bradykinin-mediated and different from histamine-mediated angioedema. A century ago, angioedema was often seen in response to the then popular 'serum therapy' and allergic mechanisms were newly discovered. As a consequence, angioedema became widely held to be an allergy, induced by anaphylactic mechanisms, rather than 'angioneurotic' responses. This may explain why it took 50 years after the Crowders' description of the autosomal-dominant pattern of inheritance in HAE before Donaldson and Evans [20] discovered, in 1963, that HAE, which, as we know today, is bradykinin-mediated, to be caused by a deficiency or defect of C1INH, the inhibitor of the complement component C1.

References

1 Schadewaldt H: Geschichte der Allergie. Munich, Dustri, 1983, vol 3, chapt 2, 3.
2 Neijing H: The Su Wen of the Huangdi Neijing (Inner Classic of the Yellow Emperor). Jin dynasty, 1115–1234.
3 Cullen W: Synopsia Nosologiae Methodicae. Edinburgh, Kincaid & Creech, 1769.
4 More T: The history of King Richard III; in Campbell WE (ed): The English Works of Sir Thomas More. London, Eyre and Spottiswoode, 1931, p 426.
5 Czarnetzki BM: Urticaria. Berlin, Springer, 1986, chapt 1.
6 Heberden W: On the nettle-rash. Med Trans Coll Phys (London) 1767, p 185.
7 Gull W: On factitious urticaria. Guys Hospital Reports 1859;5:316.
8 Falk H: Beitrag zum Studium des Dermographismus. Med Diss München, 1901.
9 Borsch JF: De purpura urticata, quam vocant 'die Nesselsucht'; med diss, Halle, 1719.
10 Veiel T: Über einen Fall von Eczema solare. Arch Derm Syph (Berlin) 1887;19:1113.
11 Frank JP: De curandis hominum morbis epitome. Mannheim, Schwan & Goetz, 1792, vol 3, p 104.
12 Duke WW: Urticaria caused specifically by the action of physical agents. J Am Med Assoc 1924;83:3.
13 Urbach E, Fasal P: Mechanische Urtikaria. Ein weiterer Beitrag zur physikalischen Allergie der Haut. Klin Wochenschr 1929;8: 2368.
14 Shelley WB, Rawnsley HM: Aquagenic urticaria: contact sensitivity to water. JAMA 1964;189:895.
15 Donati M: De medica historia mirabile. Mantua, Osana, 1586, vol 7, chapt 3, p 304.
16 Quincke HI: Über akutes umschriebenes Hautödem. Hamburg, Monatshefte für Praktische Dermatologie, 1882, vol 1, pp 129–131.
17 Török L: Urticaria; in Jadassohn J, Marchionini A (eds): Handbuch der Haut- und Geschlechtskrankheiten. Berlin, Springer, 1928, vol 6, part 2, pp 145–215.
18 Crowder JR, Crowder TR: Five generations of angioneurotic edema. Arch Intern Med 1917;20:840–852.
19 Osler W: Hereditary angio-neurotic oedema. Am J Med Sci 1888;95:362–367.
20 Donaldson VH, Evans RR: A biochemical abnormality in heredity angioneurotic edema: absence of serum inhibition of C1-esterase. Am J Med 1963;35:37–44.

Prof. Marcus Maurer
Department of Dermatology and Allergy
Charité – Universitätsmedizin Berlin, Charitéplatz 1
DE–10117 Berlin (Germany)
E-Mail marcus.maurer@charite.de

Bergmann K-C, Ring J (eds): History of Allergy. Chem Immunol Allergy. Basel, Karger, 2014, vol 100, pp 105–108
DOI: 10.1159/000358615

Allergy and the Eye

Sergio Bonini

Department of Medicine, Second University of Naples, Naples, and Institute of Translational Pharmacology, Italian National Research Council, Rome, Italy

Abstract

This review of the major milestones in the history of ocular allergy and immunology shows how significantly this subdiscipline has contributed to the tremendous progress in the understanding of mechanisms of allergic and immunologic diseases, as well as in their better management. It also indicates unmet needs and priority areas for future research.

Although the eye was reported to be the first organ involved in the allergic reaction described in the original case of hay fever reported by John Bostock almost 200 years ago, ocular allergy has never received the same attention that has been given to respiratory or skin allergy. On the contrary, in view of the peculiar anatomy and the prominent representation of the immune system in the ocular tissues, the eye has always represented an extremely useful model to study the immune and allergic response to environmental or endogenous stimuli, as well as the peripheral localization of systemic immune diseases.

There are several reasons for ocular allergy being the Cinderella of allergic diseases, even from a historical perspective. First is the attitude of allergists to focus mainly on respiratory and skin manifestations of the allergic response, meaning eye symptoms are often considered only a 'complication' of rhinitis under the unacceptable term of rhinoconjunctivitis. Second, the participation of ocular tissues in several autoimmune and systemic diseases has often been considered as a prominent competence of other disciplines, such as internal medicine or rheumatology. Finally, the prevalent surgical commitment of ophthalmologists has so far not enabled the needed collaboration with allergists to focus on diseases usually considered of minor priority in pharmacological and clinical research and practice, thus making ocular allergists a small group of segregated subspecialists.

While drawing attention to the fact that eye involvement in the allergic and immunologic response represents one of the major causes of a poor quality of life and may often be serious enough to affect vision, I would like to focus this chapter on how studies of ocular allergy have significantly contributed to the tremendous progress in knowledge of the mechanisms leading to symptoms and disease in the allergic patient, as well as on how the history of allergy in the eye may indicate unmet needs and suggest new approaches for allergy research and practice.

The Contribution of Ocular Allergy to a Better Understanding of Mechanisms of the Immune Reaction

In 1819, John Bostock [1], presenting his 'Case of a periodical affection of the eyes and chest', wrote:

> About the beginning or middle of June in every year the following symptoms make their appearance, with a greater or less degree of violence.
> A sensation of heat and fullness is experienced in the eye, first along the edges of the lids, and especially in the inner angles ... there is a slight degree of redness and a discharge of tears. This state gradually increases, until the sensation becomes converted into what may be characterized as a combination of the most acute itching and smarting ... This state of the eyes comes on the paroxysm, at uncertain intervals ...
> ... to this succeeds irritation of the nose, producing sneezing, which occurs in fits of extreme violence ...
> ... to the sneezing are added a further sensation of tightness of chest, and difficulty of breathing, with a general irritation of fauces and trachea ...
> ... to these local symptoms are at length added a degree of general indisposition, a great degree of languor, an incapacity of muscular exertion, loss of appetite, emaciation, restless night, often attended with profuse perspirations, the extremities, however, being generally cold.

Therefore, ocular symptoms appear to have been the first manifestation of hay fever since its original description.

However, in order to have conclusive evidence of a causal relationship between allergen exposure and ocular allergy symptoms, we had to wait for the work of Charles Blackley [2] and his book entitled *Experimental Researches on the Causes and Nature of Catarrhus Aestivus* published in 1873.

Charles Blackley reported in this way the first conjunctival auto-provocation test:

> A decoction of the pollen *Gladiolus* was made by boiling a portion of this with one hundred times its weight of distilled water. One drop of this liquid was placed in contact with the conjunctiva of the right eye. The effect was almost instantaneous. The first sensation was that of intense burning and smarting, coupled with a feeling such as might be imagined to be caused by fine sand being blown into the eye. The photophobia was so severe that for some minutes the eye could not be opened than more for a single second at a time. In about thirty seconds the capillary vessels of the conjunctiva were seen to be greatly distended.

Interestingly enough, the occurrence of a late-phase reaction is also accurately described, since the author continues the description of his experiment as such:

> In six hours the eye still felt uneasy, but there was very little pain on moving the eyeball, although the vessels of the conjunctiva were still injected. The chemosis still remained as severe as before. In eighteen hours there was scarcely any congestion of the vessels remaining, but the chemosis was still very distinct. In thirty-two hours all traces of the derangement had disappeared.

Charles Blackley also explained the discrepancy between eye symptoms and respiratory symptoms induced by allergen challenge in sensitized individuals by providing the first report on the relevance of the sensitivity of target organs and of the dose of allergen used for provocation in causing clinical symptoms:

> The difference between the quantity of pollen inhaled and that which is thrown against the eyeball by the force of the wind, may be judged by the results of the experiments just quoted. In one sense it is a fortunate thing for the patient that this difference does exist, for if the same quantity of pollen that is inhaled came in contact with the eyeball his condition would be almost unbearable.

These pioneer observations [3] found a more structured explanation in the description of a type I hypersensitivity reaction in the framework of the categorization of allergic reactions made by Coombs and Gell [4] in the early 1970s, and mainly through the studies of Mathea Allansmith showing the peculiar preferential distribution of mast cells within the ocular tissues [5]. In the following years, our group provided the first description of the cells and mediators participating in the early and late phase of the ocular allergic reaction [6, 7], as well as the role of a non-specific conjunctival hyperreactivity in influencing the appearance and severity of clinical symptoms of a red eye in allergic and non-allergic individuals [8].

The pathophysiology of allergic eye diseases is now extended to include a vast array of cells and cytokines [9], and largely contributes to a more advanced comprehension of the complex mechanisms that lead from sensitization to tissue inflammation and remodeling.

However, the contribution of the eye to the history of allergy and clinical immunology is not confined to immunoglobulin (Ig) E-mediated diseases. In his overview of the history of immunology and of the birth of ocular immunology as a new discipline, Arthur Silverstein [10] drew attention to the relevant contribution of the eye to a better understanding of autoimmune phenomena.

While sympathetic ophthalmia and endophthalmitis phacoanaphylactica or phacoantigenic uveitis have represented interesting models for understanding the role of autoantibodies in causing inflammation and symptoms, the eye's participation in Sjögren's syndrome, Graves' disease, Behçet's disease and Vogt-Koyanagi-Harada's disease have provided an important contribution to the understanding of the complex cell interactions and human leukocyte antigen associations involved in autoimmune phenomena and systemic diseases. Finally, the immunological privilege of the cornea involving both the afferent and efferent limbs of the immune response has represented an important paradigm for understanding the cellular mechanisms responsible for success or failure of organ and tissue transplantation [10]. Therefore, in their 'view from the eye', McGonagle and Georgouli [11] used the example of eye inflammation to show how the eye's pathophysiological responses can be used to better conceptualize all aberrant immunological reactions.

The Contribution of Ocular Allergy to Clinical Practice in Allergy and Clinical Immunology

The evidence of a participation of the eye in most diseases with a derangement of the immune system requests the inclusion of an accurate eye examination in allergic and immunologic diseases. Moreover, some ocular diagnostic tests, such as the Schirmer test, represent an important contribution that ophthalmologists may provide to the diagnosis of systemic diseases.

The conjunctival provocation test, although less relevant than skin tests in revealing a sensitization, may provide significant advantages versus other provocation tests for a better understanding of cells and mediators involved in the allergic reaction, as well as for evaluating the efficacy of antiallergic drugs [12]. In fact, the conjunctival provocation test is safely performed, permits a visual monitoring of symptoms elicited and allows an easy collection of cells and mediators present in tears, with the advantage of using the contralateral eye as an internal control [13].

With reference to treatment, in the last 30 years the eye has represented a primary target for most antiallergic drugs introduced onto the market, from the aspirin derivatives and first-generation antihistamines to the new antiallergic molecules with multiple actions and immunomodulators [14]. It is relevant to note that the effects on eye symptoms were the primary outcome in the original introduction to immunotherapy by Leonard Noon [15].

At present, eye symptoms are usually included in the total symptom score in clinical trials not only of ocular allergic diseases, but also of allergic diseases affecting other organs, such as allergic rhinitis. Moreover, the conjunctival allergen provocation is considered in the USA as a valid surrogate marker to evaluate the effects of antiallergic treatments.

How Ocular Allergy Can Contribute to a Continuing Progress of Allergy and Clinical Immunology

Looking at history has no value if it is not associated with the learning of elements that improve our vision of unmet needs and pathways for further progress. There are several areas of ocular allergy where further research is needed, with potential translational impact on other fields of allergy and clinical immunology.

While the pathophysiology of seasonal and perennial conjunctivitis is sufficiently elucidated, vernal and atopic keratoconjunctivitis represent severe orphan diseases still awaiting a better understanding of the pathogenetic mechanisms involved and effective and safe treatment. Vernal and atopic keratoconjunctivitis represent examples of eosinophilic inflammation often associated with polyclonal IgE activation, but not necessarily with detectable and clinically relevant specific IgE. Therefore, studies of vernal and atopic keratoconjunctivitis may provide significant information on other allergic diseases with a similar pathological and clinical picture, such as NARES, nasal polyps, aspirin asthma and atopic eczema.

Clinical research in ocular allergy still appears inadequate for the standards required for the registration and study of new drugs. A systematic review of clinical trials of allergic conjunctivitis performed since 1965 showed that only a minority of them fulfilled the criteria for a proper design with reference to population sample selection, interventions, comparators and mainly standardized outcome measures [16]. Without correcting these limitations it will be difficult for both regulators and professionals to achieve a level of evidence that can guarantee the efficacy and safety of new antiallergic treatments.

Conclusions

This brief overview of the history of ocular allergy over the past 200 years highlights several milestones that have significantly contributed to progress in allergy and clinical immunology. This should prompt the inclusion of ocular allergy and immunology in the future research agenda of allergists and clinical immunologists in order to answer unmet needs and knowledge gaps. These still need to be addressed for the continued development of our discipline and a better global management of the allergic patient.

References

1 Bostock J: Case of a periodical affection of the eyes and chest. Med Chir Trans 1819;10: 161–165.
2 Blackley C: Experimental Researches on the Causes and Nature of Catarrhus Aestivus. London, Balliere & Tindall, 1873.
3 D'Amato G, Bonini S, Bousquet J, Durham SR, Platts-Mills TAE (eds): Pollenosis 2000: Global Approach. Naples, JGC Editions, 2001.
4 Coombs RRA, Gell PGH: The classification of allergic reactions underlying disease; in Gell PGH, Coombs RRA (eds): Clinical Aspects of Immunology. Philadelphia, Davis, 1963, p 317.
5 Allansmith MR: The Eye and Immunology. St Louis, Mosby, 1982.
6 Bonini S, Bonini S, Berruto A, Tomassini M, Carlesimo S, Bucci MG, Balsano F: Conjunctival provocation test as a model for the study of allergy and inflammation in humans. Int Arch Allergy Appl Immunol 1989;88:144–148.
7 Bonini S, Bonini S, Bucci MG, Berruto A, Adriani E, Balsano F, Allansmith MR: Allergen dose response and late symptoms in a human model of ocular allergy. J Allergy Clin Immunol 1990;86:869–876.
8 Bonini S, Bonini S, Schiavone M, Centofanti M, Allansmith MR, Bucci MG: Conjunctival hyperresponsiveness to ocular histamine challenge in patients with vernal conjunctivitis. J Allergy Clin Immunol 1992;89: 103–107.
9 Bielory L, Bonini S, Bonini S: Allergic eye disorders; in Zweiman B, Schwartz LB: (eds): Inflammatory Mechanisms in Allergic Disease. New York, Dekker, 2002, pp 311–323.
10 Silverstein AM: Ocular immunology: on the birth of a new discipline. Cell Immunol 1991;136:504–518.
11 McGonagle D, Georgouli T: The importance of the 'Mechnikov's thorn' for an improved understanding of 21st century medicine and immunology: a view from the eye. Scand J Immunol 2008;68:129–139.
12 Abelson MB: Conjunctival allergen challenge: models in the investigation of ocular allergy. Curr Allergy Asthma Rep 2003;3: 363–368.
13 Bonini S, Bonini S, Vecchione A, Naim DM, Allansmith MR, Balsano F: Inflammatory changes in conjunctival scrapings after allergen provocation in humans. J Allergy Clin Immunol 1988;82:462–469.
14 Bielory L: Allergic conjunctivitis: the evolution of therapeutic options. Allergy Asthma Proc 2012;17:129–139.
15 Noon L: Prophylactic inoculation against hayfever. Lancet 1911;i:1572–1574.
16 Mantelli F, Lambiase A, Bonini S, Bonini S: Clinical trials of allergic conjunctivitis: a systematic review. Allergy 2011;66:919–924.

Prof. Sergio Bonini
Institute of Translational Pharmacology
Italian National Research Council
Via Ugo De Carolis 55
IT–00136 Rome (Italy)
E-Mail se.bonini@gmail.com

Bergmann K-C, Ring J (eds): History of Allergy. Chem Immunol Allergy. Basel, Karger, 2014, vol 100, pp 109–119
DOI: 10.1159/000358616

History of Food Allergy

2

Brunello Wüthrich

Faculty of Medicine, University of Zurich, Zurich, Switzerland

Abstract

In this chapter we will first consider whether there is real evidence on the basis of literature for early descriptions in antiquity of pathogenic reactions after food intake that could be comparable to allergy, for instance in the scriptures of Hippocrates or Lucretius. On this topic we are skeptical, which is in agreement with the medical historian Hans Schadewaldt. We also assert that it is unlikely that King Richard III was the first food-allergic individual in medical literature. Most probably it was not a well-planned poisoning ('allergy') with strawberries, but rather a birth defect ('... his harm was ever such since his birth') that allowed the Lord Protector to bring Mylord of Ely to the scaffold in the Tower, as we can read in *The History of King Richard III* by Thomas More (1478–1535; published by his son-in-law, Rastell, in 1557). In 1912, the American pediatrician Oscar Menderson Schloss (1882–1952) was probably the first to describe scratch tests in the diagnosis of food allergy. Milestones in the practical diagnosis of food allergy are further discussed, including scratch tests, intradermal tests, modified prick tests and prick-to-prick tests. False-negative results can be attributed to the phenomenon of a 'catamnestic reaction' according to Max Werner (1911–1987), or to the fermentative degradation of food products. Prior to the discovery of immunoglobulin E, which marked a turning point in allergy diagnosis, and the introduction of the radioallergosorbent test in 1967, several more or less reliable techniques were used in the diagnosis of food allergy, such as pulse rate increase after food intake according to Coca, the leukopenic index, drop in basophils or drastic platelet decrease. The 'leukocytotoxic test' (Bryan's test), today called the 'ALCAT' test, shows no scientific evidence. The double-blind placebo-controlled food challenge test remains the gold standard in the diagnosis of food allergy. For the future, component-resolved diagnostics with the use of recombinant molecular allergens or chip arrays, such as the ISAC technique, hold a lot of promise. With regard to the clinical situation, a subjective selection is given, touching on the pollen-associated food allergies ('birch-mugwort-celery-spice syndrome'), as well as the new phenomenon of lethal food allergies that have appeared since the 1980s. Finally, rare ways of elicitation of a 'derivative allergy', first described by Erich Fuchs (1921–2008), for example by kissing, as well as 'oral allergy syndrome' and oral hyposensitization are considered.

Food Allergy in Antiquity and the Middle Ages: Myth or Reality?

In classic antiquity the teaching of the four humors led to the term 'idiosyncrasy', which was probably used for unexpected allergic reactions. In this context, Hippocrates and Lucretius are quoted as first descriptors of 'idiosyncratic' reactions to food. This will be briefly discussed here.

Hippocrates (460–375 BC), the father of medicine, is assumed to have given the first description of cheese allergy. In chapter 20 of the *Corpus Hippocraticum* ('About Antique Medicine') from the 5th century BC, we can read, according to Hans Schadewaldt:

> Cheese occasionally could be a 'dangerous food', because it causes discomfort in those who fill themselves with it. [1]

And the following:

> Also wine in high amounts consumed might usually cause complaints. But with the cheese there is the special situation that it causes pain only in certain individuals whose constitution of humors is not compatible with cheese, who so to speak are enemies to cheese.

Unfortunately there is no description of the nature of the complaints suffered by individuals after the consumption of cheese or wine. It is impossible to really evaluate whether these conditions were allergic or due to enzymatic intolerance (lactase deficiency or histamine intolerance). Most likely it was an exaggerated dose that led to the symptoms. The therapy of this condition was clear-cut and effective: 'Don't eat cheese.'

The following often-quoted verse from Titus Lucretius Carus (109–150 BC) is usually taken as the first description of food allergy:

> What is normal food for one, may be strong poison for another one. [2]

However, when we read literally the corresponding verses in his epos *De natura rerum* [3], the quotation is:

> Nunc aliis alius qui sit cibus ut
> videamus expediam, quareve aliis quod
> triste et amarum est; hoc tamen esse
> aliis possit perdulce videri. Tantaque in
> his rebus distantia differitasque est, ut
> quod aliis cibus est aliis fiat acre
> venenum, at capris adipes et
> cocturni cibus auget!

Again, according to Schadewaldt [4], Lucretius made note of an observation that certain animals are able to eat certain weeds without damage to their health, but the same plants are poisonous to other animals. In detail, he describes that hemlock, for example, is a poison for humans, but provides good nutrition for goats and quails, probably due to different enzymatic metabolic processes in different species. Furthermore, Lucretius describes differences in taste between animals and human beings – 'the leaves of olive trees obviously are delicious food for bearded goats, but for humans of utter bitterness':

> Quippe videre licet pinquescere saepe
> cicuta barbigeras pecudes, homini quae
> est acre venenum.

Now we turn to Shakespeare and the character of Richard III, purportedly the first food-allergic individual in medical literature (fig. 1); but what is the truth? We read in act 3, scene 4:

> My lord of Ely, when I was last in
> Holborn I saw good strawberries in your garden there.
> I do beseech you send for some of them.
> Marry and will, my lord, with all my heart.
> Where is my lord the Duke of Gloucester?
> I have sent for these strawberries.

After the herald arrived, the monarch ostentatiously ate one of the strawberries and continued with the trial. One hour later he caused consternation among the assembly of lords when he revealed his arm by pushing back the sleeve of his shirt, and said:

> I pray you all, tell me what they deserve
> That do conspire my death with devilish plots
> Of damned witchcraft, and that have prevail'd
> Upon my body with their hellish charms? ...
> Then be your eyes the witness of their evil.
> Look how I am bewitch'd; behold, mine arm
> Is like a blasted sapling wither'd up.

Obviously, it was not an acute strawberry-induced urticaria that afflicted King Richard III, as we allergists like to claim, but was probably a birth defect that brought Mylord of Ely to the scaffold of the Tower.

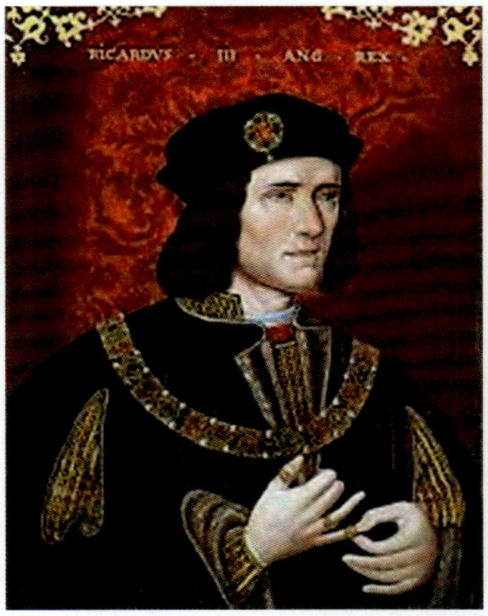

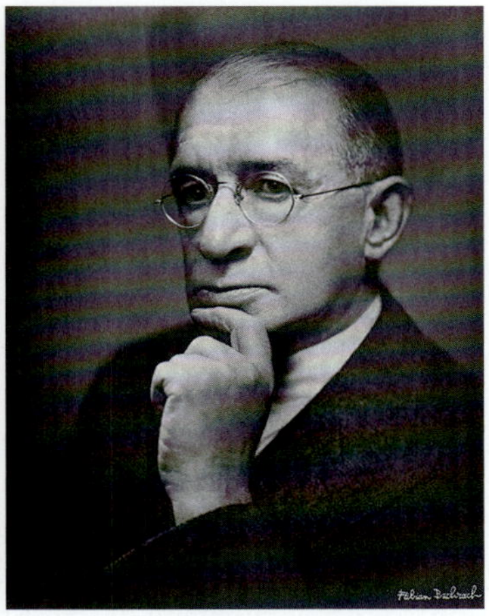

Fig. 1. King Richard III of England (1452–1485). He probably was not the first documented patient with strawberry allergy.
Fig. 2. Oscar Menderson Schloss (1882–1952), the first author to describe the 'scratch test' and the first documented case of food allergy.

First Documentation of Food Allergy – Skin Test as Diagnostic Routine Method

The first scientific report of food allergy can be found from the beginning of the 20th century [5]. In 1912, the American pediatrician Oscar Menderson Schloss [6] (1882–1952; fig. 2) was the first to diagnose food allergy by skin tests. He could prove that a case of allergy was due to the consumption of egg, since a scarification test (scratch test) with hen's egg white was positive. He was also able to test isolated fractions of hen's egg white and to note that ovomucoid apart from ovoglobulin and ovomucin were the strongest elicitors of allergic skin reactions. He also tested oatmeal and almonds. His paper is a milestone in the history of allergy. Following a further publication [7], the scratch test, which was originally introduced by Blackley in 1873 for the detection of pollen allergy [5], became the routine method in the diagnosis of food allergy.

In 1908, Mendel and Mantoux introduced the intradermal test as a tuberculin test, which was then used by Cooke and van der Veer in 1916 for testing aeroallergens [5]. With this method, Karl Prausnitz (1876–1963) and Heinz Küstner (1897–1963) succeeded in passively transferring fish allergy using the serum of an allergic individual [8]. Soon it became apparent that intradermal tests with foods could be false negative, either with exclusively gastrointestinal symptoms because the skin was not the 'shock organ', or because the relevant allergens were denatured during the extract production. Some authors mentioned that fermentative metabolites could have sensitizing properties [9–11]. The observation of Max Werner (1911–1987) is of interest when he stated a 'catamnestic skin reaction' [12] where intradermal tests with food allergens only became positive after a 10- to 14-day elimination diet, an observation which was confirmed by other authors [13].

The modified prick test was developed by Helmtraut Ebruster and published in 1959 in relation to aeroallergens [14]. Using the knowledge of the 1970s that skin tests with commercial extracts from foods and vegetables often yielded false-negative results, in the examination of these allergens the prick-to-prick test method was increasingly used besides scratch tests with native material [15, 16]. The test needle was first pricked into the fresh fruit or vegetable and then pricked into the skin of the patient (fig. 3).

Other Test Methods for Food Allergy Prior to the Discovery of Immunoglobulin E

Since cutaneous testing with food allergens often remained unreliable (either false negative or false positive), besides attempts at re-exposure, other test methods were employed. However, these were also not totally reliable. Examples include the increase in pulse rate according to Coca after food exposure

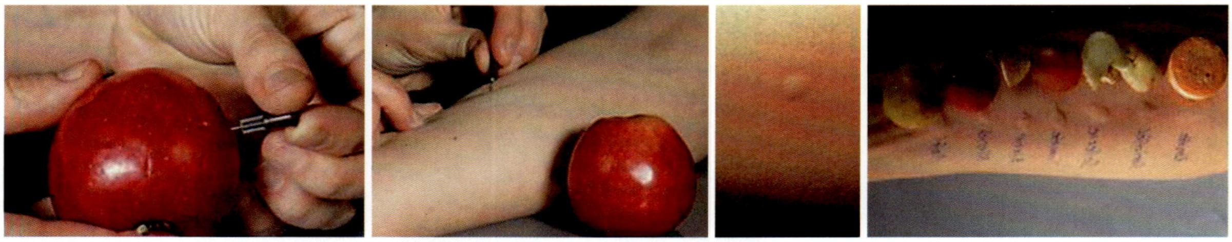

Fig. 3. Prick-to-prick tests with raw apples and vegetables.

[17], the leukopenic index [18], drop in basophil leukocytes [19], the platelet drop [20, 21] and – in patients with exclusively gastrointestinal symptoms – complex exposure tests at the small intestine [22]. At the end of the 1950s, Black and Bryan developed a leukocytotoxic test (Bryan's test) for the detection of allergies against foods and additives based on the microscopic evaluation of activation-induced alterations or autolysis of leukocytes after adding food or food extracts to the blood. This test was not registered for proving allergies in the USA because of unreliability [23, 24]. The ALCAT test (antigen leukocyte cellular antibody test) or leukocyte activation test, which even nowadays is still advertised as a diagnostic method for qualitative determination of food intolerances, is nothing more than a modified Bryan test. Many national and international societies state that this test cannot be used in the diagnosis of food allergy [25, 26].

Radioallergosorbent Test – Significant Progress in the Diagnosis of Immunoglobulin E-Mediated Food Allergies

The discovery of immunoglobulin (Ig) E as a new class of immunoglobulins with reagin activity and the development of sensitive and quantitative in vitro methods like the radioimmunosorbent test for the determination of total serum IgE [27], or the radioallergosorbent test (RAST) for detection of circulating antibodies with IgE specificity [28], without doubt represents a major advancement in allergy diagnosis, including food allergy. By using highly purified cod fish allergen extracts in children with allergic symptoms after fish consumption, 100% concordance between history, RAST and skin test was found [29]. The spectrum of available food species for IgE determination was gradually extended; however, it was also recognized that the diagnostic reliability of RAST as a skin test is limited. Positive IgE detection only measures sensitization against the food, but does not prove clinical relevance, indicating the occurrence of allergy symptoms after exposure. In contrast, the lack of detection of serum IgE antibodies against foods by RAST or other modified in vitro techniques, such as the ImmunoCAP FEIA (fluor enzyme immunoassay), cannot exclude a certain kind of food as the cause of the elicitation of symptoms. Many food extracts are poorly standardized. Degradation of allergenic proteins during the extraction process represents a common phenomenon, resulting in too low concentrations of allergens in the final extracts. On the other hand, similar molecular structures in foods and aeroallergens (pollen, house dust mite, latex, etc.) give rise to multiple positive results in skin tests and RASTs due to cross-reacting IgE antibodies [30].

Component-Resolved Diagnostic Techniques

A new promising strategy to distinguish cross-reactions from genuine co-sensitizations as possible therapeutic consequences can be seen in the use of recombinant allergens which are already available for the ImmunoCAP System (Phadia, Thermo Fisher, Uppsala, Sweden). The component-resolved diagnostics, namely the detection of the specific IgE against molecular marker proteins within foods, is able to distinguish relevant from irrelevant sensitizations [31]. At the same time, allergologic research in recent decades has identified marker allergens for certain disease conditions, respective of clinical symptoms, for example wheat-dependent exercise-induced anaphylaxis (WDEIA) with s-IgE against rTri-α-omega-5-gliadin. With the immuno solid-phase allergen chip (ISAC), we now have a test system for in vitro diagnosis that allows the analysis of a large number of allergen components in a single step. Using the ISAC technology, many relevant allergy elicitors can be measured in one analysis with a rather small volume of patient serum [32]. Due to the magnitude of the results and relatively high costs, the ISAC test should only be used by allergists or physicians with special knowledge in the field.

Double-Blind Placebo-Controlled Food Challenge – The Gold Standard and the Diagnosis of Food Allergy

Oral provocation tests are often the last diagnostic opportunity to detect actual food allergy or intolerance. The so-called double-blind placebo-controlled food challenge (DBPCFC) is regarded as the only scientifically accepted detection method of food allergy or intolerance [30]. Even if the DBPCFC is the gold standard of clinical studies, this procedure is rather complex for routine diagnosis and only used in special allergy centers since provocation tests can always implicitly lead to generalized anaphylactic reactions.

Fatal Food Allergies

A fatal reaction after a food challenge was published in 1926 [33]: an 18-month-old infant with atopic eczema and three episodes of generalized allergic reaction after the consumption of a few spoons of pease pudding was tested under in-patient conditions at a pediatric hospital during the lunch break when the head nurse gave a carrot/pea mixture to the infant. Immediately after the application the child developed angioedema, cyanosis and shock, and died in spite of intensive emergency treatment. The first case of a spontaneous fatal allergic food reaction was published 25 years ago [34]. A 24-year-old female patient with peanut allergy died after eating a cake. The Canadian patient had repeatedly eaten and tolerated hazelnut cake with marzipan and almond icing. However, a short time after eating a few bites of the cake she suddenly developed a severe allergic reaction leading to suffocation and death. The forensic autopsy of this extraordinary case revealed that the paste used for the icing of the cake contained 'arachides', a name for peanuts that was not known to the English-speaking baker.

Fatal or potentially fatal or life-threatening allergic reactions to foods in infants and children are unfortunately no rarity any more, especially in adolescents and young adults. Since the end of the 1990s, a series of fatal cases have been published in the USA, mostly after exposure to hidden food allergens, commonly peanuts, but also other tree nuts, Brazil nut and cashew nut, and also cow's milk, hen's egg, fish and crustacea (lobster, crabs) [35–37]. The lay press regularly reports such fatalities [38]. It is estimated that in the USA approximately 120 fatal cases occur each year due to anaphylactic reactions against foods. Hidden allergens, for example peanut allergens in sweets or chocolate, often make avoidance strategies difficult or impossible in spite of improved declaration rules.

Pollen-Associated Food Allergies and the 'Oral Allergy Syndrome'

At the end of the 1970s, Scandinavian allergists reported that 30–50% of patients with pollinosis against birch, hazel or alder pollen suffer from untoward symptoms like itch in the lips or the palate after eating raw apples. Similar symptoms were reported after consumption of other fruits, raw carrots or celery [39, 40]. A sensitization was proven by scratch or prick-to-prick tests with fresh materials [15, 16, 40, 41]. The most common symptoms in this oral 'contact urticaria syndrome' [42] or 'oral allergy syndrome' [43, 44] often start immediately after contact with certain foods, especially apples, raw vegetables, celery, nuts, hazel nuts and almonds. They are not necessarily only itch or swelling of the lips and tongue, or in the cavum oris or the palate, but can also be hoarseness due to discrete laryngeal edema, difficulties in swallowing and dyspnea. Furthermore, sneezing, rhinorrhea, obstruction of the nose ventilation and conjunctivitis can be observed.

Classical immediate symptoms of gastrointestinal food allergy like gastric cramps, vomitus, nausea, abdominal pain, colic or diarrhea are rare in patients with oral allergy syndrome [13, 45]. Recent investigations using molecular allergens in patients with oral allergy syndrome showed that a sensitization to birch pollen often reflects the thermolabile major antigen Bet v 1 [46, 47]. Birch pollen-associated food allergy has been shown to occur in 40–93% of birch pollen-allergic individuals in various studies.

At the beginning of the 1980s, several authors from Finland [45], Sweden [48], Germany [49], Austria [50], France [51, 52] and Switzerland [13, 53] independently reported anaphylactic reactions or shock fragments after the consumption of celery in association with birch, mugwort pollen or spice allergy. The term, 'celery-mugwort-spice syndrome' or 'celery-carrot-mugwort-spice syndrome' was proposed [53–56]. It was stressed that in these patients the consumption of celery root (celeriac), either boiled, raw or used as a spice in soups, was able to elicit severe reactions in contrast to cases of birch pollen-associated celery allergy, in which only raw celery, and not cooked celery, induced symptoms, mainly oral allergy syndrome. The first publication of a celery allergy comes from Zurich [57] and was proven for the first time using DBPCFC in 2000 [58]. In 1926, Werner Jadassohn and Margarete Zaruski described a young woman who developed urticaria, dyspnea and fever at three different times after eating celery. Other 'idiosyncrasies' were unknown, except for a mild hay fever [57]. After application of celery juice to the skin treated with abrasive paper or scratching, wheals with red flares occurred, while the application of the same celery juice to healthy skin did not induce reactions. The allergen was regarded as 'coctostabile' since the affect was not diminished after 5 min of boiling. The pellets developed during boiling and dialysis were as effective in the skin test as the supernatants. According to Prausnitz and Küstner the transfer was positive in 18 out of 20 volunteers, including with celery dialysate, while when the serum was heated for over half an hour to 56°C the sensitizing properties were lost. The authors postulated that: 'our antigen most likely is not a protein and probably not a very high molecular substance and that the substance apiol from celery is not the urticariogenic substance, because it did not yield any reaction.'

While the first botanic taxonomical associations with Rosaceae (the rose family) and Apiaceae (or Umbelliferae; known as carrot or parsley family) were suspected, it soon became apparent that several allergens, especially Bet v 1 and Bet v 2 (profilin), in birch pollen were responsible for these cross-reactivities [59–61] (fig. 4). The thermostable allergen in mugwort pollen and celery is yet to be identified; however, a lipid-transfer protein is most likely [62].

'Derivative Allergy' – A Rare Pathway of Elicitation of Food Allergy

The elicitation of food allergy via a mediator in the form of a second person (mother, partner) was described as the phenomenon of 'derivative allergy' in 1954 by Erich Fuchs [63]. The first report of a kiss-induced oral allergy syndrome described a birch pollen-allergic woman who developed symptoms after kissing her boyfriend, who had eaten an apple. An even more severe reaction occurred in a highly sensitized peanut-allergic man after kissing his girlfriend, who again had eaten a few peanuts 2 h previously [55, 64–68]. In one case it was possible to use the saliva of a man, who had eaten a suspected fruit, to elicit positive skin prick tests in his birch and grass pollen-allergic girlfriend, but only when the saliva was used within 5 min after the consumption of the fruit (e.g. kiwi), probably due to the instability of the birch pollen cross-reactive kiwi allergen [66]. This phenomenon is not at all rare: out of 379 allergic individuals with severe life-threatening reactions to peanuts and tree nuts, 20 (5.3%, 4 males, 16 females) reported to have suffered from a reaction after kissing. The symptoms ranged from oral allergy syndrome, lip swelling, massive angioedema and lid swelling to dyspnea with expiratory wheezing in 4 cases [68]. In most cases the symptoms occurred between less than 1 min and 30 min after the kiss, but occasionally also after some hours (indicating the stability of peanut and tree nut allergens). Recently, the media reported a fatal anaphylaxis in a 15-year-old Canadian girl with severe peanut allergy after kissing a friend who had eaten a peanut butter sand-

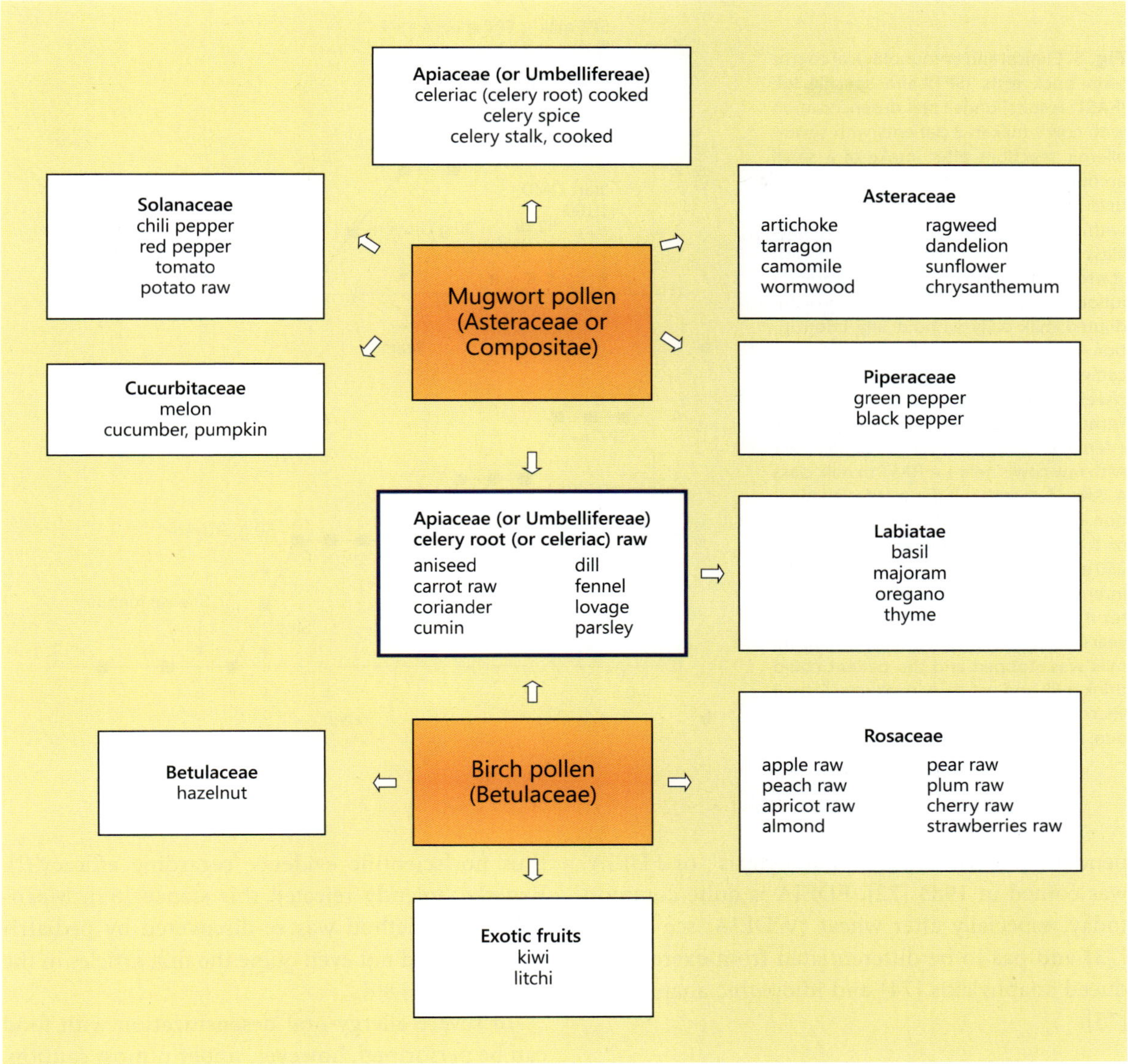

Fig. 4. Birch and mugwort pollen-associated food allergy.

wich [69]. Also, a case of food allergy elicited by sexual intercourse was reported as 'connubial allergy' [70]. The eliciting allergen was from Brazil nuts which had been eaten by a man prior to intercourse with his girlfriend, who was severely allergic to nuts. Prick tests with sperm were negative before and positive after Brazil nut consumption. Thus, foods eaten by other persons can endanger the life or the quality of life of food-allergic individuals.

Food-Induced/Food-Dependent Exercise-Induced Anaphylaxis

In 1979, American authors observed a phenomenon in which an allergic sensitization was elicited in a marathon runner only after the concomitant exposure of physical exercise and food, while exercise alone or consumption of the food alone were each tolerated without reaction [71]. The term 'food-de-

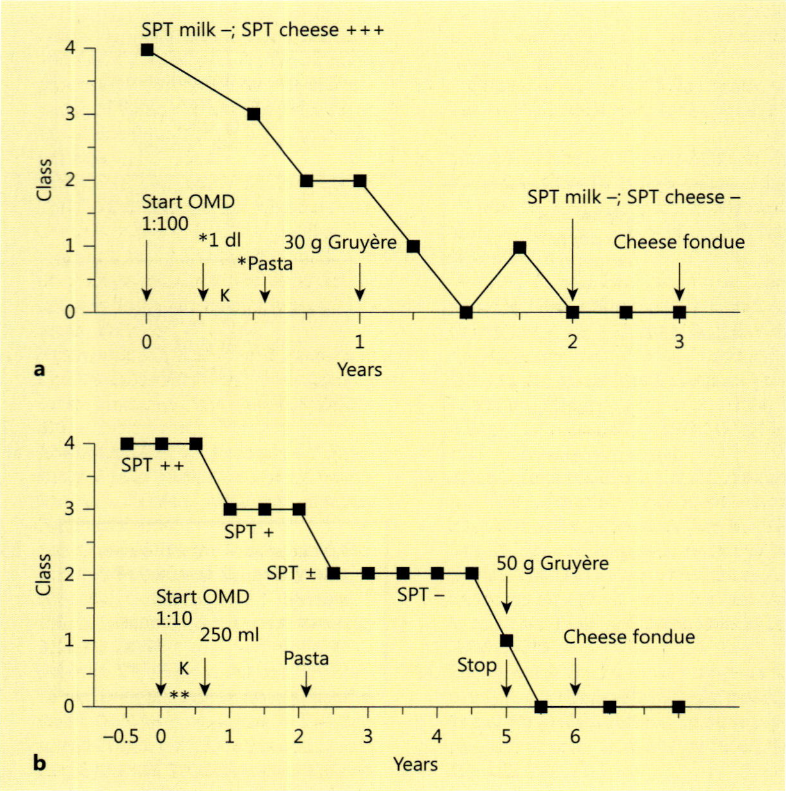

Fig. 5. Clinical and immunological course [skin prick tests (SPT) and specific IgE (RAST) results] under oral desensitization with cow's milk in 2 patients with severe allergic reactions after intake of a small amount of cheese or hidden diary products. **a** Case 1, 29-year-old female: SPT with cheese (Gruyère) +++; RAST to milk class 4. Oral milk desensitization (OMD) started with a drop of 1:100 milk:water dilution, increasing the dose to 250 ml of undiluted milk daily without any interruption. After 2 years the SPT and RAST became negative and the patient could eat a cheese fondue and other dairy products without any problems. * = Dyspnea, eyelid edema. **b** Case 2, 45-year-old female: SPT with raw cow's milk ++; RAST to milk class 4. After 6 months under a strict elimination diet, OMD was started with a drop of 1:10 milk:water dilution, increasing to 250 ml of undiluted milk daily without any interruption. The SPT became negative after 4 years, and the RAST only after 5.5 years, so that the daily intake of 250 ml milk was stopped and the patient could drink milk and eat dairy products. After 6 years, the patient could eat a cheese fondue. ** = Urticaria, cramps; K = ketotifen.

pendent exercise-induced anaphylaxis', or FDEIA, was coined in 1983 [72]. FDEIA is quite common today, especially after wheat (WDEIA; see above) [73] and has to be differentiated from exercise-induced anaphylaxis [74] and idiopathic anaphylaxis [75].

Oral Desensitization – Long Controversial, but Now Established

On several occasions since the 1980s we have published, initially in the German literature [13, 76–79] and later in international medical literature [80, 81], the possibility of oral desensitization in food allergy, especially with untreated cow's milk. Some authors have repeated our results [82–84]. However, the European Academy of Allergy and Clinical Immunology, EAACI, did not accept this technique, since there were no placebo-controlled studies and thus no 'scientific evidence regarding efficacy'(!). Experts violently rejected this stance [85]. Meanwhile, the method was re-discovered by pediatricians who did not even quote the first articles in the literature [86–89].

In severe allergy oral desensitization with food can be performed, however, under utmost caution: the treatment has to be started with adequate dilutions of the allergen and under emergency conditions. Lack of success may be explained by very low tolerance thresholds on the one hand, or a too rapid increase on the other hand. After reaching the maintenance dose it is important that the tolerated food is consumed every day since even short intervals can break the tolerance. This first phase may be called tolerance induction; the later application over months or years then leads to true desensitization and can be proven in negative test results in skin tests and RAST against milk proteins such as casein (fig. 5). In a series of 16 patients with IgE-mediated cow's milk allergy, in 50% of cases complete tolerance to cow's milk and cheese was induced after a 3- to 5-year treatment program [80]. In 4 patients (25%) partial tolerance could be induced; these patients were able to consume at least 1 dl of cow's milk every day together with some cheese, but not hard cheese. In 4 patients (25%) oral hypersensitization had to be stopped because of repeated allergic reactions occurring even with low doses and concomitant therapy with antihistamines or ketotifen [80].

Acknowledgement

I would like to thank Johannes Ring for the English translation.

2

References

1 Schadewaldt H: Magen-Darmallergie; in Schadewaldt H (ed): Geschichte der Allergie. Deisenhofen, Dustri, 1983, vol 4, pp 37–51.

2 Panzani R: Cypress and food allergy: was it suspected in antiquity? J Asthma 1985;22; 223–226.

3 Lucretius TC: De natura rerum; in Güthling O (ed): Von der Natur der Dinge, ed 2, revised. Leipzig, Reclam, 1927.

4 Schadewaldt H: Geschichte der Allergie. Deisenhofen, Dustri, 1983, vol 1, p 22.

5 Schadewaldt H: Geschichte der Allergie. Deisenhofen, Dustri, 1983, vol 1, pp 403–404.

6 Schloss O: A case of food allergy. Idiosyncrasy to eggs, almonds and oats, due to anaphylaxis. Arch Paediat 1912;29:219.

7 Schloss OM: Allergy to common food. Arch Paediat 1915;32:349.

8 Prausnitz K, Küstner H: Studien über die Überempfindlichkeit. Zbl Bakt 1921;86: 160.

9 Cooke RA: Protein derivatives as factors in allergy. Ann Int Med 1942;16:71.

10 Blamoutier P: Allergie digestive: sensibilisation à un produit de désintégration de la protéine alimentaire. Presse Méd 1945;53: 162.

11 Wüthrich B, Schwarz-Speck M: Milch- und Hühnerei-Eiweiss-Allergie: Ausfall der Hautteste mit Gesamtextrakten und mit Hydrolysaten. Dermatologica 1970;141: 102–112.

12 Werner M: Über die katamnestische Hautreaktion. Acta Allergol 1959;14:51–65.

13 Wüthrich B: Nahrungsmittelallergie. Allergologie 1981;4:320–328.

14 Bergmann KC, Aberer W: Aus der Geschichte der Allergologie: Frau Helmtraut Ebruster – die vergessene Autorin des modifizierten Pricktests. Allergologie 2011; 34:599–600.

15 Storck H, Wüthrich B: Allergie-Diagnostik (in vivo) bei allergischen Erkrankungen der Haut und innerer Organe; in Braun-Falco O, Marghescu S (eds): Fortschritte der praktischen Dermatologie und Venerologie. Berlin, Springer, 1976, vol 8, pp 99–107.

16 Wüthrich B: Allergologische Diagnostik bei atopischen Erkrankungen; in Braun-Falco O, Burg G (eds): Fortschritte der praktischen Dermatologie und Venerologie. Berlin, Springer, 1983, vol 10, pp 112–120.

17 Coca AF: Familial Nonreaginic Food Allergy. Springfield, Thomas, 1945.

18 Vaughan WT: Food allergens. 3. The leukopenic index. J Allergy 1934;5:601.

19 Juhlin J, Westphal O: Degranulation of basophil leukocytes in a case of milk allergy. Acta Derm Venereol 1962;42:273.

20 Storck H, Hoigné R, Koller F: Thrombozytenabfall als Hilfsmittel zur Allergiediagnose; in Grumbach AS, Rivkine A (eds): First International Congress for Allergy. Basel, Karger, 1952, pp 739–744.

21 Much T, Wüthrich B: Erfahrungen mit dem Thrombozytopenietest in der spezifischen Diagnostik der Nahrungsmittel-Allergie. Schweiz Med Wochenschr 1977;107:267–271.

22 Werner M: Der intestinale Expositionstest bei Nahrungsmittelallergien. Internist 1960;1:202.

23 American Academy of Allergy: Position statements – controversial techniques. J Allergy Clin Immunol 1981;67:333–338.

24 New York Academy of Medicine Committee on Public Health: Statement on cytotoxic testing for food allergy (Bryan's test). Bull NY Acad Med 1988;64:117–119.

25 Ortolani C, Bruijnzeel-Koomen C, Bengtsson U, Bindslev-Jensen C, Björkstén B, Host A, Ispano M, Jarish R, Madsen C, Nekam K, Paganelli R, Poulsen LK, Wüthrich B: Controversial aspects of adverse reactions to food. Allergy 1999;54:27–45.

26 Wüthrich B: Unproven techniques in allergy diagnosis. J Invest Allergol Clin Immunol 2005;15:86–90.

27 Johansson SGO, Bennich H, Wide L: A new class of immunoglobulin in human serum. Immunology 1968;14:265–272.

28 Wide L, Bennich H, Johansson SGO: Diagnosis of allergy by an in vitro test for allergen antibodies. Lancet 1967;ii:1105–1107.

29 Aas K, Lundvist U: The radioallergosorbent test with a purified allergen from cod fish. Clin Allergy 1973;3:255.

30 Bruijnzeel-Koomen C, Ortolani C, Aas K, Bindslev-Jensen C, Björstén B, Moneret-Vautrin D, Wüthrich B: Adverse reactions to food. Allergy 1995;50:623–635.

31 Ballmer-Weber BK, Scheurer S, Fritsche P, Enrique E, Cistero-Bahima A, Haase T, Wüthrich B: Component-resolved diagnosis with recombinant allergens in patients with cherry allergy. J Allergy Clin Immunol 2002;110:167–173.

32 Ott H, Baron JM, Heise R, Ocklenburg C, Stanzel S, Merk HF, Niggemann B, Beyer K: Clinical usefulness of microarray-based IgE detection in children with suspected food allergy. Allergy 2008;63:1521–1528.

33 von Stark K: Primäre spezifische Allergie und idiosynkratrischer Schock. Monatsschr Kinderheilkd 1926;32:119–127.

34 Evans S, Skea D, Dolovitch J: Fatal reaction to peanut antigen in almond icing. Can Med Assoc J 1988;139:232–233.

35 Yunginger JW, Sweeney KG, Sturner WQ, Giannandrea LA, Teigland JD: Fatal food-induced anaphylaxis. JAMA 1988;260: 1450–1452.

36 Sampson HA, Mendelson L, Rosen JP: Fatal and near-fatal anaphylactic reactions to food in children and adolescents. N Engl J Med 1992;327:380–384.

37 Wüthrich B: Lethal or life-threatening allergic reactions to food. Invest Allergol Clin Immunol 2000;10:59–65.

38 Wüthrich B: Lethal or life-threatening food anaphylaxis: notes from the 'lay press'. Allergy Clin Immunol Int 2003;15: 175–180.

39 Hannuksela M, Lahti A: Immediate reactions to fruits and vegetables. Contact Dermatitis 1977;3:79–84.
40 Lahti A, Hannuksela M: Hypersensitivity to apple and carrot can be reliably detected with fresh material. Allergy 1978;33:143–146.
41 Kleinhans D: Apfel-Allergie: Vergleichende Hauttestungen mit kommerziellen Testlösungen und der nativen Frucht. Akt Dermatol 1978;4:71–75.
42 Kremser M, Lindemayr W: Zur Häufigkeit sogenannter 'Apfelallergie' ('Apfelkontakt-Urtikariasyndrom') bei Patienten mit Birkenpollenallergie. Z Hautkr 1983;58:543–552.
43 Amlot PL, Kemeny DM, Zachary C, Parkes P, Lessof MH: Oral allergy syndrome (OAS): symptoms of IgE-mediated hypersensitivity to foods. Clin Allergy 1987;17:33–42.
44 Ortolani C, Ispano M, Pastorello E, Bigi A, Ansaloni R: The oral allergy syndrome. Ann Allergy 1988;61:47–52.
45 Kauppinen K, Kousa M, Reunala T: Aromatic plants – a cause of severe attacks of angioedema and urticaria. Contact Dermatitis 1980;6:251–254.
46 Ebner C, Birkner T, Valenta R, Rumpold H, Breitenbach M, Scheiner O, Kraft D: Common epitopes of birch pollen and apples: studies by Western and Northern blot. J Allergy Clin Immunol 1991;88:588–594.
47 Ebner C, Hirschwehr R, Bauer L, Breiteneder H, Valenta R, Ebner H, Kraft D: Identification of allergens in fruits and vegetables: IgE cross-reactivities with the important birch pollen allergens Bet v 1 and Bet v 2 (birch profilin). J Allergy Clin Immunol 1995;95:962–969.
48 Forsbeck M, Ros AM: Anaphylactoid reaction to celery. Contact Dermatitis 1979;5:191.
49 Thiel C, Fuchs E: Über korrelative Beziehungen bei Kräuterpollen- und Gewürzallergenen. Berichtsband. 3. Kölner RAST Symposium. Berlin, Grosse, 1981, pp 178–185.
50 Kremser M, Lindemayer JW: Sellerieallergie (Sellerie-Kontakturtikaria Syndrom) und Zusammenhänge mit Allergien gegen Pflanzenallergene. Wiener Klin Wochenschr 1983;23:838–843.
51 Déchamp C, Michel J, Deviller P, Perrin LF: Anaphylactic shock to celery and sensitization to ragweed and mugwort: crossed or concomitant allergy? (in French). Presse Med 1984;13:871–874.
52 Pauli G, Bessot JC, Dietermann-Molard A, Braun PA, Thierry R: Celery sensitivity: clinical and immunological correlations with pollen allergy. Clin Allergy 1985;15:273–279.
53 Wüthrich B, Hofer T: Nahrungsmittelallergie: das 'Sellerie-Beifuss-Gewürz-Syndrom': Assoziation mit einer Mangofrucht-Allergie? Dtsch Med Wochenschr 1984;109:981–986.
54 Wüthrich B, Dietschi R: Das 'Sellerie-Karotten-Beifuss-Gewürz-Syndrom': Hauttest- und RAST-Ergebnisse. Schweiz Med Wochenschr 1985;115:358–364.
55 Stäger J, Wüthrich B: Association de l'allergie au céleri à l'allergie aux épices. Résultats des RAST aux épices chez des patients présentant une allergie au céleri. Rev Fr Allergol 1987;27:137–141.
56 Wüthrich B, Stäger J, Johansson SGO: Celery allergy associated with birch and mugwort pollinosis. Allergy 1990:45:566–571.
57 Jadassohn W, Zaruski M: Idiosynkrasie gegen Sellerie. Arch Derm Syph 1926;151:93–97.
58 Ballmer-Weber BK, Vieths S, Luttkopf D, Heuschmann P, Wuthrich B: Celery allergy confirmed by double-blind, placebo-controlled food challenge: a clinical study in 32 subjects with a history of adverse reactions to celery root. J Allergy Clin Immunol 2000;106:373–378.
59 Bauer L, Ebner C, Hirschwehr R, Wüthrich B, Pichler W, Fritsch R, Scheiner O, Kraft D: IgE cross-reactivity between birch pollen, mugwort pollen and celery is due to at least three distinct cross-reacting allergens: immunoblot investigation of the birch-mugwort-celery syndrome. Clin Exp Allergy 1996;26:1161–1170.
60 Jensen-Jarolim E, Leitner A, Hirschwehr R, Kraft D, Wüthrich B, Scheiner O, Graf J, Ebner C: Characterization of allergens in Apiaceae spices: anise, fennel, coriander and cumin. Clin Exp Allergy 1997;27:1299–1306.
61 Leitner A, Jensen-Jarolim E, Grimm R, Wüthrich B, Ebner H, Scheiner O, Kraft D, Ebner C: Allergens in pepper and paprika: immunologic investigation of the celery-birch-mugwort-spice syndrome. Allergy 1998;53:36–41.
62 Ballmer-Weber BK, Hoffmann A, Wüthrich B, Lüttkopf D, Pompei C, Wangorsch A, Kästern M, Vieths S: Influence of food processing on the allergenicity of celery: DBPCFC with celery spice and cooked celery in patients with celery allergy. Allergy 2002;57:228–235.
63 Fuchs E: Durch Zwischenträger vermittelte Kontaktallergie: 'derivative Allergie'. Dtsch Med Wochenschr 1954;79:473.
64 Wüthrich B: Oral allergy syndrome to apple after a lover's kiss. Allergy 1997;52:235–236.
65 Wüthrich B, Däscher M, Borelli S: Kiss-induced allergy to peanut. Allergy 2001;56:913.
66 Mancuso G, Berdondini RM: Oral allergy syndrome from kiwi fruit after a lover's kiss. Contact Dermatitis 2001;45:41.
67 Steensma DP: The kiss of death: a severe allergic reaction to a shellfish induced by a good-night kiss. Mayo Clin Proc 2003;78:221–222.
68 Hallett R, Haapanen LA, Teuber SS: Food allergies and kissing. N Engl J Med 2002;346:1833–1834.
69 Boyfriend's kiss causes girl's death: 15-year-old had allergy to the peanut butter he had eaten. Edmonton J, Nov 26, 2005.
70 Bansal AS, Chee R, Nagendran V, Warner A, Hayman G: Dangerous liaison: sexually transmitted allergic reaction to Brazil nuts. J Invest Allergol Clin Immunol 2007;17:189–191.
71 Maulitz RM, Pratt DS, Schocket AL: Exercise-induced anaphylactic reaction to shellfish. J Allergy Clin Immunol 1979;63:433–434.
72 Kidd JM, Cohen SH, Sosman AJ, Find J: Food-dependent exercise-induced anaphylaxis. J Allergy Clin Immunol 1983;71:407–411.
73 Wüthrich B, Hofer T: Nahrungsmittelbedingte, anstrengungsinduzierte Anaphylaxie bei starker Sensibilisierung auf Getreideproteine, insbesondere auf Omega-5-Gliadin, und bei fraglichem Hausstaubmilben-Krustazeen-Syndrom. Allergologie 2010;33:205–210.
74 Sheffer AL, Austen KF: Exercise-induced anaphylaxis. J Allergy Clin Immunol 1984;73:699—703.
75 Lenchner K, Grammer LC: A current review of idiopathic anaphylaxis. Curr Opin Allergy Clin Immunol 2003;3:305–311.
76 Wüthrich B, Hofer T: Nahrungsmittelallergien. 3. Therapie: Eliminationsdiät, symptomatische, medikamentöse Prophylaxe und spezifische Hyposensibilisierung. Schweiz Med Wochenschr 1986;116:1401–1410, 1446–1449.
77 Wüthrich B: Therapie von Nahrungsmittel-Allergien; in Braun-Falco O, Schill WB (eds): Fortschritte der Praktischen Dermatologie und Venerologie. Berlin, Springer, 1987, vol 11, pp 439–440.
78 Wüthrich B: Neuere Aspekte zur Diagnostik und Therapie der Nahrungsmittelallergie. Dargestellt anhand ausgewählter Fallbeispiele von Milchallergie. Allergologie 1987;10:370–376.
79 Wüthrich B, Stäger J: Allergie au lait de vache chez l'adulte et désensibilisation spécifique au lait par voie orale. Méd Hyg 1988;46:1899–1905.

80 Wüthrich B: Oral desensitization with cow's milk in cow's milk allergy. Pro!; in Wüthrich B, Ortolani C (eds): Highlights in Food Allergy. Basel, Karger, 1996, pp 236–240.
81 Bucher C, Wüthrich B: Oral desensitization in cow's milk allergy. Ital J Allergy Clin Immunol 2000;10:119–120.
82 Bauer A, Ekanayake Mudiyanselage S, Wigger-Alberti W, Elsner P: Oral rush desensitisation to milk. Allergy 1999;54:894–895.
83 Patriarca G, Nucera E, Roncallo C, Pollastrini E, Bartolozzi F, De Pasquale T, Buonomo A, Gasbarrini G, Di Campli C, Schiavino D: Oral desensitizing treatment in food allergy: clinical and immunological results. Aliment Pharmacol Ther 2003;17:459–465.
84 Meglio P, Bartone E, Plantamura M, Arabito E, Giampietro PG: A protocol for oral desensitization in children with IgE-mediated cow's milk allergy. Allergy 2004;59:980–987.
85 Bahna SL: Oral desensitization with cow's milk in IgE-mediated cow's milk allergy. Contra!; in Wüthrich B, Ortolani C (eds): Highlights in Food Allergy. Basel, Karger, 1996, pp 233–235.
86 Niggemann B, Staden U, Rolinck-Werninghaus C, Beyer K: Specific oral tolerance induction in food allergy. Allergy 2006;61:808–811.
87 Staden U, Rolinck-Werninghaus C, Brewe F, Wahn U, Niggemann B, Beyer K: Specific oral tolerance induction in food allergy in children: efficacy and clinical patterns of reaction. Allergy 2007;62:1261–1269.
88 Staden U, Blumchen K, Blankenstein N, Dannenberg N, Ulbricht H, Dobberstein K, Ziegert M, Niggemann B, Wahn U, Beyer K: Rush oral immunotherapy in children with persistent cow's milk allergy. J Allergy Clin Immunol 2008;122:418–419.
89 Nowak-Wegrzyn A, Bloom KA, Sicherer SH, Shreffler WG, Noone S, Wanich N, Sampson HA: Tolerance to extensively heated milk in children with cow's milk allergy. J Allergy Clin Immunol 2008;122:342–347.

Prof. em. Dr. med. Brunello Wüthrich
Im Ahorn 18
CH–8125 Zollikerberg (Switzerland)
E-Mail bs.wuethrich@bluewin.ch

Bergmann K-C, Ring J (eds): History of Allergy. Chem Immunol Allergy. Basel, Karger, 2014, vol 100, pp 120–131
DOI: 10.1159/000358617

Drug Hypersensitivity

Andreas J. Bircher

Allergy Unit, Department of Dermatology, University Hospital, Basel, Switzerland

Abstract

Before the arrival of modern pharmacotherapy, drug hypersensitivity reactions were virtually unknown. Toxicity from the many plant-, animal- and inorganic material-derived remedies must have been much more common. One famous example is the intoxications from mercury, which has been used in many ailments, but particularly for the treatment of syphilis. It was only in the 19th century when more and more active principles from e.g. plants were identified, and when the observations of skin reactions became more prevalent. In 1877, Heinrich Köbner used for the first time the term 'drug exanthema' (Arznei-Exanthem). Since then, many different types of exanthemas from the mild macular-papular forms to the severe life-threatening bullous exanthemas such as toxic epidermal necrolysis have been observed from numerous drugs. The systematic investigation of severe drug reactions has only started in the second half of the 20th century, parallel to the increasing knowledge in immunology. Drug hypersensitivity reactions still remain one of the most challenging problems in allergology due to their manifold clinical manifestations and their very diverse pathophysiology. The introduction of new drugs and in turn the emergence of new hypersensitivity reactions will remain a challenge in the future.

Drug Hypersensitivity – The Emergence of New Disorders

Primum non nocere.

Above all, do no harm! This famous aphorism is often attributed to the Hippocratic school based on the statement in the Hippocratic Oath 'to abstain from doing harm' (in Greek: ἐπὶ δηλήσει δὲ καὶ ἀδικίῃ εἴρξειν). It is still valid and often used today. A detailed investigation of its origins was published by Smith [1]. Rather than being of ancient origin as usually assumed, the specific expression, and its even more distinctive associated Latin term, can be more likely traced back to Thomas Sydenham (1624–1689), as mentioned in a book by Thomas Inman (1820–1876). Pharmacotherapy is inherently associated with adverse drug effects and represents a paradigm for this statement.

This review on some historical aspects of drug hypersensitivity is far from complete and contains some personal reflections and points of view. Apart from the early beginnings of drug hypersensitivity, first descriptions of some important drug-induced syndromes and some major drug groups are briefly discussed. Among many articles, it is also based on the indispensable four volumes *Geschichte der Aller-*

gie (History of Allergy) by Hans Schadewaldt [2], and some general books on historical aspects of allergy and medicine.

Drug hypersensitivities have a special significance as they belong to the major iatrogenic diseases [3]. Often, but not always, they are caused by the physician himself or his prescribed medications and frequently feed the immanent fear of patients towards 'chemical agents' and intoxication. They belong to the most complex hypersensitivity disorders based on immunoallergic and non-immunologic mechanisms, appearing with a wide variety of clinical manifestations. This has led to Goldberg's [4] statement that drug reactions have replaced syphilis and tuberculosis as the great imitator of diseases.

Reading through the older literature, it is interesting and astonishing how exact and detailed the clinical descriptions were, often even better and clearer than today with all the diagnostic, technical and imaging possibilities at hand. More than 100 years ago medical doctors were astute observers, had an impressive knowledge on clinical manifestations and, despite limited insights into pathomechanisms, they made observations, drew conclusions and formulated hypotheses that are still valid today.

Terminology – An Ongoing Controversy

This topic is discussed in detail in another chapter of this book [Ring, this vol., pp. 46–52]. Unwanted effects of drugs are generally named adverse drug reactions. They include toxic as well as hypersensitivity reactions and long-term effects, such as carcinomas induced by arsenic. Until today the terminology of allergic reactions and particularly drug hypersensitivity reactions has remained a controversial issue.

When Clemens von Pirquet [5] (1874–1929) coined the term 'allergy', he described a concept of changed or altered reactivity of an organism towards a foreign substance which could include protective immunity as well as hypersensitivity in the current sense [6, 7]. It was only later that the term 'allergy' was applied and limited to hypersensitivity reactions to innocuous agents – the so-called allergens. Recently it has been confined to immunologically mediated reactions, called immunoglobulin (Ig) E-mediated, or non-IgE-mediated mechanisms [8].

The proposal of Coombs and Gell [9] in 1963 was a major step forward into the classification of immunologically mediated reactions [10]. For didactic and clinical purposes it is still in use, although it has been far overtaken by the current knowledge of the immune system. In their fundamental paper on classifications of immunologic reactions they used the concept of von Pirquet [10] and tried in vain to reestablish its original meaning.

Hypersensitivity reactions from drugs, with their diverse pathophysiology and clinical manifestations, have especially led to many different terms that are often used in different ways. 'Idiosyncrasy', the oldest term, goes back to the Hippocratic school and is still used today to describe an individual disposition to develop a particular clinical manifestation, be it based on an enzymatic variation, a particular human leukocyte antigen (HLA) type, or other still unknown causes. 'Pseudoallergy' was coined in 1987 by Kallos and Schlumberger [11] to describe hypersensitivity to acetyl salicylic acid and NSAIDs, a topic also discussed in detail elsewhere. 'Intolerance' has been used for pharmacologically explained toxic drug reactions as well as for drug hypersensitivity with unexplained pathogenesis. The term 'toxicodermia' for drug exanthemas or fixed toxic eruption for fixed drug eruption is also still in use, although an immunological pathomechanism has been elucidated in many instances.

Early History – Poisons and Placebos

> All ding sind gifft und nichts on gifft, alleyn die dosis macht dass eyn ding on gifft ist.
> *Paracelsus* (1493–1541)

Philippus Aureolus Theophrastus Bombastus von Hohenheim, called Paracelsus (1493–1541), is credited as the father of toxicology and modern pharmacotherapy based on his proposal to use not only plant-derived medicine, but also inorganic material, particularly metals [12]. As an alchemist he postulated a theory based on three elements: salt (representing stability), sulfur (representing combustibility) and mercury (representing liquidity).

2

He challenged the generally accepted and still applied humoral theory of Galen on which contemporary medicine was based, and even publicly burned the old textbooks of Galen and Avicenna. Therefore, he had many enemies in the medical establishment. Following an incident, he had to leave Basel clandestinely by night where he had been the municipal physician and a professor at the university [12]. He is credited as being the first to have drawn attention to the relation between dose and toxicity, expressed in his famous proverb: 'All things are poison, and nothing is without poison; only the dose permits something not to be poisonous.' [13]

In previous centuries it was certainly difficult for physicians to distinguish toxic symptoms from hypersensitivity reactions, although the toxicity of many plants, extracts and metals was already known in antiquity. Theophrastus (370–286 BC), influenced by Aristotle, mentioned many poisonous plants in *De Historia Plantarum*. Dioscorides, a Greek physician of the Roman emperor Nero, made the first attempt at classifying poisons into plant, animal and mineral categories in his book *De Materia Medica,* which contains references to some 600 plants [13].

The organic plant-, animal- and even human tissue-derived drugs and inorganic elements used, such as metals, were far from standardized, and inefficacy, overdose and intoxications must have been very common. Astute observers such as William Withering (1741–1799) already recognized the problem of overdosing foxglove extracts:

> When given in very large and quickly repeated doses occasions sickness, vomiting, purging, giddiness, confused vision, objects appearing green and yellow, increased secretion of urine, with frequent motions to part with it, and sometimes inability to retain it, slow pulse, even as slow as 35 in a minute, cold sweats, convulsions, syncope, death. [14]

One of the first observations of an idiosyncratic reaction was mentioned in the 2nd century by an unknown colleague of Galen, describing an unexpected event to a small non-toxic drug dose [2].

Ipecacuanha was recognized in the 16th century as a cause of asthma in pharmacists and may be the first occupational allergen [2]. Jesuit's bark from the cinchona tree was brought back from Peru. It contains alkaloids and quinine, the active principle for treatment of malaria and digestive disorders. The first accounts of eczemas and exanthemas appeared relating to the popular use of topical sulfur and mercury ointments and mercury vapors, particularly in the treatment of syphilis. However, differentiation from toxic effects due to acute or chronic overdose is not always possible [2]. For centuries the symptoms of mercury intoxication were thought to be necessary to treat syphilis; many patients were more likely to die from the remedies than from the disease. The depiction of the physicians in Molière's (1622–1673) 'Le malade imaginaire' and a quotation from Matthew Prior in 1714: 'Yesterday healed from my disease, I died last night from my physician' [15], reflects drastically the contemporary recognition of medical knowledge and proficiency.

19th Century – The Dawn of Drug Hypersensitivity

> … throw out a few specifics which our art did not discover, and it is hardly needed to apply; throw out wine, which is a food, and the vapors which produce the miracle of anaesthesia, … and I firmly believe that if the whole materia medica [medical drugs], as now used, could be sunk to the bottom of the sea, it would be all the better for mankind, – and all the worse for the fishes.
> *Oliver Wendell Holmes Sr.* (1860)

In the 19th century, an empirical approach of pharmacotherapy was still common and the concepts of humoral pathology according to Galen continued to be applied. The recognition of elements as components of all matter was the basis of the isolation and chemical synthesis of drugs, and more and more specific substances were isolated and characterized. This was closely associated with the identification of dyes, which were also able to stain biological tissues. The increasing use and development of germicides resulted from this knowledge, in parallel with the detection of the infectious origin of many diseases. In the first half of the century, among many others, morphine, codeine and salicin from willow, and quinine from cinchona tree bark were isolated [16]. Attempts to synthesize these substances led to the derivatives of the toxic aniline, phenacetin and many other pyrazolones.

Medications that were available encompassed topical ointments, in particular plant-derived drugs, and the first chemically synthesized agents became available. However, they often caused more harm than good. One of the most distinguished critics was Oliver Wendell Holmes, professor at Harvard University and Dartmouth College. His quotation on the uselessness of the contemporary medications became famous, but as he stated himself: 'Some of the old doctors, I fear, never pardoned me for saying that if a ship, loaded with an assorted cargo of the drugs which used to be considered the natural food of sick people, went to the bottom of the sea, it would be all the better for mankind – and all the worse for the fishes.' Holmes was repeatedly attacked by the medical establishment for this statement. However, in the second half of the century continuous progress was made in the detection and on the development of new drugs [16], and also on their drawbacks. As a consequence, observations on new types of skin manifestations became more prevalent. In 1814, Antoine de Montègre reported on the observation of urticaria to Copaiva balm, which eventually led to the term 'urticaria balsamica', coined by Römhild [2], because it was initially thought to be specific for this balm only [17, 18]. In 1792, Dejean reported on 'roses' upon topical application of mercury, and George Alley reported on a vesicular exanthema in a boy [2]. In 1823, Kahleis observed exanthemas, fever and swellings after internal administration of mercury, and in 1827 Ferdinand Ascherson reported urticaria upon topical application of mercury. Von Kussmaul was probably the first to differentiate the symptoms of secondary and tertiary syphilis from the toxic and possibly allergic reaction due to a mercury treatment [2]. A case with a scarlatiniform exanthema (fig. 1) from calomel [mercury(I) chloride] was reported; the patient previously had the same manifestation from mercury pills and upon inhalation of mercury vapors [19].

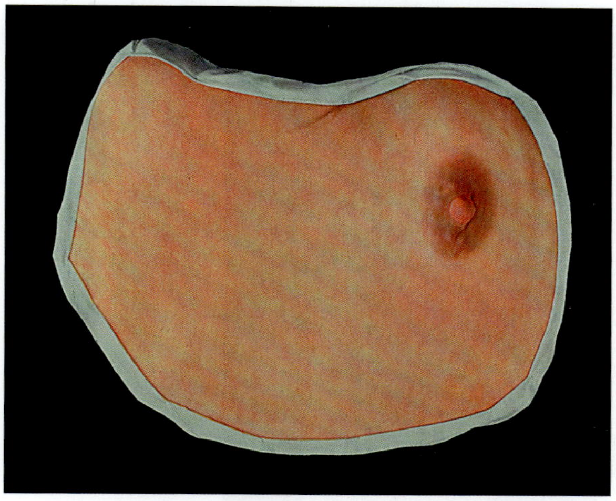

Fig. 1. Mercury exanthema (toxicodermia mercurialis). Mercury was used in ointments for many skin disorders and played an eminent role in the treatment of syphilis, often resulting in toxicity.

Several patients with exanthemas from quinine were independently reported in 1853 by the French investigators Rilliet, Barthez and Briquet; however, they were attributed to underlying typhoid fever. In 1869, Edward Garraway observed an exanthema to quinine, which he thought to be of toxic origin. However, when his patient received a quinine-containing tonic she suffered from the same manifestation. On making the diagnosis herself she told him: 'Oh, You have poisoned me with quinine again.' [2]

In 1877, Heinrich Koebner (1838–1904) published an analysis on drug exanthema from quinine in 2 patients, with a detailed account of the small dose necessary and the faster reappearance at re-exposure [20]. He discussed other cases from the literature and, in detail, the manifestations of erysipelas and scarlet fever, two often confused differential diagnoses. He also mentioned that the appearance was often similar in exanthemas from other drugs, such as chloral hydrate and digitalis, separated toxic effects from this skin manifestation and used the term 'drug exanthema' ('Arznei-Exanthem') for the first time.

In 1879, Gustav Behrend (1847–1925) described a case of exanthema from opium and discussed in detail the possible pathogenesis [17, 18]. He correctly recognized that minute doses may elicit exanthemas, which could vary among individuals. Upon reexposure the exanthema possibly appeared earlier, but was always identical in a given individual. Two similar cases of opium exanthemas were soon thereafter published in the same journal [21].

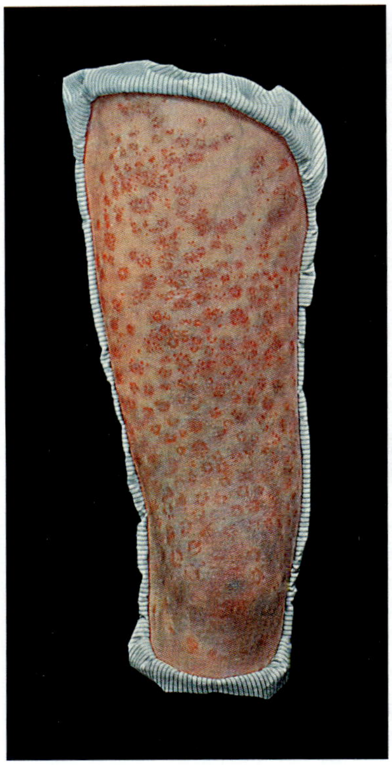

Fig. 2. Exanthema from Copaiva balm (toxicodermia ex usu balsami Copaivae). Copaiva was used to treat gonorrhea.

In a second article [22] he further discussed the clinical diagnosis and evolution of the drug exanthemas, as he now called them, as a distinct entity of skin disorders arising from different drugs, such as Copaiva balm (fig. 2), digitalis, quinine, mercury and opium. He had already mentioned the variable atypical manifestations of drug-induced exanthemas and the reproducibility upon re-exposure. A particular case of an epileptic boy could be the common bromoderma or could represent the description of a fixed drug eruption from potassium bromate. On the lateral leg a livid non-itching plaque of the size of a hand with exudation and crusts was present. After stopping the drug, hyperpigmentation persisted for more than 2 years.

These publications stimulated more reports and studies by Arthur van Harlingens (1845–1936), Prince A. Morrow (1846–1913) and T. Colcott Fox (1848–1916) [14]. Morrow recognized that percutaneous absorption of such drugs as mercury can cause an eruption similar to that seen by ingestion. He pointed out that 'the same eruptive form may be produced by different drugs, and that the same drug may produce a variety of eruptive forms'. However, he brought forward a hypothesis of idiosyncrasy and concluded neuropathic origin [14]. It was already clear that the same drug may cause various manifestations, such as urticaria, anaphylaxis and exanthemas, in different individuals and that the same clinical manifestation may be caused by different drugs.

Drug-Induced Syndromes – The Bad and the Ugly

Drug-induced diseases can mimic practically every naturally occurring clinical disease. At the beginning of the 20th century syphilis was called the great simulator of diseases, so great was its incidence and so manifold its presentations. With the gradual taming of syphilis, tuberculosis took over as the great simulator. Now with the virtual conquest of tuberculosis it would seem that the adverse drug reaction is the great simulator of diseases, a constant threat to the unwary diagnostician. [4]

Maculopapular exanthemas are the most common clinical manifestation of delayed drug hypersensitivity [23, 24]. They represent a differential diagnostic challenge, their severity is usually mild, and morbidity is low. However, there are a few drug-induced syndromes which have a considerable morbidity and mortality. Up to today there is still some controversy concerning the exact definitions and terms. In addition, as was true in this case, drug syndromes are great imitators of other diseases and represent a considerable diagnostic and therapeutic challenge. The other large group of manifestations includes the immediate hypersensitivity reactions angioedema, urticaria, bronchospasm and anaphylaxis. The latter is discussed in detail in another chapter of this book [pp. 54–61].

Stevens-Johnson Syndrome and Toxic Epidermal Necrolysis

The severe bullous disorders Stevens-Johnson syndrome (SJS) and toxic epidermal necrolysis (TEN), or Lyell's syndrome, are the most severe delayed-occurring adverse drug reactions. They represent a continuum of severe to lethal manifestations, mostly dependent on the extent of the epidermolysis and comorbidities [25].

SJS was first described in 1922 in 2 children who presented with 'an extraordinary, generalized eruption with continued fever, inflamed buccal mucosa and severe purulent conjunctivitis' [26]. An association between the development of SJS/TEN and drugs has often been established; however, an association with antecedent infection is less clear, but may be present [25].

A nearly fatal pemphigus-like rash to sulfadiazine involving the eyes and oral mucosa was reported in 1942 in a 10-year-old girl [27]. A fatal case involving sulfadiazine was described in a 20-year-old man. After 10 days of treatment the patient first suffered a morbilliform rash, followed by a pemphigus-like eruption with positive Nikolski's sign, involvement of mucosae and a high fever [28]. In 1948, Ruskin [29] described in detail another fatal case of a fulminating dermatitis bullosa medicamentosa due to methylphenylethyl hydantoin in a 10-year-old girl. Lyell [30] reported on 4 cases and coined the term 'toxic epidermal necrolysis' in 1956. Butazolidin, a pyrazolone, was suspected in a second recurrent case involving Dover's powder containing aspirin. This clinical picture was later referred to as Lyell's syndrome for some time; today the neutral term TEN is preferred.

Staphylococcal toxin-associated variants were later separated. Staphylococcal scalded skin syndrome was identified as the earlier known dermatitis exfoliativa von Rittershain and was attributed to toxin-producing staphylococci [31].

At the beginning of the 1990s, severe erythema multiforme, SJS and TEN were understood to be a continuum of diseases with different severity and extension, ranging from mild forms with typical target lesions to more than 30% detachment of the epidermis. In 1994, five categories were separated to encompass the spectrum of disease [32].

Great progress on the epidemiology and clinical manifestations was made, first when the French dermatologists Jean Revuz and Jean-Claude Roujeau [33, 34] and then German dermatologists on the initiative of Erwin Schöpf started national registries of SJS and TEN, and later also included other severe drug hypersensitivity reactions [35]. Currently there is still some controversy surrounding the classification, and particularly concerning the treatment of these severe adverse drug reactions. There is agreement that erythema multiforme of the major type; SJS and TEN are possibly the milder and more severe variant of a continuum reaction spectrum. Besides a genetic predisposition for some drugs, immunological factors also seem to play a role [36].

2

Ampicillin Rash

All had a discharge diagnosis of infectious mononucleosis. None of these patients had any previously recognized allergy. A characteristic and pruritic skin rash was noted in all those who had received ampicillin for whatever reason. Onset of rash occurred 5 to 8 days after the drug was started.

This is an excerpt of the description of the typical exanthema from aminopenicillins in patients with acute EBV infections made and published by a carefully observing pediatric resident in 1967 [37]. It was probably the first time that the association of a viral infection and an exanthema from a drug was made.

Today it is known that some of these patients later tolerate amoxicillin whereas others have become apparently sensitized during the acute illness [38]. This should be ruled out by a complete allergological work-up.

Drug Hypersensitivity Syndrome

Meritt and Putnam are credited with first reporting the drug hypersensitivity syndrome (DHS) in 1938. They published a large series of patients treated with phenytoin. Besides mild morbilliform eruptions that healed when phenytoin was withdrawn, more severe febrile exanthemas were also observed. Their patient had no other systemic symptoms and no blood changes. His nephropathy could have been due to a severe hypertension. He was later treated without problems with phenobarbital, a potentially cross-reactive drug [39]. Chaiken et al. [40] described the systemic implications with lymphadenopathy and multivisceral involvement, such as hepatitis. Many reports followed, particularly for anticonvulsants, sulfonamides and later also allopurinol, and most recently abacavir and nevirapine [41]. The terminology included DHS and often the name of the eliciting drug, such as phenytoin or allopurinol hypersensitivity syndrome. Many cases may have been reported under other terms, e.g. when hepatitis was a more prominent feature than the skin eruption or eosinophilia.

Since the early 1940s, drug eruptions from hydantoin and derivatives imitating lymphoma have been reported. In 1959, Saltzstein [42] discussed the literature and reported 7 additional cases of lymphadenopathy induced by anticonvulsant drugs. Of these patients, 4 had cutaneous eruption, fever and eosinophilia associated with lymphadenopathy; the other 3 had lymphadenopathy with a mild eosinophilia and, in 1 case, hepatosplenomegaly. The histology of the lymph nodes showed a lymphoma-like pattern, therefore the term 'pseudolymphoma' was used because with cessation of therapy there was remission of all symptoms.

Bocquet et al. [43] were the first to separate pseudolymphoma from the DHS, and proposed the acronym DRESS (drug rash with eosinophilia and systemic symptoms) for the latter.

Currently there is still some controversy surrounding the terminology DHS, DRESS and drug-induced hypersensitivity syndrome. Less controversial is the emerging role of viruses, particularly from the herpes group. Initially thought to be reactivated during the inflammatory process they seem to play an important pathophysiological role in this syndrome [41]. Patel [37] made an important contribution when he first reported Epstein-Barr virus-associated exanthemas from antibiotics.

Acute Generalized Exanthematous Pustulosis

In 1968, Baker and Ryan [44] reported on 104 patients with pustular psoriasis. Five patients without a previous history of psoriasis had an acute transient pustular eruption in which drugs or infections were suspected as the trigger. The term exanthematic pustular psoriasis was proposed for this subgroup [45]. Later terms like pustular drug rash [46] or toxic pustuloderma [47] were used for patients with such drug-induced pustular diseases. The term 'pustulose exanthématique aiguë généralisée' was first coined in 1980 in the French literature by Beylot et al. [48], and found its way into the English literature as acute generalized exanthematous pustulosis [49]. It is a morphological reaction pattern – mainly caused by drugs, rarely from viral infections – whose hallmark is the occurrence of a highly febrile disseminated non-follicular pustular rash.

Hoigné Syndrome

The first descriptions of Hoigné syndrome date back to 1951, including 8 cases receiving higher doses of procaine penicillin and presenting only emotional symptoms without signs of anaphylaxis [50]. Five of them received the same drug again without reactions, indicating an accidental intravascular injection. In 1959, Hoigné and Schoch [51] and Hoigné and Krebs [52] meticulously described particular symptoms upon the injection of procaine penicillins. They separated these from anaphylactic reactions based on a different symptomatology and time pattern. Symptoms mostly include neuropsychiatric signs such as dizziness, vision and hearing disturbances, and feeling of impending doom [52]. Currently, Hoigné's syndrome is considered a pseudoanaphylactic or pseudoallergic reaction following intramuscular and intravenous aqueous procaine penicillin administration. This disorder is characterized predominantly by neuropsychiatric alterations, including severe psychomotor agitation with confusion, sensations of disintegration, perceived changes of body shape, visual and auditory hallucinations, panic-like anxiety, including fear of death, as well as alterations of consciousness and seizures. Beside the 'classic' immediate manifestation of Hoigné's syndrome, subacute forms as well as reactions of the so-called latent type are also known [53]. The pathogenesis is thought to be embolic-toxic reaction or a form of kindling phenomenon in the limbic system. The

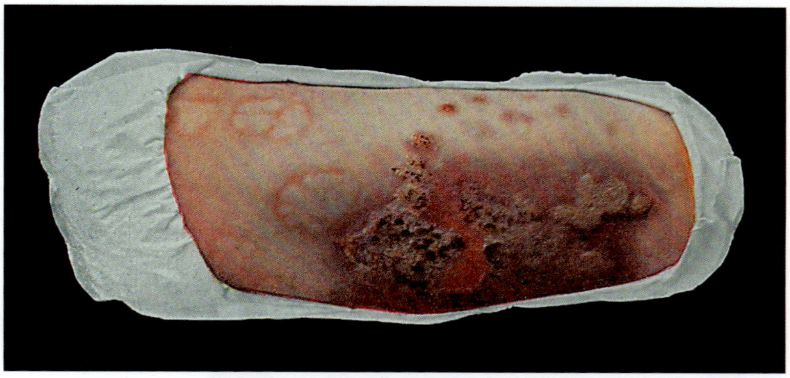

Fig. 3. Tuberous bromoderma (toxicodermia ex usu bromi). Bromine was used in the treatment of epilepsy.

differentiation from anaphylaxis is justified because it allows the treatment of the patient with penicillin again, whereas in the case of anaphylaxis this is contraindicated [54].

Selected Drugs

Wo viel Licht ist, ist starker Schatten
[Where there is light, there is also shadow].
From Götz von Berlichingen, J.W. Goethe

Although modern pharmacotherapy has become much safer, it is still inherently associated with adverse effects. In former times with less knowledge on pharmacokinetics and dynamics, problems arising from drugs were undoubtedly much more common. Particularly the toxic effects must have presented a considerable portion of adverse drug reactions. The recognition of the often new, previously unseen hypersensitivity manifestations was certainly a challenge for the physicians and may often have not been recognized. In the following sections a selected number of drugs are briefly reviewed.

Halogenated Drugs – Iodine and Bromides

The halogens iodine and bromine were used in different compositions in the treatment of syphilis and epilepsy, and caused the often very extensive fungating granulomas (fig. 3) called tuberous iododerma and bromoderma [14]. Today these reactions are rarely seen in patients with renal insufficiency receiving high doses of iodinated contrast media. However, exanthemas to iodoform have also already been reported [55]. Bruck had thought that he had achieved passive transfer of this idiosyncratic reaction. However, Bruno Bloch, at that time head of the Dermatology Section at Basel University, Switzerland, was unable to demonstrate passive transfer by serum, and postulated a cell-bound reaction. He demonstrated later by patch tests and careful observations that the idiosyncrasy to iodine was a cellular phenomenon. He also described that the reactivity was dependent on methane groups, a view that was later disproved [56].

Analgesics

The first analgesic and antipyretic drugs were actually byproducts of the industry and were based on aniline. One of the first was called 'antipyrine'; however, it caused quite severe gastric irritations [57]. Thereafter, acetanilide was detected to have antipyretic qualities and was introduced as 'antifebrine'. When phenacetin was produced again from a byproduct of the dye industry in 1888 it was one of the first big successes of drug marketing. These pyrazolones caused not only gastric irritation, but also idiosyncratic reactions such as urticarial exanthemas and the unusual fixed drug eruptions (fig. 4). By 1853, it had been reported that ace-

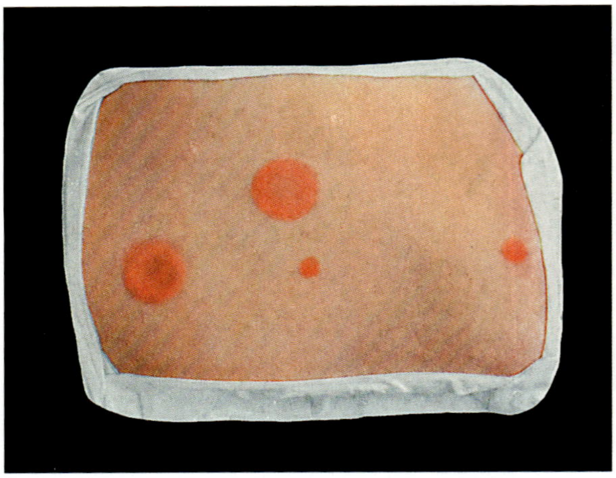

Fig. 4. Fixed drug eruption from Antipyrine® (phenazone; toxicodermia ex usu Antipyrini). Antipyrin was used as an antipyretic and analgetic drug.

tyl salicylic acid was less irritating for the gastric mucosa than salicylic acid. It was Felix Hoffmann at Bayer who found an easy way of producing acetyl salicylic acid. In 1899, it was introduced onto the market under the name Aspirin and became one of the most successful drugs. It took, however, another 60 years until its mechanism of action was identified. Soon thereafter, in 1902, the first report of an idiosyncrasy was published by Geheimer Sanitätsrat V.G.S. Hirschfeld. About 3 h after one grain of aspirin, a male patient developed angioedema of the face and throat and few urticarial lesions on the upper trunk and the leg [58, 59]. In 1922, Fernand Widal et al. [60] published their landmark paper 'Anaphylaxie et idiosyncrasie' [61]. It describes the complex case of a 37-year-old female with chronic urticaria triggered by cold, and later rhinitis associated with nasal polyps and asthma episodes. She had acute urticaria after about 11 years and upon provocation also asthma to Aspirin and Antipyrine® (phenazone). Interestingly, Pyramidone® (aminophenazone), quinine and other drugs were tolerated. She was finally successfully desensitized with aspirin.

Bruno Bloch, who was by that time director of the dermatology clinic in Zurich, often used an analgesic drug (Allonal®, containing aprobarbital and amidopyrine) in patients being treated with Salvarsan® for syphilis in order to ameliorate fever and headaches [62]. He also used the drug quite often himself. Recurrent neutropenia was detected on one occasion; however, no link was made to the drug. It was only after he died in 1933 from the consequences of agranulocytosis that the first description of this severe adverse effect was published [63] – unfortunately too late to save his life [Michael Geiges, Zurich, pers. commun.].

Salvarsan

Salvarsan was the first anti-infectious drug, which was developed based on the concept of the chemical reactivity of dyes followed by numerous experimental trials. The development took many years based on the previous work of Paul Ehrlich, whose knowledge of dyes by using them in histology resulted in the concept of using them to destroy microorganisms. In 1913, it was applied in syphilis as the first chemotherapeutic agent. However, Salvarsan had many adverse effects, many of which were toxic, including urticaria, dermatitis and toxic erythema.

Anticonvulsants

In 1916, ethylphenylhydantoin (Nirvanol) was introduced in the treatment of chorea minor. In 1926, Bernhard D. Rütter [2] first described peripheral eosinophilia, and 2 years later the adverse reactions from Nirvanol were interpreted as an allergic phenomena. The disorder was so frequent when it was used over prolonged periods that it received the term 'Nirvanol sickness' [64]. The typical eruption from Nirvanol was seen after a delay of 9–12 days, whereas fever generally developed from day 6 to 9. Generally, after this first eruption, the exanthema faded within about 4 days, but in other patients a second exanthema and enanthema arose. Rarely, agranulocytosis, nephritis (with lethal outcome) and other complications were observed [64].

Diphenylhydantoin was introduced for the symptomatic treatment of epilepsy by Merritt and Putnam in 1938. In 5% of patients morbilliform erythemas and, more rarely, SJS and DHS have been observed.

Sulfonamides

It was again the investigation of azo-dyes that led to the detection and preparation of the first sulfonamides in 1908 by Paul Gelmo [14]. However, it took another 24 years until the therapeutic value of sulfonamides was recognized by Gerhard Domagk (1895–1964). Soon thereafter, the first adverse effects, such as exanthemas with fever, exfoliative dermatitis and SJS were reported. Sulfonamides may also cause a variety of other disorders, such as urticaria, anaphylaxis, photodermatitis and vasculitis.

Penicillin

Penicillin was discovered in 1928 by Alexander Fleming (1881–1955). However, it was the work of the pathologist Howard Walther Florey (1898–1968) and the chemist Ernest Chain (1906–1979) and their colleagues that brought penicillin into clinical use. In the USA in 1941, during the Second World War, it was the second most important project after the Manhattan project – the development of the atomic bomb – and revolutionized the treatment of bacterial diseases. Penicillin was primarily thought to be rather non-toxic. In 1943, urticarial eruptions were reported in 14 out of 500 cases. Their cause often remained obscure since in some of the cases the urticaria did not appear for several days after penicillin was discontinued. In others it did not recur when penicillin was again injected, and in others it developed during the exhibition of it. Whether these reactions have been due to some impurity in the penicillin cannot be stated at present. In several cases in which penicillin has been given after an attack of urticaria there have been no signs of recurrence. The urticaria usually disappears temporarily following the injection of epinephrine. The uncritical use of penicillin as a topical, oral or parenteral drug resulted in sensitization and a considerable number of accidents [65].

The incidence of allergic reactions which were not further outlined was studied in 1,303 patients. Among 598 patients receiving aqueous crystalline penicillin the rate was 1.2%, among 557 patients receiving crystalline penicillin in oil and beeswax it was 2.7%, and among 148 patients receiving procaine penicillin in oil it was 1.4%. In patients receiving very large doses of the aqueous preparation the reaction rate was high (7.8%). Reactions were more frequent when a product was administered for a longer period of time. Reactions were more frequent among patients who gave a history of previous allergy or who had previous known contact with penicillin [66].

Although penicillin was estimated to be a rather non-toxic drug, the first fatal reactions were reported [67]. A 39-year-old female patient with severe bronchial asthma was under desensitization and had previously received several courses of penicillin. She again received intramuscular penicillin and within a very short time suffered a severe reaction, including flush, swelling of the throat, cyanosis, collapse and instant death. A previous report of a delayed anaphylactic shock was more likely a serum disease from penicillin [68]. A lethal outcome of severe exfoliative dermatitis from penicillin was also published [69].

p-Amino Benzoic Acid

p-Amino benzoic acid was recognized as a member of the vitamin B complex by Stefan Ansbacher in 1941. Its sun-protective effect was detected and it was commonly used in lotions and creams. Then its potential to elicit allergic contact dermatitis was identified [14]. *p*-Amino benzoic compounds are an example of cross-reactivity because positive patch tests to benzocaine and *p*-phenylenediamine are often found. In some patients cross-reactivity also extended to the aromatic sulfonamides and to other local anesthetics from the ester type. The potential of cross-reactivity is still relevant although it has become less frequent, possibly because *p*-amino benzoic compounds are not used as often as UV filters anymore, and because the use of ester local anesthetics has declined.

Outlook

Do not rashly use every new product of which the peripatetic siren sings. Consider what surprising reactions may occur in the laboratory from the careless mixing of unknown substances. Be as considerate of your patient and yourself as you are of the test tube.
Sir William Osler (1849–1919)

The success of modern medicine would be impossible without the achievements of pharmacotherapy. Several thousand pharmaceutical agents are available, and the knowledge on their adverse effects and potentials has greatly increased. Still, unexpected hypersensitivity reactions, ranging from mild exanthemas to the very severe bullous disorders, are an immanent feature of pharmacotherapy. For some drugs, pharmacogenetic typing is available to prevent most severe adverse effects in patients with, for example, a particular HLA type, such as nevirapine-induced hypersensitivity.

The development of new drug classes, such as the biologics [70], has led, on the one hand, to the recognition of new adverse events such as so-called cytokine storms, which had not previously been observed, but also to the resurrection of old syndromes such as serum sickness disease due to the formation of anti-drug antibodies. Today, the recognition and also reporting of adverse effects from drugs should be as established and part of patient management as the detailed description of the success and the follow-up of the treated disease itself. Uncritical widespread use of new drugs in an off-label manner should be avoided since rare side effects of drugs are often only detected during an extended post-marketing phase. Also, the combination of new drugs could lead again to new adverse effects with potentially deleterious consequences. Therefore, the statement by Schimmel [3], that the physician may sometimes better represent a pathogen than a benefactor, has kept at least some of its truth.

References

1 Smith CM: Origin and uses of primum non nocere – above all, do no harm! J Clin Pharmacol 2005;45:371–377.
2 Schadewaldt H: Geschichte der Allergie. Munich, Dustri, 1983.
3 Schimmel EM: The physician as pathogen. J Chronic Dis 1963;16:1–4.
4 Goldberg A: Foreword to the third edition; in Davies DM (ed): Textbook of Adverse Drug Reactions. Oxford, Oxford University Press, 1985, pp xi–xii.
5 von Pirquet C: Klinische Studien über Vakzination und vakzinale Allergie. Münch Med Wochenschr 1906;53:1457–1458.
6 Kay AB: 'Allergy. The History of a Modern Malady' by Mark Jackson. Clin Exp Allergy 2006;36:1350.
7 Jamieson M: Imagining 'reactivity': allergy within the history of immunology. Stud Hist Philos Biol Biomed Sci 2010;41:356–366.
8 Johansson SGO, Bieber T, Dahl R, Friedmann PS, Lanier BQ, Lockey RF, Motala C, Ortega Martell JA, Platts-Mills TAE, Ring J, Thien F, Van Cauwenberge P, Williams HC: Revised nomenclature for allergy for global use: report of the Nomenclature Review Committee of the World Allergy Organization, October 2003. J Allergy Clin Immunol 2004;113:832–836.
9 Gell PGH, Coombs RRA: Clinical Aspects of Immunology. Oxford, Blackwell, 1963.
10 Coombs RRA: The Jack Pepys Lecture. The hypersensitivity reactions – some personal reflections. Clin Exp Allergy 1992;22:673–680.
11 Kallós P, Schlumberger HD: Pseudo-allergic reactions – PAR. Int Archs Allergy Appl Immun 1987;82:1–3.
12 Borzelleca JF: Profile in toxicology. Toxicol Sci 2000;53:2–4.
13 Gallo MA: History and scope of toxicology; in Klaassen CD, Watkins JBI (eds): Casarett and Doull's Essentials of Toxicology. New York, McGraw-Hill, 2003, p 3 ff.
14 Laughlin S, Jackson R: A brief history of drug reactions. Clin Dermatol 1986;4:1–14.
15 Porter R: Die Kunst des Heilens. Heidelberg, Hohe Spektrum Akademischer, 2007.
16 Dousset J-C: Histoire des médicaments des origines à nos jours. Paris, Payot, 1985.
17 Behrend G: Über ein diffus-entzündliches Opiumexanthem nebst Bemerkungen über die Pathogenese der Arzneiausschläge. Berl Klin Wochenschr 1879;16:626–629.
18 Behrend G: Über ein diffus-entzündliches Opiumexanthem nebst Bemerkungen über die Pathogenese der Arzneiausschläge (Schluss). Berl Klin Wochenschr 1879;16:644–647.
19 Engelmann F: Fall von Erythema universale nach Gebrauch von Calomel. Berl Klin Wochenschr 1879;16:647–648.
20 Köbner H: Über Arznei-Exantheme, insbesondere über Chinin-Exanthem. Berl Klin Wochenschr 1877;14:305–309.
21 Brand: Zwei Fälle von Opium-Exanthem. Berl Klin Wochenschr 1879;16:718.
22 Behrend G: Zur allgemeinen Diagnostik der Arzneiausschläge. Berl Klin Wochenschr 1879;16:714–718.
23 Bircher AJ: Arzneimittelallergie und Haut. Stuttgart, Georg Thieme, 1996.
24 Bircher AJ: Uncomplicated drug-induced disseminated exanthemas; in French LE (ed): Adverse Cutaneous Drug Eruptions. Basel, Karger, 2012, pp 79–97.
25 Parrillo S: Stevens-Johnson syndrome and toxic epidermal necrolysis. Curr Allergy Asthma Rep 2007;7:243–247.
26 Stevens AM, Johnson FC: A new eruptive fever associated with stomatitis and ophthalmia: report of two cases in children. Arch Ped Adolesc Med 1922;24:526–533.
27 Raffetto JF, Nichols S: A nearly fatal reaction to sulfadiazine in a ten year old girl involving skin, eyes and oropharynx. J Pediatr 1942;20:753.

28 Greenberg SI, Messer AL: Fatal bullous dermatitis following administration of sulfadiazine. J Am Med Assoc 1943;122:944–944.
29 Ruskin DB: Fulminating dermatitis bullosa medicamentosa due to 'mesantoin'. J Am Med Assoc 1948;137:1031–1035.
30 Lyell A: Toxic epidermal necrolysis: an eruption resembling scalding of the skin. Br J Dermatol 1956;68:355–361.
31 Tyson RG, Ushinski SC, Kisilevsky R: Toxic epidermal necrolysis (the scalded skin syndrome): its association in two cases with pathogenic staphylococci and its similarity in infancy to Ritter's disease. Am J Dis Child 1966;111:386–392.
32 Roujeau JC: The spectrum of Stevens-Johnson syndrome and toxic epidermal necrolysis: a clinical classification. J Invest Dermatol 1994;102:28S–30S.
33 Roujeau J, Guillaume J, Fabre J, Penso D, Fléchet M, Girre J: Toxic epidermal necrolysis (Lyell syndrome): incidence and drug etiology in France, 1981–1985. Arch Dermatol 1990;126:37–42.
34 Roujeau JC: Lyell syndrome and its attributability to medications: methodological problems (in French). Allerg Immunol (Paris) 1990;22:217–221.
35 Schöpf E, Stühmer A, Rzany B, Victor N, Zentgraf R, Kapp J: Toxic epidermal necrolysis and Stevens-Johnson syndrome: an epidemiologic study from West Germany. Arch Dermatol 1991;127:839–842.
36 Harr T, French LE: Stevens-Johnson syndrome and toxic epidermal necrolysis; in French LE (ed): Adverse Cutaneous Drug Eruptions. Basel, Karger, 2012, pp 149–166.
37 Patel BM: Skin rash with infectious mononucleosis and ampicillin. Pediatrics 1967;40:910–911.
38 Jappe U: Amoxicillin-induced exanthema in patients with infectious mononucleosis: allergy or transient immunostimulation? Allergy 2007;62:1474–1475.
39 Merritt H, Putnam TJ: Sodium diphenyl hydantoinate in the treatment of convulsive disorders. J Am Med Assoc 1938;111:1068–1073.
40 Chaiken BH, Goldberg BI, Segal JP: Dilantin sensitivity. N Engl J Med 1950;242:897–898.
41 Shiohara T, Kano Y, Takahashi R, Ishida T, Mizukawa Y: Drug-induced hypersensitivity syndrome: recent advances in the diagnosis, pathogenesis and management; in French LE (ed): Adverse Cutaneous Drug Eruptions. Basel, Karger, 2012, pp 122–138.
42 Saltzstein SL, Ackerman LV: Lymphadenopathy induced by anticonvulsant drugs and mimicking clinically pathologically malignant lymphomas. Cancer 1959;12:164–182.
43 Bocquet H, Bagot M, Roujeau JC: Drug-induced pseudolymphoma and drug hypersensitivity syndrome (drug rash with eosinophilia and systemic symptoms: DRESS). Semin Cutan Med Surg 1996;15:250–257.
44 Baker H, Ryan TJ: Generalized pustular psoriasis: a clinical and epidemiological study of 104 cases. Br J Dermatol 1968;80:771–793.
45 Sidoroff A: Acute generalized exanthematous pustulosis; in French LE (ed): Adverse Cutaneous Drug Eruptions. Basel, Karger, 2012, pp 139–148.
46 Macmillan AL: Generalised pustular drug rash. Dermatologica 1973;146:285–291.
47 Staughton RC, Payne CM, Harper JI, McMichen H: Toxic pustuloderma – a new entity? J R Soc Med 1984;77(suppl 4):6–8.
48 Beylot C, Bioulac P, Doutre MS: Acute generalized exanthematic pustuloses (four cases) (in French). Ann Dermatol Venereol 1980;107:37–48.
49 Roujeau J-C, Bioulac-Sage P, Bourseau C, Guillaume J-C, Bernard P, Lok C, Plantin P, Claudy A, Delavierre C, Vaillant L, Wechsler J, Danan G, Benichou C, Beylot C: Acute generalized exanthematous pustulosis: analysis of 63 cases. Arch Dermatol 1991;127:1333–1338.
50 Batchelor RCL, Horne GO, Rogerson HL: An unusual reaction to procaine penicillin in aqueous suspension. Lancet 1951;258:195–198.
51 Hoigné R, Schoch K: Anaphylaktischer Schock und akute nicht-allergische Reaktionen nach Procain-Penicillin. Schweiz Med Wochenschr 1959;89:1350–1356.
52 Hoigné R, Krebs A: Kombinierte anaphylaktische und embolisch-toxische Reaktionen durch akzidentelle intravasculäre Injektion von Procain-Penicillin. Schweiz Med Wochenschr 1964;18:610–614.
53 Dill-Müller D: Ausgewählte Notfälle nach Injektionen und Infusionen. Hautarzt 2006;57:195–201.
54 Schmied C, Schmied E, Vogel J, Saurat JH: Hoigné's syndrome or pseudo-anaphylactic reaction to procaine penicillin G: a still current classic (in French). Schweiz Med Wochenschr 1990;120:1045–1049.
55 Neisser A: Über Jodoform-Exantheme. Dtsch Med Wochenschr 1884;10:467–468.
56 Bloch B: Experimentelle Studien über das Wesen der Jodoformidiosynkrasie. Z Exp Pathol Ther 1911;9:509–538.
57 Jeffreys D: Aspirin: The Remarkable Story of a Wonder Drug. New York, Bloomsbury, 2004.
58 Hirschberg VGS: Mitteilung über einen Fall von Nebenwirkungen des Aspirin. Dtsch Med Wochenschr 1902;28:416.
59 Hirschberg VGS: Anaphylactoid reaction to aspirin. Allergy Proc 1990;11:249–250.
60 Widal F, Abrami P, Lermoyez J: Anaphylaxie et idiosyncrasie. Presse Med 1922;30:189–193.
61 Anonymous: Treasure hunt: pertinent excerpts from past literature. J Asthma 1987;24:297–300.
62 Rufli T: Die Geschichte der Dermatologen und der Dermatologie an der Universität Basel 1460–1913. Basel, Schwabe, 2008.
63 Stone CH, Margolis J: Granulopenia following allonal. J Am Med Assoc 1934;103:1933.
64 Madden JF: Nirvanol eruptions. Arch Dermatol 1932;26:1065–1073.
65 Keefer CS, Blake FG, Marshall EKJ, Lockwood JS, Wood WBJ: Penicillin in the treatment of infections: a report of 500 cases. J Am Med Assoc 1943;122:1217–1224.
66 Lepper MH, Dowling HF, Robinson JA, Stone TE, Brickhouse RL, Caldwell ER, Whelton RL: Studies on hypersensitivity to penicillin. I. Incidence of reactions in 1,303 patients. J Clin Invest 1949;28:826–831.
67 Waldbott GL: Anaphylactic death from penicillin. J Am Med Assoc 1949;139:526–527.
68 Wilensky AO: Fatal delayed anaphylactic shock after penicillin. J Am Med Assoc 1946;131:1384–1384.
69 Rabinovitch J, Snitkoff MC: Acute exfoliative dermatitis and death following penicillin therapy. J Am Med Assoc 1948;138:496–498.
70 Scherer K, Spoerl D, Bircher AJ: Unerwünschte Arzneimittelreaktionen auf Biologika. J Dtsch Dermatol Ges 2010;8:411–427.
71 Jacobi E: Atlas der Hautkrankheiten, ed 3. Berlin, Urban & Schwarzenberg, 1907.

Prof. Andreas J. Bircher
Allergy Unit, Department of Dermatology
University Hospital, Petersgraben 4
CH–4031 Basel (Switzerland)
E-Mail andreas.bircher@unibas.ch

Most Common Allergic Diseases: Historical Reflections in Understanding

Bergmann K-C, Ring J (eds): History of Allergy. Chem Immunol Allergy. Basel, Karger, 2014, vol 100, pp 132–139
DOI: 10.1159/000358618

Aspirin Hypersensitivity

Mario Sánchez-Borges

Allergy and Clinical Immunology Department, Centro Médico-Docente 'la Trinidad' and Clínica El Avila, Caracas, Venezuela

Abstract

Hypersensitivity reactions to acetylsalicylic acid and non-steroidal anti-inflammatory drugs constitute a major medical concern worldwide. This article presents an overview of the observations that led to the discovery of cyclooxygenase inhibitors, as a prerequisite to better understand the basic concepts supporting seminal investigations carried out in order to elucidate the clinical features, pathogenic mechanisms, diagnosis and modern management of these common conditions. There are some unmet needs in this clinical area which will have to be solved in the future, especially concerning the pathogenesis of these reactions and the availability of novel in vitro diagnostic methods sparing both patient and physician of the risks inherent to in vivo provocation tests.

Aspirin is one of the most widely used drugs in the world and hypersensitivity reactions to aspirin and non-steroidal anti-inflammatory drugs (NSAIDs) are, after β-lactam antibiotics, the second most common cause of drug hypersensitivity. Natural salicylates such as salicin and salicylic acid are present in the bark and leaves of willow and poplar trees, and these compounds constitute the ancestry to aspirin.

Since a knowledge of the pharmacology of aspirin and NSAIDs is relevant to the understanding of adverse reactions to these drugs, we will first present an overview of the observations that resulted in the discovery of aspirin, the first synthetic drug available for use in human beings, and will then review the most important findings allowing us to obtain a better understanding of these common adverse reactions.

The Discovery of Aspirin

Ancient Times

Natural salicylates present in the bark of white willow and other trees are mentioned in texts from ancient Sumer, Egypt, Mesopotamia, Lebanon and Assyria. Around 3000 BC, ancient Egyptians recorded the medicinal value of willow bark and myrtle.

The decoction of sheets of willow is mentioned in a famous Egyptian papyrus, *Ebers Papyrus*, a medical text from around 1543 BC. The Romans also knew its medical properties, and Chinese and Greek civilizations employed willow bark more than 2,000 years ago.

Hippocrates of Kos, the Greek physician considered as the father of modern medicine, described 'a bitter powder that came from the bark and leaves of the willow tree which eases pain and reduces fever'. The active extract of the bark was called salicin after the Latin name of the white willow tree *(Salix alba)*, a member of the Salicaceae family, salicin being the glycoside of salicylic acid. Celsus, Pliny the Elder, Dioscorides and Galen also used these natural remedies.

The Roman encyclopedist Celsus, in his *De Medicina* of circa 30 BC suggested willow leaf extracts to treat inflammation. Willow treatments also appeared in the Greek physician Dioscorides' *De Materia Medica*, and Pliny the Elder's *Natural History*. By the time of Galen, willow was commonly used throughout the Roman and Arab worlds. In the Middle Ages Hildegard of Bingen, a nun, and Henrik Harpestreng used salicylates for fever and rheumatism. The Cherokee and other Native Americans and the Hottentots of South Africa used an infusion of the bark for fever and other medicinal purposes for centuries.

From Willow Bark to Salicin to Salicylic Acid

The first clinical trial on the therapeutic use of willow bark against fever was reported to the Royal Society of Medicine on April 25, 1763, by Reverend Edward (Edmund) Stone, a vicar from Chipping Norton in Oxfordshire, England. This investigator noted that it was effective in reducing malarial fever ('agues'). Stone had tasted the bark in 1758 and noticed an astringent taste reminiscent of the standard ague cure of Peruvian bark. He collected, dried and powdered a substantial amount of willow bark, and over the next 5 years tested it on a number of people sick with fever and agues, involving an ill-defined constellation of symptoms, including intermittent fever, pain and fatigue that primarily referred to malaria. Lewis and Clark used willow bark tea for fever in 1803–1806. In 1824, Bartolomeo Rigartelli used a willow bark extract as a therapeutic agent, denominating it 'salino amarissimo antifebrile' (very bitter antipyretic salts). In 1828, Johann Andreas Buchner, professor of pharmacology at the University of Munich, isolated a tiny amount of bitter-tasting yellow needle-like crystals from willow tree which he called 'salicina' (salicin). Brugnatelli and Fontana had obtained salicin in a highly impure form in 1826.

In 1829, French pharmacist Henri Leroux isolated salicin in crystalline form. He boiled the powder of white willow bark in water and, while trying to concentrate the preparation, obtained the soluble crystals that he named salicylic acid. At around the same time, Löwig, a German chemist, found salicylic acid in meadowsweet. This compound had an unpleasant taste and caused gastric irritation and nausea. In 1830, the Swiss pharmacist Johann Pagenstecher discovered what he thought was a new pain-reducing substance isolated from meadowsweet *(Spiraea ulmaria)*, and in 1838 Rafaelle Piria, an Italian chemist then working at the Sorbonne in Paris, was able to convert salicin to salicylic acid. He split salicin into a sugar and an aromatic component (salicylaldehyde) and converted the latter by hydrolysis and oxidation to an acid of crystalized colorless needles which he named salicylic acid.

From Natural to Synthetic Acetylsalicylic Acid

A major breakthrough occurred in 1853 when Charles Frédéric Gerhardt, a French chemist, first synthesized acetylsalicylic acid (ASA) by buffering salicylic acid with acetyl chloride and sodium salicylate. The resulting product was unstable and impure, and Gerhardt called it acetosalicylic anhydride. In 1859, Hermann Kolbe, a chemistry professor at Marburg University, prepared salicylic acid from sodium phenate and carbon dioxide, and in the same year von Gilm created ASA again, calling it acetylated salicylic acid. In 1869, Schröder, Prinzhorn and Kraut were the first to assign the correct structure of ASA with the acetyl group connected to phenolic oxygen. In 1876, the antirheumatic effect of salicin was described by Thomas MacLagan, a Scottish physician from Dundee, and that of salicylic acid by S. Stricker and L. Riess.

In 1880, the German chemical industry was investigating the potential of new tar-derived medicines and, in 1886, Kalle & Co. discovered by accident the antipyretic properties of the dye derivative acetanilide, which was called Antifebrin. Afterwards, Carl Duisberg, head of research at the small dye firm Friedrich Bayer & Co., Elberfeld, Germany, developed phenacetin (acetophenetidin). On August 10, 1897, Felix Hoffman, a German chemist working at Friedrich Bayer & Co., discovered a better method for synthesizing pure, stable and palatable ASA, the first modern, truly synthetic drug. He neutralized salicylic acid by buffering it with sodium and acetyl chloride. He was looking for a medicine for his father who suffered with chronic rheumatism. The disgusting sweet taste of sodium salicylate was refined by acetylation of the free phenolic hydroxyl group of salicylic acid through substitution of the hydrogen atom with a methyl group. Hoffman clearly understood that aspirin was an effective pain reliever that did not have the unpleasant side effects of salicylic acid. Apparently, Arthur Eichengrün, Hoffman's boss, was the one that envisioned the idea to synthesize the drug.

In 1899, Heinrich Dreser, Bayer's head of pharmacology laboratories, set up animal experiments and showed the anti-inflammatory and analgesic effects of ASA, and Bayer & Co. patented it on March 6, 1899. The beneficial effect of ASA on pain and rheumatic fever was then recognized by K. Witthauer and Julius Wohlgemuth. Aspirin was first sold as a powder, and in 1900 aspirin tablets were produced. In 1915, the tablets became available to the public without a prescription. The name aspirin comes from 'a' in acetyl chloride, 'spir' from Spirsäure (salicylic acid) in *S. ulmaria* (the plant they derived the salicylic acid from) and 'in', a familiar name ending for medicines. In fact, ASA had been manufactured by the Chemische Fabrik von Heyden & Co. since 1897 without a brand name. Aspirin's popularity declined after the development of acetaminophen/paracetamol in 1956 and ibuprofen in 1962.

Mechanisms of Action

In regard to its mechanisms of action, Heinrich Dreser proposed that aspirin relieved pain by acting on the central nervous system. In 1958, Harry Collier, a biochemist in the London Laboratory of Parke Davis & Co., began investigating the relationship between kinins and the effects of aspirin. In tests in guinea pigs he found that pretreatment with aspirin inhibited the bronchoconstriction induced by bradykinin. Cutting the vagus nerve did not affect the action of bradykinin or the inhibitory effect of aspirin, evidence that ASA worked locally to inhibit pain and inflammation, rather than on the central nervous system. John Robert Vane, a British pharmacologist and his graduate student Priscilla Piper, from London's Royal College of Surgeons, found that aspirin inhibited the release of an unidentified chemical generated by guinea pig lungs that caused rabbit tissue to contract. By 1971, Vane had identified the chemical (which he called 'rabbit-aorta contracting substance' or RCS) as a prostaglandin. In June 1971, Vane and Piper suggested that aspirin and similar drugs (the NSAIDs) worked by blocking the production of prostaglandins. Later on it was shown that NSAIDs worked by inhibiting cyclooxygenase, the enzyme responsible for converting arachidonic acid into a prostaglandin, which was described in 1976. For this discovery, Vane received the Nobel Prize in Physiology and Medicine in 1982 and was knighted in 1984 for his contributions to science.

Cyclooxygenase Isoenzymes

Other than cyclooxygenase-1 (COX-1), the constitutive enzyme present in all cells, there are at least two other COX isoforms, designated as COX-2 and COX-3. COX-2, the inducible isoenzyme, was discovered in 1988 by Daniel Simmons and his team at Brigham Young University. The mouse COX-2 gene was cloned by UCLA scientist Harvey Herschman. COX-3 was discovered due to the observation that the COX-1/COX-2 model did not explain the antipyretic and analgesic properties of acetaminophen. Although its effects could be due to inhibition of COX-2, it was clear that paracetamol is not an effective anti-inflammatory. Simmons and his team suggested that a variant of COX-1, which they named COX-3, was especially sensitive to acetaminophen and related compounds (phenacetin, antipyrine, dipyrone).

Table 1. Historical chronology of aspirin discovery

Date	Discovery
Around 1543 BC	Egyptians mention the medicinal value of a decoction of willow bark and myrtle leaves in the *Ebers Papyrus*
460 BC	Hippocrates prescribes the bark and leaves of the white willow tree *(S. alba)* for pain, including labor pain, and fever
100 AD	Dioscorides, a Greek surgeon, uses willow leaves for pain relief
200	Pliny the Elder alludes to willow leaves in his writings
1763	Edward (Edmund) Stone reports the successful treatment of malarial fever (agues) with willow bark
1826	Brugnatelli and Fontana obtained impure salicin
1828	Johann Andreas Buchner, a pharmacologist from Munich, isolated pure salicin from willow bark
1829	Henri Leroux, a French pharmacist, isolates salicin
1830	Johann Pagenstecher, a Swiss pharmacist, discovers a new analgesic isolated from meadowsweet *(S. ulmaria)*
1835	Karl Löwig, a German chemist, finds salicylic acid in meadowsweet flowers
1838	Raffaele Piria, an Italian chemist, converts salicin (salicoside) into salicylic acid
1853	Charles Frédéric Gerhardt, a French chemist, synthesizes impure ASA
1859	H. von Gilm also prepares impure ASA
1869	Kraut, Schröder and Prinzhorn describe the molecular structure of ASA
1874	Herman Kolbe prepares salicylic acid from coal tar
1876	Thomas MacLagan, a Scottish physician, describes the antirheumatic effect of salicin, and S. Stricker and L. Riess that of salicylic acid
1897	Felix Hoffman, a German chemist, prepares the first pure and stable sample of ASA on August 10. He realizes that ASA is devoid of the gastric side effects of salicylic acid
1899	Heinrich Dreser shows the anti-inflammatory and analgesic effects of ASA
1900	Bayer & Co. introduces aspirin in water-soluble tablet form
1915	Aspirin becomes available to the public without prescription
1969	Aspirin is included in the self-medication kits taken to the moon by the Apollo astronauts
1948	Lawrence Craven, a family physician from California, describes the potential of aspirin to prevent heart attacks
1971	John Vane, a British pharmacologist, discovers the mechanism of action of aspirin as an inhibitor of the cyclooxygenase pathway
1980	US FDA approves the use of aspirin to reduce the risk of stroke
1982	John Vane is awarded the Nobel Prize in Physiology and Medicine
1985	US FDA approves the use of aspirin for prevention of heart attacks and strokes
1999	COX-3 is discovered by Simmons and co-workers

Antithrombotic Effects of Aspirin

The antiplatelet effects of aspirin were first noticed by Lawrence Craven, a family doctor from California. He gave his tonsillectomy patients chewable Aspergum, an aspirin-laced chewing gum, and found that an unusual number of patients had to be hospitalized for severe bleeding. In the 1960s, Harvey Weiss found that aspirin had an antiaggregation effect on blood platelets. John O'Brien and Peter Elwood showed in 1973 a modest but not statistically significant reduction in heart attacks among patients taking aspirin. A meta-analysis by Richard Peto convinced the US Food and Drug Administration (FDA) of aspirin's effectiveness for the prevention of myocardial infarction. The chronology of aspirin development is summarized in table 1.

Hypersensitivity Reactions to ASA and NSAIDs

Early Observations

The first description of a hypersensitivity reaction triggered by aspirin was made only 3 years after the introduction of the drug for therapeutic use, by Hirschberg [1] in 1902. This author described a patient with acute angioedema and urticaria occurring immediately after aspirin intake [1]. Gilbert recognized for the first time an asthmatic reaction to ASA in 1911 [2], whereas Reed and Cookes repeated the same observation in 1919. In 1920, Van der Veer described the first ASA-induced fatal asthmatic reaction.

M. Fernand Widal, Pierre Abrami and Jacques Lermoyez observed in 1922 the association between aspirin sensitivity, aspirin-induced asthma and nasal polyposis, the ASA triad, which was rediscovered more than 40 years later by Samter (see below) [3]. In modern times this disease is designed as a tetrad that also includes chronic hyperplastic eosinophilic sinusitis. These investigators also described for the first time the phenomenon of aspirin desensitization.

Samter's Disease

In 1968, Max Samter proposed the concept of aspirin triad (Samter's triad) as a distinct clinical entity [4]. This disease has also been mentioned in the literature as the Widal-Abrami-Lermoyez triad, Widal-Lermoyez syndrome and Widal's syndrome. Different terminologies are used by various authors for aspirin-induced asthma, including the following: aspirin-intolerant asthma, aspirin sensitivity, aspirin-sensitive asthma, aspirin-exacerbated asthma. Presently, the designation of aspirin-exacerbated respiratory disease (AERD) is the most commonly accepted because it includes the wider involvement of both the upper and lower airways, and also due to the fact that the disease progresses independently of any aspirin or NSAID exposure. In order to harmonize the nomenclature, we have recently proposed that cross-reactive urticaria/angioedema observed in patients with underlying chronic spontaneous urticaria be designated aspirin-exacerbated cutaneous disease, AECD [5]. In 1997, we reported the association of cutaneous aspirin sensitivity (urticaria/angioedema) with allergic rhinitis and severe systemic reactions to mite-contaminated foods, and we proposed this clinical picture as a 'new aspirin triad' [6].

Classification of Hypersensitivity Reactions to ASA and NSAIDs

Since there were discrepancies in the literature in regard to the terminology used by different investigators, Stevenson [7] proposed the first classification system for ASA hypersensitivity in 1993. A further step followed in 2001 when Stevenson et al. [8] published a second classification system for reactions that inhibit cyclooxygenase enzymes. Recently, a more comprehensive classification including immediate and delayed reactions to NSAIDs has been proposed by EAACI/ENDA and GA2LEN/HANNA [9].

Pathogenesis

Aspirin and NSAIDs that inhibit COX-1 cross react to induce reactions in all patients with AERD and AECD, and in patients with multiple NSAID-induced urticaria and angioedema, as recognized early by Vanselow [10]. Reactions, including asthma, are observed when NSAIDs are administered by diverse routes, including oral, parenteral, topical in the skin or even conjunctival [11].

In the 1970s, the link between precipitation of asthma attacks and inhibition of cyclooxygenase by aspirin and other NSAIDs was described. Later on, other alterations in arachidonic acid metabolism were discovered, and also found to be common in aspirin-induced angioedema and urticaria [12]. This observation led Szczeklik [13] to propose the cyclooxygenase theory.

Overproduction of cysteinyl leukotrienes, increased expression of CysLTR1 in the airways mucosa [14], decreased production of prostaglandin E_2, which acts like a break on the uncontrolled synthesis of cysteinyl leukotrienes, and reduced lipoxin synthesis are also involved in the pathogenesis of ASA/NSAIDs reactions. In this regard, Picado et al. [15] found a decreased expression of COX-2 mRNA in nasal polyps from subjects suffering from AERD.

The hypothesis that aspirin-induced asthma results from a persistent, latent rhinovirus infection of the respiratory tract giving origin to alterations in arachidonate metabolism, as proposed by Szczeklik [16], has not been substantiated.

Reactions to a single NSAID, where drug-specific immunoglobulin (Ig) E antibodies are thought to be involved, are rarely observed. These allergic reactions have been reported more often for the pyrazolone group of NSAIDs [17].

Table 2. Milestones in the history of aspirin hypersensitivity

Date	Discovery
1902	Hirschberg describes the first case of aspirin hypersensitivity
1911	Gilbert recognizes aspirin-induced asthmatic reaction
1919	Reed and Cookes again observe that aspirin could provoke asthma attacks
1920	Van der Veer describes the first aspirin-induced fatal asthmatic reaction
1922	M. Fernand Widal, Pierre Abrami and Jacques Lermoyez observe the association of aspirin sensitivity, aspirin-induced asthma and nasal polyposis
1967	Samter and Beers propose the concept of aspirin triad
1967	Vanselow reports on asthma induced by indomethacin
1973	Zeiss and Lockey propose that aspirin-induced asthma is inherited as autosomal recessive
1976	Stevenson develops oral aspirin challenges for aspirin-sensitive asthma
1977	Stevenson implements aspirin desensitization as a treatment for aspirin-induced asthma
1977	Bianco introduces the aspirin inhalation test
1977	Milewski describes the nasal provocation test with lysine-aspirin
1989	Settipane reports respiratory reactions to increased doses of acetaminophen
1990	Szczeklik [13] proposes the cyclooxygenase theory to explain aspirin-intolerant asthma
1997	A new aspirin triad of allergic rhinitis, severe allergic reaction to ingested aeroallergens and aspirin sensitivity is proposed by Sánchez-Borges et al. [6]
1999	IgE-mediated reactions to pyrazolones reported by Kowalski et al. [26]
2000	Sánchez-Borges and co-workers show that atopy is a risk factor for NSAID hypersensitivity reactions
2000	Picado demonstrates a decrease of COX-2 mRNA in nasal polyps from patients with aspirin triad
2001	A new classification of reactions to NSAIDs is proposed by Stevenson, Sánchez-Borges and Szczeklik
2001	Selective COX-2 inhibitors are tolerated by patients with ASA-intolerant asthma and urticaria
2004	Mastalerz et al. [12] propose that the pathogenesis of aspirin-induced urticaria is due to inhibition of cyclo-oxygenase
2006	Intravenous desensitization with aspirin is proposed
2009	Sánchez-Borges et al. [30] propose the concept of the 'high-risk' phenotype for reactions to NSAIDs
2010	The concept of AECD is proposed
2011	A new classification system for NSAID-induced hypersensitivity reactions is developed by Kowalski et al. [9]

Genetics

In 1973, Lockey et al. [18] described four members of a Mennonite family who suffered with ASA-induced asthma, three of whom were first cousins. The presence of the disease in relatives, influenced by the presence of consanguinity, suggested an autosomal recessive mode of inheritance.

More recently, progress in molecular genetics has permitted the study of a number of genetic polymorphisms associated with reactions to NSAIDs [reviewed in 19]. In AERD the following genetic variants have been recognized: HLADPB1*0301, LTC4S-444A>C, ALOX5, CysLTR1 and CysLTR2, PGE2 receptor subtype 2 (EP2), TBXA2R and TBX21. For aspirin-induced urticaria and angioedema the following genetic variants have been reported: HLA-DRB1*1302 and HLA-DQB1*0609, LTC4S-444A>C and FcεRIα-344C>T. It has to be mentioned that these genetic markers are applicable only for the populations under study, and sometimes are not reproducible in other populations of a different genetic background. Presently, its usefulness for diagnostic purposes has not been validated.

Developments in Diagnostic Methods

Provocation tests with aspirin and other NSAIDs constitute the gold standard to confirm the diagnosis of NSAID hypersensitivity. Challenges can be performed by different routes, such as oral [20], bronchial [21] and nasal [22]. For reactions to a single NSAID, presumably IgE-mediated, immediate-type prick and intradermal skin tests have been recommended, although sensitivity and specificity are variable [23].

In vitro methods to avoid the undesirable and potentially risky effects of in vivo challenges have been proposed, but presently they are not widely used and require further validation. They include the sulfidoleukotriene release assay [24], the basophil activation test [25], and the 15-HETE generation assay (ASPITest) [26].

Advances in Patient Management

The avoidance of all classic COX-1 inhibitors is usually recommended for patients with cross-reactive NSAID hypersensitivity, together with the use of weak COX inhibitors, especially acetaminophen. However, Settipane and Stevenson [27] observed more than 20 years ago that acetaminophen can cause bronchoconstriction at doses greater than 1,000 mg in 34% of individuals with AERD.

With the incorporation of new drugs that are highly selective for COX-2, the safety of such NSAIDs in patients with respiratory or cutaneous disease was investigated. Stevenson and Simon [28] found that selective COX-2 inhibitors may be used safely in the majority of aspirin-sensitive patients with asthma. Similar results were observed in patients with aspirin-induced urticaria and angioedema [29]. It is worth mentioning that a small number of NSAID-sensitive patients will not tolerate the above-mentioned alternative drugs (weak COX inhibitors and selective COX-2 inhibitors). We have proposed that these patients are considered as the 'high-risk phenotype' of NSAID hypersensitivity [30].

In patients who require NSAIDs for chronic conditions such as rheumatic diseases and ischemic coronary disease, desensitization is an option. In 1976, Zeiss and Lockey [31] described the paradoxical finding that ASA-intolerant patients revealed a 3-day refractory period after oral aspirin challenge resulted in respiratory symptoms. This observation constituted the basis for the oral desensitization protocols that have been preconized by Stevenson et al. [32], who demonstrated that oral administration by means of an initial desensitization with gradually ascending doses of aspirin could be followed safely by a daily maintenance dose. The first randomized, double-blind, placebo-controlled crossover trial of oral desensitization was published by the same investigators in 1984 [33]. Desensitization has also been performed with lysine-aspirin by other routes, such as bronchial [34], nasal [35] and intravenous [36]. The milestones in the study of aspirin and NSAID hypersensitivity reactions are shown in table 2.

Conclusions

Adverse hypersensitivity reactions to aspirin and NSAIDs are a major cause of consultation in general medical practice as well as in specialized allergy clinics. Major advances in the understanding of the clinical features of these reactions have permitted to design better diagnostic and management efforts for patients suffering from these conditions. This has been possible thanks to the dedication of a number of pioneer clinical and basic investigators led by Prof. Max Samter, Prof. Sir John Vane, Prof. Donald D. Stevenson, Prof. Andrej Szczeklik, Prof. Alain De Weck and Prof. Richard Lockey, and a whole new generation of professionals that includes Marek Kowalski, Cesar Picado and Hae Sim Park, among others. In spite of the huge amount of knowledge presently available on these reactions there are some loopholes in the understanding of their pathogenesis. New and improved in vitro diagnostic methods sparing the affected patients of the risks of challenge tests are dearly needed at the present time.

References

1 Hirschberg SR: Mitteilung über einen Fall von Nebenwirkung des Aspirin. Dtsch Med Wochenschr 1902;28:416.
2 Gilbert GB: Unusual idiosyncrasy to aspirin. J Am Med Assoc 1911;56:1262.
3 Widal MF, Abrami P, Lermoyez J: Anaphylaxie et idiosyncrasie. Presse Med 1922;30: 189–192.
4 Samter M, Beers RF: Intolerance to aspirin: clinical studies and consideration of its pathogenesis. Ann Intern Med 1968;68: 975–983.
5 Sánchez-Borges M: NSAID hypersensitivity (respiratory, cutaneous and generalized, anaphylactic symptoms). Med Clin North Am 2010;94:853–864.
6 Sánchez-Borges M, Capriles-Hulett A, Capriles-Behrens E, Fernandez-Caldas E: A new triad: sensitivity to aspirin, allergic rhinitis, and severe allergic reaction to ingested aeroallergens. Cutis 1997;59:311–314.

7 Stevenson DD: Challenge procedures in detection of reactions to aspirin and nonsteroidal anti-inflammatory drugs. Ann Allergy 1993;71:417–418.
8 Stevenson DD, Sánchez-Borges M, Szczeklik A: Classification of allergic and pseudoallergic reactions to drugs that inhibit cyclooxygenase enzymes. Ann Allergy Asthma Immunol 2001;87:177–180.
9 Kowalski ML, Makowska JS, Blanca M, Bavbek S, Bochenek G, Bousquet J, Bousquet P, Celik G, Demoly P, Gomes ER, Nizankowska-Mogilnicka E, Romano A, Sánchez-Borges M, Sanz M, Torres MJ, De Weck A, Szczeklik A, Brockow K: Hypersensitivity to nonsteroidal anti-inflammatory drugs (NSAIDs) – classification, diagnosis and management: review of the EAACI/ENDA and GA2LEN/HANNA. Allergy 2011;66:818–829.
10 Vanselow H: Bronchial asthma induced by indomethacin. Ann Intern Med 1967;66:568–572.
11 Sitenga GL, Ing EB, Van Dellen RG, Younge BR, Leavitt JA: Asthma caused by topical application of ketorolac. Ophthalmology 1996;103:890–892.
12 Mastalerz L, Setkowicz M, Sanak M, Szczeklik A: Hypersensitivity to aspirin: common eicosanoid alterations in urticaria and asthma. J Allergy Clin Immunol 2004;113:771–775.
13 Szczeklik A: The cyclooxygenase theory of aspirin-induced asthma. Eur Respir J 1990;3:588–593.
14 Souza AR, Parikh A, Scadding G, Corrigan CJ, Lee TH: Leukotriene-receptor expression on nasal mucosal inflammatory cells in aspirin-sensitive rhinosinusitis. N Engl J Med 2002;347:1493–1499.
15 Picado C, Fernandez-Morata JC, Juan M, Roca-Ferrer J, Fuentes M, Xaubet A, Mullol J: Cyclooxygenase-2 mRNA is down-expressed in nasal polyps from aspirin-sensitive asthmatics. Am J Respir Crit Care Med 1999;160:291–296.
16 Szczeklik A: Aspirin-induced asthma as a viral disease. Clin Allergy 1988;18:15–20.
17 Kowalski ML, Bienkiewicz B, Wosczek G, Iwaszkiewicz J, Poniatowska M: Diagnosis of pyrazolone drug sensitivity: clinical history versus skin testing and in vitro testing. Allergy Asthma Proc 1999;20:347–352.
18 Lockey RF, Rucknagel DL, Vanselow NA: Familial occurrence of asthma, nasal polyps and aspirin intolerance. Ann Intern Med 1973;78:57–63.
19 Kim S-H, Park H-S: Genetic markers for differentiating aspirin-hypersensitivity. Yonsei Med J 2006;47:15–21.
20 Stevenson DD, Arroyave CM, Bhat KN, Tan EM: Oral aspirin challenges in asthmatic patients: a study of plasma histamine. Clin Allergy 1976;6:493–505.
21 Bianco S, Robuschi M, Petrigni G: Aspirin induced tolerance in aspirin-asthma detected by a new challenge test. J Med Sci 1977;5:129–130.
22 Schapowal A, Schmitz-Schuman M, Szczeklik A, Bruijnzeel P, Hansel T, Virchow C: Lysine-aspirin nasal provocation and anterior rhinomanometry for the diagnosis of aspirin-sensitive asthma. Atemw Lungenkrkh 1990;16:S1–S5.
23 Himly M, Jahn-Schmid B, Pittertschatscher K, Bohle B, Grubmayr K, Ferreira F, Ebner H, Ebner C: IgE-mediated immediate-type hypersensitivity to the pyrazolone drug propyphenazone. J Allergy Clin Immunol 2003;111:882–888.
24 Sanz ML, Gamboa P, De Weck AL: A new combined test with flowcytometric basophil activation and determination of sulfidoleukotrienes is useful for in vitro diagnosis of hypersensitivity to aspirin and other nonsteroidal anti-inflammatory drugs. Int Arch Allergy Immunol 2005;136:58–72.
25 Gamboa P, Sanz ML, Caballero MR, Urrutia I, Antepara I, Esparza R, de Weck AL: The flow-cytometric determination of basophil activation induced by aspirin and other non-steroidal anti-inflammatory drugs (NSAIDs) is useful for in vitro diagnosis of the NSAID hypersensitivity syndrome. Clin Exp Allergy 2004;34:1448–1457.
26 Kowalski ML, Bienkiewicz B, Woszczek G: Diagnosis of pyrazolone drug sensitivity: clinical history versus skin testing and in vitro testing. Allergy Asthma Proc 1999;20:347–352.
27 Settipane RA, Stevenson DD: Cross-sensitivity with acetaminophen in aspirin-sensitive subjects with asthma. J Allergy Clin Immunol 1989;84:26–33.
28 Stevenson DD, Simon RA: Lack of cross reactivity between rofecoxib and aspirin-sensitive patients with asthma. J Allergy Clin Immunol 2001;108:47–51.
29 Sánchez-Borges M, Capriles-Hulett A, Caballero-Fonseca F, Perez CR: Tolerability to new COX-2 inhibitors in NSAID-sensitive patients with cutaneous reactions. Ann Allergy Asthma Immunol 2001;87:201–204.
30 Sánchez-Borges M, Capriles-Hulett A, Caballero-Fonseca F: A novel phenotype of nonsteroidal anti-inflammatory drug hypersensitivity: the high-risk patient. World Allergy Organ J 2009;2:17–19.
31 Zeiss CR, Lockey RF: Refractory period to aspirin in a patient with aspirin-induced asthma. J Allergy Clin Immunol 1976;57:440–448.
32 Stevenson DD, Simon RA, Mathison DA: Aspirin-sensitive asthma: tolerance to aspirin after positive oral aspirin challenges. J Allergy Clin Immunol 1980;66:82–88.
33 Stevenson DD, Pleskow WW, Simon RA, Mathison DA, Lumry WR, Schatz M: Aspirin-sensitive rhinosinusitis asthma: a double-blind crossover study of treatment with aspirin. J Allergy Clin Immunol 1984;73:500–507.
34 Schmitz-Schumann M, Schaub E, Virchow C: Inhalation provocation test with lysine-acetylsalicylic acid in patients with analgetics-induced asthma (in German). Prax Klin Pneumol 1982;36:17–21.
35 Patriarca G, Schiavino D, Nucera E, Papa G, Schinco G, Fais G: Prevention of relapse in nasal polyposis. Lancet 1991;337:1488.
36 Pfaar O, Spielhaupter M, Wrede H: Aspirin desensitization on patients with aspirin intolerance and nasal polyps: a new therapeutic approach by the intravenous route. Allergologie 2006;8:322–331.

Dr. Mario Sánchez-Borges
Allergy and Clinical Immunology Department
Centro Médico-Docente 'la Trinidad'
6a transversal Urbanización Altamira, piso 8, consultorio 803
Caracas 1060 (Venezuela)
E-Mail sanchezbmario@gmail.com

Most Common Allergic Diseases: Historical Reflections in Understanding

Bergmann K-C, Ring J (eds): History of Allergy. Chem Immunol Allergy. Basel, Karger, 2014, vol 100, pp 140–147
DOI: 10.1159/000358619

Bradykinin-Mediated Diseases

Allen P. Kaplan

Department of Medicine, Medical University of South Carolina, Charleston, S.C., USA

Abstract

Diseases which have been demonstrated to be caused by increased plasma levels of bradykinin all have angioedema as the common major clinical manifestation. Angioedema due to therapy with angiotensin-converting enzyme (ACE) inhibitors is caused by suppressed bradykinin degradation so that it accumulates. This occurs because ACE metabolizes bradykinin by removal of Phe-Arg from the C-terminus, which inactivates it. By contrast, angioedema due to C1 inhibitor deficiency (either hereditary types I and II, or acquired) is caused by bradykinin overproduction. C1 inhibitor inhibits factor XIIa, kallikrein and activity associated with the prekallikrein-HK (high-molecular-weight kininogen) complex. In its absence, uncontrolled activation of the plasma bradykinin cascade is seen once there has been an initiating stimulus. C4 levels are low in all types of C1 inhibitor deficiency due to the instability of C1 (C1r, in particular) such that some activated C1 always circulates and depletes C4. In the hereditary disorder, formation of factor XIIf (factor XII fragment) during attacks of swelling causes C4 levels to drop toward zero, and C2 levels decline. A kinin-like molecule, once thought to be a cleavage product derived from C2 that contributes to the increased vascular permeability seen in hereditary angioedema (HAE), is now thought to be an artifact, i.e. no such molecule is demonstrable. The acquired C1 inhibitor deficiency is associated with clonal disorders of B cell hyperreactivity, including lymphoma and monoclonal gammopathy. Most cases have an IgG autoantibody to C1 inhibitor which inactivates it so that the presentation is strikingly similar to type I HAE. New therapies for types I and II HAE include C1 inhibitor replacement therapy, ecallantide, a kallikrein antagonist, and icatibant, a B2 receptor antagonist. A newly described type III HAE has normal C1 inhibitor, although it is thought to be mediated by bradykinin, as is an antihistamine-resistant subpopulation of patients with 'idiopathic' angioedema. The mechanism(s) for the formation of bradykinin in these disorders is unknown.

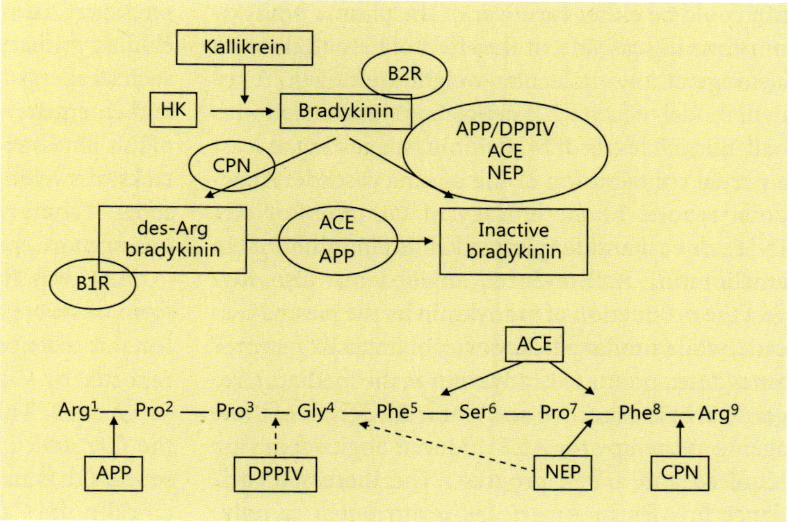

Fig. 1. Degradation of bradykinin. Bradykinin, produced by kallikrein digestion of high-molecular-weight kininogen (HK), activates the B2 receptor (B2R) to cause vasodilation and to increase vascular permeability. Digestion of bradykinin by ACE removes C-terminal Phe-Arg, and then Ser-Pro, to inactivate it. Removal of the C-terminal arginine by carboxypeptidase N (plasma) or carboxypeptidase M (endothelial cells) produces des-Arg, which is far less active on the B2 receptor but can stimulate B1 receptors (B1R). Sites of cleavage by aminopeptidase P (APP), dipeptidyl peptidase IV (DPPIV) and neutral endopeptidase (NEP) are shown.

The lability of the bradykinin-forming cascade is actually an impediment in understanding its role in human disease, i.e. it always seems somewhat activated due to the trauma of virtually any procedure, as well as infection, dilution of plasma, exposure to certain negatively charge macromolecules, etc. Presently, disorders manifest by severe angioedema appear to be the ones where the role of bradykinin is assured. These include hereditary angioedema (HAE), acquired C1 inhibitor deficiency, angioedema due to inhibitors of angiotensin-converting enzyme (ACE), and possibly a subpopulation of antihistamine-resistant patients with 'idiopathic' angioedema. This review will focus on angioedema due to ACE inhibitors and types I and II HAE as prototypic bradykinin-mediated diseases. The history by which our understanding of the pathogenesis of HAE evolved is particularly instructive.

Inhibition of Bradykinin Degradation by Angiotensin-Converting Enzyme Inhibitors

Severe bradykinin-mediated angioedema can be seen in patients taking ACE inhibitors. Swelling has a predilection for facial structures and huge tongue and pharyngeal swelling can occur so that patients may choke on secretions. Bona fide laryngeal edema can also be seen leading to inspiratory stridor and asphyxiation. The overall incidence of angioedema in those taking the drug is approximately 0.1–0.2%, with an incidence that is 5-fold increased in the African-American population.

ACE (also known as plasma kininase II) is a key protein required for bradykinin degradation. It removes C-terminal Phe-Arg (which is sufficient to inactivate bradykinin completely) followed by a second cleavage of Ser-Pro, leaving the Arg-Pro-Pro-Gly-Phe pentapeptide [1]. If the C-terminal Arg is first removed by plasma kininase I (i.e. carboxypeptidase N) or cell surface carboxypeptidase M, the product des-Arg^9 bradykinin loses its ability to stimulate the B2 receptor. The B2 receptor is constitutively present and is responsible for the permeability-enhancing properties of bradykinin. However, des-Arg^9 bradykinin may then stimulate B1 receptors which can be induced during the inflammatory response. The ACE enzyme will cleave the tripeptide Ser-Pro-Phe^2 from des-Arg^9 bradykinin so that it is inactive and can no longer interact with the B1 receptor (fig. 1) [2].

The fact that bradykinin accumulates when degradation is inhibited suggests that there is a baseline rate of production at all times and, if this equilibrium is upset between production and destruction, serious angioedema can result. The source of bradyki-

2

nin could be either turnover of the plasma bradykinin-forming cascade, or the effect of tissue kallikrein cleavage of low-molecular-weight kininogen. A rodent model of factor XII deficiency is associated with half-normal levels of bradykinin, suggesting at least a partial contribution of the plasma cascade. Anecdotal reports of the efficacy of C1 inhibitor (C1 INH), or ecallantide (plasma kallikrein inhibitor) in ameliorating ACE-induced angioedema, also suggest the production of bradykinin by the plasma cascade, while similar efficacy of icatibant, a B2 receptor antagonist, points to bradykinin as the mediator, regardless of the mechanism. Controlled trials of these agents as therapy for ACE-induced angioedema are required and are in progress. The increased incidence in African-Americans is attributed to polymorphisms in additional plasma proteins that contribute to bradykinin degradation, which may become critical when ACE is inhibited [3]. These include aminopeptidase P, neutral endopeptidase, and dipeptidyl peptidase IV.

Hereditary Angioedema

HAE is now considered to be the prototypic bradykinin-mediated disease with manifestations consisting of peripheral attacks of swelling (hands, feet, face, genitalia), gastrointestinal attacks (severe abdominal pain, vomiting, diarrhea) and oropharyngeal attacks, including laryngeal edema, and severe tongue and pharyngeal swelling. Episodes average 3 days in duration and can be precipitated by trauma, infection, estrogen and anxiety, although a cause for most episodes is not evident. Gastrointestinal attacks resemble acute bowel obstruction or an acute abdomen often leading to emergency room visits, while asphyxiation due to laryngeal edema was commonplace prior to the advent of therapies that could treat or prevent attacks of swelling. The first episode typically occurs in a young person (90% occur between the ages of 1 and 20 years) but a delay in diagnosis of many years is not uncommon, even though the requisite tests for diagnosis are readily available. Performance of a complement C4 level and C1 INH level measurement by protein and function in every patient with recurrent angioedema in the absence of urticaria is required by all physicians caring for patients with angioedema, including primary care physicians, as well as specialists such as allergists, dermatologists, gastroenterologists and emergency room physicians. During the course of this illness 95–100% of patients have peripheral attacks of swelling, 90% will have gastrointestinal episodes at some point in the illness, and 50% will have one or more episodes of laryngeal edema.

HAE was first described by Osler as a familial form of severe angioedema, and the underlying defect, an absence or dysfunction of the C1 INH, was reported by Virginia Donaldson and Richard Evans [4] in 1963. This protein inhibits the active form of the C1r and C1s subcomponents of C1. In its absence, C1 is unstable and autoactivates. More specifically, the C1r subcomponent of C1 autoactivates [5], the active enzyme activates C1s, and the activated C1s cleaves and activates its substrates, C4 and C2. However, C4 is a more sensitive substrate of activated C1s, which accounts for its low level in 95% of HAE patients even when they are asymptomatic. Thus, a C4 level is a good screening test, but confirmation of the diagnosis requires measurement of C1 INH by protein and function. Over 300 mutations of the C1 INH protein have been described and these are spread throughout all 8 exons of the C1 INH gene. Eighty-five percent of patients have a mutation which severely compromises protein synthesis and/or secretion (e.g. a stop codon, insertion, deletion), and have a very low protein level and commensurately low function. This is called type I HAE. Fifteen percent of patients have a normal protein level but abnormal function and are designated type II HAE. Here the mutation is more commonly a point mutation manifested as single amino acid substitutions (often within exon 8 near the inhibitory site of the protein) so that the mRNA is translated into protein, but the protein is non-functional [6]. HAE is transmitted as an autosomal dominant disorder, so there is one normal C1 INH gene. Yet the functional level often varies from 0 to 35% in symptomatic patients, much less than the 50% predicted if the one normal gene functioned optimally. This has been attributed to consumption of C1 INH by circulating active enzymes and/or trans-inhibition of the normal gene by the mutant gene at the transcriptional or perhaps translational level [7].

C1 Inhibitor as Inhibitor of the Bradykinin-Forming Cascade

Soon after C1 INH was described as a complement inhibitor, it was found to inhibit plasma kallikrein [8], followed in succession by inhibitor activity for factor XIIa, factor XIIf, factor XII autoactivation [9], prekallikrein cleavage of high-molecular-weight kininogen (HK) [10], and HSP-90-dependent conversion of prekallikrein to kallikrein [11]. In its absence one would anticipate persisting activation of the bradykinin-forming cascade once it had been instituted. C1 INH is the only significant inhibitor of factor XIIa and factor XIIf, as well as the site within the prekallikrein-HK complex.

Plasma kallikrein is inhibited by α_2-macroglobulin [12] as well as C1 INH, and the percent contribution of each is about 70% C1 INH and 30% α_2-macroglobulin at body temperature. At colder temperatures, inhibition by α_2-macroglobulin becomes progressively more prominent [12]. Nevertheless, the definition of C1 INH as a complement inhibitor and observed consumption of C4 and then C2 [13] (during attacks of swelling) focused attention on the possibility of a vasoactive mediator of swelling derived from the complement cascade, and C2 in particular.

The Myth of C2-Kinin

The early studies of the pathogenesis of HAE focused on the complement component C2 since it is normal when HAE patients are asymptomatic and decreases as attacks of swelling proceed. In 1972, Donaldson et al. [14] demonstrated that plasmin digestion of the products of C2 activation (C2a and C2b) liberates a peptide with kinin-like activity that is distinguished from bradykinin by its inactivation by trypsin but with comparable properties of causing smooth muscle contraction and increased vascular permeability. Additional studies appeared consistent with this observation, for example injection of activated C1 into HAE patients caused a skin permeability reaction in excess of that seen in normal patients [15]. One might consider that the trauma of the injection simply produced bradykinin; however, in an animal model, vasopermeability was seen with injected C1, but not in an animal lacking C2 [16]. During the decade between 1972 and 1983, there was considerable evidence of C1 INH being the key control protein of the bradykinin-forming cascade, but no confirmation of the experiments relating to C2-kinin by other laboratories, and no molecular identification of the kinin.

In 1983, we attempted to reproduce the experiments describing C2-kinin as a contractile activity and reported that activation of C1, C4 and C2 followed by plasmin digestion of the products did not produce any kinin-like activity [17] (fig. 2a). Furthermore, HAE plasma drawn in EDTA, when incubated without any additional activating surface, produced progressively more bradykinin with time [17] (fig. 2b). We concluded that HAE plasma is unstable and that, of the two possibilities being considered at that time, C-kinin as the answer was untenable, leaving the remaining choice, bradykinin, as the answer. Other workers tried to produce a kinin from the second component of complement and also failed. Yet one publication described an amino acid sequence within C2 that has permeability properties [18], but no known enzyme cleaves C2 to release it.

Additional data accumulated during the decade from 1983 to 1993 until bradykinin was finally accepted to be the mediator of the swelling of HAE. To date, there is no other paper that directly addresses the existence or non-existence of a C2-kinin; all subsequent articles provide evidence in favor of bradykinin, but one could then propose that both molecules are important and contributory. That is the reason why the demonstration that bradykinin is the mediator of HAE (prior to treatment with drugs that specifically target the bradykinin-forming cascade) required an attempt to reproduce the data demonstrating C2-kinin.

Bradykinin Is the Mediator of Hereditary Angioedema

Curd et al. [19] studied induced skin blisters in normal patients versus those with HAE, and found plasma kallikrein levels within the blisters to be far in excess of that seen in normal controls. Decreased prekallikrein and HK levels were found in HAE pa-

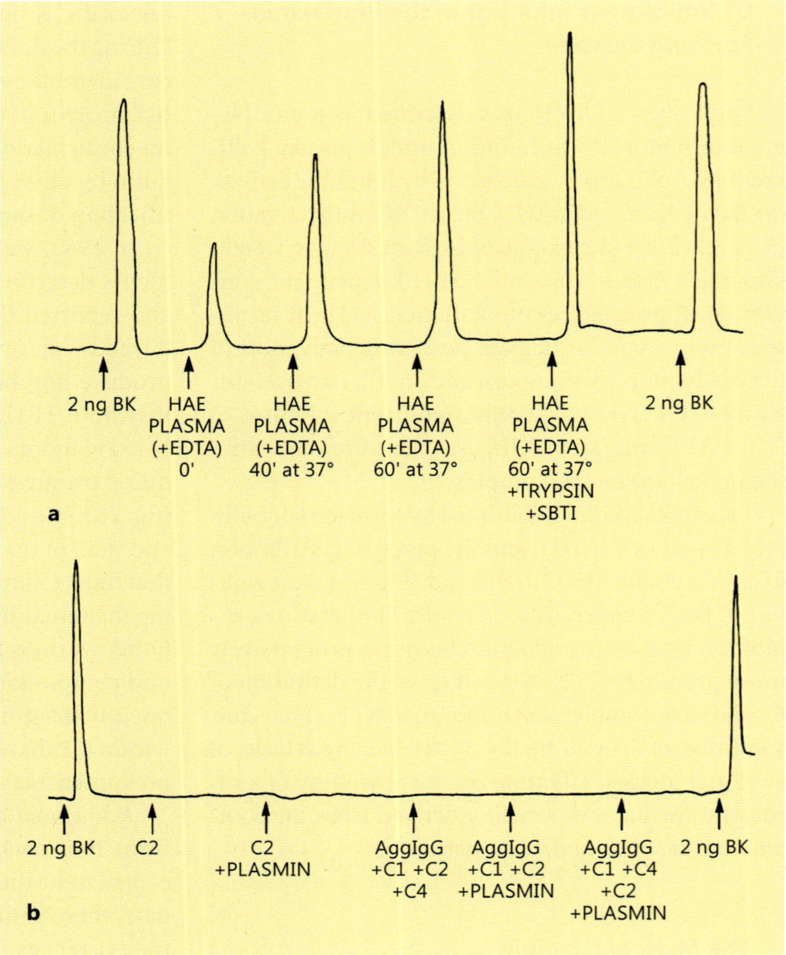

Fig. 2. Bradykinin production by plasma from patients with HAE. A bioassay recording of the contraction of a guinea pig ilium. Standard 2-mg contractions are shown at the beginning and end. HAE plasma in plastic test tubes was incubated and assayed at 0, 40 and 60 min, and a duplicate 60-min sample was incubated for an additional 30 min with trypsin. A progressive increase in bradykinin formation is seen which is unaffected by tryptic digestion (the putative C2-kinin was trypsin sensitive). Normal plasma, assayed under the same conditions, has no detectable bradykinin at any time point.

tients during attacks of swelling, as well as factor XII activation and cleavage of HK. Subsequently, a family was described in which a C1 INH mutation was found that failed to inhibit C1, so that C4 levels were diminished, but the inhibitory activity on factor XIIa and kallikrein was present [20, 21]. None of the family members had a history of swelling. A number of authors of the original publications dealing with C2-kinin then re-examined plasma activation. Bradykinin was measured by radioimmunoassay and permeability studies were included. Activation of HAE plasma was shown to generate bradykinin, permeability effects were attributable to bradykinin, and plasma deficient in C2 behaved in exactly the same way, i.e. the only vasoactive mediator was bradykinin and the presence or absence of C2 was irrelevant [22]. The authors held out the possibility that some other kinin might still be important but not demonstrable in vitro employing plasma experiments, despite the fact that some of the original experiments could not be reproduced.

Bradykinin levels were found to be elevated at the site of swelling in patients with HAE [23] followed by the development of a rodent model by Han et al. [24] with the C1 INH gene knocked out, which demonstrated a prominent cutaneous blueing reaction with Evans blue dye indicative of increased permeability. This reaction was prevented by knockout of the B2 receptor gene. Rodents lacking C1 INH do not have angioedema, but this model is consistent

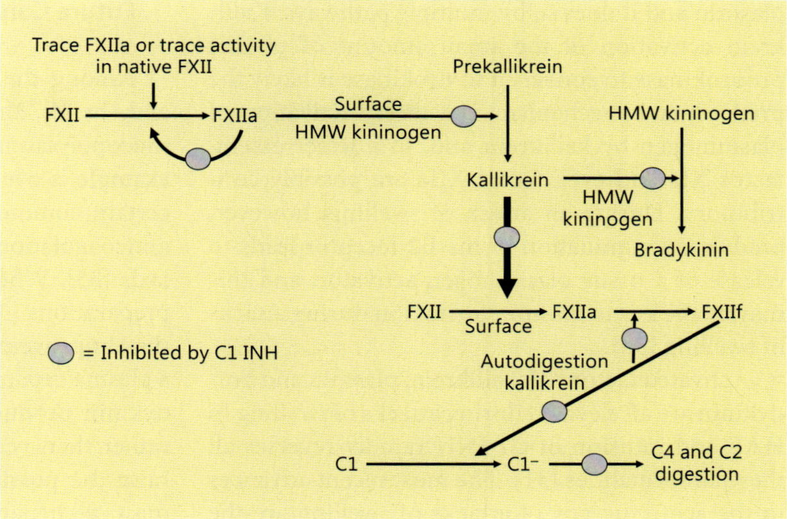

Fig. 3. Bradykinin production in HAE. The sites of C1 INH action to inhibit proteases requisite for bradykinin formation are shown. It inhibits factor XII autoactivation, factor XIIa activation of prekallikrein, kallikrein digestion of HK to produce bradykinin, kallikrein feedback activation of factor XII to produce factor XIIa, further digestion of factor XIIa to produce factor XIIf, and factor XIIf activation of C1 and inhibition of activated C1 to cleave C4 and C2.

with bradykinin as the permeability factor released when C1 INH is absent. During this decade, review articles continued to have C2-kinin included in diagrams of the pathogenesis of HAE. In response to this we wrote an editorial asserting that not only is bradykinin the only vasoactive substance demonstrated to cause the swelling of HAE, but also questioning the existence of any kinin derived from C2 [25].

It is important to note that a C4 level (which is diminished in 95% of HAE patients when they are asymptomatic) and C1 INH by protein and function should be measured in all patients with recurrent angioedema without urticaria to screen for types I and II HAE. During attacks of swelling, C4 levels approach zero and C2 levels diminish. This appears to be due to activation of C1r and then C1s by factor XIIf [26] and perhaps plasmin. A diagrammatic representation of the control of the bradykinin-forming cascade by C1 INH is shown in figure 3, including its role in controlling C1 activation.

Treatment of Hereditary Angioedema

Numerous publications in recent years have dealt with the therapy of HAE. Replacement with C1 INH, available in Europe and Australia for the past 25 years, can be used acutely to abort attacks of swelling (Berinert), including laryngeal edema, or can be given on a regular basis for prophylaxis (Cinryze). These have become available in the USA since 2008, but prior to that the treatment of choice was attenuated androgens such as danazol or stanazolol [27, 28]. Once instituted, these agents dramatically improved patients' lives even though numerous side effects are possible because treatment is prolonged and resistant patients required particularly high doses.

Mention should be made of the use of epsilon aminocaprioc acid, or tranexamic acid for prophylaxis in HAE, particularly in children, where androgens should be avoided. These agents are still occasionally employed but are not as effective as the androgenic compounds. They act to inhibit plasmin or, more importantly, conversion of plasminogen to plasmin. The main interaction of plasmin with the bradykinin cascade is the activation of factor XII to factor XIIa and factor XIIf, i.e. it functions in a similar fashion to the kallikrein feedback activation of factor XII. In fact the original discovery of factor XIIf employed plasmin as the enzyme to produce it. Plasmin cannot activate prekallikrein and its effect on HK is minimal. It may degrade C1 INH to further lower levels [29]. The factor XII-dependent cascade does lead to the conversion of plasminogen to plasmin and it does so by multiple pathways. Kallikrein activation of the small amount of plasma prourokinase to convert it to urokinase is likely the predominant mechanism, but direct activation of plasminogen by kallikrein and, to a lesser extent, factor XIa and even factor XIIa are possibly contributory. During an attack of swelling, however, bradykinin stimulation of the B2 receptor leads to release of a tissue plasminogen activator, and this may be the key to plasmin formation during attacks of swelling [30].

Activated factor XII, kallikrein, plasmin and bradykinin are all elevated during attacks of swelling in HAE and infusion of C1 INH rapidly reverses all these abnormalities [31]. The most recent advances in the acute therapy of attacks of swelling are the subcutaneous injection of either a plasma kallikrein inhibitor, ecallantide [32], or a B2 receptor antagonist, icatibant [33], and the efficacy of these compounds have expanded the treatment options for patients. Together with C1 INH [34], they provide considerable efficacy without the potential side effects of androgenic components. Proof of bradykinin as the mediator of the swelling of HAE is not possible without a demonstration that inhibiting its production or inhibiting its action provides specific therapy that blocks the process, and this has been achieved [33].

Future Considerations

Among the interesting activators of factor XII and, hence, the bradykinin-forming cascade, are mucopolysaccharides that are oversulfated. A prime example is oversulfated heparin that contaminated certain commercial heparin preparations used for anticoagulation and caused symptoms of anaphylaxis [35]. When factor XIIf contaminates albumin preparations [36] it leads to profound shock rather than improvement in hypotensive patients requiring a plasma expander, emphasizing the potency of bradykinin production when it occurs in the arterial rather than venous circulation. These occurrences raise the possibility that release of bradykinin by mast cell heparin (which is also oversulfated) could be a major contributor to the hypotension of anaphylaxis. Perhaps there is an analogous effect in the skin in patients with antihistamine-resistant chronic urticaria.

Another factor XII-dependent initiator of bradykinin formation appears to be aggregated proteins such as is seen in amyloidosis or the β-protein of Alzheimer's disease [37]. In each instance, the monomeric protein is inactive while the aggregate functions as a surface upon which factor XII activation can proceed [38]. Perhaps there are physiologic consequences beyond the interesting biochemistry.

References

1 Sheikh I, Kaplan A: Mechanism of digestion of bradykinin and lysylbradykinin (kallidin) in human serum: role of carboxypeptidase, angiotensin-converting enzyme and determination of final degradation products. Biochem Pharmacol 1989;38:993–1000.

2 Sheikh I, Kaplan A: Studies of the digestion of bradykinin, Lys-bradykinin, and des-Arg^9-bradykinin by angiotensin-converting enzyme. Biochem Pharmacol 1986;35: 1951–1956.

3 Blais CJ, Rouleau J, Brown N, et al: Serum metabolism of bradykinin and des-Arg^9-bradykinin in patients with angiotensin-converting enzyme inhibitor-associated angioedema. Immunopharmacology 1999;43: 293–302.

4 Donaldson V, Evans R: A biochemical abnormality in hereditary angioneurotic edema. Am J Med 1963;35:37–44.

5 Ziccardi RJ: Spontaneous activation of the first component of human complement (C1) by an intramolecular autocatalytic mechanism. J Immunol 1982;128:2500–2504.

6 Cugno M, Zanichelli A, Foieni F, et al: C1-inhibitor deficiency and angioedema: molecular mechanisms and clinical progress. Trends Mol Med 2009;15:69–78.

7 Quastel M, Harrison R, Cicardi M, et al: Behavior in vivo of normal and dysfunctional C1 inhibitor in normal subjects and patients with hereditary angioneurotic edema. J Clin Invest 1983;71:1041–1046.

8 Gigli I, Mason JW, Colman RW, et al: Interaction of plasma kallikrein with the C1 inhibitor. J Immunol 1970;104:574–581.

9 Weiss R, Silverberg M, Kaplan AP: The effect of C1 inhibitor upon Hageman factor autoactivation. Blood 1986;68:239–243.

10 Joseph K, Tholanikunnel B, Kaplan A: Factor XII-independent cleavage of high-molecular-weight kininogen by prekallikrein and inhibition by C1 inhibitor. J Allergy Clin Immunol 2009;124:143–149.

11 Joseph K, Tholanikunnel B, Kaplan A: Heat shock protein 90 catalyzes activation of the prekallikrein-kininogen complex in the absence of factor XII. Proc Natl Acad Sci USA 2002;99:896–900.

12 Harpel P, Lewin M, Kaplan A: Distribution of plasma kallikrein between C1 inactivator and α_2-macroglobulin in plasma utilizing a new assay for α_2-macroglobulin-kallikrein complexes. J Biol Chem 1985;260:4257–4263.

13 Austen K, Sheffer A: Detection of hereditory angioneurotic edema by demonstration of a reduction in the second component of human complement. N Engl J Med 1965;272: 649–656.

14 Donaldson VH, Rosen FS, Bing DH: Role of the second component of complement (C2) and plasmin in kinin release in hereditary angioneurotic edema (H.A.N.E.) plasma. Trans Assoc Am Physicians 1977;90:174–183.
15 Willms K, Rosen F, Donaldson V: Observations on the ultrastructure of lesions induced in human and guinea pig skin by C1 esterase and polypeptide from hereditary angioneurotic edema (HANE) plasma. Clin Immunol Immunopathol 1975;4:174–188.
16 Strang C, Auerbach H, Rosen F: C1s-induced vascular permeability in C2-deficient guinea pigs. J Immunol 1986;137:631–635.
17 Fields T, Ghebrehiwet B, Kaplan AP: Kinin formation in hereditary angioedema plasma: evidence against kinin derivation from C2 and in support of 'spontaneous' formation of bradykinin. J Allergy Clin Immunol 1983;72:54–60.
18 Strang CJ, Cholin S, Spragg J, et al: Angioedema induced by a peptide derived from complement component C2. J Exp Med 1988;168:1685–1698.
19 Curd J, Prograis LJ, Cochrane C: Detection of active kallikrein in induced blister fluids of hereditary angioedema patients. N Engl J Med 1980;152:742–747.
20 Wisnieski J, Knauss T, Yike I, et al: Unique C1 inhibitor dysfunction in a kindred without angioedema. 1. A mutant C1 INH that inhibits C1-s but not C1-r. J Immunol 1994;152:3199–3209.
21 Zahedi R, Bissler J, Davis AE, et al: Unique C1 inhibitor dysfunction in a kindred without angioedema. 2. Identification of an Ala443→Val substitution and functional analysis of the recombinant mutant protein. J Clin Invest 1995;95:1299–1305.
22 Shoemaker L, Schurman S, Donaldson V, et al: Hereditary angioneurotic oedema: characterization of plasma kinin and vascular permeability-enhancing activities. Clin Exp Immunol 1994;95:22–28.
23 Nussberger J, Cugno M, Cicardi M, et al: Local bradykinin generation in hereditary angioedema. J Allergy Clin Immunol 1999;104:1321–1322.
24 Han E, MacFarlane R, Mulligan A, et al: Increased vascular permeability in C1 inhibitor-deficient mice mediated by the bradykinin type 2 receptor. J Clin Invest 2002;8:1057–1063.
25 Kaplan A, Ghebrehiwet B: Does C-2 kinin exist? J Allergy Clin Immunol 2004;115:876.
26 Ghebrehiwet B, Randazzo B, Dunn J, et al: Mechanisms of activation of the classical pathway of complement by Hageman factor fragment. J Clin Invest 1983;71:1450–1456.
27 Gelfand JA, Sherins RJ, Alling DW, et al: Treatment of hereditary angioedema with danazol: reversal of clinical and biochemical abnormalities. N Engl J Med 1976;295:1444–1448.
28 Sheffer AL, Fearon DT, Austen KF: Clinical and biochemical effects of stanozolol therapy for hereditary angioedema. J Allergy Clin Immunol 1981;68:181–187.
29 Wallace EM, Perkins SJ, Sim RB, et al: Degradation of C1-inhibitor by plasmin: implications for the control of inflammatory processes. Mol Med 1997;3:385–396.
30 Zhao Y, Qiu Q, Mahdi F, et al: Assembly and activation of HK-PK complex on endothelial cells results in bradykinin liberation and NO formation. Am J Physiol Heart Circ Physiol 2001;280:H1821–H1829.
31 Joseph K, Tholanikunnel T, Kaplan A: Treatment of episodes of hereditary angioedema with C1 inhibitor: serial assessment of observed abnormalities of the plasma bradykinin-forming pathway and fibrinolysis. Ann Allergy Asthma Immunol 2010;104:50–54.
32 Cicardi M, Levy R, McNeil D: Ecallantide for the treatment of acute attacks in hereditary angioedema. N Engl J Med 2010;363:523–531.
33 Cicardi M, Banerji A, Bracho F, et al: Icatibant, a new bradykinin receptor antagonist in hereditary angioedema. N Engl J Med 2010;363:532–541.
34 Zuraw B, Busse P, White M: Nanofiltered C1 inhibitor concentrate for treatment of hereditary angioedema. N Engl J Med 2010;363:513–522.
35 Kishimoto T, Viswanathan K, Ganguly T, et al: Contaminated heparin associated with adverse clinical events and activation of the contact system. N Engl J Med 2008;358:2457–2467.
36 Alving BM, Hojima Y, Pisano JJ, et al: Hypotension associated with prekallikrein activator (Hageman-factor fragments) in plasma protein fraction. N Engl J Med 1978;299:66–70.
37 Shibayama Y, Joseph K, Nakazawa Y, et al: Zinc-dependent activation of the plasma kinin-forming cascade by aggregated β amyloid protein. Clin Immunol 1999;90:89–99.
38 Maas C, Govers-Riemslay J, Bouma B, et al: Misfolded proteins activate factor XII in humans, leading to kallikrein formation without initiating coagulation. J Clin Invest 2008;118:3208–3218.

Dr. Allen P. Kaplan
Department of Medicine
Medical University of South Carolina
171 Ashley Avenue
Charleston, SC 29425-2220 (USA)
E-Mail kaplana@musc.edu

3 Mechanisms of Allergy: Important Discoveries

Bergmann K-C, Ring J (eds): History of Allergy. Chem Immunol Allergy. Basel, Karger, 2014, vol 100, pp 150–154
DOI: 10.1159/000358621

The Discovery of Immunoglobulin E and Its Role in Allergy

S.G.O. Johansson

Department of Medicine, Clinical and Immunology Unit, Karolinska Institute, and Department of Clinical Immunology and Transfusion Medicine, Karolinska University Hospital, Stockholm, Sweden

Abstract

Immunoglobulin E (IgE) was discovered in 1967. Today, more than 40 years after the discovery, the normal beneficial function in the body of this enigmatic immunoglobulin still remains unclear. However, ever since the discovery new knowledge about allergic diseases and allergens, new treatments and new diagnostic tools have continued to emerge as a direct result of our ability to identify and measure IgE and IgE antibodies.

The immunoglobulin E (IgE) molecule is a single four-chain unit with a molecular weight above 190,000 Da and a carbohydrate content of about 11% [1]. It shares the general characteristics of all immunoglobulins, but with two salient features. One is the unique ability of the IgE system to respond to extremely minute amounts of specific proteins – the annual dose of pollen allergen has been calculated to be just 1 μg [2] – and then activate basophils and mast cells, mediating the release of histamine and other mediators in response to the exposure to these small amounts of protein. The other is the extremely low concentration in normal serum [3, 4]. The latter feature was of course the main reason why it took so long before it was discovered.

The Search for the Elusive Factor

The first connection between allergic symptoms and a serum factor was made in 1919, when M.A. Ramirez reported a case of asthma caused by allergy being passively transferred by blood transfusion [5], which was recently documented experimentally [6]. In 1921, Prausnitz and Küstner [7] reported their famous passive transfer of a positive skin test, the PK test. Coca and Cooke [8] coined the term 'atopy' in 1923 and linked this hereditary trait to the presence of 'bodies' in serum which they called 'reagins'.

However, it would take several decades before any significant steps towards exploring this connection were taken. It was only in the 1960s that sufficiently sensitive techniques for the separation and identification of proteins became available, and it became possible to look in earnest for a factor, i.e.

the reagin, in the blood that could mediate such responses.

The discovery of the immunoglobulin that later became known as IgE resulted from the work of two independent research teams. In Denver (Colo., USA), Kimishige and Teruko Ishizaka were specifically searching for a serum factor through structured laboratory work, although for a long time with only limited success. In 1966–1967, they had an antiserum that could precipitate a serum fraction, resulting in a decrease in PK activity [9]. They postulated that this represented a new immunoglobulin class, which they called γE-globulin. However, as the proposed γE-globulin was not isolated, it was not possible to demonstrate that it was a homogeneous immunoglobulin rather than a complex of inflammatory factors.

In Uppsala, Sweden, myself and Hans Bennich approached the problem from another direction. The starting point was the discovery of a serum with an atypical myeloma protein.

The M component could not be identified as belonging to any of the then established immunoglobulin classes IgG, IgM or IgA; nor was it IgD, which had recently been discovered [10]. Our investigations confirmed that it had unique antigens and unique biochemical/physiochemical properties that distinguished it from the other immunoglobulins, so we first called it IgX.

A radioimmunoassay based on antibodies to antigens on the Fc fragment of IgX was developed, and sera of blood donors inhibited the assay in a dose-response manner. Thus, IgX had all the properties needed for the definition of a new immunoglobulin class; it was a unique biochemical structure carrying unique antigens generally present in the population. In addition, it was shown that the new immunoglobulin [11], and later its Fc fragment [12], blocked the PK test. The new immunoglobulin was provisionally named IgND, using the initials of the patient from whom the original blood sample came, as was the routine at that time.

Further studies revealed that the serum IgND concentration was increased in about 60% of the cases with allergic asthma [3]. A radioimmunoassay for IgND antibodies to common allergens was developed. This, which became the groundbreaking RAST test, gave results that correlated well with clinical allergy diagnoses [13].

In early 1967, reagents were exchanged between the Uppsala and Denver groups and it was found that antiserum to γE-globulin reacted with isolated IgND, and that purified IgND could block the reaction of anti-γE in a biological test system for reaginic activity. γE and IgND shared antigenic determinants and biological activity. The official declaration of the new immunoglobulin class IgE was made in 1968 by the World Health Organization Immunoglobulin Reference Center in Lausanne [14].

Knowledge about IgE and the immune and inflammatory mechanism behind clinical allergy had a most positive impact on the allergy specialty and the respect for allergic patients in society. However, changes take time and it was not until just after the turn of the millennium that the European Academy of Allergology and Clinical Immunology [15] and the World Allergy Organization [16] tried to clean up the communication and understanding within the field of allergy by promoting a common nomenclature for allergy.

IgE and the Allergic Inflammation

Early studies of the mechanisms of allergy used the basophil granulocytes as representatives of the cell system involved in the allergic inflammation [17, 18]. The results from the Johns Hopkins group are still both relevant and important. The importance of the IgE antibody link in the inflammatory cascade chain reaction has been highlighted. Recently, the basophil allergen threshold sensitivity has been 'rediscovered' as a most interesting alternative to allergen provocations [6], for example bronchial allergen challenge testing [19].

Allergy Diagnosis

The discovery of IgE had its first major impact in clinical practice in the form of reliable and safe in vitro tests for allergy. The in vivo skin tests that had long been used suffered from severe drawbacks in terms of accuracy and safety. They still do today [20–

22], whereas the in vitro IgE tests have gone through a process of continuous development and refinement.

The first method developed was to measure the total amount of circulating IgE in the blood ('total IgE') [3]. The first commercial total IgE test, the Pharmacia IgE Test (Pharmacia, Uppsala, Sweden) was introduced in 1972.

However, it is the IgE antibodies, specific to the relevant allergens, that are involved in the mediation of histamine release and, thus, responsible for the allergic symptoms. The first test capable of measuring these allergen-specific IgE antibodies was reported in 1967 [13]. It was the RAST test which became generally available in 1974 (Phadebas RAST, Pharmacia). Since then, continued development work has resulted in increasingly sensitive and accurate test systems, enabling the detection and measurement of IgE antibodies to many hundreds of allergens.

In recent years, a clear relationship has been shown to exist between the concentration of antibodies in the patient's serum and the likelihood of developing allergic symptoms, and the severity of the symptoms [23, 24]. The ability to make quantitative measurements of IgE antibody concentrations is thus of great importance when evaluating the prognosis of an allergic disease, and also before starting immunotherapy.

We now also see an increasing scientific and clinical interest in the individual proteins that make up an allergen, i.e. a foodstuff. As some of these allergen components may be cross-reacting with rather innocent allergens, for example from pollens, while others seem to carry the major allergenic property of the allergen source in question, knowledge of the individual patient's sensitization to different components can be of great clinical interest [25].

However, the daily work of the practicing physician is hardly made easier by the large amounts of detailed information made available by 'component-resolved diagnostics'. Since prevalences of asthma, allergic rhinoconjunctivitis and food allergy as high as 25–35% have been reported [26, 27], it is obvious that the great majority of allergic patients are managed in primary care. Thus, there is a need for simple tools that can help the primary care physician diagnose allergy and identify the patients that should be referred to an allergy specialist. Near-patient tests for IgE antibodies are now also available for this purpose.

Treatment

The first basic step in the management of allergic patients should be elimination, if possible, or avoidance of the source of the allergens triggering the symptoms. This, of course, requires the identification of the source, and the ability to test for IgE antibodies in the patient's blood is a crucial step.

A most remarkable example of this is the 'pholcodine story' [28]. In some countries a high prevalence of anaphylaxis caused by neuromuscular blocking agents during anesthesia is reported, while in others such reactions are very rare. In Norway, such reactions were 10–20 times more common than in Sweden, a neighbor country with a similar health care system and living habits. Investigations of the IgE sensitization to different drugs and common household chemicals showed that the most likely reason was that many individuals in Norway were sensitized to a cough syrup that was not marketed in Sweden. This contained pholcodine, which shares allergenic determinants with the neuromuscular blocking agents. When the cough syrup was withdrawn from the Norwegian market, the annual number of cases decreased from around 20 to just 2–3 cases per year [29].

Allergen-specific immunotherapy has also benefited greatly from the ability to measure IgE antibodies as this has made it possible to characterize the allergen extracts used, both in terms of content and potency. Using the allergens that are relevant for the individual patient is, of course, crucial in this form of treatment. The recently developed tests for antibodies to specific allergen components also offers new tools for identifying the patients that will respond well to allergen-specific immunotherapy.

A new form of treatment of IgE-mediated allergic asthma is based on the use of anti-IgE monoclonal antibodies (anti-IgE-specific immunotherapy), for example omalizumab (Xolair; Novartis, Basel, Switzerland) [30], introduced in 2003. By binding to IgE and eliminating it from serum, the monoclonal antibodies interrupt the signals that may trigger the allergic inflammatory cascade. This treatment is currently prescribed based on the serum level of IgE ('total IgE'). However, recommendations should be given concerning anti-IgE dosage in relation to the concentration of IgE antibodies [31, 32].

Basophil allergen threshold sensitivity [33], referred to by us as CD-sens [6], has been shown to be a most useful approach to evaluating the patient's allergen sensitivity, i.e. the link in the allergy chain to which anti-IgE treatment is targeted. A correlation was found between CD-sens and the percentage of IgE antibodies of IgE [34]. In a recent study using CD-sens, we evaluated the importance of the size of the IgE antibody fraction in patients undergoing anti-IgE treatment, and found that if the percentage of IgE antibodies was higher than 3.8%, none of the patients responded with a 'turning off' of the triggering IgE [31]. A recent study of patients with allergic rhinitis confirmed these findings [32].

An increase of the anti-IgE dosage given to such patients should therefore be considered. Obviously, to obtain a good response by anti-IgE-specific immunotherapy the presence and concentration of clinically relevant IgE antibodies must be duly taken into consideration, which might be of special importance in the 'real atopics' with low IgE concentrations but large IgE antibody fractions [35].

The Beneficial Function of IgE

Although the role of IgE in allergic diseases has been well established, the normal beneficial function of the immunoglobulin in the body remains unclear. Speculations as to the primary role of IgE in the immune defense have included a possible role in the defense against parasitic infections. However, as one of the unique features of IgE is its ability to detect extremely small amounts of proteins, it does not seem likely that its main function would be to defend against organisms secreting large amounts of proteins. Another area that has been in focus is allergy and cancer. Here different hypotheses have been proposed which are in fact quite contradictory. It has been suggested that IgE may have a protective effect against cancer by enhancing immune surveillance. However, it has also been suggested that allergy could mean an increased risk for cancer as a result of the chronic stimulation of the immune system. No real scientific proof for any of these hypotheses has been produced.

Animal studies have shown that an IgE sensitization can promote the IgG antibody response to the same antigen [36, 37], indicating that the IgE system is involved in and communicates with the regular immune defense system. The involvement in immunoglobulin synthesis is also illustrated by the close to 100-fold polyclonal increase in IgE occurring after a minute exposure, i.e. 1 ml per day during a week, to a pholcodine-containing over-the-counter cough syrup in individuals who are IgE sensitized to pholcodine [38]. A similar increase is seen in graft-versus-host disease following bone marrow transplantation [39].

I personally believe that the answer to the beneficial function of IgE should be looked for in another direction. Given the ability of IgE to detect minute amounts of foreign proteins, and its ability to activate other parts of the immune system, it seems likely that its main function is to raise the alarm when a foreign protein enters the body, recruiting and activating other antibodies and cells that can attack and defeat the intruder. Maybe allergic symptoms like sneezing and diarrhea are actually primary attempts to get rid of a foreign, potentially harmful intruder.

If this is the case, the next logical question is what causes this mechanism to malfunction in the case of allergy? Why do harmless substances initiate an IgE-mediated disease reaction? Also, why is this occurring to such an extent in the western world that allergic diseases have become some of our most common diseases? There are many theories but so far no definitive answers. Despite all the progress in the past decades, many questions surrounding IgE remain to be answered.

References

1 Bennich H, Johansson SGO: Studies on a new class of human immunoglobulins. 2. Chemical and physiological properties; in Killander J (ed): Gamma Globulins. Structure and Control of Biosynthesis. Nobel Symposium 3. Stockholm, Almqvist & Wiksell, 1967, p 199.

3

2 Marsh DG: Allergens and the genetics of allergy; in Sela M (ed): The Antigens. New York, Academic Press, 1975, vol 3, pp 271–359.
3 Johansson SGO: Raised levels of a new immunoglobulin class (IgND) in asthma. Lancet 1967;ii:951–953.
4 Johansson SGO: Serum IgND levels in healthy children and adults. Int Arch Allergy 1968;34:1–8.
5 Ramirez MA: Horse asthma following blood transfusion: report on a case. JAMA 1919; 73:984.
6 Johansson SGO, Nopp A, van Hage M, Olofsson N, Lundahl J, Wehlin L, Söderström L, Stiller V, Öman H: Passive IgE-sensitization by blood transfusion. Allergy 2005;60:1192–1199.
7 Prausnitz C, Küstner H: Studien über die Überempfindlichkeit. Zentralbl Bakteriol I Abt Orig 1921;86:160.
8 Coca AF, Cooke RA: On the classification of the phenomenon of hypersensitiveness. J Immunol 1923;8:163–182.
9 Ishizaka K, Ishizaka T: Identification of γE-antibodies as a carrier of reaginic activity. J Immunol 1967;99:1187.
10 Rowe DS, Fahey JL: A new class of human immunoglobulins. 2. Normal serum IgD. J Exp Med 1965;121:185–199.
11 Stanworth DR, Humphrey JH, Bennich H, Johansson SGO: Specific inhibition of the Prausnitz-Küstner reaction by an atypical human myeloma protein. Lancet 1967;ii: 330–332.
12 Stanworth DR, Humphrey JH, Bennich H, Johansson SGO: Inhibition of Prausnitz-Küstner reaction by proteolytic-cleavage fragments of a human myeloma protein of immunoglobulin class E. Lancet 1968;i:17–18.
13 Wide L, Bennich H, Johansson SGO: Diagnosis of allergy by an in-vitro test for allergen antibodies. Lancet 1967;ii:1105–1107.
14 Bennich HH, Ishizaka K, Johansson SGO, Rowe DS, Stanworth DR, Terry WD: Immunoglobulin E, a new class of human immunoglobulin. Bull World Health Organ 1968; 38:151–152.
15 Johansson SGO, Hourihane JO, Bousquet J, Bruijnzeel-Koomen C, Dreborg S, Haahtela T, et al: A revised nomenclature for allergy: an EAACI position statement from the EAACI nomenclature task force. Allergy 2001;56:813–824.
16 Johansson SGO, Bieber T, Dahl R, Friedmann PS, Lanier BQ, Lockey RF, et al: Revised nomenclature for allergy for global use: report of the Nomenclature Review Committee of the World Allergy Organization, October 2003. J Allergy Clin Immunol 2004;113:832–836.
17 Lichtenstein LM, Osler AGJ: Studies on the mechanisms of hypersensitvity phenomena. 9. Histamine release from leukocytes by ragweed pollen allergen. J Exp Med 1964; 120:507–530.
18 Conroy MC, Adkinson NF Jr, Lichtenstein LM: Measurement of IgE on human basophils: relation to serum IgE and anti-IgE-induced histamine relese. J Immunol 1977; 118:1317–1321.
19 Dahlén B, Nopp A, Johansson SGO, Eduards M, Skedinger M, Adédoyin J: Basophil allergen threshold sensitivity, CD-sens, is a measure of allergen-sensitivity in asthma. Clin Exp Allergy 2011;41:1091–1097.
20 Vohlonen I, Terho EO, Koivikko A, Vanto T, Holmén A, Heinonen OP: Reproducibility of the skin prick test. Allergy 1989;44:525–531.
21 Nelson H: Variables in allergy skin testing. Allergy Proc 1994;15:265–268.
22 Lockey RF, Benedict LM, Turkeltaub PC, Bukantz SC: Fatalities associated with immunotherapy and skin testing. J Allergy Clin Immunol 1987;79:660–677.
23 Sampson HA, Ho DG: Relationship between food-specific IgE concentrations and the risk of positive food challenges in children and adolescents. J Allergy Clin Immunol 1997;100:444–451.
24 Sampson HA: Utility of food-specific IgE concentrations in predicting symptomatic food allergy. J Allergy Clin Immunol 2001; 107:891–896.
25 Valenta R, Lidholm J, Niederberger V, et al: The recombinant allergen-based concept of component-resolved diagnostics and immunotherapy (CRD and CRIT). Clin Exp Allergy 1999;29:896–904.
26 Beasley R, Keil U, von Mutius E, Pearce N: Worldwide variation in prevalence of symptoms of asthma, allergic rhinoconjunctivitis, and atopic eczema: ISAAC. Lancet 1998;351:1225–1232.
27 Mills ENC, Mackie AR, Burney P, Beyer K, Frewer L, Madsen C, Botjes E, Crevel RWR, van Ree R: The prevalence, cost and basis of food allergy across Europe. Allergy 2007;62: 717–722.
28 Florvaag E, Johansson SGO: The pholcodine story. Immunol Allergy Clin North Am 2009;29:419–427.
29 Florvaag E, Johansson SGO, Irgens Å, de Pater GH: IgE-sensitization to the cough suppressant pholcodine and the effects of its withdrawal from the Norwegian market. Allergy 2011;66:955–960.
30 Holgate ST, Chuchalin AG, Herbert J, Lotvall J, Persson GB, Chung KF, et al: Efficacy and safety of a recombinant anti-IgE antibody (omalizumab) in severe allergic asthma. Clin Exp Allergy 2004;34:632–638.
31 Johansson SGO, Nopp A, Öman H, Ankerst J, Cardell LO, Grönneberg R, Matsols H, Rudblad S, Strand V, Stålenheim G: The size of the disease relevant IgE antibody fraction in relation to 'total-IgE' predicts the efficacy of anti-IgE (Xolair®) treatment. Allergy 2009;64:1472–1477.
32 Eckman JA, Sterba PM, Kelly D, Alexander V, Liu MC, Bochner BS, et al: Effects of omalizumab on basophil and mast cell responses using an intranasal cat allergen challenge. J Allergy Clin Immunol 2010; 125:889–895.
33 Kleine-Tebbe J, Erdmann S, Knol EF, MacGlashan DW, Poulsen L, Gibbs B: Diagnostic tests based human basophils: potentials, pitfalls and perspectives. Int Arch Allergy Clin Immunol 2006;141:79–90.
34 Nopp A, Johansson SGO, Ankerst J, Bylin G, Cardell LO, Grönneberg R, et al: Basophil allergen threshold sensitivity: a useful approach to anti-IgE treatment efficacy evaluation. Allergy 2006;61:298–302.
35 Johansson SGO, Öman H, Nopp A, Pettersson S: The importance of IgE antibody levels in anti-IgE treatment. Allergy 200;61: 1216–1219.
36 Heyman B, Tianmin L, Gustavsson S: In vivo enhancement of the specific antibody response via the low-affininty receptor for IgE. Eur J Immunol 1993;23:1739–1742.
37 Getahun A, Hjelm F, Heyman B: IgE enhances antibody and T cell responses in vivo via CD23⁺ B cells. J Immunol 2005;175: 1473–1482.
38 Florvaag E, Johansson SGO, Öman H, Harboe T, Nopp A: Pholcodine stimulates a dramatic increase of IgE in IgE-sensitized individuals: a pilot study. Allergy 2006;61:49–55.
39 Ringdén O, Persson U, Johansson SGO: Are increased IgE-levels a signal of an acute graft-versus-host reaction? Immunol Rev 1983;71:57–75.

Dr. S.G.O. Johansson
Department of Medicine, Clinical and Immunology Unit
Karolinska Institute and University Hospital
SE–104 01 Stockholm (Sweden)
E-Mail s.g.o.johansson@ki.se

Bergmann K-C, Ring J (eds): History of Allergy. Chem Immunol Allergy. Basel, Karger, 2014, vol 100, pp 155–164
DOI: 10.1159/000358622

T Cell Subpopulations

Sergio Romagnani

Department of Internal Medicine, University of Florence, Florence, Italy

3

Abstract

The role of allergen-specific CD4+ effector type 2 helper (Th2) cells in the pathogenesis of allergic disorders is an established fact. Th2 cells produce interleukin (IL)-4 and IL-13, which induce immunoglobulin E production by B cells, and IL-5 that allows recruitment of eosinophils. Two main mechanisms control the Th2-mediated allergic inflammation: immune deviation (or Th1 redirection) and immune regulation. Regulatory T (Treg) cells exhibit a CD4+ phenotype and include Foxp3-positive thymic and induced Tregs, as well as Foxp3-negative IL-10-producing cells. Both immune deviation and immune regulation evoked by the maternal and newborn microbial environment probably operate in preventing allergen-specific Th2 responses. However, microbe-related protection from allergy seems to mainly depend on epigenetically controlled acetylation of the IFNG promoter of CD4+ T cells. Even Th17 and Th9 cells, as well as invariant NKT cells, have been implicated in the pathogenesis of allergic disorders, but their role is certainly more limited. Recently, innate lymphoid type 2 cells (ILC2) have been found to be able to produce high amounts of IL-5 and IL-13 in response to stimulation with IL-25 and IL-33 produced by non-immune cells. Together with Th2 cells, ILC2 may contribute to the induction and maintenance of allergic inflammation.

CD4+ T cells play a fundamental role in the function of the immune system. They help B cells to produce antibodies, to enhance and maintain the responses of cytotoxic CD8+ T cells, and regulate macrophage functions. Finally, CD4+ T cells are important mediators of immunologic memory. Because of all these activities, CD4+ T cells not only orchestrate immune responses against a variety of pathogenic microorganisms, but also regulate immune responses both to adjust the magnitude and persistence of protective responses and to control autoimmunity. From a functional point of view CD4+ T cells can be subdivided into two main categories, which are defined as effector and regulatory.

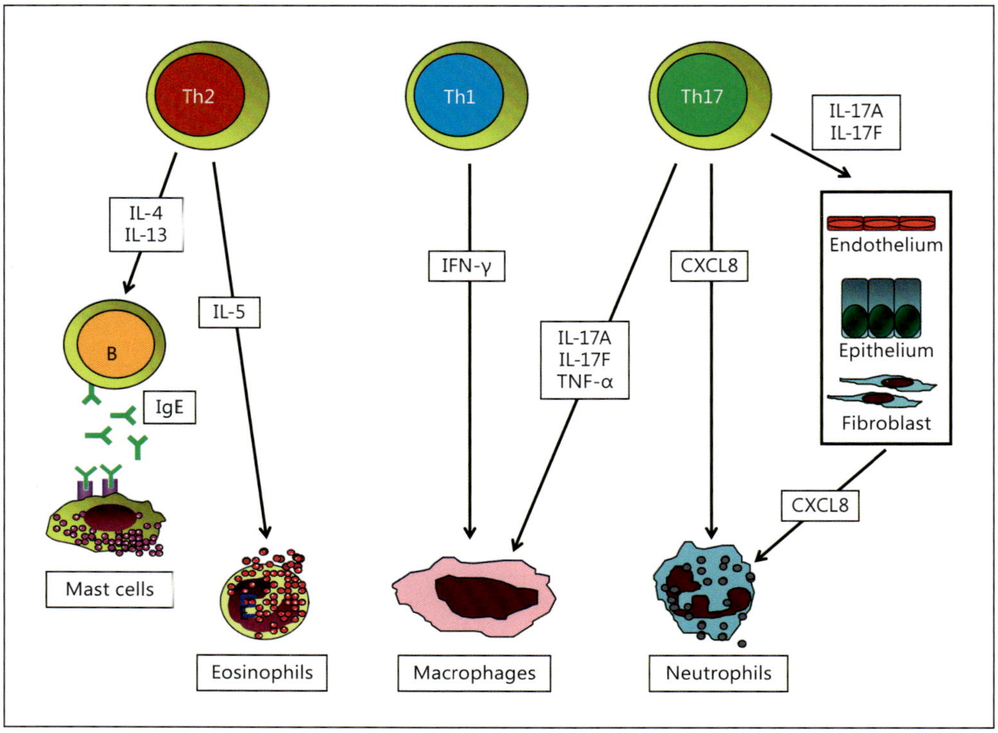

Fig. 1. The three major subpopulations of CD4+ effector T cells, their cytokines and the non-specific cells of the immune system they are able to activate. Th2 cells produce IL-4 and IL-13, which allow B lymphocytes to switch to the IgE production, and IL-5, which favors the activation and survival of eosinophil granulocytes. Th1 cells are the major activators of macrophages via the production of IFN-γ. Th17 cells can activate macrophages via the production of IL-17A, IL-17F and TNF-α, and also neutrophil granulocytes via the direct production of CXCL8 or its production by endothelial cells, epithelial cells and fibroblasts stimulated by IL-17A and IL-17F.

Effector CD4+ T Cells

The different effector functions of CD4+ T cells are achieved through the differentiation of naive CD4+ T cells as they are stimulated by their cognate antigen. This is presented by competent antigen-presenting cells to become effector and/or memory cells of specialized phenotypes.

The Th1/Th2 Paradigm

The initial understanding of the existence of distinctive populations of differentiated CD4+ T cells came from the analysis of mouse T cell clones that were shown to be divisible into two major groups designated T helper (Th)1 and Th2 cells [1], which were subsequently described even in humans [2]. In both mice and humans, Th1 and Th2 cells could be distinguished mainly by the cytokines they produce, but also because of the expression of distinct transcription factors and chemokine receptors. With regard to cytokine production, Th1 cells make interferon (IFN)-γ their signature cytokine and uniquely produce lymphotoxin, also named tumor necrosis factor (TNF)-β, but they can additionally produce TNF-α and interleukin (IL)-2. Because of these activities, Th1 cells display the peculiar ability of activating macrophages (fig. 1). By contrast, Th2 cells fail to produce IFN-γ or lymphotoxin and their signature cytokines are IL-4, IL-5 and IL-13. Th2 cells also produce TNF-α and some of them produce IL-9. On the other hand, Th2 cells were initially found to be able to produce IL-10, at least in the mouse, but subsequently this cytokine appeared to be produced by both Th1 and Th2 cells in humans and mice. The cytokine pathway of Th2 cells enabled the explanation of the activation of immunoglobulin E (IgE)-producing B cells (via IL-4 and IL-13), the recruitment of eosinophil granulocytes (via IL-5) and the growth of mast cell/basophils (via IL-9, IL-10; fig. 1). Human Th1 cells originate from naive Th cells in the presence of IL-12 [3], whereas Th2 cells develop in the presence of IL-4 [4]. Subsequent studies showed that Th1 and Th2 cells really represent distinct T cell lineages because they express different and mutually exclusive transcription factors. Th1, but not Th2 cells, express T-bet, whereas Th2 cells, but not Th1 cells, express GATA-binding protein-3 (GATA-3) and c-maf [5]. Finally, human Th1 cells were found to express distinct chemokine receptors, such as CCR5 and CXCR3, whereas Th2 cells mainly expressed CCR4 and CCR8 [6]. A series of studies performed in both experimental animal models and humans demonstrated that Th1 responses were prevalent in organ-specific autoimmune disorders and other cases of chronic inflammation, whereas allergic (atopic) disorders were found to be mainly dominated by Th2 responses against allergens. This dichotomy was named the Th1/Th2 paradigm [7] and maintained its validity for many years.

Beyond the Th1/Th2 Paradigm

In 2003, a third major effector population of murine CD4+ T cells was shown to exist. These cells, designated Th17 cells, were characterized by the production of IL-17A, IL-17F and IL-22 as signature cytokines, molecules not produced by Th1 or Th2 cells. IL-17 was found to be a strong activator of both macrophages and neutrophil granulocytes (fig. 1). Moreover, Th17 expressed a transcription factor distinct from those of Th1 (T-bet) and Th2 (GATA-3) cells, called ROR(γ)t [8]. Subsequent studies showed that IL-22 could also be produced by a subset of skin memory CD4+ T cells even in the absence of IL-17, IL-4 and IFN-γ production. Th22 cells mainly play a protective role in the skin and liver. These cells were claimed to be an independent and stable lineage of Th cells because they did not change their phenotype even under all polarizing conditions and the expression of the transcription factors BNC-2 and FOXO4 in the presence of reduced RORC, GATA-3 and T-bet [9]. However, whether Th22 cells originate as an independent lineage or result from Th17 cells that lost the ability to produce IL-17 is not yet surely established.

A major function of Th1, Th2 and Th17 cells is to help B cells produce IgM, IgG and IgA (and also IgE for Th2 cells) antibody in response to T-dependent antigens, as well as to control immunoglobulin class switching and somatic hypermutation. These events mainly occur within germinal centers, and the CD4+ T cells that enter the germinal centers to mediate their helper function for antibody production have been termed T follicular helper (Tfh) cells [10]. The possibility that Tfh cells represent an independent lineage, essentially parallel to Th1, Th2 and Th17 cells, has been suggested. However, whether these cells reflect the phenotypic state of each of the three major effector lineages remains uncertain.

IL-9, cloned more than 20 years ago, was initially found to be a Th2-specific cytokine. However, CD4+ T cells able to produce IL-9 were also generated from naive Th cells in the presence of both TGF-β and IL-4. Recently, it was reported that transforming growth factor (TGF)-β can induce Th2 cells to maintain the production of IL-9 alone, and these cells were designated as Th9 cells [11]. However, the conditions used to stimulate IL-17 production from human memory CD4+ T cells can also promote IL-9 expression. Thus, the fact that Th9 cells represent a stable and independent lineage remains to be proven.

Regulatory CD4+ T Cells

Besides exerting pro-inflammatory functions, CD4+ T cells can also exert regulatory functions. These cells were first discovered in 1995 when a subset of CD4+ T cells constitutively expressing high amounts of the IL-2 receptor α-chain (CD25) was identified. These cells, then termed regulatory T (Treg) cells, were highly enriched in suppressor activity [12]. Treg cells were able to prevent autoimmunity upon transfer into thymectomized mice and, in various other experimental models of autoimmunity, inhibit transplant rejection and thwart tumor immunity [12].

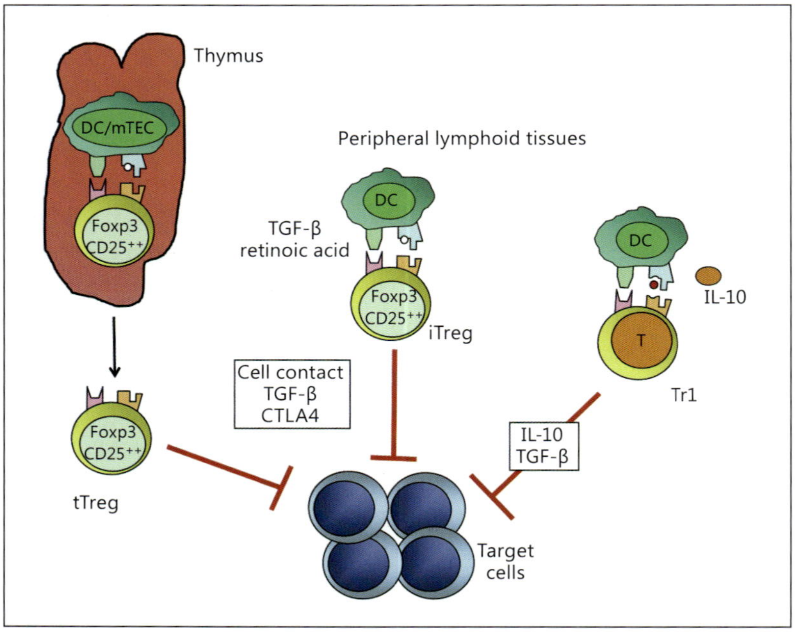

Fig. 2. The three major subpopulations of CD4+ Treg cells, their origin and mechanisms of regulatory activity. Foxp3+CD25+ Treg cells can be generated directly from the thymus (tTreg) or are induced in the periphery (iTreg) when naive T cells interact with DC producing TGF-β and retinoic acid. Both tTreg and iTreg exert their regulatory activity through direct contact with the target cell, but the nature of the molecules involved in this activity is still debated.

Foxp3+ Regulatory T Cells

Foxp3 is the master gene for Treg cell differentiation that occurs at the thymic level in both mice and humans (fig. 2). These cells have also been defined as natural or thymic Treg (tTreg) cells. The genetic loss of Foxp3 results in the loss of immunological tolerance and induction of multiorgan autoimmune disease in both mice ('scurfy', an X-linked recessive mouse mutant) and humans (immunodysregulation, polyendocrinopathy and enteropathy; X-linked syndrome IPEX) [13]. In addition to tTreg, there is another category of Foxp3-expressing Treg cells which do not derive from the thymus but originate from naive T cells in the periphery (fig. 2). These cells have been defined as adaptive or induced Treg (iTreg) cells [14]. While the differentiation of tTreg cells in the thymus is promoted by increased affinity interactions with self-peptide-MHC complexes, differentiation of iTreg cells likely occurs in response to non-self antigens, e.g. allergens, food and commensal microbiota [14], as a result of high-affinity T cell receptor (TCR) signaling together with suboptimal co-stimulation (increased CTLA-4 and decreased CD28 signaling) which favor Foxp3 induction and, therefore, iTreg cell generation. In addition, both in vitro and in vivo studies have demonstrated that, besides strong TCR signaling and suboptimal co-stimulation, induction of Foxp3 expression in naive T cells is facilitated by high amounts of TGF-β [14]. IL-2 is also required for TGF-β-mediated induction of Foxp3 in peripheral T cells in vitro [14]. Generation of iTreg mainly occurs in particular environments or tissues, such as the gut-associated lymphoid tissues and mesenteric lymph nodes. The understanding of molecular mechanisms of suppression by both tTreg and iTreg is still limited. Several cell surface molecules were proposed to play a role as mediators of Treg cell-mediated suppression: CD25, CTLA-4, membrane TGF-β, CD39, CD73, LAG-3, TIGIT, but none of the aforementioned mechanisms of suppression can singly account for Treg cell-mediated control of immune responses [14]. Whether Treg cells implement a universal hard-wired program to limit different types of immunity or modular programs of suppression, tailored to inhibit a particular class of the immune response, is still unclear. The possibility that Th1, Th2 and Th17 responses are regulated by specific classes of Treg cells has recently been suggested [14].

Type 1 Regulatory T Cells

In addition to Foxp3+ Treg cells, another category of iTreg cells has been described and defined as type 1 Treg (Tr1) cells (fig. 2). Tr1 cells do not express Foxp3 and suppress via the production of cytokines, such as IL-10 and TGF-β [15]. However, although Tr1 cells can be differentiated from naive T cells under conditions characterized by the presence of IL-10 or IL-27, the lack of consensus regarding their phenotype and differentiation factors, as well as the inability to expand these cells in large quantities in vitro have hampered progress in understanding their biology. Since Tr1 cells are orphans of a specific marker, they probably do not represent a specific lineage, but rather a transient status of different effector T cells.

Role of T Cell Subsets in Allergic Disorders

Both effector and regulatory CD4+ T cells certainly play an important role in the pathogenesis of allergic disorders.

Th2 Cells in Allergic Disorders

Soon after the discovery that IL-4 produced by T cells was involved in the production of IgE by B cells [16], and the demonstration of the existence of human Th1 and Th2 subsets [2], the hypothesis was postulated that allergy could be defined as a Th2-driven hypersensitivity to innocuous environmental antigens (allergens) [17]. Indeed, IL-4-producing T cells had been detected in the bronchial biopsies of asthmatic subjects [18]. In the subsequent years, the Th2 hypothesis in allergy rapidly became an established fact based on the results obtained in experimental animal models of asthma and allergy, as well as on the ex vivo studies performed in humans on the target organs of allergic disorders. This complex series of studies enabled the suggestion that virtually all the pathophysiological manifestations of allergic asthma could be explained by the activity of cytokines directly or indirectly related to Th2 cell responses (fig. 3). Th2-related cytokines (IL-4, IL-5, IL-13), Th2-specific transcription factors (GATA-3, c-maf) and Th2-related chemoattractant receptors (CCR4, CCR8, CRTH2) were clearly demonstrated by several studies in the bronchi, nose and skin of allergic patients, whereas no evidence of Th1-related cytokines, transcription factors or chemoactrattants were reported [19].

Regulation of the Th2 Response in Allergy

Following the discovery that allergen-specific Th2 responses may be responsible for the triggering of allergic inflammation, the question of the nature of the mechanisms that regulate such a type of response has been debated for many years. Their definition is essential for understanding the role of environmental factors in the genesis of allergic disorders, as well as for developing novel immunotherapeutic strategies.

Immune Deviation or Redirection

For many years, the only regulatory mechanism of allergen-specific Th2 responses has been thought to be the antagonistic activity of Th1 responses. In both mice and humans, the major Th1-polarizing cytokines, such as IFNs and IL-12, were found to be able to redirect the allergen-specific Th2 responses towards the Th1 phenotype. This process has been termed 'immune deviation' or 'redirection' [20]. The immune deviation has been well demonstrated in studies performed in both experimental animal models and in vitro in humans. Allergen-specific Th2 cells can be redirected to the Th0 and even to the Th1 phenotype by IL-12, inasmuch as these cells still express the β2 chain of the IL-12 receptor. Since many bacterial and viral microbial components, defined as pathogen-associated molecular patterns, or PAMPs, are able to induce Toll-like receptor (TLR) stimulation and IL-12 production by dendritic cells (DC), they are also capable of inducing the shifting of Th2 into Th1 cells. These findings have provided the basis for a first interpretation of the so-called 'hygiene hypothesis'. According to this hypothesis, the increased prevalence of allergy that has become evident in the last decade in 'westernized' countries could be explained by the reduced microbial burden in the environment of children during childhood, due to the different style of life in comparison with previous decades and with people living in developing countries. The high microbial burden present in the environment before birth and during early childhood induces strong IL-12 production by DC, thus

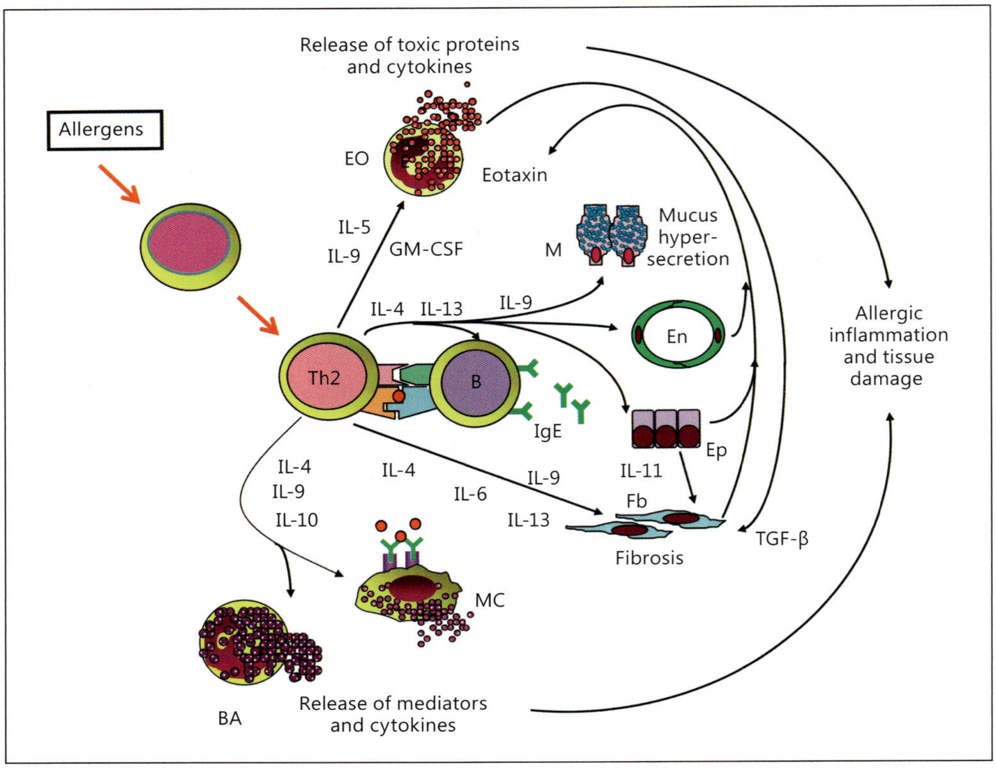

Fig. 3. Cytokines produced by activated allergen-specific Th2 cells may account for virtually all the pathophysiological manifestations of allergic asthma. EO = Eosinophil; M = mucous cells; B = B lymphocytes; En = endothelial cells; Ep = epithelial cells; Fb = fibroblasts; MC = mast cells; BA = basophils.

favoring microenvironmental conditions in which the Th2-type response to allergens is impaired and there is a shifting of this response towards the Th1 phenotype ('immune deviation' or 'redirection'). Based on this concept, a lot of studies have been undertaken devoted to identifying novel therapeutic strategies based on adjuvants able to redirect the allergen-specific Th2 response towards the Th1 or even a less polarized phenotype. Among these, CpG motifs containing oligonucleotides received great attention for some time. However, the results of clinical studies have been partially disappointing insofar as it is difficult to modify in a definite way an already established Th2 response because memory Th2 cells are much less sensitive than naive Th cells to the influence of cytokines in their differentiation process. Moreover, because of their ability to stimulate not only DC, but also B cells, these adjuvants may have the disadvantage of inducing B cell proliferation and autoantibody production. For this reason, other adjuvants are now under study.

Immune Suppression or Regulation

The theory of the mechanism of 'immune deviation' being responsible for the explanation of the hygiene hypothesis, and also useful as a method for the development of novel specific immunotherapeutic strategies in allergic disorders, was almost completely removed following the discovery of Treg cells [12], and all previous experiments demonstrating its validity have been 'cancelled'. Taking into account the epidemiological observations that in the last decades there has been an increased prevalence of not only Th2-mediated allergic disorders, but also of Th1-mediated chronic inflammatory disorders (multiple sclerosis, type 1 diabetes mellitus, Crohn's disease) in the more developed countries, it was claimed that the reduction of the microbial burden does not favor the development of allergic disorders because of a missing immune deviation, but because of a minor activation of Treg cells. This view is now prevalent despite the validity of previous reports, as well as the strong evidence derived from more recent epidemiological and molecular studies, particularly those performed in children living on farms. The possible role of Tr1 cells has been demonstrated in bee keepers who become tolerant to bee venom through multiple stings during the months spent tending their bees, whereas tolerance wanes rapidly during the winter months [21]. However, since in some murine experimental models IL-10 favors rather than protects from allergy, whether or not preventive tolerance can be achieved by inducing memory IL-10-producing Treg cells remains to be established. Moreover, bee keepers clearly represent a population different from atopic subjects.

Impaired Immune Deviation and Reduced Immune Suppression Account for Reduced Prevalence of Allergy, but the Role of Impaired Immune Deviation Is Prevalent

A series of studies performed in the last few years in children living on farms has clearly shown the protective role against the development of allergy played by their microbial exposure during both fetal life in the maternal uterus and during the early months of their lives [22]. In addition, part of this protection is also due to the consumption by these children of unpasteurized milk, containing several non-pathogenic bacteria, such as *Acinetobacter lwoffii* and *Lactococcus lactis*, which induce the Th1-polarizing program (via the induction of the Delta, instead of the Jagged, Notch ligand in DC). *A. lwoffii* is also able to give prenatal asthma protection via maternal TLR signaling. Finally and most importantly, the inhibitory effects of *A. Lwoffii* on allergic responsiveness was found to be dependent on IFN-γ and to be epigenetically controlled though chromatin histone 4 acetylation of the IFNG promoter of CD4+ T cells; conversely, inhibition of histone 4 acetylation abolishes the Th2-protective phenotype [23]. Taken together, these findings provide clear evidence that even if a reduced activation of Treg cells may partially explain the immunologic alterations responsible for the increased prevalence of allergy, there is no doubt that the missing immune deviation from Th2 to Th1 remains the prevalent mechanism (fig. 4), as initially proposed in the hygiene hypothesis [24].

Possible Pathogenic Role in Allergy of CD4+ Effectors other than Th2 Cells

Following the discovery of Th17 and Th9 cells, a possible role for these subsets in the pathogenesis of allergic disorders has also been hypothesized. In particular, T cells able to produce both IL-17 and IL-4 have been found to be increased in the circulation of patients with severe asthma. IL-17 can indeed play a role in those forms of severe steroid-resistant bronchial asthma characterized by the presence of neutrophil instead of eosinophil granulocytes. This is due to the peculiar activity of recruitment of these cells by Th17 cells via the stimulation of CXCL8 production by epithelial cells, endothelial cells and fibroblasts, as well as direct CXCL8 production. In addition, Th22 cells may play a role in atopic dermatitis. As mentioned above, under certain conditions relevant to chronic disease (IL-4 and TGF-β production), a distinct population of Th9 cells may appear. However, although it has been reported that IL-9 can promote mucus production in the epithelium and airway remodeling, the contribution of Th9 cells in allergic disease is currently unknown.

Possible Pathogenic Role of Natural Killer T Cells

Invariant natural killer T (iNKT) cells are characterized by an invariant variable region of the TCR α-chain 14-joining region 18, which selectively recognizes the glycolipid α-galactosylceramide presented to the TCR by the antigen-presenting cells CD1d. A role for iNKT cells in asthma has been suggested by extensive studies in animal (mostly mouse) models of lung inflammation driven by allergen, viral infection, ozone exposure or bacterial components. The idea requires that in causing airway hyperreactivity, iNKT cells function together with Th2 cells or independently of adaptive immunity. However, regardless of whether the mouse studies are highly suggestive, the role of CD1d-restricted iNKT cells in human asthma remains controversial [25].

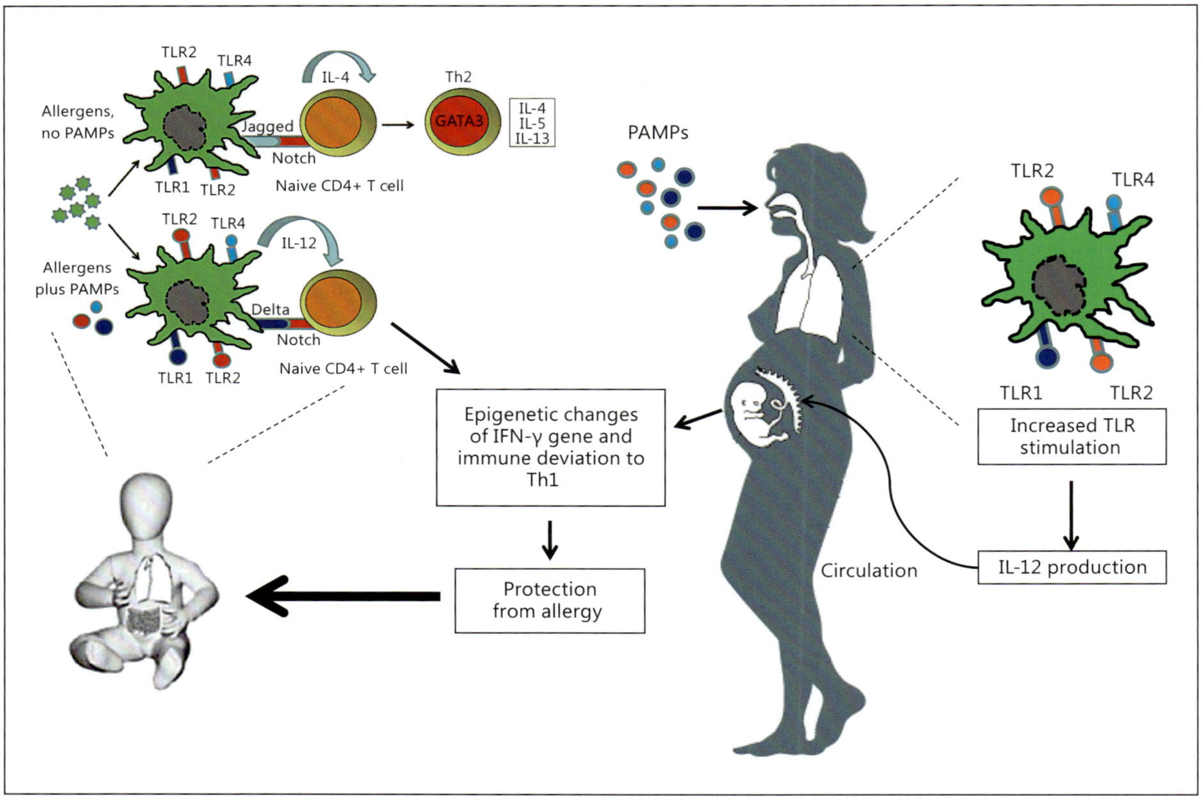

Fig. 4. The immune deviation induced by the environmental microbial burden during both pregnancy and early childhood is the main explanatory mechanism for the protective role from the development of allergy. The high microbial burden in the maternal environment results in persistent TLR stimulation and consequently increased production of IL-12 that can reach the fetus through the circulation together with allergenic molecules inhaled or ingested by the mother. After birth, allergen inhalation and ingestion in the absence of maternal IL-12 production, as well as missing newborn TLR stimulation by environmental PAMPs, results in the Notch ligand Jagged expression by DC and Th2 polarization of allergen-specific naive Th cells. By contrast, allergen inhalation and ingestion by the newborn in the presence of prolonged TLR stimulation results in the Notch ligand Delta expression by DC and IL-12 production. Persistently high IL-12 levels, due to both maternal and newborn TLR stimulation, allow epigenetic changes of the IFN-γ gene and allergen-specific Th1 polarization, which can protect from the development of allergy.

Role of Innate Immunity in Allergic Disorders

In the last few years, a novel population of immune cells that may be involved in the pathogenesis of allergic disorders has been described. These cells are lymphocytes but they do not possess the TCR and have been variably termed nuocytes, natural helper cells, innate helper cells and, more recently, type 2 innate lymphoid cells (ILC2) [26]. ILC2 express GATA-3 as an exclusive marker and display the ability to produce both IL-5 and IL-13, and lower amounts of IL-4 and IL-9. These cells may be important in the protection against worms, but it has been suggested that they can also play a pathogenic role in asthma and other allergic disorders. ILC2 are stimulated by the cytokines IL-25 and IL-33 (fig. 5). The major source of IL-25 in asthma are the lung epithelium, DC, eosinophils, mast cells and basophils. IL-33 is produced by macrophages and epithelial cells in the lung, and epithelial expression of IL-33 increases in asthmatics. However, the respective role of – and the possible interaction between – classic Th2 and ILC2 in the pathogenesis of allergic disorders remains to be established.

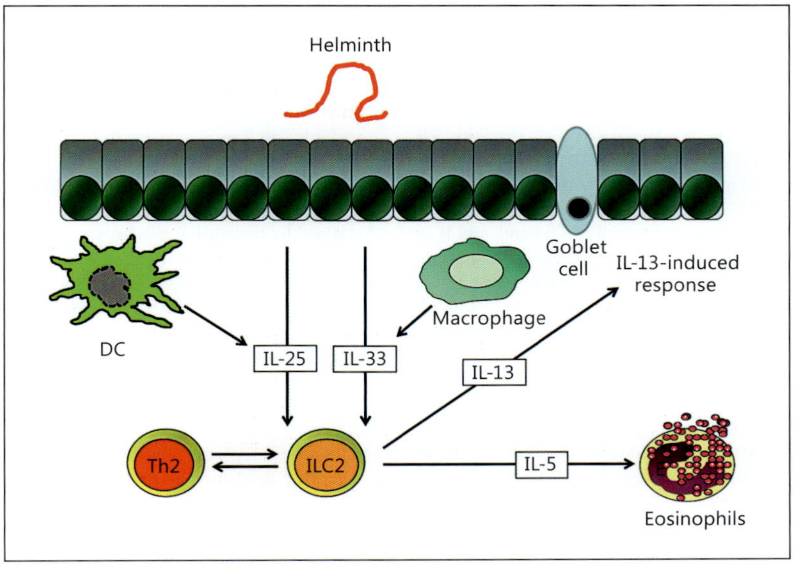

Fig. 5. ILC2, together with Th2 cells, may contribute not only to protection against worms, but also to the pathogenesis of allergic disorders. In response to helminths (and probably to some allergens), mucosal epithelial cells, DC and macrophages produce IL-25 and/or IL-33, which stimulate ILC2 to produce IL-5 and IL-13, and also favor the development of Th2 cells.

Concluding Remarks

The essential role of adaptive immunity and particularly of allergen-specific CD4+ Th2 cells in the pathogenesis of allergic disorders is clearly established. Th2 cells produce cytokines, such as IL-4 and IL-13 that can switch B cells to produce IgE. They also produce IL-5 that is essential for eosinophil granulocyte recruitment and survival. The mechanisms that regulate the Th2-mediated allergic inflammation have also been largely investigated and two main mechanisms of regulation have been described. The development of Th2 cells is counteracted by the Th1-related cytokines, such as IL-12 and IFNs (redirection or immune deviation) and can be suppressed by Treg cells. Different types of Treg cells have been described, such as the Foxp3+ tTreg and iTreg, and the Foxp3- and IL-10-producing Tr1 cells. Both Th1 and Treg cells may be important in preventing and/or inhibiting allergen-specific Th2 responses, but the more recent data favor the view that the protective mechanisms of the allergic responsiveness is dependent on IFN-γ and is epigenetically controlled though chromatin histone 4 acetylation of the IFNG promoter of CD4+ T cells.

More recently, in addition to Th1 and Th2 cells, other CD4+ T cell subsets, such as Th17 and Th9, have been discovered. Th17 cells may play some role in severe chronic asthma, probably through their ability to recruit neutrophil granulocytes, whereas the contribution of Th9 cells in allergic disorders is presently unknown. Likewise, although the possible pathogenic role of iNKT cells in murine models of asthma has been demonstrated, their possible importance in the pathogenesis of human asthma remains controversial. By contrast, the importance of ILC2, which represent the innate counterpart of the Th2 cells, in contributing to the inflammation in allergic disorders is highly probable. These cells indeed produce high amounts of IL-5 and IL-13 in response to IL-25 and IL-33, two cytokines that can be released by different cell types of immune and non-immune cells, including lung epithelial cells.

References

1 Mosmann TR, Coffman RL: Heterogeneity of cytokine secretion patterns and functions of helper T cells. Adv Immunol 1989;119: 382–392.
2 Romagnani S: Human TH1 and TH2 subsets: doubt no more. Immunol Today 1991; 12:256–257.

3 Manetti R, Parronchi P, Giudizi MG, Piccinni MP, Maggi E, Trinchieri G, Romagnani S: Natural killer cell stimulatory factor (interleukin 12 [IL-12]) induces T helper type 1 (Th1)-specific immune responses and inhibits the development of IL-4-producing Th cells. J Exp Med 1993;177:1199–2004.
4 Maggi E, Parronchi P, Macchia D, Piccinni MP, Simonelli C, Romagnani S: Reciprocal regulatory effects of IFN-gamma and IL-4 on the in vitro development of human Th1 and Th2 clones. J Immunol 1992;148:2142–2147.
5 Hwang ES, Szabo SJ, Schwartzberg PL, Glimcher LH: T helper cell fate specified by kinase-mediated interaction of T-bet and GATA-3. Science 2005;307:430–433.
6 D'Ambrosio D, Iellem A, Bonecchi R, Mazzeo D, Sozzani S, Mantovani A, Sinigaglia F: Selective up-regulation of chemokine receptors CCR4 and CCR8 upon activation of polarized human type 2 Th cells. J Immunol 1998;161:5111–5115.
7 Romagnani S: The Th1/Th2 paradigm. Immunol Today 1997;27:1751–1755.
8 Weaver CT, Harrington LE, Mangan PR, Gavrieli M, Murphy KM: Th17: an effector CD4 T cell lineage with regulatory T cell ties. Immunity 2006;24:677–688.
9 Eyerich S, Eyerich K, Pennino D, Carbone T, Nasorri F, Pallotta S, Cianfarani F, Odorisio T, Traidl-Hoffmann C, Beherendt H, Durham SR, Schmidt-Weber CB, Cavani A: Th22 cells represent a distinct human subset involved in epidermal immunity and remodeling. J Clin Invest 2009;119:3573–3585.
10 King C, Tangye SG, Mackay CR: T follicular helper (THF) cells in normal and dysregulated immune response. Annu Rev Immunol 2008;26:741–766.
11 Veldhoen M, Uyttenhove C, van Snick J, Helmby H, Westendorf A, Buer J, Martin B, Wihelm C, Stokinger B: Transforming growth factor-β 'reprograms' the differentiation of T helper 2 cells and promotes an interleukin 9-produing subset. Nat Immunol 2008;9:1341–1346.
12 Sakaguchi S, Sakaguchi N, Asano M, Itoh M, Toda M: Immunologic self-tolerance maintained by activated T cells expressing IL-2 receptor alpha chains (CD25): breakdown of a single mechanism of self-tolerance causes various autoimmune disaeases. J Immunol 1995;155:1151–1164.
13 Notarangelo LD, Gambineri E, Badolato R: Immunodeficiencies with autoimmune consequences. Adv Immunol 2006;89:321–370.
14 Josefowicz SZ, Lu LF, Rudensky AY: Regulatory T cells: mechanisms of differentiation and function. Annu Rev Immunol 2012;30:531–564.
15 Roncarolo MG, Gregori S, Battaglia M, Bacchetta R, Fleischhauer K, Levings MK: Interleukin 10-secreting type 1 regulatory T cells in rodents and humans. Immunol Rev 2006;212:28–50.
16 Del Prete GF, Maggi E, Parronchi P, Chrètien I, Tiri A, Macchia D, Ricci M, Banchereau J, De Vries J, Romagnani S: IL-4 is an essential factor for IgE synthesis induced in vitro by human T cell clones and their supernatants. J Immunol 1988;140:4193–4198.
17 Romagnani S: Lymphokine production by human T cells in disease states. Annu Rev Immunol 1994;12:227–257.
18 Robinson DS, Hamid Q, Bentley A, Ying S, Tsicopoulos A, Barkans J, Bentley AM, Corrigan C, Durham SR, Kay AB: Predominant TH2-like bronchoalveolar T-lymphocyte population in atopic asthma. N Engl J Med 1991;94:189–193.
19 Romagnani S: The role of lymphocytes in allergic disease. J Allergy Clin Immunol 2000;195:399–408.
20 Coffman RL, Romagnani S: Redirection of Th1 and Th2 Responses. Berlin, Springer, 1999.
21 Meiler F, Zumkehr J, Klunker S, Ruckert B, Akdis CA, Akdis M: In vivo switch to IL-10-secreting T regulatory cells in high dose allergen exposure. J Exp Med 2008;205: 2887–2898.
22 Debarry J, Garm H, Hanusskiewicz A, Dickgreber N, Blumer N, von Mutius E, Bufe A, Gatermann S, Renz H, Holst O, Heine H: *Acinetobacter lwoffii* and *Lactococcus lactis* strains isolated from cowsheds possess strong allergy-protective properties. J Allergy Clin Immunol 2007;119:1514–1521.
23 Brand S, Teich R, Dicke T, Harb H, Yildirim AO, Tost J, Schneider-Stock R, Waterland RA, Bauer UM, von Mutius E, Garn H, Pfefferle PI, Renz H: Epigenetic regulation in murine offspring as a novel mechanism for transmaternal asthma protection induced by microbes. J Allergy Clin Immunol 2012; 128:618–625.
24 Romagnani S: The increased prevalence of allergy and the hygiene hypothesis: missing immune deviation, reduced immune suppression, or both? Immunology 2004;112: 352–363.
25 Holgate ST: Innate and adaptive immune responses in asthma. Nat Med 2012;18: 673–683.
26 Spits H, Cupedo T: Innate lymphoid cells: emerging insights in development, lineage relationships, and function. Annu Rev Immunol 2012;30:647–675.

Dr. Sergio Romagnani
Department of Internal Medicine, University of Florence
Laboratorio di Immunoallergologia e Terapie cellular
Complesso Polivalente, viale Pieraccini, 6
IT–50139 Florence (Italy)
E-Mail s.romagnani@dmi.unifi.it

Bergmann K-C, Ring J (eds): History of Allergy. Chem Immunol Allergy. Basel, Karger, 2014, vol 100, pp 165–171
DOI: 10.1159/000358733

Mast Cell Research

Hirohisa Saito

National Research Institute for Child Health and Development, Tokyo, Japan

Abstract

The role of mast cells in allergy remained unrevealed until the observation that they contained histamine in 1953, and then the discovery of immunoglobulin E (IgE) in 1966, nearly a century after Ehrlich's first publication. After the discovery of IgE, myeloma-derived IgE from Peter Shackford, who made a great contribution to mankind by providing 40 liters of plasma in the year prior to his death, was distributed to many researchers. This accelerated the exploration of the mechanisms involved in allergic reactions, especially regarding the role of mast cells in IgE-mediated reactions. The identification of mast cells as a progeny of a bone marrow hematopoietic stem cell in 1977 led us to the successful in vitro culture of mast cells. Along with the development of molecular biological techniques, the structure of the high-affinity IgE receptor (FcεRI) was determined in 1989. Thus, we now understand the whole molecules the expression of which is changed when mast cells are activated via FcεRI cross-linking. However, the physiological and pathological roles of mast cells, especially where IgE is not involved, are not yet fully understood. It will be necessary to determine the mechanisms involved in the 'non-IgE-mediated' steps of mast cell activation in allergic or other diseases.

As was first described in 1878 by Paul Ehrlich, mast cells are present throughout connective tissues and mucosal surfaces, particularly at the interface with the external environment such as the skin, respiratory tract and gastrointestinal tract. On the basis of their unique staining characteristics, such as metachromasia for basic/aniline dyes, and large granules, it was mistakenly believed that mast cells existed to nourish the surrounding tissue. It took almost a century after the discovery of mast cells until we understood the important role of mast cells in allergy or immunity, i.e. the presence of histamine [1] in their granules and the functional high-affinity immunoglobulin E (IgE) Fc receptors (FcεRI) on their surfaces (fig. 1) [2–4]. Since then, our knowledge about the role of mast cells in allergic diseases has rapidly progressed. Now, IgE-sensitized mast

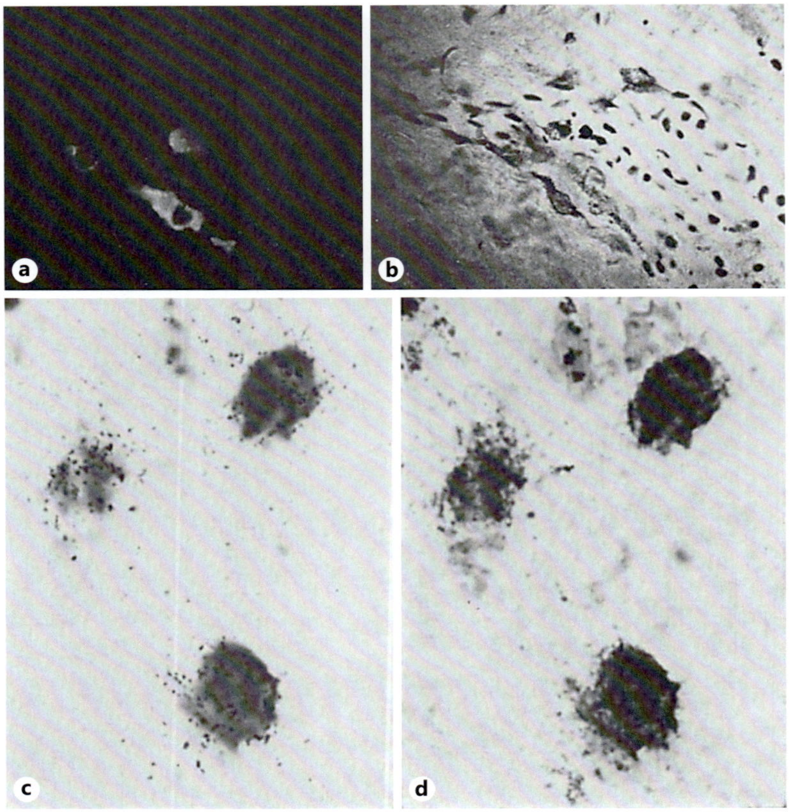

Fig. 1. First identification of IgE molecules bound to mast cells. **a** Fluorescence micrograph of a paraffin section from a monkey skin biopsy incubated with ragweed-allergic serum and stained for bound antigen E. **b** Light microscope micrograph of the same area counterstained with toluidine blue [adapted from 2, fig. 8]. Binding of ^{125}I-anti-IgE with mast cells – the microscope was focused on radioactive grains (**c**) or the cells (**d**). Mast cells in sensitized monkey skin bound ^{125}I-anti-IgE [adapted from 4, fig. 1A, B]. Panels **a** and **b**, adapted from Hubscher et al. [2], demonstrate that some mast cells can bind allergen-specific antibody, and panels **c** and **d**, adapted from Tomioka and Ishizaka [4], confirm that mast cells can bind IgE antibody.

cells are known to immediately release a variety of biological mediators such as histamine or leukotrienes in response to allergen stimulation. They also synthesize and release cytokines several hours after this allergen stimulation. In this chapter, the history of mast cell research is chronologically described, mainly with reference to articles that can be obtained electronically.

Discovery of Histamine in Mast Cells/Basophils

Histamine has been suspected to cause anaphylaxis since the studies by Dale and Laidlaw were published in 1910. However, anaphylactic shock was also recognized to be associated with a decrease in the histamine content of blood. This controversy was, of course, interpreted by the later discovery that histamine is stored in basophils, rapidly degenerated when it is released in vivo into blood, and that basophils also release histamine during serum separation in vitro, as well as allergic reactions in vivo.

Soon after the discovery of histamine in mast cells in 1953, Fawcett [5] reported that rat mast cells can release histamine when stimulated with compound 48/80, which was known as a histamine liberator. Related to histamine release in allergic reactions, in 1964 Lichtenstein and Osler [6] first demonstrated in vitro the release of histamine from human leukocytes obtained from hay fever patients by the specific antigen. Following the discovery of IgE in 1966 [7], it was confirmed that human leukocytes [8], and later basophils [9] among leukocytes, can release histamine in an IgE-dependent manner. Knowledge regarding the molecular characterization of human IgE made it possible for us to identify the IgE of other species. Thus, IgE-sensitized mast cells were demonstrated for the first time to release histamine after challenge with allergen using rat peritoneal mast cells [3].

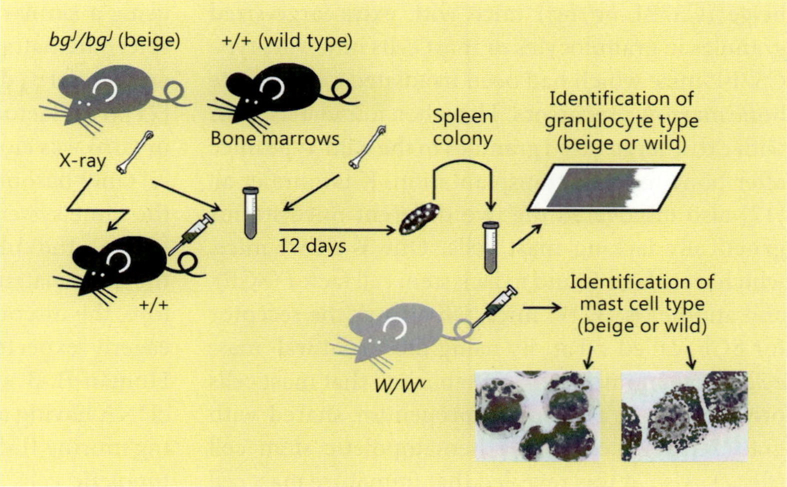

Fig. 2. Identification of mast cells as a progeny of a multipotent hematopoietic stem cell. Mixed bone marrow cells obtained from a beige *(bg^J/bg^J)* mouse and a wild-type mouse *(+/+)* were injected to an irradiated wild-type mouse, following which single hematopoietic cell-derived spleen colonies were obtained after 12 days. Cells obtained from a single colony were injected to a mast cell-deficient *(W/W^V)* mouse. Each colony gave rise to either mast cells and granulocytes with large-sized granules (beige) or those with normal granule size (wild type).

As has been nicely reviewed elsewhere [10], in 1942, H_1-antihistamines, which stabilize the inactive conformation of the H_1-receptor as inverse agonists, were introduced for clinical use. Now, more than 45 H_1-antihistamines are available worldwide, comprising the largest class of medications used in the treatment of allergic diseases such as allergic rhinoconjunctivitis and urticaria.

Discovery of IgE Receptors on Mast Cells/Basophils

Myeloma-derived IgE from Mr. Peter Shackford, who made a great contribution to mankind by providing 40 liters of plasma until his death, was purified by Kimishige Ishizaka. It was then distributed to many researchers, which accelerated the exploration of the mechanisms involved in allergic reactions, especially regarding the role of mast cells [11] and basophils [8] in IgE-mediated reactions. Metzger's group started to identify the structural features of IgE receptors present on basophils and mast cells [12]. IgE molecules alone do not normally activate mast cells after binding to their receptors. This phenomenon seemed unique, and certainly unlike other ligand-receptor interactions. It was revealed that multivalent antigens/molecules are usually capable of activating IgE-sensitized mast cells whereas univalent antigens/molecules in general cannot [13].

In 1989, along with the development of molecular biological techniques, the structure of FcεRI was finally determined [14]. Today, we understand that FcεRI is a tetrameric structure comprised of an α-chain (FcεRIα) which binds IgE, a β-chain-signaling subunit (FcεRIβ), and two γ-subunits which exist as a homodimer-signaling subunit (FcεRIγ) [15]. The molecular cloning of FcεRI and the development of techniques to make mice deficient of the targeted genes have accelerated our understanding of the signal transduction pathway in IgE-dependent mast cell activation.

Discovery of Mast Cell Origin and the Culture Methods

Regarding the origin of mast cells, Ehrlich suggested the source to be fibroblasts present in connective tissue. He could not imagine, of course, that these cells might derive from precursors of the hematopoietic lineage. It took 99 years until Kitamura demonstrated hematopoietic stem cells to be the origin of mast cells in 1977. Even in 1976, a textbook of hematology was published in which it was described that mast cells are derived from tissue. Kitamura et al. [16] transplanted bone marrow cells of beige (C57BL-bg^J/bg^J) mice with extra-large-sized granules in granulocytes or mast cells into wild-type C57BL mice which had been irradiated to eliminate bone marrow precursors. They then found mast cells with extra-large-sized granules in the wild-type mice after bone marrow transplantation. Kitamura et al. [17] also discovered the two different mice strains genetically lacking mast cells. One is *Sl/Sl^d* mice, which were later found to lack stem cell factor (SCF), and another is *W/W^v* mice, which lack the receptor for SCF, called c-Kit. By using these 'natural' mast cell-deficient mice, it was established that mast cells originate from a common progenitor shared with granulocytes, i.e. from a hematopoietic stem cell (fig. 2). Also, it was revealed that immature mast cell progenitors migrate from bone marrow into the tissue through blood circulation, unlike immature granulocytes which are kept in the bone marrow.

Ginsburg and Lagunoff [18] first reported the development of mast cells in vitro in the early 1960s. However, from mouse lymph node cells, but not from bone marrow cells, mast cell growth was obtained on fibroblast layers. Since the identification of mast cells was based only on morphology, controversy ensued as to whether these cells are mast cells. Then, in 1976, Ishizaka et al. [19] confirmed mast cell growth in the long-term culture of rat thymus cells on fibroblast monolayers by demonstrating the presence of IgE receptors on the cultured cells. These observations were interpreted by the later discovery that a very small number of hematopoietic cells, which are present even in lymphoid tissues, develop into mast cells when stimulated with a lymphocyte-derived mast cell growth factor, interleukin (IL)-3. Also, fibroblast layers would have presumably provided growth factors such as SCF to support the full maturation of mast cells.

Identification of mast cells as a progeny of a hematopoietic stem cell in 1977 [16] prompted us to utilize hematopoietic tissues for obtaining mast cells. In 1980, Denburg et al. [20] succeeded in obtaining guinea pig basophils (basophils are a dominant cell type compared to mast cells in guinea pig) in vitro by culturing bone marrow cells in the presence of supernatant derived from antigen-activated lymphocytes. Then, culture of mouse mast cells was reported by several groups almost simultaneously using a similar system: culture of bone marrow or spleen hematopoietic cells in the presence of supernatants derived from antigen-activated lymphocytes [21]. This factor supporting murine mast cell growth in vitro was cloned and termed as IL-3 [22].

Only basophil growth was obtained when using the same system for murine mast cell development [23], i.e. the culture of human hematopoietic cells in the supernatant of activated lymphocytes. Therefore, the discovery and cloning of human IL-3 was eagerly expected for culturing human mast cells. Human IL-3 was cloned based on the sequence of cDNA having a significant homology to that encoding murine IL-3. However, even by culturing hematopoietic cells with recombinant human IL-3, human mast cells did not grow [24]. These results disappointed all mast cell investigators at that time.

In fact, human IL-3 has a significant sequence homology with murine IL-3. However, the degree of homology between human and murine IL-3 is almost similar (approximately 26–28% at amino acid sequence) to that between human IL-3 and granulocyte-macrophage colony-stimulating factor (GM-CSF). Also, the receptor structure for IL-3 is distinct between human and mouse. The human has a common β-subunit that does not bind any cytokine by itself, but forms high-affinity receptors for GM-CSF, IL-3 and IL-5 with the respective α-subunit. In contrast, the mouse has two distinct β-subunits: one is specific for the IL-3 receptor and exists only on mast cells, and the other is equivalent to the human common β-subunit [25].

As was suggested in earlier studies [18, 19], Levi-Schaffer et al. [26] demonstrated that fibroblasts were able to support the development of IL-3-dependent cultured murine mast cells into the mature connective-type mast cell phenotype. They also reported that mature human lung mast cells can be maintained in vitro when co-cultured with fibroblasts. Then, in 1989, Furitsu et al. [27] finally succeeded in identifying the development of human mature mast cells from hematopoietic cells when co-cultured with the mouse 3T3 fibroblast cell line.

In 1990, a fibroblast-derived growth factor for mast cells was cloned, termed SCF, and the results were published almost simultaneously in more than 10 original papers by different researchers. While

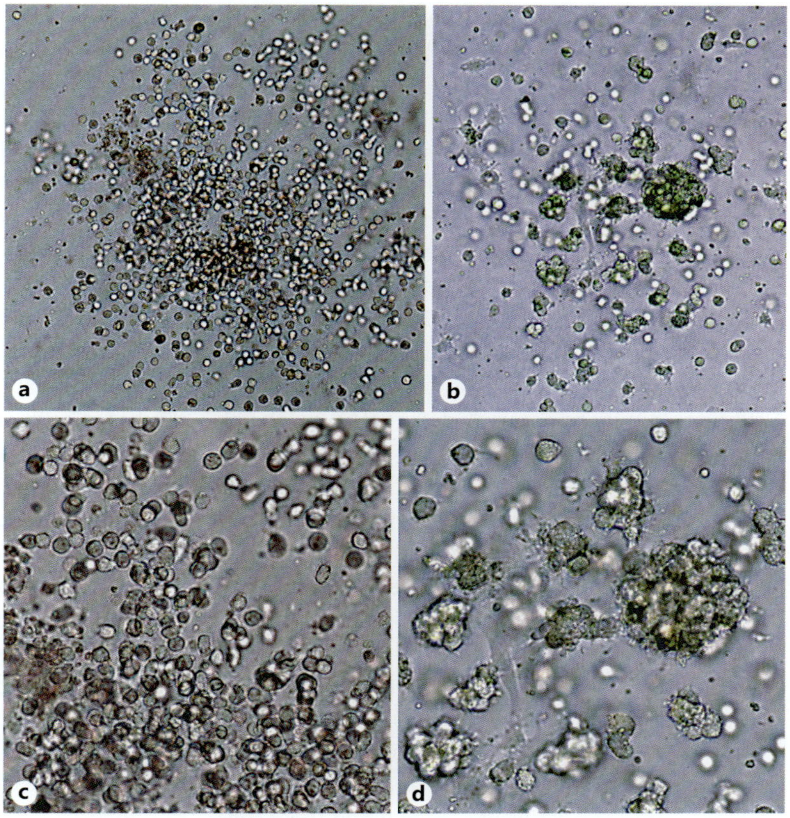

Fig. 3. A human mast cell colony grown in methylcellulose medium. Mast cell colonies (**a**, **c**) and macrophage colonies (**b**, **d**) were observed in the methylcellulose medium when adult peripheral blood cells were cultured for 6 weeks in the presence of SCF, IL-6 and IL-3. The mast cells look refractile and equally round, while macrophages look extra-large and irregularly shaped. Objective lenses were used. Original magnification ×10 (**a**, **b**), ×20 (**c**, **d**).

3

one of these articles was regarding the cloning of human SCF [28], mouse or rat SCF was found to similarly support human mast cell development. Although SCF could support the development of human mast cells, a substantial number of functionally mature mast cells were not always obtained. In fact, SCF expands more hematopoietic stem cells than mast cells. IL-6, another fibroblast-derived factor [29], is capable of supporting the self-renewal of hematopoietic stem cells as well as SCF, while most other cytokines, such as GM-CSF, suppress it. Therefore, SCF and IL-6 were employed for human mast cell culture [30]. IL-6 was later found to stimulate human mast cell maturation. Thus, for preventing the production of stem cell self-renewal-suppressive cytokines such as GM-CSF by macrophages, PGE_2 [30], the methylcellulose culture system [31] (fig. 3) or purification of mast cell progenitors [32] are used together with SCF and IL-6. When highly purified mast cell progenitors are used, IL-3 or IL-5, but not GM-CSF, increases the number of cultured mast cells in addition to SCF and IL-6 [32].

Mast Cell Phenotypes

Phenotypically distinct subsets of mast cells are present in rodents based on their distinct staining characteristics, T cell dependency and functions, namely connective tissue mast cells and mucosal mast cells [33]. In humans, two types of mast cells have been recognized based on the neutral proteases they express. TC-type mast cells (MC_{TC}) contain tryptase together with chymase and other neutral proteases, whereas T-type mast cells (MC_T) contain tryptase but lack the other neutral proteases present in MC_{TC} [34]. MC_{TC} preferentially dwell in connective tissue such as skin, while MC_T are often found in mucosa such as airway epithelium. MC_{TC} can respond to various non-immunological stimuli such as C5a or substance P, while MC_T do not.

Asthma can be divided into 2 subgroups ('Th2-high' and 'Th2-low' asthma), based on epithelial cell gene signatures for the activity of Th2 cytokines such as IL-13. Patients with Th2-high asthma have more infiltration of mast cells into the airway epithelium. These intraepithelial mast cells express both tryptase and carboxypeptidase A3 (CPA3), but not chymase [35]. According to the classical definition [34], MC_T were not supposed to express CPA3. However, according to public microarray data (http://www.nch.go.jp/imal/GeneChip/public.htm), all types of mast cells and basophils express the CPA3 transcript. Therefore, we can consider these epithelial mast cells at least as a sort of MC_T. Mast cells exposed to conditioned media from IL-13-activated epithelial cells showed downregulation of chymase, but no change in tryptase or CPA3 expression [35]. This may be the reason why MC_T are preferentially found in mucosa and are deficient in immunodeficiency patients [34]. This is in contrast to results demonstrating that human mast cell phenotypes, such as chymase expression, are retained over weeks, even when these mast cells are cultured in standard mast cell culture condition (supplemented with SCF and IL-6) [36].

Discovery of Cytokine Production by Mast Cells

Activated mast cells can release various protein cytokines as well as low-molecular-weight mediators such as histamine. It was described in 1987 that activated mast cells express and release cytokines such as tumor necrosis factor, TNF [37]. Later, mast cell-derived TNF was shown to play a significant role in airway hyperreactivity, T cell development (enhancement) and bacterial infection (protection).

IL-4 production seems reproducible when using mouse mast cells. However, so far only a few groups have succeeded to immunohistochemically demonstrate the presence of IL-4 on human mast cells. In any case, at least in humans, basophils are more potent producers of IL-4, and IL-4 potently activates human mast cell function and maturation. Interestingly, human mast cells can produce a substantial amount of another Th2 cytokine, IL-13, in response to IgE-mediated stimuli when mast cells are pre-incubated with IL-4 [38]. Through the development of molecular biological techniques, such as microarray, and the establishment of the human mast cell culture system, we now understand that both human and mouse mast cells can express and release a variety of cytokines (mainly Th2 cytokines) and chemokines (mainly CC-chemokines and IL-8) in response to IgE- and non-IgE-associated stimuli (http://www.nch.go.jp/imal/GeneChip/public.htm) [38, 39].

Future Perspective

Today we even understand the whole molecular pattern, the expression of which is changed when mast cells are activated via FcεRI cross-linking. However, the physiological and pathological roles of mast cells, especially where IgE is not involved, are not fully understood yet. It will be necessary to determine the mechanisms involved in the 'non-IgE-mediated' phase of mast cell activation in allergic or other diseases. Also, we need to understand the relative role of mast cells in allergic or innate-type inflammation compared to the roles of other immune and tissue-derived cells.

References

1 Riley JF, West GB: The presence of histamine in tissue mast cells. J Physiol 1953; 120:528–537.

2 Hubscher T, Watson JI, Goodfriend L: Target cells of human ragweed-binding antibodies in monkey skin. 1. Immunofluorescent localization of cellular binding. J Immunol 1970;104:1187–1195.

3 Bach MK, Bloch KJ, Austen KF: IgE and IgGa antibody-mediated release of histamine from rat peritoneal cells. 1. Optimum conditions for in vitro preparation of target cells with antibody and challenge with antigen. J Exp Med 1971;133:752–771.

4 Tomioka H, Ishizaka K: Mechanisms of passive sensitization. 2. Presence of receptors for IgE on monkey mast cells. J Immunol 1971;107:971–978.

5 Fawcett DW: Cytological and pharmacological observations on the release of histamine by mast cells. J Exp Med 1954;100:217–224.

6 Lichtenstein LM, Osler AG: Studies on the mechanisms of hypersensitivity phenomena. 9. Histamine release from human leukocytes by ragweed pollen antigen. J Exp Med 1964;120:507–530.
7 Ishizaka K, Ishizaka T, Hornbrook MM: Physico-chemical properties of human reaginic antibody. 4. Presence of a unique immunoglobulin as a carrier of reaginic activity. J Immunol 1966;97:75–85.
8 Ishizaka T, Ishizaka K, Johansson SG, Bennich H: Histamine release from human leukocytes by anti-γE antibodies. J Immunol 1969;102:884–892.
9 Ishizaka T, De Bernardo R, Tomioka H, Lichtenstein LM, Ishizaka K: Identification of basophil granulocytes as a site of allergic histamine release. J Immunol 1972;108:1000–1008.
10 Simons FER, Simons KJ: Histamine and H_1-antihistamines: celebrating a century of progress. J Allergy Clin Immunol 2012;128:1139–1150.
11 Ishizaka T, Ishizaka K, Orange RP, Austen KF: The capacity of human immunoglobulin E to mediate the release of histamine and slow reacting substance of anaphylaxis (SRS-A) from monkey lung. J Immunol 1970;104:335–343.
12 Kulczycki A Jr, Isersky C, Metzger H: The interaction of IgE with rat basophilic leukemia cells. 1. Evidence for specific binding of IgE. J Exp Med 1974;139:600–616.
13 Ishizaka K, Ishizaka T: Immune mechanisms of reversed type reaginic hypersensitivity. J Immunol 1969;103:588–595.
14 Blank U, Ra C, Miller L, White K, Metzger H, Kinet JP: Complete structure and expression in transfected cells of high affinity IgE receptor. Nature 1989;337:187–189.
15 Gilfillan AM, Tkaczyk C: Integrated signalling pathways for mast-cell activation. Nat Rev Immunol 2006;6:218–230.
16 Kitamura Y, Shimada M, Hatanaka K, Miyano Y: Development of mast cells from grafted bone marrow cells in irradiated mice. Nature 1977;268:442–443.
17 Kitamura Y, Yokoyama M, Matsuda H, Ohno T, Mori KJ: Spleen colony-forming cell as common precursor for tissue mast cells and granulocytes. Nature 1981;291:159–160.
18 Ginsburg H, Lagunoff D: The in vitro differentiation of mast cells: cultures of cells from immunized mouse lymph nodes and thoracic duct lymph on fibroblast monolayers. J Cell Biol 1967;35:685–697.
19 Ishizaka T, Okudaira H, Mauser LE, Ishizaka K: Development of rat mast cells in vitro. 1. Differentiation of mast cells from thymus cells. J Immunol 1976;116:747–754.
20 Denburg JA, Davison M, Bienenstock J: Basophil production. J Clin Invest 1980;65:390–399.
21 Schrader JW, Lewis SJ, Clark-Lewis I, Culvenor JG: The persisting (P) cell: histamine content, regulation by a T cell-derived factor, origin from a bone marrow precursor, and relationship to mast cells. Proc Natl Acad Sci USA 1981;78:323–327.
22 Ihle JN, Keller J, Oroszlan S, Henderson LE, Copeland TD, Fitch F, Prystowsky MB, Goldwasser E, Schrader JW, Palaszynski E, Dy M, Lebel B: Biologic properties of homogeneous interleukin 3. 1. Demonstration of WEHI-3 growth factor activity, mast cell growth factor activity, p cell-stimulating factor activity, colony-stimulating factor activity, and histamine-producing cell-stimulating factor activity. J Immunol 1983;131:282–287.
23 Razin E, Rifkind AB, Cordon-Cardo C, Good RA: Selective growth of a population of human basophil cells in vitro. Proc Natl Acad Sci USA 1981;78:5793–5796.
24 Saito H, Hatake K, Dvorak AM, Leiferman KM, Donnenberg AD, Arai N, Ishizaka K, Ishizaka T: Selective differentiation and proliferation of hematopoietic cells induced by recombinant human interleukins. Proc Natl Acad Sci USA 1988;85:2288–2292.
25 Miyajima A: Molecular structure of the IL-3, GM-CSF and IL-5 receptors. Int J Cell Cloning 1992;10:126–134.
26 Levi-Schaffer F, Austen KF, Caulfield JP, Hein A, Gravallese PM, Stevens RL: Co-culture of human lung-derived mast cells with mouse 3T3 fibroblasts: morphology and IgE-mediated release of histamine, prostaglandin D2, and leukotrienes. J Immunol 1987;139:494–500.
27 Furitsu T, Saito H, Dvorak AM, Schwartz LB, Irani AM, Burdick JF, Ishizaka K, Ishizaka T: Development of human mast cells in vitro. Proc Natl Acad Sci USA 1989;86:10039–10043.
28 Martin FH, Suggs SV, Langley KE, Lu HS, Ting J, Okino KH, Morris CF, McNiece IK, Jacobsen FW, Mendiaz EA, Birkett NC, Smith KA, Johnson MJ, Parker VP, Flores JC, Patel AC, Fisher EF, Erjavec HO, Herrera CJ, Wypych J, Sachdev RK, Pope JA, Leslie I, Wen D, Lin CH, Cupples RL, Zsebo KM: Primary structure and functional expression of rat and human stem cell factor DNAs. Cell 1990;63:203–211.
29 Van Damme J, Cayphas S, Van Snick J, Conings R, Put W, Lenaerts JP, Simpson RJ, Billiau A: Purification and characterization of human fibroblast-derived hybridoma growth factor identical to T-cell-derived B-cell stimulatory factor-2 (interleukin-6). Eur J Biochem 1987;168:543–550.
30 Saito H, Ebisawa M, Tachimoto H, Shichijo M, Fukagawa K, Matsumoto K, Iikura Y, Awaji T, Tsujimoto G, Yanagida M, Uzumaki H, Takahashi G, Tsuji K, Nakahata T: Selective growth of human mast cells induced by Steel factor, IL-6, and prostaglandin E_2 from cord blood mononuclear cells. J Immunol 1996;157:343–350.
31 Saito H, Kato A, Matsumoto K, Okayama Y: Culture of human mast cells from peripheral blood progenitors. Nat Protoc 2006;1:2178–2183.
32 Kirshenbaum AS, Goff JP, Semere T, Foster B, Scott LM, Metcalfe DD: Demonstration that human mast cells arise from a progenitor cell population that is $CD34^+$, c-kit^+, and expresses aminopeptidase N (CD13). Blood 1999;94:2333–2342.
33 Enerbäck L: Mast cells in rat gastrointestinal mucosa. 1. Effects of fixation. Acta Pathol Microbiol Scand 1966;66:289–302.
34 Irani AMA, Schecter NM, Craig SS, DeBlois G, Schwartz LB: Two types of human mast cells that have distinct neutral protease compositions. Proc Natl Acad Sci USA 1986;83:4464–4469.
35 Dougherty RH, Sidhu SS, Raman K, Solon M, Solberg OD, Caughey GH, Woodruff PG, Fahy JV: Accumulation of intraepithelial mast cells with a unique protease phenotype in T_H2-high asthma. J Allergy Clin Immunol 2010;125:1046–1053.
36 Kashiwakura J, Yokoi H, Saito H, Okayama Y: T cell proliferation by direct cross-talk between OX40 ligand on human mast cells and OX40 on human T cells: comparison of gene expression profiles between human tonsillar and lung-cultured mast cells. J Immunol 2004;173:5247–5257.
37 Young JD, Liu CC, Butler G, Cohn ZA, Galli SJ: Identification, purification, and characterization of a mast cell-associated cytolytic factor related to tumor necrosis factor. Proc Natl Acad Sci USA 1987;84:9175–9179.
38 Bischoff SC: Role of mast cells in allergic and non-allergic immune responses: comparison of human and murine data. Nat Rev Immunol 2007;7:93–104.
39 Nakajima T, Inagaki N, Tanaka H, Tanaka A, Yoshikawa M, Tamari M, Hasegawa K, Matsumoto K, Tachimoto H, Ebisawa M, Tsujimoto G, Matsuda H, Nagai H, Saito H: Marked increase in CC chemokine gene expression in both human and mouse mast cell transcriptomes following Fcε receptor I cross-linking: an interspecies comparison. Blood 2002;100:3861–3868.

Prof. Hirohisa Saito
National Research Institute for Child Health and Development
2-10-1 Okura, Setagaya-ku
Tokyo, 157-8535 (Japan)
E-Mail saito-hr@ncchd.go.jp

Mechanisms of Allergy: Important Discoveries

Bergmann K-C, Ring J (eds): History of Allergy. Chem Immunol Allergy. Basel, Karger, 2014, vol 100, pp 172–192
DOI: 10.1159/000358734

Basophils: Historical Reflections and Perspectives

Gianni Marone · Francesco Borriello · Gilda Varricchi · Arturo Genovese · Francescopaolo Granata

Department of Translational Medical Sciences and Center for Basic and Clinical Immunology Research (CISI), School of Medicine, University of Naples Federico II, Naples, Italy

Abstract

Basophils were discovered by Paul Ehrlich in 1879 and account for less than 1% of blood leukocytes, which suggests a tightly controlled regulation of basopoiesis. The conservation of basophils in a wide spectrum of the animal kingdom suggests a non-redundant role in innate and adaptive immunity. In the early 1990s, it was demonstrated that murine and human basophils synthesize interleukin (IL)-4 and IL-13, thereby suggesting that these cells are important for Th2 polarization and IgE synthesis. Human basophils also synthesize IL-3, VEGFs and other pro-angiogenic molecules. Recently, various groups have introduced the use of basophil-depleting antibodies or have developed transgenic mice that constitutively lack basophils by more than 90%. These models have highlighted previously unrecognized roles of basophils, distinct from those played by mast cells, in innate and adaptive immunity. Although the physiologic role of basophils remains unknown, there is now compelling evidence that basophils, despite their small numbers in peripheral blood and inflamed tissues, are critically involved in a wide spectrum of immunologic disorders (allergic, autoimmune and infectious diseases, immunodeficiencies and cancer). It is not inconceivable that basophils and/or their products could be promising therapeutic targets for such disorders.

Basophils were discovered in human peripheral blood and named by Paul Ehrlich in 1879 [1]. They account for less than 1% of blood leukocytes, which suggests a tightly controlled regulation of basopoiesis. Basophils are found in a wide spectrum of the animal kingdom [2], which suggests a non-redundant role in innate and adaptive immunity. However, the physiologic role of basophils remains unknown.

Basophils are characterized by the surface expression of the high-affinity receptor for IgE (FcεRI) and by the release of inflammatory mediators such

G.M. and F.B. contributed equally to this work.

as histamine and cysteinyl leukotrienes [3]. These characteristics are shared with tissue-resident mast cells, thereby leading to the long-standing but erroneous conclusion that basophils are surrogates of mast cells. In fact, despite some similarities, there are striking differences in the roles played by mast cells and basophils in innate and adaptive immunity [4, 5]. In addition, basophils mature in the bone marrow whereas mast cells leave the bone marrow as progenitors and mature in the peripheral tissues, where they presumably reside for the duration of their life span. By contrast, the life span of circulating basophils is much shorter (several days) and basophils do not proliferate after they mature. Under certain pathological conditions, basophils are recruited to peripheral tissues [6, 7]. The detection of basophils in human tissues is difficult given their low numbers and the fact that activated basophils are often degranulated. Monoclonal antibodies that recognize basogranulin (BB1), a cytoplasmic protein (2D7), or pro-major basic protein 1 (J175-7D4) can be used to stain basophils in human tissues [8–10]. The study of human and murine basophils has been hampered by both their rarity and, until recently, the lack of tools such as basophil-deficient mice.

The Different Eras of Basophil Biology

The history of basophil biology can be tentatively distinguished by three different eras. The first period of pioneers of basophil biology started around the 1970s, when it was discovered that IgE, the effector immunoglobulin of allergic disorders, binds with high affinity to human basophils and that cross-linking of their receptors with antigens or anti-IgE can induce the release of histamine [11–13]. This straightforward in vitro reaction was extensively studied by Lichtenstein's group, which made seminal observations correlating the release of histamine from basophils to the symptoms in allergic patients [14]. They also introduced the concept of basophil releasability (the ability of a basophil to release a given percentage of mediator in response to an immunological stimulus), which was associated with a number of allergic and immune disorders [15].

In the subsequent decades, basophils episodically attracted the attention of immunologists and only few groups active in this field kept alive the interest in these cells. The lack of enthusiasm for basophils at that time was also illustrated by the few lectures given at international immunology meetings.

The era of the resurrection of interest in basophils began with the seminal observation that mouse basophils are an important source of T helper 2 (Th2)-type cytokines such as interleukin (IL)-4 [16]. This observation was extended to human basophils which rapidly produce large quantities of IL-4 in response to various stimuli, including signaling through FcεRI [17–19]. It was subsequently demonstrated that human basophils produce a restricted profile of cytokines such as IL-4, IL-13 [20–23] and, more recently, IL-3 [24]. These findings suggested that basophils could be involved in the pathogenesis of allergic disorders and immunity to helminths. However, at that time researchers carrying out biochemical studies of basophils faced the difficulty of purifying them in sufficient numbers, as well as the lack of relevant cell lines.

The third era of basophil biology, a real renaissance, started in 2007 when different groups introduced the use of basophil-depleting antibodies (MAR-1 and Ba103, respectively specific for FcεRIα and CD200R3) [25, 26]. In addition, conditional basophil-deficient mouse strains based on a basophil-specific differentiation marker (mouse mast cell protease 8, mMCP-8, encoded by the *Mcpt8* gene) [27–29] or basophil-specific *Il4* enhancer elements [30] have recently been established.

With the use of these new tools, recent studies have now highlighted previously unrecognized roles for basophils in both innate and adaptive immunity [4]. It should be emphasized that marked discrepancies have already emerged by using different models to deplete mouse basophils [25–30]. Whatever the results, there is no doubt that we are facing an extraordinary era of increasing interest in the role of basophils in human and experimental models. This review will discuss the roles of basophils in innate and adaptive immunity.

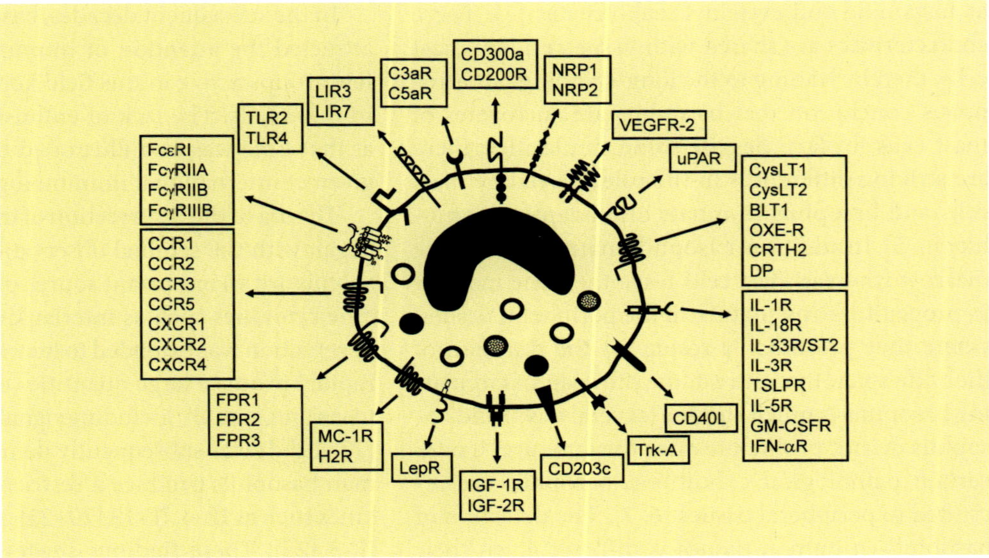

Fig. 1. Surface receptors expressed by human basophils. Basophils express the tetrameric high-affinity receptor for IgE, FcεRI. These cells also express the activating FcγRIIA, the inhibitory FcγRIIB and minute amounts of the GPI-anchored low-affinity receptor FcγRIIIB. Basophils express TLR2 and TLR4, as well as various receptors for chemokines (CCR1, CCR2, CCR3, CCR5, CXCR1, CXCR2 and CXCR4) and cytokines (IL-1R, IL-18R, IL-33R/ST2, IL-3R, IL-5R, GM-CSFR, TSLPR, IFN-αR, Trk-A and LepR), the activation of which modulates chemotaxis and/or mediator release. Basophils express both receptors for PGD_2, DP and CRTH2. They also express at least two receptors for cysLTs (CysLT1 and CysLT2), the receptor for LTB_4 (BLT1), the receptor for 5-oxo-HETE (OXE-R) and three formyl peptide receptors (FPR1, FPR2 and FPR3). Basophils express receptors for anaphylatoxins (C3aR and C5aR) and for IGF-1R and IGF-2R. Basophils express the receptor (VEGFR-2) and the co-receptors (NRP1 and NRP2) for the pro-angiogenic molecule VEGF-A. The uPA induces chemotaxis through engagement of the uPA receptor (uPAR). Human basophils express H_2R, the activation of which inhibits the release of mediators. Basophils express low levels of LIR3 and LIR7; cross-linking of LIR7 induces the secretion of mediators, whereas co-ligation of LIR3 and FcεRI inhibits the release of mediators. Basophils express MC-1R, the receptor for the neuropeptide α-melanocyte-stimulating hormone, and they also express the activation-linked marker CD203c. Ligation of CD40L by CD40-expressing B cells induces IL-4 production from basophil and IgE class switching in B cells. Immunoreceptor tyrosine-based inhibition motif-containing inhibitory receptors CD300a and CD200R have been detected on human basophils.

Activating Receptors on Human Basophils

Basophils express on the cytoplasmic surface a variety of receptors and can therefore respond to numerous immunologic and non-immunologic signals that regulate their development, homeostasis and effector functions (fig. 1). They express a complete FcεRI ($\alpha\beta\gamma_2$), the surface expression of which correlates with free IgE concentrations [31]. IgE itself upregulates the expression of FcεRI on both mouse and human basophils [31–33]. Aggregation of FcεRI bound to IgE by multivalent antigens, anti-IgE or immunoglobulin superantigens leads to basophil activation and mediator release [11–13, 34, 35]. The number of FcεRI on human basophils ranges from a few thousand to one million, with the median levels among non-atopic and atopic subjects being approximately 100,000 and 250,000, respectively [7, 36]. The overall receptor number is not the only factor regulating the sensitivity of a basophil to an IgE-dependent stimulus. MacGlashan [37] has demonstrated that human basophil releasability is influenced by a complex series of intracellular biochemical steps.

Both in vivo and in vitro studies point to IL-3 playing an important role in the development of basophils [38–40]. Human and mouse basophils retain high levels of IL-3 receptor (CD123) throughout their life span, accounting for the fact that IL-3 represents the most potent basophil-activating cytokine. IL-3 essentially augments every function of these cells, including mediator release [41, 42], survival [43], motility [44], adhesiveness to the endothelium, and expression of activation markers [45].

IL-3 is likely not the only growth factor for these cells. The first indication that growth factors other than IL-3 might regulate basophil development arose from studies showing that these cells persist in IL-3-deficient mice [40]. The exact cytokines regulating human and mouse basophil development, in addition to IL-3, remains to be determined, although thymic stromal lymphopoietin (TSLP) has been suggested as playing a role in the mouse [46]. TSLP acts directly on bone marrow-resident basophil precursors (BaPs) to induce their proliferation, maturation and subsequent exit into the periphery in both IL-3/IL-3R-sufficient and -deficient environments. However, basophil development in a steady-state condition was not impaired in mice deficient for both IL-3R and TSLPR, suggesting that neither IL-3 nor TSLP is strictly required for basophil development. TSLP-elicited basophils are phenotypically and functionally different from IL-3-elicited basophils. TSLP-elicited basophils express higher levels of CD123, IL-33R and IL-18Rα, and produce significantly more cytokines and chemokines in response to IL-3, IL-33 and IL-18. IL-3-elicited basophils exhibit elevated expressions of CD11b and CD62L, and higher β-hexosaminidase release in response to IgE cross-linking. Moreover, transcriptomic analysis revealed divergent gene expression profiles between TSLP- and IL-3-elicited basophils. TSLP-elicited basophils have been suggested to play a major role in the development of Th2 cytokine-mediated inflammation associated with both helminth infection and an atopic dermatitis model [47–49].

The heterogeneity of mouse basophils has also been suggested for human basophils. More than 70% of human basophils stimulated overnight with IL-3 expressed TSLPR, and basophils isolated from the peripheral blood of patients with eosinophilic esophagitis exhibited higher levels of IL-33R [48, 49]. However, the ability of TSLP to modulate human basophil functions needs to be fully elucidated. Moreover, it remains to be determined whether TSLP- and IL-3-elicited basophils represent distinct subsets of basophils or more simply different states of activation.

IL-1 family members, IL-5 and GM-CSF, as well as several chemokines, play an important role in the regulation of homeostasis and effector functions of basophils in an IgE-dependent and -independent manner [50]. IL-33, a member of the IL-1 family, activates basophils through the ST2 receptor, resulting in IL-4, IL-8 and IL-13 production and potentiation of IgE-mediated degranulation [51, 52]. Furthermore, IL-33 induces CD11b expression on human basophils and thus can enhance their transmigration into tissues [52]. Human basophils express receptors for IL-1 and IL-18, but are not activated by these cytokines, whereas IL-18 induces IL-4 and IL-13 production by mouse bone marrow-derived basophils and promotes their survival [51, 52].

Basophils express C3aR and C5aR and can be activated by their ligands C3a and C5a [53]. IL-3-primed human basophils readily respond to C3a with the release of histamine and the production of LTC_4 [54]. C5a induces histamine release even in the absence of IL-3, while LTC_4 production in response to C5a requires IL-3 priming [42]. Moreover, IL-3-primed human basophils secrete IL-13 (and to a lesser extent IL-4) in response to C5a [22].

Leptin, a member of the IL-6 cytokine family, has metabolic effects as an adipokine and participates in the modulation of several aspects of the immune response [55]. Human basophils express leptin receptor, LepR, and its expression is upregulated by IL-33. Leptin enhances the survival and induces degranulation, cytokine synthesis and migration of human basophils [56]. Interestingly, serum levels of leptin are elevated in patients with allergic disorders and obesity increases their prevalence [57].

Nerve growth factor (NGF), a neurotrophic cytokine discovered by Rita Levi-Montalcini [58], regulates the survival and functions of neuronal cells [59]. Human basophils express functional Trk-A, the high-affinity receptor for NGF, but not the other neurotrophin receptors (LNGFR, Trk-B and Trk-C). NGF, like IL-3, exerts a priming effect on human basophils, as measured by histamine secretion and cytokine production (IL-4 and IL-13) in response to various stimuli, including anti-IgE. At high concentrations, NGF alone, as well as IL-3, can release cytokines but little histamine [60–63].

Human basophils express LIR7 on their surface, an activating member of the leukocyte immunoglobulin-like receptor (LIR) family. LIR7 cross-linking elicits the release of histamine, LTC_4 and IL-4 both in the presence and in the absence of IL-3 [64].

Human basophils express receptors for different bacterial products. These cells express Toll-like receptor (TLR) 2 and TLR4 at both the mRNA and protein level, but only TLR2 ligands (e.g. peptidoglycan) induce IL-4 production and potentiate IgE- and non-IgE-induced activation [65]. Human basophils express low levels of TLR9 and TLR10 mRNAs, although their role in modulating basophil functions is still unclear [66]. All three N-formyl-methionyl-leucyl-phenylalanine (fMLP) receptors (FPR1, FPR2 and FPR3) are expressed at the mRNA level in human basophils. fMLP induces migration and degranulation of human basophils through the engagement of the fMLP receptors [67].

Human basophils display a large number of chemokine receptors on their surface, some of which induce mediator release (CCR2) and many others (CXCR1, CXCR2, CXCR4, CCR1, CCR3 and CCR5) elicit basophil chemotaxis. In addition, human basophils express several α- and β-integrins that modulate basophil adhesion to endothelium and extravasation [68]. The expression of both integrins and chemokine receptors can be modulated by several factors. For example, IL-3 upregulates the expression of β2-integrins thereby potentiating the β2-integrin-mediated adherence of basophils to the endothelium [45]. Moreover, surface CXCR4 expression was not detected in fresh- and whole-blood basophils, but it became apparent gradually during short-term incubation. CXCR4 expression was completely abrogated by IL-3 and downregulated by IL-5, GM-CSF and IL-4. SDF-1/CXCL12, a specific ligand for CXCR4, induced a strong migratory response in basophils cultured for 24 h [69]. Thus, transient or inducible expression of integrins and chemokine receptors significantly modify the recruitment of basophils at inflammatory sites.

Several other receptors besides those for chemokines exert a chemotactic effect on basophils. The urokinase plasminogen activator (uPA) binds to a specific high-affinity GPI-anchored surface receptor, uPAR [70]. Human basophils express uPAR at both mRNA and protein levels. uPA induces the chemotaxis of basophils through the exposure of the chemotactic uPAR epitope $uPAR_{84-95}$, which is an endogenous ligand for FPR2 and FPR3 [67].

VEGF-A, a key regulator of blood vessel growth, signals through the tyrosine kinase receptors VEGFR-1 and VEGFR-2, which are expressed on endothelial cells [71, 72]. Human basophils express VEGFR-2 as well as neuropilin (NRP) 1 and NRP2, and VEGF-A induces their chemotaxis through the engagement of VEGFR-2 [73].

Insulin-like growth factor (IGF)-2 stimulates the chemokinesis of basophils and synergizes with eotaxin-1/CCL11 in basophil chemotaxis. Recombinant IGF-1 exhibits similar basophil-selective effects as IGF-2, and both growth factors were detected in human nasal polyp extracts [74]. In addition, IGF-1 enhances histamine release induced by IgE and certain non-IgE-mediated stimuli. IGF-2 and insulin, both of which have high amino acid sequence homology with IGF-1, also prime basophils [75].

Basophils express several receptors for lipid mediators. In particular, human basophils express transcripts for both receptors of PGD_2, DP and CRTH2 [76, 77]. CRTH2 is a 7-transmembrane G protein-coupled receptor highly expressed on Th2 cells, basophils and eosinophils [77, 78]. PGD_2 induces chemotaxis of Th2 cells, eosinophils and basophils through the activation of CRTH2 [76]. CRTH2 engagement is responsible for the pro-inflammatory effects of PGD_2 on human basophils (CD11b upregulation, chemotaxis and enhanced degranulation), whereas DP receptor activation exerts a negative signal antagonizing the effects of CRTH2 in these cells [79, 80].

Human basophils express receptors (cysLT1 and cysLT2) for cysteinyl leukotrienes (LTC_4/LTD_4/LTE_4) and BLT1 receptor for LTB_4. LTD_4 and LTB_4 induce a transient increase in cytosolic calcium, whereas LTB_4 stimulates degranulation of IL-3-primed basophils [81, 82].

OXE-R is a 7-transmembrane G protein-coupled receptor activated by 5-oxo-ETE, a product of the 5-lipoxygenase pathway [83]. 5-oxo-ETE is produced by inflammatory cells and is a potent chemoattractant for basophils [82, 84, 85].

Inhibitory Receptors on Human Basophils

Besides high-affinity IgE receptors, human basophils express activating (FcγRIIA) and inhibitory (FcγRIIB) low-affinity IgG receptors. Human basophils also express minute amounts of the GPI-anchored low-affinity IgG receptor FcγRIIIB [86], the biological properties of which are not clear. They express neither FcγRIIIA nor high-affinity IgG receptors (FcγRI) and, unlike human mast cells [87], FcγRI was not inducible by IFN-γ in human basophils [88]. The possibility that FcγRs can negatively regulate human basophil activation was suggested by showing that bifunctional molecules, which coligated FcεRI with FcγRII, inhibited IgE-induced basophil activation [89].

As indicated above, a DP-selective agonist inhibits basophil migration in response to eotaxin or DK-PGD_2 (a CRTH2-selective agonist), and reduces IgE-dependent histamine release [80], probably by increasing intracellular cAMP levels [76].

Human basophils express LIR3, an inhibitory member of the LIR family. Co-ligation of LIR3 to LIR7 or to FcεRI significantly inhibited histamine release, cysLTs production and IL-4 generation [64].

Several groups have reported the expression of the immunoreceptor tyrosine-based inhibition motif-containing inhibitory receptors CD300a and CD200R on human basophils [90–92]. Viral CD200 homologues as well as human CD200 downregulated the activation of basophils in response to anti-FcεRI, but not IL-3 [92]. Moreover, IgE-mediated activation of human basophils rapidly increased the expression of both CD300a and CD200R. The activation of these receptors induced by anti-CD300a/c and anti-CD200R monoclonal antibodies inhibited IgE-dependent histamine release and CD63 expression (a granule-associated protein that is induced on the surface of basophils during activation as a result of granule membranes fusing with the plasma membrane) [7, 93]. Interestingly, basophils from allergic patients constitutively expressed less CD300a than those from non-allergic individuals, suggesting an in vivo relevance for this pathway [90, 91].

Recently, it has been shown that the melanocortin receptor MC-R1 is expressed on human basophils and that α-melanocyte-stimulating hormone inhibits the release of cytokines from basophils activated by fMLP [94]. Basophils purified from patients undergoing specific venom immunotherapy exhibited rapid upregulation of histamine H_2 receptor (H_2R) and H_4R mRNA [95]. Stimulation of basophils by the H_2R agonist dimaprit inhibited their IgE-mediated release of histamine, LTC_4 and IL-4. The latter findings extend the original observation made by Lichtenstein and Gillespie [96] demonstrating the inhibition of mediator release from human basophils by histamine engagement of H_2R. Therefore, there is the possibility that autocrine histamine released from activated basophils represents a relevant negative feedback pathway in vivo.

3

Mediators

Mediators produced by human basophils can be divided into preformed pro-inflammatory mediators, newly synthesized lipid mediators, cytokines, chemokines and angiogenic molecules (fig. 2). The major pre-formed mediator in cytoplasmic granules of basophils is histamine (approx. 1 pg/cell) [7]. Histamine in these granules complexes with chondroitin sulfate and dissociates after exocytosis by ion exchange and changes in pH. The secretory granules of human basophils also contain BB1, recognized by the monoclonal antibody BB1 [10]. Activated basophils rapidly produce LTC_4 [97]; this is of particular importance because cysLTs are potent bronchoconstrictors and increase vascular permeability [98]. Activated human basophils can synthesize platelet-activating factor (PAF) and its 1-acyl analogue, 1-acyl-2-acetyl-sn-glycero-3-phosphocholine, AAGPC [99].

Murine [16] and human basophils activated by IgE-mediated stimuli rapidly synthesize IL-4 [19, 100]. Basophils expressing IL-4 and CD40L have been suggested to be important for the amplification of IgE synthesis [101, 102]. Subsequently, it was demonstrated that the secretion of IL-13 from human basophils peaks after approximately 20 h as opposed to the production of IL-4, which is essentially over after 4–6 h [21–23]. Schroeder et al. [24] demonstrated that human basophils produce IL-3 fol-

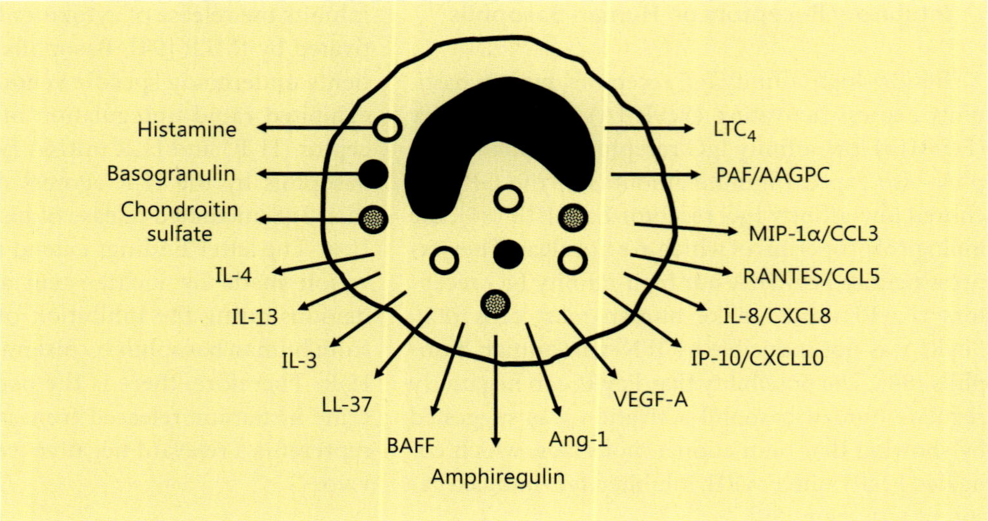

Fig. 2. Mediators synthesized by human basophils. Basophils contain histamine (~1 pg/cell) stored in secretory granules complexed with chondroitin sulfate. Secretory granules contain BB1, a specific protein recognized by the monoclonal antibody BB1, and tryptase at levels of less than 1% of those of mast cells. IgE-mediated and non-IgE-mediated activation of basophils leads to the release of histamine, BB1 and the production of cysteinyl leukotrienes (LTC_4, LTD_4 and LTE_4), IL-3, IL-4 and IL-13. Activated basophils also synthesize PAF and its 1-acyl analogue AAGPC. IgD-mediated activation of human basophils induces the release of IL-4, IL-13, BAFF, IL-8/CXCL8 and IP-10/CXCL10, but not histamine. BAFF secretion is not induced by anti-IgE. Moreover, anti-IgD induces the expression of antimicrobial factors such as cathelicidin LL-37. Basophils produce and release several pro-angiogenic molecules (VEGF-A and Ang-1) and tissue remodeling factors (amphiregulin). There is some evidence that basophils from normal and particularly from atopic subjects express IL-25 (IL-17E) mRNA, and their activation by IL-3 alone or IL-3 plus anti-IgE produces IL-25, which promotes angiogenesis in asthma.

lowing IgE-dependent activation. IL-3 is the most important growth factor for human basophils and potentiates the release of mediators and cytokines from activated basophils. In addition, basophils from normal and atopic subjects can secrete IL-25 (IL-17E), which augments the functions of Th2 memory cells [103]. However, there is little evidence that human basophils produce additional Th2-like cytokines, which is in contrast with what has been published for their murine counterpart [7, 26].

Recent evidence suggests that activated human basophils release VEGF-A [73], angiopoietin-1 [Prevete et al., unpubl. observations] and amphiregulin [104], which implicate these cells as having a role in angiogenesis and tissue remodeling. Human basophils release several chemokines, namely IL-8/CXCL8, RANTES/CCL5 and MIP-1α/CCL3 upon stimulation with anti-IgE [105, 106]. IL-3 priming augments IgE-dependent MIP-1α/CCL3 secretion [105].

IgD-mediated activation of human basophils induces the release of IL-4, IL-13, BAFF, IL-8/CXCL8 and IP-10/CXCL10, but not histamine. Interestingly, BAFF secretion was not induced by anti-IgE. Moreover, anti-IgD induced the expression of antimicrobial factors such as β-defensin 3, cathelicidin LL-37 and PTX3 [107].

Histamine-Releasing Factor

Since Grant and collaborators [108] described an activity from cultured peripheral blood mononuclear cells that induced histamine release from basophils, histamine-releasing activities have been studied for more than 30 years [109]. In addition to several cytokines/chemokines with this activity, an unrelated protein termed histamine-releasing factor (HRF) was purified and molecularly cloned in 1995

[110]. HRF, also known as translationally controlled tumor protein (TCTP) and fortilin, is a highly conserved protein with both intracellular and extracellular functions. HRF is secreted by macrophages and other cell types and can stimulate histamine release and IL-4 and IL-13 production from IgE-sensitized basophils and mast cells [109, 111]. HRF has been implicated in late-phase allergic reactions and chronic allergic inflammation [112]. Despite considerable efforts, researchers have failed for several decades to identify an HRF receptor. In a combined effort different groups have recently demonstrated that HRF can dimerize and bind to immunoglobulins via interactions of its N-terminal and internal regions with the Fab region of immunoglobulins [113]. They have also demonstrated that HRF exerts pro-inflammatory roles in mouse models of allergic disorders, suggesting that HRF is a potential therapeutic target.

Basophils as Potential Inducers of Type 2 Immunity

The rapid and robust IL-4 production by activated mouse and human basophils [16, 19, 100] led to the hypothesis that these cells provide the initial burst of IL-4 used by CD4 T cells in their differentiation to the Th2 phenotype [114]. Consistent with this possibility, naive CD4 T cells stimulated in vitro in the presence of basophils preferentially differentiate into IL-4-producing Th2 cells even in the absence of exogenous IL-4 [115]. Moreover, basophils from healthy individuals produce IL-4 upon stimulation with *Schistosoma* egg antigens. This suggests that IL-4 produced by activated basophils induces parasite-specific naive T cells to become Th2 cells [116]. Basophils may also play a role in immunoglobulin class switching to IgE in vitro [101, 102]. Whether basophils exert any role in Th2 differentiation and immunoglobulin class switching in vivo, however, remains to be fully demonstrated. Indeed, an elegant study by Voehringer and colleagues [27], using Mcpt8Cre mice that constitutively lack basophils by more than 90% compared to control mice, demonstrated that differentiation and accumulation of Th2 cells, induction of eosinophilia, and increase in serum IgE or IgG1 induced by allergens or by infection with the helminth *Nippostrongylus brasiliensis* is basophil independent.

Basophils as Antigen-Presenting Cells: An Unsettled Controversy

In the summer of 2009, *Nature Immunology* published a unique back-to-back set of three papers describing a breakthrough regarding the role of basophils as antigen-presenting cells (APCs). Sokol et al. [117] showed that basophils activated by papain express MHC-II less than dendritic cells (DCs), but similar to macrophages. They also found that basophils transiently enter lymph nodes after papain challenge and endocytose, process and present soluble antigens. They concluded that basophils are sufficient for Th2 differentiation in vivo and function as APCs. Perrigoue et al. [46] studied Th2 responses induced via infection with the parasite *Trichuris muris*. They showed that basophils present the antigenic peptide of the parasite on MHC-II molecules to naive T cells. Basophil depletion with an anti-FcεRI antibody (MAR-1) impaired immunity against helminth infection. Finally, Yoshimoto et al. [118] suggested that basophils take up and process ovalbumin (OVA) and can induce Th2 cells in vivo. The administration of MAR-1 induced partial depletion (~90%) of basophils and reduced Th2 cell development.

Tang et al. [119] studied the role of DCs and basophils in initiating Th2 responses to papain. Subcutaneous immunization with papain plus antigen induced reactive oxygen species (ROS) in lymph node DCs, dermal DCs and epithelial cells of the skin. ROS induced the production of TSLP by epithelial cells and induction of DC-derived chemokine CCL7, which mediated recruitment of IL-4^+ basophils to the lymph node. Interestingly, DCs or basophils alone were insufficient to polarize a papain-induced Th2 response. Although DCs were proficient in inducing T cell proliferation, basophils were a critical source of IL-4 required for Th2 differentiation in response to papain. The authors concluded that Th2 response to papain requires DC-basophil cooperation via ROS signaling.

3

Two recent studies have challenged the hypothesis that basophils are fundamental APCs. MacDonald and colleagues [120] used a murine model of *Schistosoma mansoni* infection and demonstrated that depletion of DCs dramatically impaired T cell production of Th2 cytokines, whereas basophil depletion using MAR-1 antibody had no effect on Th2 induction. Using another murine model of house dust mite inhalation, Lambrecht and colleagues [121] demonstrated that depletion of basophils only partially reduced Th2 immunity. Moreover, basophils did not take up inhaled antigens, present them to T cells, or express antigen presentation machinery, whereas a population of FcεRI⁺ DCs readily did.

These apparently conflicting results might imply that antibody-mediated depletion of basophils may cause bystander effects including depletion of FcεRI-expressing DCs and monocytes [121], activation of mast cells and macrophages, formation of immune complexes, and activation of the complement system. To address these issues, Voehringer and colleagues [27] established a murine model (Mcpt8Cre mice) in which basophils were not depleted by monoclonal antibodies, but were constitutively ablated. They observed that Mcpt8Cre mice developed a normal Th2 cell response after immunization with OVA-papain, OVA-alum, or infection with *N. brasiliensis*, while constitutive deletion of DCs impaired the development of a Th2 cell response against OVA-papain despite normal basophil recruitment to lymph nodes. Thus, Th2 polarization under the tested conditions was dependent on DCs rather than basophils.

Locksley and collaborators [28] developed the Basoph8 × DTα mouse strain in which basophils express the gene encoding the diphtheria toxin-α chain and, thus, are selectively depleted. They found no defect in Th2 response after challenging these mice with *S. mansoni* eggs or papain. Moreover, using the Basoph8 reporter mouse strain, they confirmed that basophils can enter into inflamed lymph nodes in response to soluble and particulate stimuli. However, they demonstrated that basophils apparently did not produce IL-4 in lymphoid tissues and did not interact with CD4 T cells in a manner consistent with their proposed role as APCs.

Using another approach, Kubo and colleagues [30] achieved selective basophil depletion by expressing human diphtheria toxin receptor gene under the control of basophil-specific *Il4* enhancer elements (Bas-TRECK mice). Although basophils were dispensable for the differentiation of IL-4-producing CD4 T cells after OVA-papain immunization, the Th2 response was significantly reduced in basophil-depleted mice. The latter results were further extended by Artis and collaborators [47] using Bas-TRECK mice. They found that basophils contribute to optimal Th2 cytokine responses after *Trichinella* infection. In summary, although the results obtained with different mouse models tend to exclude the role of basophils as fundamental APCs, the contribution of these cells to the polarization of Th2 lymphocytes (maybe as a source of IL-4 or other polarizing factors) cannot be fully ruled out and needs further investigation.

Two recent studies have investigated the role of human basophils as APCs in allergic patients. The group of Bohle [122] demonstrated that basophils from allergic donors do not internalize specific allergens. In addition, human basophils show limited expression of MHC-II and co-stimulatory molecules. They demonstrated that human basophils did not activate allergen-reactive CD4 effector T cells. Other authors from the same institution similarly concluded that basophils are not the key APC in allergic patients [123]. In addition, basophils stimulated with Asp f 1 (an *Aspergillus fumigatus* allergen) or a TLR2 ligand did not upregulate HLA-DR and Asp f 1-pulsed basophils did not promote Th2 differentiation [124]. These three papers indicate that it is unlikely that circulating human basophils can act as major APCs.

A number of technical reasons could explain, at least in part, these discrepancies. First, it should be considered that basophils purified from peripheral blood could behave differently to tissue-dwelling basophils. Moreover, the purification of basophils from peripheral blood can provoke the selective loss of basophil subset(s). Whatever the results, the role of basophils in the modulation of different aspects of Th2 responses both in mice and in humans remains of great interest and requires additional experiments.

Human Basophils and Angiogenesis

Angiogenesis and lymphangiogenesis, the formation of new blood and lymphatic vessels respectively, are important aspects of tumor growth and inflammatory diseases [71, 125]. Both angiogenesis and lymphangiogenesis rely on the production of vascular endothelial growth factors (VEGFs). The VEGF family includes VEGF-A, -B, -C, -D and PlGF. VEGF-A and VEGF-B are key regulators of blood vessel growth, whereas VEGF-C and VEGF-D regulate primarily lymphangiogenesis. VEGFs signal through three tyrosine kinase VEGF receptors: VEGFR-1, -2 and -3 [72, 125].

Human basophils express mRNAs for the three isoforms of VEGF-A (121, 165 and 189) and two isoforms of VEGF-B (167 and 186) [73]. VEGF-A has been localized in cytoplasmic granules of basophils and their immunologic activation induces the rapid release of VEGF-A. These cells also express on their surface VEGFR-2 and the co-receptors NRP1 and NRP2. Activation of VEGFR-2 by VEGF-A induces basophil chemotaxis. The latter observations suggest that VEGF-A can exert a dual effect: it can modulate inflammatory and possibly tumor angiogenesis and can exert a chemotactic effect on basophils, presumably through the engagement of VEGFR-2, NRP1 and NRP2. In addition, it is conceivable that VEGFs produced by other resident immune cells such as macrophages [126] and mast cells [127] or neoplastic cells [128] might contribute to basophil infiltration in a variety of chronic inflammatory and neoplastic disorders. Although these in vitro findings should be extended in vivo, it has been demonstrated that basophils infiltrating nasal polyps stained for VEGF-A [73].

There is some evidence that basophils from normal and particularly from atopic subjects constitutively express IL-25 (IL-17E) mRNA, and their activation by IL-3 alone or by IL-3 plus anti-IgE produces IL-25, which augments the functions of Th2 memory cells [103]. It should be noted that IL-25, a distinct member of the IL-17 cytokine family, has the potential to promote angiogenesis in asthma [129].

Angiopoietins are a family of growth factors essential for endothelial cell survival and vascular maturation [130]. Ang-1 and Ang-2 are the best characterized angiopoietins in humans. The angiopoietin receptor system consists of two type 1 tyrosine kinase receptors (Tie1 and Tie2) primarily expressed on endothelial cells. Ang-1 is a Tie2 agonist and is essential for the maturation of blood vessels [131], whereas Ang-2 was initially described as a Tie2 antagonist [132]. Tie1, which is still an orphan receptor, binds Tie2 and regulates its activity [133]. Angiopoietins are involved not only in tumor angiogenesis [134], but also in human inflammatory diseases [135, 136]. We recently found that human basophils constitutively express Ang-1 and Ang-2 mRNAs [137]. Immunoelectron microscopy demonstrated that Ang-1 resides in cytoplasmic vesicles of basophils. Interestingly, protein kinase C activators stimulated basophils to release Ang-1, which induced migration of human mast cells through the engagement of Tie2. These findings identify a novel mechanism of cross-talk between human basophils and mast cells mediated by the Ang-1/Tie2 system that might be relevant in the complex orchestration of inflammatory and neoplastic angiogenesis.

3

Basophils in Immunity against Parasites

Ticks are blood-feeding ectoparasitic arthropods that can cause serious infectious diseases in humans and animals [138]. Karasuyama and colleagues [29] elegantly demonstrated that selective ablation of basophils in Mcpt8^{DTR} mice reveals their non-redundant role in the secondary infestation of ticks. Using the anti-mMCP-8 monoclonal antibody, they identified a cluster of basophils surrounding tick mouthparts inserted into the skin during the second, but not the first infestation.

Helminths are the most common human infectious agents in developing countries. Helminth infections typically induce Th2-type immune responses characterized by high levels of IgE, eosinophilia and T cell production of Th2 cytokines [139]. In addition, basophil numbers are increased in several animal models of helminth infections [140, 141]. Basophils readily generate large quantities of IL-4 in response to parasite-derived antigens [142–144]. However, the role of basophils in the induction of Th2-type responses and worm expulsion in vivo was uncertain until recently [139]. Using mouse models of basophil deficiency, the role of these cells in various aspects of protective immunity against primary and secondary infections of different helminths has been partially clarified.

A study with constitutively basophil-ablated Mcpt8Cre demonstrated that basophils were not required for the primary immune response against *N. brasiliensis*, but were essential for protection against secondary infection [27]. By using the Basoph8 reporter mouse, Locksley and collaborators [28] demonstrated that although neither IL-4 nor IL-13 from either CD4 T cells or basophils was alone needed to expel intestinal *N. brasiliensis* after primary infection, combined deletion of IL-4 and IL-13 from both cell types resulted in a deficit in this response. These results are compatible with the hypothesis that basophil-derived cytokines contribute to this process. They also found no deficit in immunity to secondary *N. brasiliensis* infection in basophil-deficient mice. Using a model of *Trichinella spiralis* gastrointestinal infection, Artis and colleagues [47] demonstrated that TSLP rapidly elicited the expansion of TSLP-dependent, IL-3-independent basophils. TSLP-dependent basophils were rapidly recruited to the draining lymph nodes, and the depletion of basophils resulted in impaired Th2 polarization after infection. Despite great advances in our understanding of the in vivo functions of basophils in protective immunity against helminths over the past few years, it should be remembered that some basophil-depleted mouse models might have intrinsic caveats (e.g. incomplete depletion of basophils, activation/depletion of other immune cells, activation of complement, presence of immune complexes, etc.) and that each helminth species infecting different tissues could elicit specific aspects of the immune response.

Bidirectional Interactions between Bacteria and Basophils

The human intestine, skin and lung are colonized by 100 trillion microorganisms; of these, bacteria are the most abundant. Several studies have started to highlight the complexity of the bidirectional interactions between bacteria and their products and basophils and their mediators.

The term 'superantigen' was coined by the group of Philippa Marrack and John Kappler [145] to describe the ability of the staphylococcal enterotoxin B to induce a remarkable expansion of T cells. Superantigen now refers to the ability of several exogenous proteins synthesized by a variety of infectious organisms (bacterial and viral) and of an endogenous protein (protein Fv) not only to mimic, but also to exceed the activity of conventional antigens [145–149].

Autoimmune disorders, allergic diseases, neoplasia and immunodeficiencies can be associated with superantigens [148, 150–153]. There are two types of superantigens: T cell and B cell superantigens. T cell superantigens simulate the activity of conventional antigens by mediating the interaction between T cells and APCs [147]. B cell superantigens bind to the conserved regions of the variable (V) domains of either the H- or L-chain of immunoglobulins, resulting in a massive proliferation of B cells [154–156].

Protein Fv, an endogenous protein synthesized in the human liver [146], acts as an immunoglobulin superantigen by binding to IgE V_H3^+ [157] and activating human basophils and mast cells [158, 159]. Similarly, gp120 of HIV-1 and *Staphylococcus aureus* protein A (SpA) are viral and bacterial immunoglobulin superantigens, respectively, because they interact with IgE V_H3^+ [34, 160, 161]. Moreover, protein L of *Peptostreptococcus magnus* binds to the V-domain of the k light chains of immunoglobulin [35, 162, 163]. The latter results demonstrate that endogenous, viral and bacterial products can activate human basophils to release pro-inflammatory mediators and cytokines (IL-4 and IL-13) acting as immunoglobulin superantigens. In this context, the definition of immunoglobulin superantigens has been changed to 'superallergens' [148]. The role of superantigens/superallergens in the activation of basophils in vivo and in the progression of allergic and autoimmune diseases remains to be fully elucidated.

Basophil recruitment to certain peripheral tissues and their activation has been shown in association with bacterial infections. For example, basophil infiltration has been detected in the gastric mucosa of

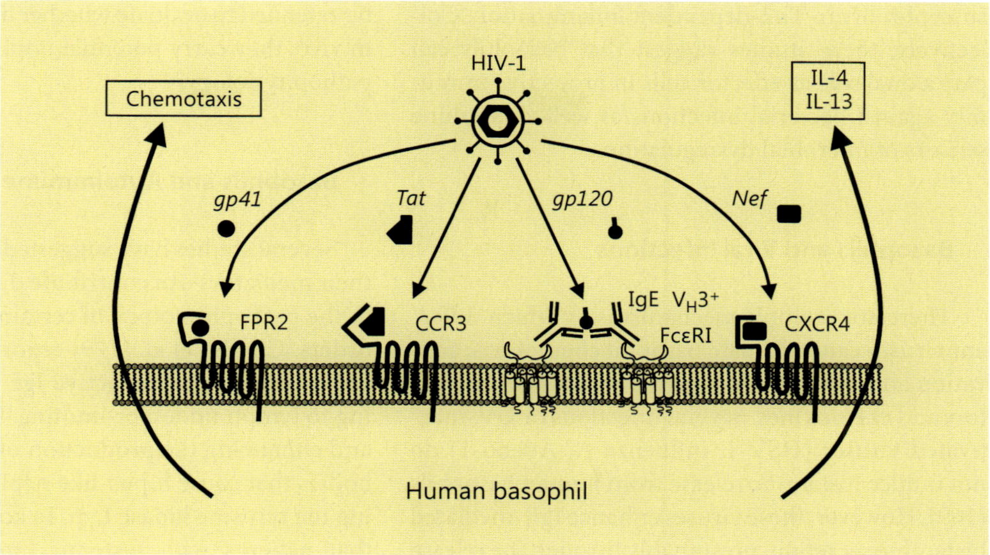

Fig. 3. Several HIV-1 products can modulate human basophil functions. The HIV-1 envelope glycoprotein gp120 from different clades induces IL-4 and IL-13 production from human basophils through the interaction with IgE V_H3^+. Tat protein, which enhances the efficiency of HIV-1 transcription, promotes basophil chemotaxis via interaction with the CCR3 receptor. Moreover, HIV-1 envelope gp41 peptides promote the migration of human basophils and inhibit IL-13 synthesis through interaction with FPR2. Finally, Nef, an HIV-1 protein critical for viral replication, induces basophil chemotaxis through the engagement of CXCR4.

Helicobacter pylori-infected patients [164]. The inflammatory component plays a fundamental role in the progression to gastric cancer [165]. *H. pylori*-derived peptide Hp(2–20) is chemotactic for basophils, as are bacterial-derived N-formyl peptides, through the engagement of FPR2 and FPR3. Moreover, Hp(2–20) promotes the migration and proliferation of gastric epithelial cells in vitro and accelerates gastric mucosal healing in vivo [166]. The role of basophils and their mediators in protective immunity or inflammatory response to *H. pylori* remains of great interest and requires additional investigation.

Cerutti and collaborators [107] have reported that human B cells from the upper respiratory mucosa generate IgD^+ IgM^- plasmablasts that produce IgD. Human basophils bind IgD on their surface through a still unidentified receptor. Microbead-bound monoclonal anti-IgD induces the release of IL-4, IL-13, BAFF, IL-8/CXCL8 and IP-10/CXCL10, but not histamine. Interestingly, BAFF secretion was not induced by anti-IgE. Moreover, anti-IgD was more effective than IgE-cross-linking in inducing the expression of antimicrobial factors such as β-defensin 3, cathelicidin LL-37 and PTX3. The authors suggested that human B cells may produce IgD to instruct basophils to monitor systemic invasion by airborne pathogens.

Recently, Artis and collaborators [167, 168] provided evidence that commensal bacterial-derived signals limit steady-state serum IgE concentration, circulating basophil number and basophil-associated inflammation. Oral antibiotic- treated mice showed an elevated serum concentration of IgE. An increased IgE concentration induced the overexpression of CD123 (IL-3R) in BaPs of germ-free and antibiotic-treated mice. Thus, BaPs from germ-free and antibiotic-treated mice were more responsive to IL-3 compared to BaPs from conventionally reared mice. Interestingly, serum IgE correlates with the number of circulating basophils in subjects with hyper-IgE syndrome. Finally, they demonstrated that basophils can contribute to the exaggerated immune responses observed in antibiotic-treated mice in response to Th2-inducing stimuli. These results indicate that commensal-derived signals can influence IgE synthesis and basophil development as well as susceptibility to Th2-dependent inflammation. Collectively, these studies suggest that basophils can play a dual role as effector cells in protective immunity against bacterial infections as well as immune sensors of microbial dysregulation.

Basophils and Viral Infections

There are multiple mechanisms by which different viruses can modulate basophil chemotaxis, activation and production of pro-inflammatory mediators and chemokines. Several infectious or UV-inactivated viruses (HSV-1, influenza A, Adeno-1) do not induce histamine release from human basophils [169]. However, these viruses enhance IgE-mediated histamine secretion, presumably through the release of interferon [170]. Furthermore, interferon enhances human basophil chemotaxis in vitro [171]. Basophils constitutively express mRNA for type I IFN receptors and IFN-α inhibits IL-3 priming of human basophil cytokine production, but not histamine release [172]. Human herpesvirus (HHV)-6, HHV-7 and HHV-8 downregulate basophil activation through the engagement of CD200R [92]. Basophils are the predominant IL-4-expressing cells in the lung of respiratory syncytial virus infection in $STAT1^{-/-}$ mice [173].

Enhanced IgE levels in adults and children with HIV-1 infection are believed to involve a switch toward a Th2-like cytokine pattern [174, 175]. Several HIV products can modulate human basophil functions (fig. 3). gp120 from different clades induces IL-4 and IL-13 production from human basophils through interaction with IgE V_H3^+ [34, 161]. Tat, another viral product, causes chemotaxis of basophils and mast cells via interaction with the CCR3 receptor [176]. Moreover, HIV-1 envelope gp41 peptides promote the migration of human basophils and inhibit IL-13 synthesis through interaction with FPR2 [177]. In addition, Nef, an HIV-1 protein critical for viral replication, induces basophil chemotaxis through the engagement of CXCR4 [de Paulis et al., unpubl. data]. Finally, there is evidence that a population of basophil/mast cell precursors in the peripheral blood of allergic donors can be infected in vitro by HIV-1 [178]. Although these in vitro results must be extended to evaluate whether these findings apply in vivo, they carry potential implications for HIV-1 pathophysiology.

Basophils and Autoimmune Disorders

Several studies have suggested that basophils and their mediators can contribute directly or indirectly to the pathophysiology of certain autoimmune disorders. Charles et al. [179] reported that activation of basophils by autoreactive IgE causes their homing to lymph nodes, promoting Th2 differentiation and enhancing the production of self-reactive antibodies that cause lupus-like nephritis in mice lacking the tyrosine kinase Lyn. In addition, they found that patients with systemic lupus erythematosus (SLE) have elevated IgE, self-reactive IgE, and activated basophils that express CD62 ligand (CD62L) and HLA-DR. Interestingly, basophils were also present in lymph nodes and spleen obtained from patients with SLE. These findings support the hypothesis that the activation of basophils by autoreactive IgE-containing immune complexes amplifies the production of autoantibodies and contributes to the pathogenesis of SLE [180]. However, another group failed to detect HLA-DR expression on circulating basophils isolated from healthy subjects or SLE patients. Basophils did not upregulate HLA-DR even when stimulated overnight with IL-3 [181]. It has been suggested that the presence of contaminating $HLA\text{-}DR^+$ $CD123^+$ $Fc\varepsilon RI^+$ plasmacytoid DCs in basophil preparations might account for these discrepancies [181].

Rheumatoid arthritis (RA) is a systemic autoimmune disease associated with anti-citrullinated protein antibodies, ACPAs. IgE-ACPAs are present in the majority of RA patients and their basophils can be activated in vitro with citrullinated proteins [182]. Moreover, histamine levels were increased in the synovial fluid of $ACPA^+$ RA patients. Interestingly, increased circulating basophils have been found in juvenile RA [183].

In summary, despite several advances, our present knowledge of the immunomodulatory and effector functions of basophils in autoimmune disorders is largely unknown. Future studies using basophil-deficient mice and/or autoimmune-prone mouse models will highlight the possible role of basophils in autoimmune diseases.

Basophils in Allergic Disorders

Basophils release preformed histamine, newly synthesized LTC_4 and PAF, as well as Th2 cytokines (IL-4, IL-13 and IL-3), all of which are involved in allergic reactions [3]. Human basophils are recruited to the site of allergic inflammation in the lungs of patients with severe and fatal asthma [184–186] and in nasal washings during the late response to antigen challenge [187]. Basophils have been detected in skin lesions of patients with urticaria, pemphigoid, atopic dermatitis and other inflammatory skin disorders [8, 188, 189]. In addition, basophils can be recruited in allergen-induced late-phase cutaneous responses in atopic subjects [190].

There are basophil phenotypic markers and functional characteristics that associate with human allergic disorders. Pioneering studies have demonstrated that basophil histamine release observed in vitro were predictive of the allergic symptoms during the pollen season in allergic rhinitis and asthma [14, 191]. The expression of CD203c (an activation-linked marker) [192, 193] is increased on basophils from asthmatics suffering an exacerbation [194]. In contrast, CD63 expression was not observed on basophils from these subjects. In addition, IgE-mediated basophil releasability is increased in asthma [195].

Human basophils are both a source and a target of angiogenic factors [73] and angiogenesis is an important feature of allergic inflammation in bronchial asthma [196]. In addition, airway vascularity is enhanced in lung biopsy specimens from children [197] and adults with asthma [196]. Finally, VEGF-A expression and vascularity correlate with asthma severity [198].

Collectively, these findings suggest that basophils play a role in the pathogenesis of allergic disorders in humans. However, the results obtained using Mcpt8Cre mice that constitutively lack basophil indicate that these cells are not required for orchestration of acute OVA-alum-induced allergic inflammation of the lung [27]. Moreover, basophils appear to be dispensable for the development of airway hyperresponsiveness and IgE production induced by systemic OVA immunization in a model of diphtheria toxin-induced basophil depletion (Bas-TRECK mice) [30]. The relevance of the latter observations to clinical asthma remains speculative at present.

Several investigators using different basophil-depleted mouse models have demonstrated that basophils play non-redundant roles in models of IgE-CAI [25, 27, 199]. A correlation between the severity of atopic dermatitis and serum IgE levels has been reported [200]. However, it is uncertain whether the IgE-CAI-type mechanism can be translated to human skin allergic disorders.

Karasuyama and colleagues [201] demonstrated that basophils, rather than mast cells, are the most important cells in IgG-mediated anaphylaxis. In this model, basophils stimulated with IgG-antigen immune complexes released PAF, which increases vascular permeability with a much higher efficacy than histamine. It should be remembered that activated human basophils can synthesize PAF [99] and that the concentration of PAF in human sera correlates with the severity of anaphylaxis [202]. Therefore, it will be interesting to investigate whether the above-mentioned PAF-mediated pathway of anaphylaxis is also operative in humans.

Conclusions and Perspectives

The history of basophil biology has passed through various distinct eras since being first identified by Paul Ehrlich in 1879. Around the 1970s it was discovered that IgE binds with a high affinity to human basophils and that their cross-linking with antigens or anti-IgE antibodies can induce the release of pro-inflammatory mediators. After this first promising period basophils fell out of favor with many immunologists, and only a few groups kept the basophil torch alive. The resurrection of interest in basophils began in the early 1990s when it was shown that mouse and human basophils produce large quantities of IL-4 and IL-13, thereby suggesting that these cells could be involved in the pathogenesis of allergic disorders and immunity against helminths. The era of basophil renaissance commenced in 2007 when several groups described different models to deplete mouse basophils in vivo. Although the results obtained with diverse experimental models, as expected, are not always consistent, these new tools have highlighted hitherto unrecognized roles for basophils in both innate and adaptive immunity. However, there are still many issues open for in vitro as well as in vivo exploration, namely the potential role of basophils in tissue remodeling, angiogenesis/lymphangiogenesis, and autoimmune, metabolic and autoinflammatory disorders, as well as in cancer.

Recently, the transcription factor P1-Runx1 was shown to play an important role in mouse basophil development [203]. A better knowledge of transcriptional networks selectively modulating human and mouse basophil development might pave the way to the identification of specific genetic tools for the depletion of basophils in vivo.

The possibility that basophils display phenotypic and functional heterogeneity needs to be explored with modern approaches. It is possible that peripheral blood basophils might differ from basophils recruited to inflamed tissues or even in lymph nodes. Elevated local concentrations of cytokines/chemokines in inflamed tissues might play a dual role, namely they may serve both to attract basophils and to modulate their reactivity. Using two-photon imaging and IL-4 reporter mice, it has been possible to study the interactions between basophils and antigen-specific CD4 T cells in lymph nodes and in lung tissue [28]. The phenotypic plasticity of mouse and human basophils upon migration into various organs remains largely unexplored. Moreover, it is possible that subpopulations of basophils, or basophils at various stages of maturation, might even play, in some cases, anti-inflammatory and/or protective roles in the pathogenesis of different disorders [204].

The study of mouse and human basophils has long been hampered by their rarity and difficult identification. Basophil-specific monoclonal antibodies for humans [8–10] and mice [203, 205] are now available for the histologic detection of basophil infiltration into tissues [73]. In addition, specific basophil surface markers allow these cells to be identified by flow cytometry. Importantly, during the last years several models of in vivo depletion of mouse basophils have been developed using basophil-depleting antibodies [25, 26] or genetically engineered mice [27–30]. The results emerging from these models have shed light on previously unrecognized roles of basophils, distinct from those played by mast cells, in innate and adaptive immunity. However, the results obtained with various mouse models have already highlighted substantial controversies due, at least in part, to different experimental approaches.

Since their identification by Paul Ehrlich, the founder of modern immunology, basophils have always been a challenge to illuminated immunologists. Recent technological advances have opened a new and exciting era in basophil research. There now remains little doubt that basophils, despite their small number in peripheral blood and in inflamed tissues, are critically involved in a wide spectrum of immunologic diseases in mouse models as well as in humans. Given this scenario, it is feasible that basophils and/or their products will represent promising therapeutic targets for certain immunological disorders.

Acknowledgements

This work was supported in part by grants from the Ministero dell'Istruzione, Università e Ricerca (MIUR), the Istituto Superiore di Sanità AIDS project 'Role of Basophils in HIV-1 Infection', the Regione Campania 'CISI-Lab Project', CRÈME Project and TIMING Project.

References

1 Ehrlich P: Beiträge zur Kenntniss der granulirten Bindegewebszellen und der eosinophilen Leukocythen. Arch Anat Physiol (Leipzig) 1879;3:166.
2 Canfield PJ: Comparative cell morphology in the peripheral blood film from exotic and native animals. Aust Vet J 1998;76:793.
3 Marone G, Triggiani M, Genovese A, De Paulis A: Role of human mast cells and basophils in bronchial asthma. Adv Immunol 2005;88:97.
4 Karasuyama H, Mukai K, Obata K, Tsujimura Y, Wada T: Nonredundant roles of basophils in immunity. Annu Rev Immunol 2011;29:45.
5 Crivellato E, Nico B, Ribatti D: The history of the controversial relationship between mast cells and basophils. Immunol Lett 2011;141:10.

6 Gurish MF, Austen KF: Developmental origin and functional specialization of mast cell subsets. Immunity 2012;37:25.

7 Schroeder JT: Basophils: emerging roles in the pathogenesis of allergic disease. Immunol Rev 2011;242:144.

8 Plager DA, Weiss EA, Kephart GM, Mocharla RM, Matsumoto R, Checkel JL, Schwartz LB, Gleich GJ, Leiferman KM: Identification of basophils by a mAb directed against pro-major basic protein 1. J Allergy Clin Immunol 2006;117:626.

9 Kepley CL, Craig SS, Schwartz LB: Identification and partial characterization of a unique marker for human basophils. J Immunol 1995;154:6548.

10 McEuen AR, Buckley MG, Compton SJ, Walls AF: Development and characterization of a monoclonal antibody specific for human basophils and the identification of a unique secretory product of basophil activation. Lab Invest 1999;79:27.

11 Ishizaka T, Ishizaka K, Johansson SG, Bennich H: Histamine release from human leukocytes by anti-γE antibodies. J Immunol 1969;102:884.

12 Ishizaka K, Tomioka H, Ishizaka T: Mechanisms of passive sensitization. 1. Presence of IgE and IgG molecules on human leukocytes. J Immunol 1970;105:1459.

13 Ishizaka T, De Bernardo R, Tomioka H, Lichtenstein LM, Ishizaka K: Identification of basophil granulocytes as a site of allergic histamine release. J Immunol 1972;108:1000.

14 Lichtenstein LM, Osler AG: Studies on the mechanisms of hypersensitivity phenomena. 9. Histamine release from human leukocytes by ragweed pollen antigen. J Exp Med 1964;120:507.

15 Marone G, Spadaro G, Patella V, Genovese A: The clinical relevance of basophil releasability. J Allergy Clin Immunol 1994;94:1293.

16 Seder RA, Paul WE, Dvorak AM, Sharkis SJ, Kagey-Sobotka A, Niv Y, Finkelman FD, Barbieri SA, Galli SJ, Plaut M: Mouse splenic and bone marrow cell populations that express high-affinity Fcε receptors and produce interleukin 4 are highly enriched in basophils. Proc Natl Acad Sci USA 1991;88:2835.

17 Brunner T, Heusser CH, Dahinden CA: Human peripheral blood basophils primed by interleukin 3 (IL-3) produce IL-4 in response to immunoglobulin E receptor stimulation. J Exp Med 1993;177:605.

18 Schroeder JT, MacGlashan DW Jr, Kagey-Sobotka A, White JM, Lichtenstein LM: IgE-dependent IL-4 secretion by human basophils. The relationship between cytokine production and histamine release in mixed leukocyte cultures. J Immunol 1994;153:1808.

19 MacGlashan D Jr, White JM, Huang SK, Ono SJ, Schroeder JT, Lichtenstein LM: Secretion of IL-4 from human basophils: the relationship between IL-4 mRNA and protein in resting and stimulated basophils. J Immunol 1994;152:3006.

20 Gibbs BF, Haas H, Falcone FH, Albrecht C, Vollrath IB, Noll T, Wolff HH, Amon U: Purified human peripheral blood basophils release interleukin-13 and preformed interleukin-4 following immunological activation. Eur J Immunol 1996;26:2493.

21 Li H, Sim TC, Alam R: IL-13 released by and localized in human basophils. J Immunol 1996;156:4833.

22 Ochensberger B, Daepp GC, Rihs S, Dahinden CA: Human blood basophils produce interleukin-13 in response to IgE-receptor-dependent and -independent activation. Blood 1996;88:3028.

23 Redrup AC, Howard BP, MacGlashan DW Jr, Kagey-Sobotka A, Lichtenstein LM, Schroeder JT: Differential regulation of IL-4 and IL-13 secretion by human basophils: their relationship to histamine release in mixed leukocyte cultures. J Immunol 1998;160:1957.

24 Schroeder JT, Chichester KL, Bieneman AP: Human basophils secrete IL-3: evidence of autocrine priming for phenotypic and functional responses in allergic disease. J Immunol 2009;182:2432.

25 Obata K, Mukai K, Tsujimura Y, Ishiwata K, Kawano Y, Minegishi Y, Watanabe N, Karasuyama H: Basophils are essential initiators of a novel type of chronic allergic inflammation. Blood 2007;110:913.

26 Sokol CL, Barton GM, Farr AG, Medzhitov R: A mechanism for the initiation of allergen-induced T helper type 2 responses. Nat Immunol 2008;9:310.

27 Ohnmacht C, Schwartz C, Panzer M, Schiedewitz I, Naumann R, Voehringer D: Basophils orchestrate chronic allergic dermatitis and protective immunity against helminths. Immunity 2010;33:364.

28 Sullivan BM, Liang HE, Bando JK, Wu D, Cheng LE, McKerrow JK, Allen CD, Locksley RM: Genetic analysis of basophil function in vivo. Nat Immunol 2011;12:527.

29 Wada T, Ishiwata K, Koseki H, Ishikura T, Ugajin T, Ohnuma N, Obata K, Ishikawa R, Yoshikawa S, Mukai K, Kawano Y, Minegishi Y, Yokozeki H, Watanabe N, Karasuyama H: Selective ablation of basophils in mice reveals their nonredundant role in acquired immunity against ticks. J Clin Invest 2010;120:2867.

30 Sawaguchi M, Tanaka S, Nakatani Y, Harada Y, Mukai K, Matsunaga Y, Ishiwata K, Oboki K, Kambayashi T, Watanabe N, Karasuyama H, Nakae S, Inoue H, Kubo M: Role of mast cells and basophils in IgE responses and in allergic airway hyperresponsiveness. J Immunol 2012;188:1809.

31 Malveaux FJ, Conroy MC, Adkinson NF Jr, Lichtenstein LM: IgE receptors on human basophils: relationship to serum IgE concentration. J Clin Invest 1978;62:176.

32 MacGlashan D Jr, McKenzie-White J, Chichester K, Bochner BS, Davis FM, Schroeder JT, Lichtenstein LM: In vitro regulation of FcεRIα expression on human basophils by IgE antibody. Blood 1998;91:1633.

33 Lantz CS, Yamaguchi M, Oettgen HC, Katona IM, Miyajima I, Kinet JP, Galli SJ: IgE regulates mouse basophil Fc epsilon RI expression in vivo. J Immunol 1997;158:2517.

34 Florio G, Petraroli A, Patella V, Triggiani M, Marone G: The immunoglobulin superantigen-binding site of HIV-1 gp120 activates human basophils. AIDS 2000;14:931.

35 Genovese A, Borgia G, Bjorck L, Petraroli A, de Paulis A, Piazza M, Marone G: Immunoglobulin superantigen protein L induces IL-4 and IL-13 secretion from human FcεRI$^+$ cells through interaction with the κ light chains of IgE. J Immunol 2003;170:1854.

36 Conroy MC, Adkinson NF Jr, Lichtenstein LM: Measurement of IgE on human basophils: relation to serum IgE and anti-IgE-induced histamine release. J Immunol 1977;118:1317.

37 MacGlashan DW Jr: Relationship between spleen tyrosine kinase and phosphatidylinositol 5′ phosphatase expression and secretion from human basophils in the general population. J Allergy Clin Immunol 2007;119:626.

38 Dvorak AM, Monahan-Earley RA, Estrella P, Kissell S, Donahue RE: Ultrastructure of monkey peripheral blood basophils stimulated to develop in vivo by recombinant human interleukin 3. Lab Invest 1989;61:677.

39 Dvorak AM, Saito H, Estrella P, Kissell S, Arai N, Ishizaka T: Ultrastructure of eosinophils and basophils stimulated to develop in human cord blood mononuclear cell cultures containing recombinant human interleukin-5 or interleukin-3. Lab Invest 1989;61:116.

40 Lantz CS, Boesiger J, Song CH, Mach N, Kobayashi T, Mulligan RC, Nawa Y, Dranoff G, Galli SJ: Role for interleukin-3 in mast-cell and basophil development and in immunity to parasites. Nature 1998;392:90.

41 Hirai K, Morita Y, Misaki Y, Ohta K, Takaishi T, Suzuki S, Motoyoshi K, Miyamoto T: Modulation of human basophil histamine release by hemopoietic growth factors. J Immunol 1988;141:3958.

42 Kurimoto Y, de Weck AL, Dahinden CA: Interleukin 3-dependent mediator release in basophils triggered by C5a. J Exp Med 1989;170:467.

43 Miura K, Saini SS, Gauvreau G, MacGlashan DW Jr: Differences in functional consequences and signal transduction induced by IL-3, IL-5, and nerve growth factor in human basophils. J Immunol 2001;167:2282.
44 Yamaguchi M, Hirai K, Shoji S, Takaishi T, Ohta K, Morita Y, Suzuki S, Ito K: Haemopoietic growth factors induce human basophil migration in vitro. Clin Exp Allergy 1992;22:379.
45 Bochner BS, McKelvey AA, Sterbinsky SA, Hildreth JE, Derse CP, Klunk DA, Lichtenstein LM, Schleimer RP: IL-3 augments adhesiveness for endothelium and CD11b expression in human basophils but not neutrophils. J Immunol 1990;145:1832.
46 Perrigoue JG, Saenz SA, Siracusa MC, Allenspach EJ, Taylor BC, Giacomin PR, Nair MG, Du Y, Zaph C, van Rooijen N, Comeau MR, Pearce EJ, Laufer TM, Artis D: MHC class II-dependent basophil-$CD4^+$ T cell interactions promote TH2 cytokine-dependent immunity. Nat Immunol 2009;10:697.
47 Giacomin PR, Siracusa MC, Walsh KP, Grencis RK, Kubo M, Comeau MR, Artis D: Thymic stromal lymphopoietin-dependent basophils promote Th2 cytokine responses following intestinal helminth infection. J Immunol 2012;189:4371.
48 Siracusa MC, Saenz SA, Hill DA, Kim BS, Headley MB, Doering TA, Wherry EJ, Jessup HK, Siegel LA, Kambayashi T, Dudek EC, Kubo M, Cianferoni A, Spergel JM, Ziegler SF, Comeau MR, Artis D: TSLP promotes interleukin-3-independent basophil haematopoiesis and type 2 inflammation. Nature 2011;477:229.
49 Siracusa MC, Wojno ED, Artis D: Functional heterogeneity in the basophil cell lineage. Adv Immunol 2012;115:141.
50 Voehringer D: Basophil modulation by cytokine instruction. Eur J Immunol 2012;42:2544.
51 Pecaric-Petkovic T, Didichenko SA, Kaempfer S, Spiegl N, Dahinden CA: Human basophils and eosinophils are the direct target leukocytes of the novel IL-1 family member IL-33. Blood 2009;113:1526.
52 Suzukawa M, Iikura M, Koketsu R, Nagase H, Tamura C, Komiya A, Nakae S, Matsushima K, Ohta K, Yamamoto K, Yamaguchi M: An IL-1 cytokine member, IL-33, induces human basophil activation via its ST2 receptor. J Immunol 2008;181:5981.
53 Ali H: Regulation of human mast cell and basophil function by anaphylatoxins C3a and C5a. Immunol Lett 2010;128:36.
54 Bischoff SC, de Weck AL, Dahinden CA: Interleukin 3 and granulocyte/macrophage-colony-stimulating factor render human basophils responsive to low concentrations of complement component C3a. Proc Natl Acad Sci USA 1990;87:6813.
55 Procaccini C, Jirillo E, Matarese G: Leptin as an immunomodulator. Mol Aspects Med 2012;33:35.
56 Suzukawa M, Nagase H, Ogahara I, Han K, Tashimo H, Shibui A, Koketsu R, Nakae S, Yamaguchi M, Ohta K: Leptin enhances survival and induces migration, degranulation, and cytokine synthesis of human basophils. J Immunol 2011;186:5254.
57 Shore SA: Obesity, airway hyperresponsiveness, and inflammation. J Appl Physiol 2010;108:735.
58 Levi-Montalcini R: The nerve growth factor 35 years later. Science 1987;237:1154.
59 Skaper SD: The neurotrophin family of neurotrophic factors: an overview. Methods Mol Biol 2012;846:1.
60 Bischoff SC, Dahinden CA: Effect of nerve growth factor on the release of inflammatory mediators by mature human basophils. Blood 1992;79:2662.
61 Burgi B, Otten UH, Ochensberger B, Rihs S, Heese K, Ehrhard PB, Ibanez CF, Dahinden CA: Basophil priming by neurotrophic factors: activation through the trk receptor. J Immunol 1996;157:5582.
62 Sin AZ, Roche EM, Togias A, Lichtenstein LM, Schroeder JT: Nerve growth factor or IL-3 induces more IL-13 production from basophils of allergic subjects than from basophils of nonallergic subjects. J Allergy Clin Immunol 2001;108:387.
63 Gibbs BF, Zillikens D, Grabbe J: Nerve growth factor influences IgE-mediated human basophil activation: functional properties and intracellular mechanisms compared with IL-3. Int Immunopharmacol 2005;5:735.
64 Sloane DE, Tedla N, Awoniyi M, Macglashan DW Jr, Borges L, Austen KF, Arm JP: Leukocyte immunoglobulin-like receptors: novel innate receptors for human basophil activation and inhibition. Blood 2004;104:2832.
65 Bieneman AP, Chichester KL, Chen YH, Schroeder JT: Toll-like receptor 2 ligands activate human basophils for both IgE-dependent and IgE-independent secretion. J Allergy Clin Immunol 2005;115:295.
66 Komiya A, Nagase H, Okugawa S, Ota Y, Suzukawa M, Kawakami A, Sekiya T, Matsushima K, Ohta K, Hirai K, Yamamoto K, Yamaguchi M: Expression and function of Toll-like receptors in human basophils. Int Arch Allergy Immunol 2006;140(suppl 1):23.
67 de Paulis A, Montuori N, Prevete N, Fiorentino I, Rossi FW, Visconte V, Rossi G, Marone G, Ragno P: Urokinase induces basophil chemotaxis through a urokinase receptor epitope that is an endogenous ligand for formyl peptide receptor-like 1 and -like 2. J Immunol 2004;173:5739.
68 Yamaguchi M, Koketsu R, Suzukawa M, Kawakami A, Iikura M: Human basophils and cytokines/chemokines. Allergol Int 2009;58:1.
69 Iikura M, Miyamasu M, Yamaguchi M, Kawasaki H, Matsushima K, Kitaura M, Morita Y, Yoshie O, Yamamoto K, Hirai K: Chemokine receptors in human basophils: inducible expression of functional CXCR4. J Leukoc Biol 2001;70:113.
70 Blasi F, Carmeliet P: uPAR: a versatile signalling orchestrator. Nat Rev Mol Cell Biol 2002;3:932.
71 Carmeliet P: Angiogenesis in life, disease and medicine. Nature 2005;438:932.
72 Ferrara N, Gerber HP, LeCouter J: The biology of VEGF and its receptors. Nat Med 2003;9:669.
73 de Paulis A, Prevete N, Fiorentino I, Rossi FW, Staibano S, Montuori N, Ragno P, Longobardi A, Liccardo B, Genovese A, Ribatti D, Walls AF, Marone G: Expression and functions of the vascular endothelial growth factors and their receptors in human basophils. J Immunol 2006;177:7322.
74 Hartnell A, Heinemann A, Conroy DM, Wait R, Sturm GJ, Caversaccio M, Jose PJ, Williams TJ: Identification of selective basophil chemoattractants in human nasal polyps as insulin-like growth factor-1 and insulin-like growth factor-2. J Immunol 2004;173:6448.
75 Hirai K, Miyamasu M, Yamaguchi M, Nakajima K, Ohtoshi T, Koshino T, Takaishi T, Morita Y, Ito K: Modulation of human basophil histamine release by insulin-like growth factors. J Immunol 1993;150:1503.
76 Boie Y, Sawyer N, Slipetz DM, Metters KM, Abramovitz M: Molecular cloning and characterization of the human prostanoid DP receptor. J Biol Chem 1995;270:18910.
77 Nagata K, Hirai H, Tanaka K, Ogawa K, Aso T, Sugamura K, Nakamura M, Takano S: CRTH2, an orphan receptor of T-helper-2-cells, is expressed on basophils and eosinophils and responds to mast cell-derived factor(s). FEBS Lett 1999;459:195.
78 Nagata K, Tanaka K, Ogawa K, Kemmotsu K, Imai T, Yoshie O, Abe H, Tada K, Nakamura M, Sugamura K, Takano S: Selective expression of a novel surface molecule by human Th2 cells in vivo. J Immunol 1999;162:1278.
79 Hirai H, Tanaka K, Yoshie O, Ogawa K, Kenmotsu K, Takamori Y, Ichimasa M, Sugamura K, Nakamura M, Takano S, Nagata K: Prostaglandin D2 selectively induces chemotaxis in T helper type 2 cells, eosinophils, and basophils via seven-transmembrane receptor CRTH2. J Exp Med 2001;193:255.

80 Yoshimura-Uchiyama C, Iikura M, Yamaguchi M, Nagase H, Ishii A, Matsushima K, Yamamoto K, Shichijo M, Bacon KB, Hirai K: Differential modulation of human basophil functions through prostaglandin D2 receptors DP and chemoattractant receptor-homologous molecule expressed on Th2 cells/DP2. Clin Exp Allergy 2004;34:1283.

81 Gauvreau GM, Plitt JR, Baatjes A, MacGlashan DW: Expression of functional cysteinyl leukotriene receptors by human basophils. J Allergy Clin Immunol 2005;116:80.

82 Iikura M, Suzukawa M, Yamaguchi M, Sekiya T, Komiya A, Yoshimura-Uchiyama C, Nagase H, Matsushima K, Yamamoto K, Hirai K: 5-Lipoxygenase products regulate basophil functions: 5-Oxo-ETE elicits migration, and leukotriene B_4 induces degranulation. J Allergy Clin Immunol 2005;116:578.

83 Grant GE, Rokach J, Powell WS: 5-Oxo-ETE and the OXE receptor. Prostaglandins Other Lipid Mediat 2009;89:98.

84 Sturm GJ, Schuligoi R, Sturm EM, Royer JF, Lang-Loidolt D, Stammberger H, Amann R, Peskar BA, Heinemann A: 5-Oxo-6,8,11,14-eicosatetraenoic acid is a potent chemoattractant for human basophils. J Allergy Clin Immunol 2005;116:1014.

85 Suzukawa M, Komiya A, Iikura M, Nagase H, Yoshimura-Uchiyama C, Yamada H, Kawasaki H, Ohta K, Matsushima K, Hirai K, Yamamoto K, Yamaguchi M: Trans-basement membrane migration of human basophils: role of matrix metalloproteinase-9. Int Immunol 2006;18:1575.

86 Meknache N, Jonsson F, Laurent J, Guinnepain MT, Daeron M: Human basophils express the glycosylphosphatidylinositol-anchored low-affinity IgG receptor FcγRIIIB (CD16B). J Immunol 2009;182:2542.

87 Okayama Y, Kirshenbaum AS, Metcalfe DD: Expression of a functional high-affinity IgG receptor, FcγRI, on human mast cells: up-regulation by IFN-γ. J Immunol 2000;164:4332.

88 Anselmino LM, Perussia B, Thomas LL: Human basophils selectively express the FcγRII (CDw32) subtype of IgG receptor. J Allergy Clin Immunol 1989;84:907.

89 Zhu D, Kepley CL, Zhang K, Terada T, Yamada T, Saxon A: A chimeric human-cat fusion protein blocks cat-induced allergy. Nat Med 2005;11:446.

90 Gibbs BF, Sabato V, Bridts CH, Ebo DG, Ben-Zimra M, Levi-Schaffer F: Expressions and inhibitory functions of CD300a receptors on purified human basophils. Exp Dermatol 2012;21:884.

91 Sabato V, Verweij MM, Bridts CH, Levi-Schaffer F, Gibbs BF, De Clerck LS, Schiavino D, Ebo DG: CD300a is expressed on human basophils and seems to inhibit IgE/FcεRI-dependent anaphylactic degranulation. Cytometry B Clin Cytom 2012;82:132.

92 Shiratori I, Yamaguchi M, Suzukawa M, Yamamoto K, Lanier LL, Saito T, Arase H: Down-regulation of basophil function by human CD200 and human herpesvirus-8 CD200. J Immunol 2005;175:4441.

93 MacGlashan D Jr: Expression of CD203c and CD63 in human basophils: relationship to differential regulation of piecemeal and anaphylactic degranulation processes. Clin Exp Allergy 2010;40:1365.

94 Bohm M, Apel M, Sugawara K, Brehler R, Jurk K, Luger TA, Haas H, Paus R, Eiz-Vesper B, Walls AF, Ponimaskin E, Gehring M, Kapp A, Raap U: Modulation of basophil activity: a novel function of the neuropeptide α-melanocyte-stimulating hormone. J Allergy Clin Immunol 2012;129:1085.

95 Novak N, Mete N, Bussmann C, Maintz L, Bieber T, Akdis M, Zumkehr J, Jutel M, Akdis C: Early suppression of basophil activation during allergen-specific immunotherapy by histamine receptor 2. J Allergy Clin Immunol 2012;130:1153.

96 Lichtenstein LM, Gillespie E: Inhibition of histamine release by histamine controlled by H2 receptor. Nature 1973;244:287.

97 MacGlashan DW Jr, Peters SP, Warner J, Lichtenstein LM: Characteristics of human basophil sulfidopeptide leukotriene release: releasability defined as the ability of the basophil to respond to dimeric cross-links. J Immunol 1986;136:2231.

98 Austen KF: The cysteinyl leukotrienes: where do they come from? What are they? Where are they going? Nat Immunol 2008;9:113.

99 Triggiani M, Schleimer RP, Warner JA, Chilton FH: Differential synthesis of 1-acyl-2-acetyl-sn-glycero-3-phosphocholine and platelet-activating factor by human inflammatory cells. J Immunol 1991;147:660.

100 Schroeder JT, Lichtenstein LM, MacDonald SM: An immunoglobulin E-dependent recombinant histamine-releasing factor induces interleukin-4 secretion from human basophils. J Exp Med 1996;183:1265.

101 Gauchat JF, Henchoz S, Mazzei G, Aubry JP, Brunner T, Blasey H, Life P, Talabot D, Flores-Romo L, Thompson J, et al: Induction of human IgE synthesis in B cells by mast cells and basophils. Nature 1993;365:340.

102 Yanagihara Y, Kajiwara K, Basaki Y, Ikizawa K, Ebisawa M, Ra C, Tachimoto H, Saito H: Cultured basophils but not cultured mast cells induce human IgE synthesis in B cells after immunologic stimulation. Clin Exp Immunol 1998;111:136.

103 Wang YH, Angkasekwinai P, Lu N, Voo KS, Arima K, Hanabuchi S, Hippe A, Corrigan CJ, Dong C, Homey B, Yao Z, Ying S, Huston DP, Liu YJ: IL-25 augments type 2 immune responses by enhancing the expansion and functions of TSLP-DC-activated Th2 memory cells. J Exp Med 2007;204:1837.

104 Qi Y, Operario DJ, Oberholzer CM, Kobie JJ, Looney RJ, Georas SN, Mosmann TR: Human basophils express amphiregulin in response to T cell-derived IL-3. J Allergy Clin Immunol 2010;126:1260.

105 Li H, Sim TC, Grant JA, Alam R: The production of macrophage inflammatory protein-1 alpha by human basophils. J Immunol 1996;157:1207.

106 Oliver JM, Tarleton CA, Gilmartin L, Archibeque T, Qualls CR, Diehl L, Wilson BS, Schuyler M: Reduced FcεRI-mediated release of asthma-promoting cytokines and chemokines from human basophils during omalizumab therapy. Int Arch Allergy Immunol 2010;151:275.

107 Chen K, Xu W, Wilson M, He B, Miller NW, Bengten E, Edholm ES, Santini PA, Rath P, Chiu A, Cattalini M, Litzman J, Bussel JB, Huang B, Meini A, Riesbeck K, Cunningham-Rundles C, Plebani A, Cerutti A: Immunoglobulin D enhances immune surveillance by activating antimicrobial, proinflammatory and B cell-stimulating programs in basophils. Nat Immunol 2009;10:889.

108 Thueson DO, Speck LS, Lett-Brown MA, Grant JA: Histamine-releasing activity (HRA). 1. Production by mitogen- or antigen-stimulated human mononuclear cells. J Immunol 1979;123:626.

109 MacDonald SM: Histamine-releasing factors. Curr Opin Immunol 1996;8:778.

110 MacDonald SM, Rafnar T, Langdon J, Lichtenstein LM: Molecular identification of an IgE-dependent histamine-releasing factor. Science 1995;269:688.

111 Schroeder JT, Lichtenstein LM, MacDonald SM: Recombinant histamine-releasing factor enhances IgE-dependent IL-4 and IL-13 secretion by human basophils. J Immunol 1997;159:447.

112 MacDonald SM: Potential role of histamine releasing factor (HRF) as a therapeutic target for treating asthma and allergy. J Asthma Allergy 2012;5:51.

113 Kashiwakura JC, Ando T, Matsumoto K, Kimura M, Kitaura J, Matho MH, Zajonc DM, Ozeki T, Ra C, MacDonald SM, Siraganian RP, Broide DH, Kawakami Y, Kawakami T: Histamine-releasing factor has a proinflammatory role in mouse models of asthma and allergy. J Clin Invest 2012;122:218.

114 Falcone FH, Zillikens D, Gibbs BF: The 21st century renaissance of the basophil? Current insights into its role in allergic responses and innate immunity. Exp Dermatol 2006;15:855.

115 Oh K, Shen T, Le Gros G, Min B: Induction of Th2 type immunity in a mouse system reveals a novel immunoregulatory role of basophils. Blood 2007;109:2921.

116 Falcone FH, Dahinden CA, Gibbs BF, Noll T, Amon U, Hebestreit H, Abrahamsen O, Klaucke J, Schlaak M, Haas H: Human basophils release interleukin-4 after stimulation with *Schistosoma mansoni* egg antigen. Eur J Immunol 1996;26:1147.

117 Sokol CL, Chu NQ, Yu S, Nish SA, Laufer TM, Medzhitov R: Basophils function as antigen-presenting cells for an allergen-induced T helper type 2 response. Nat Immunol 2009;10:713.

118 Yoshimoto T, Yasuda K, Tanaka H, Nakahira M, Imai Y, Fujimori Y, Nakanishi K: Basophils contribute to TH2-IgE responses in vivo via IL-4 production and presentation of peptide-MHC class II complexes to CD4+ T cells. Nat Immunol 2009;10:706.

119 Tang H, Cao W, Kasturi SP, Ravindran R, Nakaya HI, Kundu K, Murthy N, Kepler TB, Malissen B, Pulendran B: The T helper type 2 response to cysteine proteases requires dendritic cell-basophil cooperation via ROS-mediated signaling. Nat Immunol 2010;11:608.

120 Phythian-Adams AT, Cook PC, Lundie RJ, Jones LH, Smith KA, Barr TA, Hochweller K, Anderton SM, Hammerling GJ, Maizels RM, MacDonald AS: CD11c depletion severely disrupts Th2 induction and development in vivo. J Exp Med 2010;207:2089.

121 Hammad H, Plantinga M, Deswarte K, Pouliot P, Willart MA, Kool M, Muskens F, Lambrecht BN: Inflammatory dendritic cells – not basophils – are necessary and sufficient for induction of Th2 immunity to inhaled house dust mite allergen. J Exp Med 2010;207:2097.

122 Kitzmuller C, Nagl B, Deifl S, Walterskirchen C, Jahn-Schmid B, Zlabinger GJ, Bohle B: Human blood basophils do not act as antigen-presenting cells for the major birch pollen allergen Bet v 1. Allergy 2012;67:593.

123 Eckl-Dorna J, Ellinger A, Blatt K, Ghanim V, Steiner I, Pavelka M, Valent P, Valenta R, Niederberger V: Basophils are not the key antigen-presenting cells in allergic patients. Allergy 2012;67:601.

124 Sharma M, Hegde P, Aimanianda V, Beau R, Senechal H, Poncet P, Latge JP, Kaveri SV, Bayry J: Circulating human basophils lack the features of professional antigen presenting cells. Sci Rep 2013;3:1188.

125 Karpanen T, Alitalo K: Molecular biology and pathology of lymphangiogenesis. Annu Rev Pathol 2008;3:367.

126 Granata F, Frattini A, Loffredo S, Staiano RI, Petraroli A, Ribatti D, Oslund R, Gelb MH, Lambeau G, Marone G, Triggiani M: Production of vascular endothelial growth factors from human lung macrophages induced by group IIA and group X secreted phospholipases A2. J Immunol 2010;184:5232.

127 Detoraki A, Staiano RI, Granata F, Giannattasio G, Prevete N, de Paulis A, Ribatti D, Genovese A, Triggiani M, Marone G: Vascular endothelial growth factors synthesized by human lung mast cells exert angiogenic effects. J Allergy Clin Immunol 2009;123:1142.

128 Melillo RM, Guarino V, Avilla E, Galdiero MR, Liotti F, Prevete N, Rossi FW, Basolo F, Ugolini C, de Paulis A, Santoro M, Marone G: Mast cells have a protumorigenic role in human thyroid cancer. Oncogene 2010;29:6203.

129 Corrigan CJ, Wang W, Meng Q, Fang C, Wu H, Reay V, Lv Z, Fan Y, An Y, Wang YH, Liu YJ, Lee TH, Ying S: T-helper cell type 2 (Th2) memory T cell-potentiating cytokine IL-25 has the potential to promote angiogenesis in asthma. Proc Natl Acad Sci USA 2011;108:1579.

130 Thomas M, Augustin HG: The role of the Angiopoietins in vascular morphogenesis. Angiogenesis 2009;12:125.

131 Thurston G, Suri C, Smith K, McClain J, Sato TN, Yancopoulos GD, McDonald DM: Leakage-resistant blood vessels in mice transgenically overexpressing angiopoietin-1. Science 1999;286:2511.

132 Maisonpierre PC, Suri C, Jones PF, Bartunkova S, Wiegand SJ, Radziejewski C, Compton D, McClain J, Aldrich TH, Papadopoulos N, Daly TJ, Davis S, Sato TN, Yancopoulos GD: Angiopoietin-2, a natural antagonist for Tie2 that disrupts in vivo angiogenesis. Science 1997;277:55.

133 Milner CS, Hansen TM, Singh H, Brindle NP: Roles of the receptor tyrosine kinases Tie1 and Tie2 in mediating the effects of angiopoietin-1 on endothelial permeability and apoptosis. Microvasc Res 2009;77:187.

134 Huang H, Bhat A, Woodnutt G, Lappe R: Targeting the ANGPT-TIE2 pathway in malignancy. Nat Rev Cancer 2010;10:575.

135 Kanazawa H, Tochino Y, Asai K: Angiopoietin-2 as a contributing factor of exercise-induced bronchoconstriction in asthmatic patients receiving inhaled corticosteroid therapy. J Allergy Clin Immunol 2008;121:390.

136 Kumpers P, David S, Haubitz M, Hellpap J, Horn R, Brocker V, Schiffer M, Haller H, Witte T: The Tie2 receptor antagonist angiopoietin 2 facilitates vascular inflammation in systemic lupus erythematosus. Ann Rheum Dis 2009;68:1638.

137 Prevete N, Staiano RI, Granata F, Detoraki A, Necchi V, Ricci V, Triggiani M, De Paulis A, Marone G, Genovese A: Expression and function of Angiopoietins and their tie receptors in human basophils and mast cells. J Biol Regul Homeost Agents 2013;27:827–839.

138 de la Fuente J, Estrada-Pena A, Venzal JM, Kocan KM, Sonenshine DE: Overview: ticks as vectors of pathogens that cause disease in humans and animals. Front Biosci 2008;13:6938.

139 Voehringer D: The role of basophils in helminth infection. Trends Parasitol 2009;25:551.

140 Falcone FH, Pritchard DI, Gibbs BF: Do basophils play a role in immunity against parasites? Trends Parasitol 2001;17:126.

141 Mitre E, Nutman TB: Basophils, basophilia and helminth infections. Chem Immunol Allergy 2006;90:141.

142 Min B, Prout M, Hu-Li J, Zhu J, Jankovic D, Morgan ES, Urban JF Jr, Dvorak AM, Finkelman FD, LeGros G, Paul WE: Basophils produce IL-4 and accumulate in tissues after infection with a Th2-inducing parasite. J Exp Med 2004;200:507.

143 Mitre E, Taylor RT, Kubofcik J, Nutman TB: Parasite antigen-driven basophils are a major source of IL-4 in human filarial infections. J Immunol 2004;172:2439.

144 van Panhuys N, Prout M, Forbes E, Min B, Paul WE, Le Gros G: Basophils are the major producers of IL-4 during primary helminth infection. J Immunol 2011;186:2719.

145 White J, Herman A, Pullen AM, Kubo R, Kappler JW, Marrack P: The Vβ-specific superantigen staphylococcal enterotoxin B: stimulation of mature T cells and clonal deletion in neonatal mice. Cell 1989;56:27.

146 Bouvet JP, Pires R, Lunel-Fabiani F, Crescenzo-Chaigne B, Maillard P, Valla D, Opolon P, Pillot J: Protein F: a novel F(ab)-binding factor, present in normal liver, and largely released in the digestive tract during hepatitis. J Immunol 1990;145:1176.

147 Kotzin BL, Leung DY, Kappler J, Marrack P: Superantigens and their potential role in human disease. Adv Immunol 1993;54:99.

148 Marone G, Rossi FW, Detoraki A, Granata F, Genovese A, Spadaro G: Role of superallergens in allergic disorders. Chem Immunol Allergy 2007;93:195.

149 Marrack P, Kappler J: The staphylococcal enterotoxins and their relatives. Science 1990;248:705.

150 Bachert C, Gevaert P, Zhang N, van Zele T, Perez-Novo C: Role of staphylococcal superantigens in airway disease. Chem Immunol Allergy 2007;93:214.

151 Goodyear CS, Silverman GJ: B cell superantigens: a microbe's answer to innate-like B cells and natural antibodies. Springer Semin Immunopathol 2005;26:463.

152 Pastacaldi C, Lewis P, Howarth P: Staphylococci and staphylococcal superantigens in asthma and rhinitis: a systematic review and meta-analysis. Allergy 2011;66:549.

153 Viau M, Zouali M: B-lymphocytes, innate immunity, and autoimmunity. Clin Immunol 2005;114:17.

154 Pascual V, Capra JD: B-cell superantigens? Curr Biol 1991;1:315.

155 Silverman GJ, Goodyear CS: A model B-cell superantigen and the immunobiology of B lymphocytes. Clin Immunol 2002; 102:117.

156 Zouali M: B-cell superantigens: implications for selection of the human antibody repertoire. Immunol Today 1995;16:399.

157 Silverman GJ, Roben P, Bouvet JP, Sasano M: Superantigen properties of a human sialoprotein involved in gut-associated immunity. J Clin Invest 1995;96:417.

158 Patella V, Bouvet JP, Marone G: Protein Fv produced during vital hepatitis is a novel activator of human basophils and mast cells. J Immunol 1993;151:5685.

159 Patella V, Giuliano A, Bouvet JP, Marone G: Endogenous superallergen protein Fv induces IL-4 secretion from human FcεRI$^+$ cells through interaction with the VH3 region of IgE. J Immunol 1998;161:5647.

160 Marone G, Tamburini M, Giudizi MG, Biagiotti R, Almerigogna F, Romagnani S: Mechanism of activation of human basophils by *Staphylococcus aureus* Cowan 1. Infect Immun 1987;55:803.

161 Patella V, Florio G, Petraroli A, Marone G: HIV-1 gp120 induces IL-4 and IL-13 release from human FcεRI$^+$ cells through interaction with the VH3 region of IgE. J Immunol 2000;164:589.

162 Patella V, Casolaro V, Bjorck L, Marone G: Protein L: a bacterial Ig-binding protein that activates human basophils and mast cells. J Immunol 1990;145:3054.

163 Genovese A, Bouvet JP, Florio G, Lamparter-Schummert B, Bjorck L, Marone G: Bacterial immunoglobulin superantigen proteins A and L activate human heart mast cells by interacting with immunoglobulin E. Infect Immun 2000;68:5517.

164 de Paulis A, Prevete N, Fiorentino I, Walls AF, Curto M, Petraroli A, Castaldo V, Ceppa P, Fiocca R, Marone G: Basophils infiltrate human gastric mucosa at sites of *Helicobacter pylori* infection, and exhibit chemotaxis in response to *H. pylori*-derived peptide Hp(2–20). J Immunol 2004;172:7734.

165 Polk DB, Peek RM Jr: *Helicobacter pylori*: gastric cancer and beyond. Nat Rev Cancer 2010;10:403.

166 de Paulis A, Prevete N, Rossi FW, Rivellese F, Salerno F, Delfino G, Liccardo B, Avilla E, Montuori N, Mascolo M, Staibano S, Melillo RM, D'Argenio G, Ricci V, Romano M, Marone G: *Helicobacter pylori* Hp(2–20) promotes migration and proliferation of gastric epithelial cells by interacting with formyl peptide receptors in vitro and accelerates gastric mucosal healing in vivo. J Immunol 2009;183:3761.

167 Hill DA, Siracusa MC, Abt MC, Kim BS, Kobuley D, Kubo M, Kambayashi T, Larosa DF, Renner ED, Orange JS, Bushman FD, Artis D: Commensal bacteria-derived signals regulate basophil hematopoiesis and allergic inflammation. Nat Med 2012; 18:538.

168 Hill DA, Artis D: The influence of commensal bacteria-derived signals on basophil-associated allergic inflammation. Gut Microbes 2013;4:76.

169 Ida S, Hooks JJ, Siraganian RP, Notkins AL: Enhancement of IgE-mediated histamine release from human basophils by viruses: role of interferon. J Exp Med 1977; 145:892.

170 Busse WW, Swenson CA, Borden EC, Treuhaft MW, Dick EC: Effect of influenza A virus on leukocyte histamine release. J Allergy Clin Immunol 1983;71:382.

171 Lett-Brown MA, Aelvoet M, Hooks JJ, Georgiades JA, Thueson DO, Grant JA: Enhancement of basophil chemotaxis in vitro by virus-induced interferon. J Clin Invest 1981;67:547.

172 Chen YH, Bieneman AP, Creticos PS, Chichester KL, Schroeder JT: IFN-α inhibits IL-3 priming of human basophil cytokine secretion but not leukotriene C4 and histamine release. J Allergy Clin Immunol 2003;112:944.

173 Moore ML, Newcomb DC, Parekh VV, Van Kaer L, Collins RD, Zhou W, Goleniewska K, Chi MH, Mitchell D, Boyce JA, Durbin JE, Sturkie C, Peebles RS Jr: STAT1 negatively regulates lung basophil IL-4 expression induced by respiratory syncytial virus infection. J Immunol 2009; 183:2016.

174 Clerici M, Shearer GM: A TH1→TH2 switch is a critical step in the etiology of HIV infection. Immunol Today 1993;14: 107.

175 Vigano A, Principi N, Crupi L, Onorato J, Vincenzo ZG, Salvaggio A: Elevation of IgE in HIV-infected children and its correlation with the progression of disease. J Allergy Clin Immunol 1995;95:627.

176 de Paulis A, De Palma R, Di Gioia L, Carfora M, Prevete N, Tosi G, Accolla RS, Marone G: Tat protein is an HIV-1-encoded β-chemokine homolog that promotes migration and up-regulates CCR3 expression on human FcεRI$^+$ cells. J Immunol 2000; 165:7171.

177 de Paulis A, Florio G, Prevete N, Triggiani M, Fiorentino I, Genovese A, Marone G: HIV-1 envelope gp41 peptides promote migration of human FcεRI$^+$ cells and inhibit IL-13 synthesis through interaction with formyl peptide receptors. J Immunol 2002;169:4559.

178 Li Y, Li L, Wadley R, Reddel SW, Qi JC, Archis C, Collins A, Clark E, Cooley M, Kouts S, Naif HM, Alali M, Cunningham A, Wong GW, Stevens RL, Krilis SA: Mast cells/basophils in the peripheral blood of allergic individuals who are HIV-1 susceptible due to their surface expression of CD4 and the chemokine receptors CCR3, CCR5, and CXCR4. Blood 2001;97:3484.

179 Charles N, Hardwick D, Daugas E, Illei GG, Rivera J: Basophils and the T helper 2 environment can promote the development of lupus nephritis. Nat Med 2010;16:701.

180 Charles N, Rivera J: Basophils and autoreactive IgE in the pathogenesis of systemic lupus erythematosus. Curr Allergy Asthma Rep 2011;11:378.

181 Dijkstra D, Hennig C, Witte T, Hansen G: Basophils from humans with systemic lupus erythematosus do not express MHC-II. Nat Med 2012;18:488.

182 Schuerwegh AJ, Ioan-Facsinay A, Dorjee AL, Roos J, Bajema IM, van der Voort EI, Huizinga TW, Toes RE: Evidence for a functional role of IgE anticitrullinated protein antibodies in rheumatoid arthritis. Proc Natl Acad Sci USA 2010;107:2586.

183 Athreya BH, Moser G, Raghavan TE: Increased circulating basophils in juvenile rheumatoid arthritis: a preliminary report. Am J Dis Child 1975;129:935.

184 Nouri-Aria KT, Irani AM, Jacobson MR, O'Brien F, Varga EM, Till SJ, Durham SR, Schwartz LB: Basophil recruitment and IL-4 production during human allergen-induced late asthma. J Allergy Clin Immunol 2001;108:205.

185 Kepley CL, McFeeley PJ, Oliver JM, Lipscomb MF: Immunohistochemical detection of human basophils in postmortem cases of fatal asthma. Am J Respir Crit Care Med 2001;164:1053.

186 Guo CB, Liu MC, Galli SJ, Bochner BS, Kagey-Sobotka A, Lichtenstein LM: Identification of IgE-bearing cells in the late-phase response to antigen in the lung as basophils. Am J Respir Cell Mol Biol 1994; 10:384.

187 Bascom R, Pipkorn U, Lichtenstein LM, Naclerio RM: The influx of inflammatory cells into nasal washings during the late response to antigen challenge: effect of systemic steroid pretreatment. Am Rev Respir Dis 1988;138:406.
188 Ito Y, Satoh T, Takayama K, Miyagishi C, Walls AF, Yokozeki H: Basophil recruitment and activation in inflammatory skin diseases. Allergy 2011;66:1107.
189 Xia HZ, Zweiman B, Schwartz LB: Levels of tryptase, chymase, and FcεRIα messenger RNA in human skin are unchanged after IgE-dependent stimulation of cutaneous mast cells in vivo. J Allergy Clin Immunol 1997;99:224.
190 Ying S, Robinson DS, Meng Q, Barata LT, McEuen AR, Buckley MG, Walls AF, Askenase PW, Kay AB: C-C chemokines in allergen-induced late-phase cutaneous responses in atopic subjects: association of eotaxin with early 6-hour eosinophils, and of eotaxin-2 and monocyte chemoattractant protein-4 with the later 24-hour tissue eosinophilia, and relationship to basophils and other C-C chemokines (monocyte chemoattractant protein-3 and RANTES). J Immunol 1999;163:3976.
191 Lichtenstein LM, Norman PS, Winkenwerder WL: Clinical and in vitro studies on the role of immunotherapy in ragweed hay fever. Am J Med 1968;44:514.
192 Ebo DG, Bridts CH, Hagendorens MM, Aerts NE, De Clerck LS, Stevens WJ: Basophil activation test by flow cytometry: present and future applications in allergology. Cytometry B Clin Cytom 2008;74:201.
193 Gernez Y, Tirouvanziam R, Yu G, Ghosn EE, Reshamwala N, Nguyen T, Tsai M, Galli SJ, Herzenberg LA, Nadeau KC: Basophil CD203c levels are increased at baseline and can be used to monitor omalizumab treatment in subjects with nut allergy. Int Arch Allergy Immunol 2011;154:318.
194 Ono E, Taniguchi M, Higashi N, Mita H, Kajiwara K, Yamaguchi H, Tatsuno S, Fukutomi Y, Tanimoto H, Sekiya K, Oshikata C, Tsuburai T, Tsurikisawa N, Otomo M, Maeda Y, Hasegawa M, Miyazaki E, Kumamoto T, Akiyama K: CD203c expression on human basophils is associated with asthma exacerbation. J Allergy Clin Immunol 2010;125:483.
195 Casolaro V, Spadaro G, Marone G: Human basophil releasability. 6. Changes in basophil releasability in patients with allergic rhinitis or bronchial asthma. Am Rev Respir Dis 1990;142:1108.
196 Detoraki A, Granata F, Staibano S, Rossi FW, Marone G, Genovese A: Angiogenesis and lymphangiogenesis in bronchial asthma. Allergy 2010;65:946.
197 Barbato A, Turato G, Baraldo S, Bazzan E, Calabrese F, Panizzolo C, Zanin ME, Zuin R, Maestrelli P, Fabbri LM, Saetta M: Epithelial damage and angiogenesis in the airways of children with asthma. Am J Respir Crit Care Med 2006;174:975.
198 Chetta A, Zanini A, Foresi A, D'Ippolito R, Tipa A, Castagnaro A, Baraldo S, Neri M, Saetta M, Olivieri D: Vascular endothelial growth factor up-regulation and bronchial wall remodelling in asthma. Clin Exp Allergy 2005;35:1437.
199 Mukai K, Matsuoka K, Taya C, Suzuki H, Yokozeki H, Nishioka K, Hirokawa K, Etori M, Yamashita M, Kubota T, Minegishi Y, Yonekawa H, Karasuyama H: Basophils play a critical role in the development of IgE-mediated chronic allergic inflammation independently of T cells and mast cells. Immunity 2005;23:191.
200 Schafer T, Heinrich J, Wjst M, Adam H, Ring J, Wichmann HE: Association between severity of atopic eczema and degree of sensitization to aeroallergens in school children. J Allergy Clin Immunol 1999;104:1280.
201 Tsujimura Y, Obata K, Mukai K, Shindou H, Yoshida M, Nishikado H, Kawano Y, Minegishi Y, Shimizu T, Karasuyama H: Basophils play a pivotal role in immunoglobulin-G-mediated but not immunoglobulin-E-mediated systemic anaphylaxis. Immunity 2008;28:581.
202 Vadas P, Gold M, Perelman B, Liss GM, Lack G, Blyth T, Simons FE, Simons KJ, Cass D, Yeung J: Platelet-activating factor, PAF acetylhydrolase, and severe anaphylaxis. N Engl J Med 2008;358:28.
203 Mukai K, BenBarak MJ, Tachibana M, Nishida K, Karasuyama H, Taniuchi I, Galli SJ: Critical role of P1-Runx1 in mouse basophil development. Blood 2012;120:76.
204 Anthony RM, Kobayashi T, Wermeling F, Ravetch JV: Intravenous gammaglobulin suppresses inflammation through a novel TH2 pathway. Nature 2011;475:110.
205 Ugajin T, Kojima T, Mukai K, Obata K, Kawano Y, Minegishi Y, Eishi Y, Yokozeki H, Karasuyama H: Basophils preferentially express mouse mast cell protease 11 among the mast cell tryptase family in contrast to mast cells. J Leukoc Biol 2009;86:1417.

Prof. Gianni Marone
Department of Translational Medical Sciences and
Center for Basic and Clinical Immunology Research (CISI)
Division of Clinical Immunology and Allergy
University of Naples Federico II, via S. Pansini 5
IT–80131 Naples (Italy)
E-Mail marone@unina.it

Bergmann K-C, Ring J (eds): History of Allergy. Chem Immunol Allergy. Basel, Karger, 2014, vol 100, pp 193–204
DOI: 10.1159/000358735

Eosinophils

Susanne Radonjic-Hösli · Hans-Uwe Simon

Institute of Pharmacology, University of Bern, Bern, Switzerland

Abstract

In 1846, T. Wharton-Jones described a coarsely granular stage in the development of granulocytic cells in animal and human blood. Shortly thereafter, Max Schultze redefined the coarsely granular cells as a type distinct from finely granular cells, rather than just a developmental stage. It was, however, not until 1879, when Paul Ehrlich introduced a method to distinguish granular cells by the staining properties of their granules, that a classification became possible. An intensive staining for eosin, among other aniline dyes, was eponymous for the coarsely granular cell type, which thereupon became referred to as eosinophil granulocyte. Eosinophilia had already been described in many diseases by the late 19th century. The role of these cells, however, today remains a matter of continuing speculation and investigation. Many functions have been attributed to the eosinophil over the years, often linked to increasing knowledge about the granular and cytoplasmatic contents. A better understanding of the regulatory mechanisms of eosinopoiesis has led to the development of knock-out mice strains as well as therapeutic strategies for reducing the eosinophil load in patients. The effect of these therapeutics and the characterization of the knock-out phenotypes have led to a great increase in the knowledge of the role of the eosinophil in disease. Today we think of the eosinophil as a multifunctional cell involved in host defense, tissue damage and remodeling, as well as immunomodulation.

The Discovery

Nearly every aspect of the eosinophil has been disputed over time, beginning with its discovery. While some historians attribute this to T. Wharton-Jones, others believe the recognition should go entirely to Paul Ehrlich [1].

T. Wharton-Jones [2] described the different corpuscles of the blood in 1846 (fig. 1) as follows:

> The first-mentioned kind of corpuscle is composed of an agglomeration of granules surrounded by a cell-membrane. ... In consequence of the structure, so far as it has been described, of the corpuscle under consideration, I propose to designate it by the name of *granule blood-cell.*

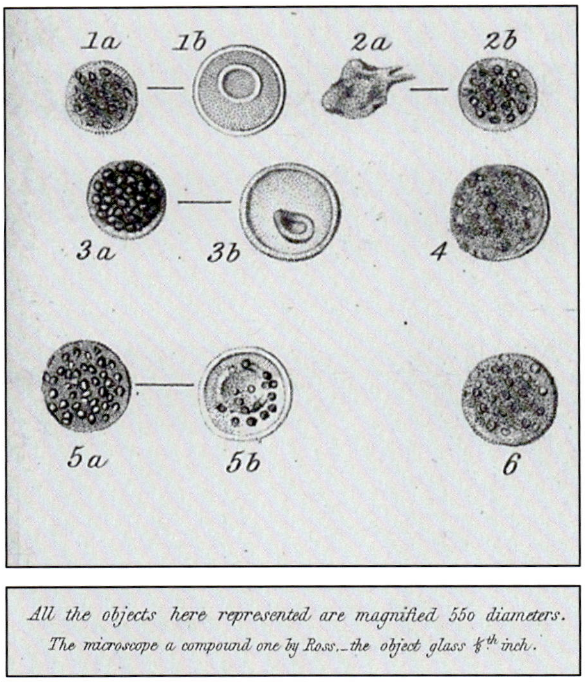

Fig. 1. The first-phase granule cell in *Man and Mammifera* illustrates what Wharton-Jones referred to as coarsely (1a, b; 3a, b; 5a, b) and finely (2, 4, 6) granular. Human (1, 2), horse (3, 4) and elephant (5, 6) cells are depicted. For better visualization he added either water (1a, 2b) or acetic acid (1b, 3b, 5b) to the cells.

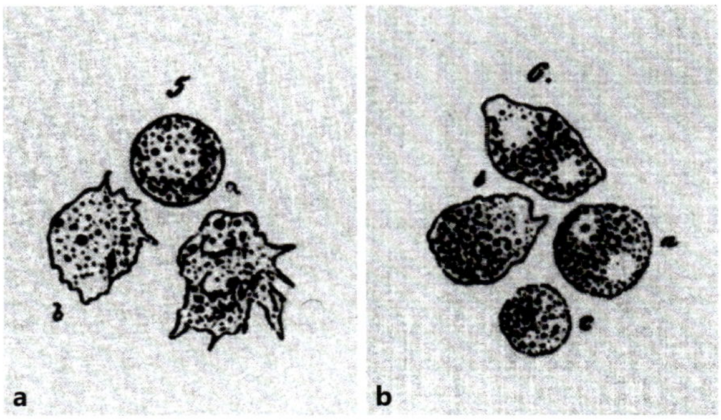

Fig. 2. Retouched drawings of Schultze's observations of the different stages of finely (**a**) and coarsely (**b**) granular white blood cells.

A few years later, Max Schultze characterized white blood cells with live microscopy and divided them further according to their phagocytosing and migratory behavior. While Wharton-Jones had described the finely and coarsely granular as different stages of the same cell type, Schultze, in 1865, described them as two distinct cell types (fig. 2) [3], as follows:

> In agreement with Wharton-Jones I will call them 'coarsely granular' in contrast to the previously described 'finely granular'. I have found in my blood and in the blood of other people scanty numbers of white cells which may be clearly distinguished from other cells by considerable numbers of small, strongly refractile, round granules, which have the brightness of small fat droplets. [transl., 3]

Thus, while Wharton-Jones and Schultze studied and morphologically characterized leukocytes, Ehrlich (fig. 3) introduced a workable cell classification based on the staining properties of their granulation [1]. The α-granules showed an intensive staining following treatment with acid dyes, such as eosin, while the basic dyes did not stain them at all [4]. A leukocyte that exhibited prominent α-granules was from then on referred to as an 'eosinophil'.

The Origin of the Eosinophil and Its Granules: Different Views over Time

The tinctorial identification of eosinophils opened up a wide spectrum of possibilities for the investigation of different diseases. The presence of eosinophils in the blood of patients with leukemia, bronchial asthma, certain skin diseases, parasitic infections and even after the injection of tuberculin had already been described by the late 19th century [5]. Because of the heterogeneity of these diseases, the origin of such cells was a matter of high debate. Many theories were put forward, mainly focusing on the origin of the granules, the latter being the property distinguishing the eosinophils from other cells. According to Biggart [6], who discussed these hypotheses in 1933, the concepts fell into the following three categories: granules were either of extrinsic, metamorphic or intrinsic origin.

The Eosinophil Granule: Extrinsic Origin

The correlation between the staining properties of eosinophil granules and red blood cells, together with the observation that in rabbits, following intraperitoneal injection of guinea pig blood, an increase in the number of local eosinophils was observed, led

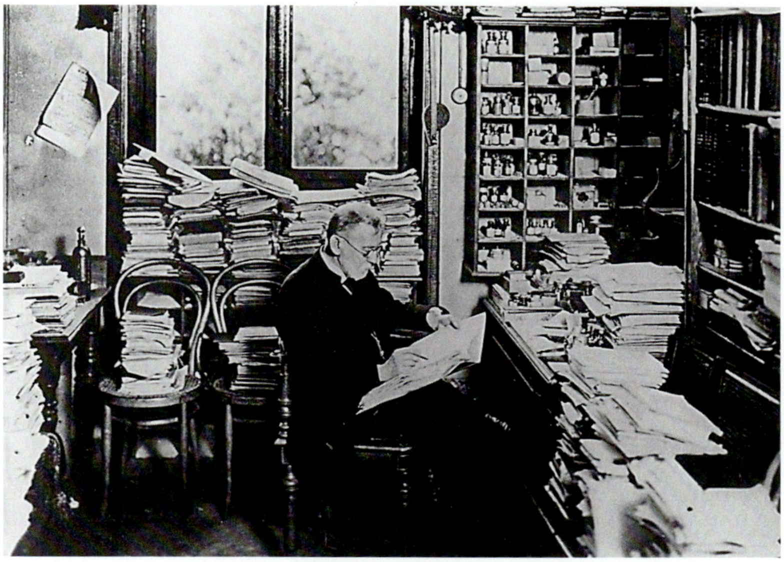

Fig. 3. A photograph of Paul Ehrlich in his office, taken in 1910 by Waldemar Titzenthaler.

3

investigators to postulate that eosinophil granules might contain degraded hemoglobin [6]. Rather imaginative scientists even believed that Charcot-Leyden crystals, observed in the spleens of leukemia patients and the sputum samples of asthmatics, recognized as deriving from eosinophils, must be erythrocyte gravestones [1].

Biggart [6] and Ehrlich [7] both refused to accept the extrinsic origin concept because eosinophils and erythrocytes could be distinguished by different stains. Furthermore, an increased number of local eosinophils could also be elicited after injection of other substances [6].

The Eosinophil Granule: Metamorphosis – Transformation from the Neutrophil Granule

At the end of the 19th century, the idea of transformation from the neutrophil into the eosinophil by a maturation process was widely accepted. However, whether it was the bone marrow or the blood that was the location of the metamorphosis was highly disputed. Brown [5] introduced an adaptation of the concept based on observations made in patients suffering from trichinosis. In muscle biopsies, he observed the following cell morphologies:

> … some of these are ordinary pus cells, neutrophiles; others show large refractile acidophilic granules in the cell body, i.e. they are eosinophiles; in some again the protoplasm, though finely granular, shows a distinct affinity for the eosin stain; in other words, the character of the cells appears to be half-way between that of neutrophiles and that of the eosinophiles.

This phenomenon, as well as the decreased numbers of neutrophils paralleling increased numbers of eosinophils in the blood of these patients, led him to believe that the transformation might take place in the tissue [5].

As has been illustrated so far, the origin of eosinophils was not at all clear. The quantity of hypotheses must have led to considerable confusion surrounding the matter of eosinophils. The following freely translated extract from a handwritten manuscript found in Paul Ehrlich's collected papers can stand as an example for the disputes of that time [1]:

> The speaker who preceded me (Grawitz) made the statement that the division of cell groups which we have suggested must be considered the cause of the enormous confusion of the current literature.
> If this opinion, offered by a hematologist, is permitted to go unchallenged, it is obviously time for me to recant and to express my regrets for confusing our knowledge of blood by introducing new techniques for staining and differentiation. If Herr Grawitz is correct in his assumption that the different types of leukocytes are derived from a single cell, that the mature neutrophil can change into eosinophils, that pus can be explained as a proliferation of 'pus cells' within an

abscess, that eosinophils are interesting, but insignificant, we might as well revert to the golden age where ... leukocytes were considered all-purpose vehicles for casual passengers. ... Perhaps stain technology, inspired by the devil, should be outlawed: who needs staining to decide whether a leukemia is unicellular or mixed? If these archaic trends prevail, let's get rid of modern science: the corpse which remains will be something to look at. [transl., 1]

The Eosinophil Granule: Intrinsic Origin

The various hypotheses belonging to this category all referred to the α-granules as products of the individual cell itself. Some put forward the idea of the granules deriving from altered mitochondria. Biggart [6], however, described the granules as true endogenous products of the cytoplasm:

When the marrow is stimulated to produce eosinophils by repeated injections of protein, it is possible to find eosinophil leucocytes at all stages of maturity. Not only do they develop by mitotic division from pre-existing myelocytes, but also from non-granular myeloblasts. In these latter, there first appear one or two small vacuoles in the cytoplasm. In the centre of each vacuole appears a small basophil dot, which gradually enlarges. As it enlarges, its staining reactions change from basophilic through azurophilic to eosinophilic. The processes of vacuolation, basophil granulation, and the ripening of basophil granules go on side by side in the same cell until the protoplasm is filled with bright refractile granules giving the typical reactions of the mature eosinophil leucocyte. ... The only apparent interpretation of such histological changes is that the eosinophil granule is a product secreted by the cell cytoplasm in response to appropriate stimuli.

Eosinopoiesis: Precursors and Transcription Factors

The following is a quotation from Ehrlich in 1904:

In man the eosinophils constitute only a few percent of the white cells. In normal blood they are always present as polymorphonuclear cells, which are very mobile and active, and participate in the process of emigration. ... They develop in the bone marrow and, as is the case with normal neutrophil polymorphonuclear cells, they develop from mononuclear precursors, which are now called eosinophil myelocytes. ... Eosinophil and neutrophil myelocytes resemble one another closely; one might say they are cousins, so to speak. [8]

In 1960, Rytömaa [9], in his study on the distribution of eosinophils in rats, confirmed Paul Ehrlich's observation that the highest density of eosinophils is indeed in the bone marrow. Owing to the morphological similarities already reported by Ehrlich, and the impossibility of distinguishing between early precursors of eosinophils, neutrophils and basophils, it had to be assumed that they originate from the same precursor [10]. A distinct precursor was, however, yet to be identified at that point [11]. In the 1980s, the hypothesis of a common precursor was opposed by some authors since several arguments seemed to contradict it: (1) normal eosinophil counts in patients with neutropenia; (2) normal levels of eosinophil peroxidase in patients showing neutrophil myeloperoxidase deficiencies and vice versa; (3) heterogeneity of the two cell types with respect to their surface markers, enzyme content and morphological aspect; (4) different rates of development for the two types of colonies (in vitro), and (5) increase in the kinetics solely of eosinophil production in experimental models to study eosinopoiesis [10, 11].

The work of Fischkoff et al. [12], published in 1984, finally showed that neutrophils and eosinophils do have the same precursor. They demonstrated the capability of the promyelocytic cell line HL-60 – from which the development of neutrophil and macrophage-like cells had been reported a few years previously – to differentiate into eosinophil-like cells under certain culture conditions.

In 1982, Vadas [13] recognized the genetic control of eosinophil production in mice. In 1998, the analysis of the eos47 gene, a gene specifically expressed by bone marrow eosinophils, revealed that a promoter region consisting of binding sites for Myb-, Ets-, c/EBP- and GATA-type transcription factors was responsible for lineage commitment. These findings have been supported in recent years with the identification of at least three classes of transcription factors, GATA-1, PU.1, an Ets family member, and c/EBP family members, which act synergistically in lineage commitment [14]. The generation of Δdbl GATA mice highlighted the importance of GATA-1 in eosinophil commitment: the deletion in the high-affinity GATA-1 binding site of the GATA-1 promoter led to the loss of the eosinophil lineage [15].

Eosinopoiesis: Cytokines and Their Receptors

The regulation of eosinopoiesis was intensively investigated at the same time as eosinopoiesis itself. Mahmoud et al. [16] identified a factor promoting eosinopoiesis in 1977. Serum from mice which had been pre-treated with anti-eosinophil serum injected into untreated recipient mice led to an increase in eosinophils both in the recipients' blood and bone marrow. These investigators correlated this eosinopoietic activity with the presence of a low-molecular-weight substance, thereafter referred to as eosinophilopoietin.

Kinetic studies performed in 1970 in which rats were injected with *Trichinella spiralis* showed a time lag of blood eosinophil augmentation [17]. Reinjection 20 days later was followed by an increased eosinophil response [18]. Two arguments, the resemblance to the 'anamnestic antibody response' observed upon re-stimulation with antigen and the inhibition of the development of eosinophilia with immunosuppressive drugs, led Boyer et al. [18] and Basten and Beeson [19] to conclude that eosinophilia had the characteristics of an immunologic phenomenon. The humoral and cellular mediators of eosinophilia were subsequently investigated. By applying different methods, such as neonatal thymectomy, adoptive transfer and anti-lymphocyte serum, these investigators were able to demonstrate that immunologically competent lymphocytes are involved in the increase of eosinophil numbers in the peripheral blood in parasitic infections [19]. The concept of 'lymphokines', soluble mediators different from antibody, secreted by antigen-activated lymphocytes, had already been introduced by Dumonde et al. [20]. The names of the lymphokines were assigned according to their activity in different bioassays [21]. Thus, it is not at all surprising that what we today call interleukin (IL)-3, received as many as a dozen different names [20]. One of the lymphokines identified, capable of replacing 'T cell helper function for normal B cells which secrete immunoglobulin' [22], was termed T cell-replacing factor (TRF). The establishment of a T cell clone producing only TRF allowed it to be distinguished from IL-1, IL-2, IL-3, IL-4 and interferon-γ [23]. Thereafter, it was re-named 'IL-5' [24].

In the meantime, the regulation of eosinopoiesis was investigated:

> ... the occurrence of eosinophils is selective, suggesting that mechanisms must exist to regulate the production of these cells independently of other members of the granulocyte-macrophage series. [25]

The stimulation of neutrophil, macrophage and eosinophil growth by granulocyte-macrophage colony-stimulating factor (GM-CSF) was described in 1979, but did not explain the selective augmentation of eosinophil counts. In 1984, a lymphokine produced by a T cell clone that selectively stimulated eosinophil differentiation was identified. It was named 'eosinophil differentiation factor', EDF [25]. Two years after the first description, Sanderson et al. [21] demonstrated that EDF showed equal activities in bioassays as a lymphokine called B cell growth factor II, BCGFII. Cloning experiments in 1986 then revealed that TRF/IL-5 and BCGFII were one and the same protein [26].

The mechanism of IL-5-mediated functions was then investigated; hence, the characterization of the IL-5 receptor (IL-5R) became of particular interest [27]. Two membrane proteins of 60 and 130 kDa could be identified as putative receptor subunits using different cross-linking strategies with murine IL-5-dependent cell lines. Furthermore, a functional IL-5 high-affinity receptor could be reconstituted upon transfection of a murine IL-3-dependent cell line using cDNA coding for the 60-kDa protein (p60 IL-5R cDNA) [28]. Then, in 1989, an antibody inhibiting the binding of IL-5 to murine IL-5-dependent cell lines (R52.120 mAb) was reported to recognize a membrane protein of 130–140 kDa, distinct from p60 [29]. A close relationship between the IL-5R and IL-3R systems was proposed by Takaki et al. [30] in 1991 owing to the following arguments: (1) a response to IL-3 could be observed in several IL-5-dependent cell lines, like T88M and B13; (2) in T88M cell phosphorylation of similar sets of proteins was induced upon IL-3 and IL-5 stimulation; (3) p60 IL-5R cDNA expression in an IL-3-dependent cell line made it responsive to IL-5 stimulation; (4) IL-3-driven proliferation of B13 was inhibited by R52.120 mAb, and (5) IL-3-dependent cell lines, non-responsive to IL-5, also expressed the R52.120 antigen. Indeed, R52.120 mAb was shown to recognize the AIC2 antigens

3

(AIC2 A and B). AIC2B had already been demonstrated to be identical to the β-chain of the GM-CSFR. The high-affinity IL-5R could be reconstituted with p60 (today IL-5Rα) and AIC2B. It was thus demonstrated that the second subunit of the IL-5R was homologous to the β-chain of the GM-CSFR and IL-3R.

The functional significance of IL-5 in vivo was highlighted by the development of IL-5 knock-out and IL-5 transgenic mouse strains, as well as anti-IL-5 antibody therapy for treatment of human disease. While the overproduction of IL-5 led to marked eosinophilia [31], the deletion of this gene reduced the eosinophil number in the blood and lungs following allergen challenge [32].

Eosinophil-Mediated Diseases

Mechanisms of Eosinophilia

The presence of eosinophilia in many diseases had already been described in the late 19th century [5]. Over the years, an explanation for the development of eosinophilia in the blood and tissues was conceived. It was proposed that the increase in cell number originated from an imbalance between cell generation and cell death towards enhanced differentiation and/or cell survival. The eosinopoietins, such as IL-5 and GM-CSF, were shown to be involved in both of these processes, as illustrated by in vitro and in vivo studies. In nasal polyposis, for example, it could be demonstrated that the pro-survival effect mediated by IL-5 was at least partially due to an inhibition of apoptosis [33].

A classification of eosinophilia based on the cause of increased differentiation/survival, either in the eosinophil lineage (intrinsic form) or mediated by cytokines (extrinsic form), was proposed in 2007. The intrinsic form results after mutations/gene fusions take place in precursors of the eosinophil lineage, and can thus be further subdivided into mutations/gene fusions in the pluripotent hematopoietic versus multipotent myeloid stem cells. The cytokines promoting eosinophil differentiation and survival in extrinsic eosinophilic disorders can originate from T cells, as in allergic diseases, or from tumor cells, as in Hodgkin's lymphoma or solid tumors of the thyroid gland, stomach, liver and bladder [34].

The hypereosinophilic syndromes (HES), first introduced in 1968 by Hardy and Anderson [35], are characterized by marked eosinophilia in the blood and peripheral tissue of unknown cause along with a variety of clinical manifestations. A subdivision of the HES into two groups, 'leukemic' and 'a hypersensitivity reaction of some type', was first proposed by Chusid et al. [36] in 1975. The increasing knowledge on specific HES identities led to an adaptation of the scheme towards a more pathogenesis-driven classification. Two major subdivisions have been proposed which contain specific entities: the lymphocytic and myeloproliferative. The former is characterized by an increased production of at least one eosinophil hematopoietin leading to a secondary polyclonal blood eosinophilia [37]. T cells with an abnormal immunophenotype could be identified in some of the patients as a source of large amounts of IL-5 [38]. A gain of function gene fusion (FIP1L1-PDGFRA) leading to a constitutively activated tyrosine kinase has been identified as an underlying cause for a subgroup of the myeloproliferative form of HES [39].

Development of Therapeutic Strategies

Today, the first-line therapy for eosinophilia is still glucocorticoid administration [40]. In 1970, Basten et al. [17] showed a pronounced effect of prednisolone on eosinophil blood levels in rats later infected with *Trichinella* larvae. Some of the known mechanisms underlying its effects are suppression of IL-5, GM-CSF, IL-3 and IL-4 gene transcription, destabilization of mRNA with reduction of the half-life of cytokines like eotaxins and inhibition of the cytokine-dependent survival of eosinophils [41].

The pathogenesis-driven characterization of HES has led to the development of a diagnostic algorithm helping to identify the subset of patients responding best to a certain therapeutic agent other than corticosteroids [40]. For example, the subset of patients with the FIP1L1-PDGFRA fusion gene shows a very good therapeutic response to the tyrosine kinase inhibitor imatinib [39]. Targeting IL-5 in patients with a lymphocytic form of HES and increased levels of IL-5, with the anti-IL-5 monoclonal antibody mepolizumab, reduced the blood eosinophil range of these patients to normal within 48 h. Tissue eosinophilia could, however, not be completely eliminated [42].

The effect of anti-IL-5 antibody treatment has been further examined in certain defined eosinophilic disorders, such as eosinophilic esophagitis, asthma and atopic dermatitis. In asthmatic patients a reduction of eosinophils in the peripheral blood and the sputum could be achieved with a single dose. However, it did not have an effect on the late asthmatic response or on hyperresponsiveness to histamine [43]. In a multicenter, placebo-controlled study, an effect of repeated infusions of mepolizumab on the rate of asthma exacerbations in patients with severe eosinophilic asthma was demonstrated, the efficacy increasing in parallel with baseline sputum eosinophil counts. However, these benefits did not correlate with a subjective increase in life quality after treatment [44]. A beneficial effect on life quality was achieved in two other studies administering mepolizumab to two subgroups of severe asthmatic patients, both exhibiting an eosinophil count greater than 3% in the sputum despite having prednisone treatment at least once [45, 46]. While in all studies performed the sputum and blood eosinophil counts could be reduced dramatically with anti-IL-5 antibody treatment, mucosal eosinophils declined only by approximately 50% [47]. Also, in eosinophil esophagitis patients, blood eosinophilia declined rapidly upon mepolizumab treatment, while tissue eosinophilia persisted at about 50% [48].

The Functions of the Eosinophil: Different Views over Time

We will now again take a step back in time to the very beginnings of eosinophil research and discuss the functions attributed to the eosinophil over the years. Especially at the beginning, the functions reflected the available knowledge about granules. The nature of the granules remained a subject of constant debate up until the 1960s. Improved microscopic techniques, such as electron microscopy, allowed the identification of a crystalline core surrounded by a homogeneous matrix. Histochemical analysis demonstrated the presence of eosinophil peroxidase. Enzymatic studies of granulocyte mixtures revealed the presence of arylsulfatase and β-glucuronidase. With the possibility to isolate entire granules, further enzyme components were identified [49].

One of the greatest difficulties the investigators faced during that period was their inability to separate a pure eosinophil fraction. In 1963, Archer and Hirsch [49] demonstrated a method to separate horse or rat eosinophils from the remaining granulocytes, allowing more precise conclusions to be drawn about eosinophil function. In 1991, Hansel et al. [50] described an immunomagnetic technique in which human blood eosinophils could be purified up to 99% based on negative selection. The availability of this technique dramatically increased the number of publications on eosinophils in the subsequent years.

The Anti-Inflammatory Role of Eosinophils

In the first years of the last century kinetic studies on the appearance of eosinophils in the blood or tissues dominated the literature. Parasitic infection models as well as the provocation of urticarial lesions upon re-stimulation with specific antigens led to a systemic or local eosinophilia. However, the increase in the eosinophil number always occurred with a certain lag in time. With regard to the time of appearance, a clearing function was attributed to the eosinophil [1].

The analysis of the enzyme contents of the cell further supported this hypothesis. Many of the enzymes identified (histaminase, kininase, arylsulfatase and phospholipidase D), have anti-inflammatory effects and are expressed at higher levels in eosinophils than in neutrophils. Additionally, the eosinophil arylsulfatase, in contrast to the neutrophil arylsulfatase, was shown to be capable of inactivating substances involved in anaphylaxis [49].

The anti-inflammatory effect of eosinophils was especially correlated with the basophil-mast cell system. The following mechanism was proposed: mast cell mediators serve as chemotactic agents for eosinophils, but, correspondingly, these contain enzymes capable of breaking down mast cell products. This hypothesis was further sustained by the fact that eosinophils were shown to be capable of phagocytosing entire mast cell granules. The ability of eosinophils to phagocytose immune complexes further supported the hypothesis of an immunoregulatory function for these cells [49]. Today, we know that eosinophils are able to express IL-10 under in vivo conditions, pointing to the possibility that eosinophils may indeed exhibit anti-inflammatory properties [51].

3

The Effector Role of Eosinophils

In 1898, Brown [5] described parasitic infections as one of the causes of eosinophilia. The role of eosinophils in parasitic infections was, however, disputed up until 1974. In 1975, the development of anti-sera specific to different inflammatory cells by Mahmoud et al. [52] established the role of eosinophils in combating *Schistosoma mansoni* infection.

> Human eosinophils initially adhere to the intact schistosomulum and then, in the presence of antibody, flatten and spread very intimately over the parasite's surface. Subsequently, dense material similar to the contents of the lysosomal granules of the eosinophils appears in the extracellular space between the eosinophil and the schistosomulum, probably following fusion of the granules with the plasma membrane of the cell. ... This release of granular material is followed by structural changes in the schistosomulum. [53]

In addition to antibody-induced cytotoxicity, complement-coating could also induce eosinophil-mediated killing of the parasites. The precise mechanism of the killing, however, remained uncertain [17].

In 1973, Gleich et al. [54] demonstrated a prominent band in an SDS-PAGE of granule extracts of guinea pig eosinophils showing a molecular weight of 11 kDa. Due to its prominence and its basic properties, it was termed the eosinophil granule major basic protein (MBP) [55]. Cytotoxic activities of this newly identified protein to intestine, spleen, skin and peripheral blood – all compartments reported to be rich in eosinophils – was described only a few years later. Furthermore, the MBP concentrations required for cytotoxicity in vitro had been shown in the blood of patients with eosinophilia [56].

> These considerations point to the possibility that the eosinophil may damage cells and impair organ function in disease states. [56]

This dramatic change in the view of eosinophil function was supported by the observation of the neurotoxicity of these cells published in the same year by Durack et al. [57]. They identified a substance with a molecular weight of 15 kDa – thus, differing from both MBP and eosinophil peroxidase – responsible for the induction of the Gordon phenomenon. The Gordon phenomenon was described as a new test for Hodgkin's disease in 1933 by an investigator of the same name. Upon injection of spleen and lymph node extracts from patients into rabbits, a paralytic disease with disequilibrium developed, histologically characterized by a loss of Purkinje cells in the cerebellum and spongiform changes in the white matter of the cerebellum, pons and spinal cord [55]. This toxic protein was called eosinophil-derived neurotoxin (EDN) [57]. At about the same time, Peterson and Venge [58] described a protein, termed eosinophil protein-X, and demonstrated the induction of the Gordon phenomenon by it, as well as other similarities to EDN. It was thus proposed that these two proteins might be identical [55].

The eosinophil cationic protein was first described by Olssen and Venge [59] in 1974. The presence of eosinophil peroxidase (EPO) had already been known many years before. The biological importance of EPO was, however, unknown until Motojima et al. [60] demonstrated that EPO by itself or in combination with H_2O_2 and halide was able to induce tracheal epithelial damage in guinea pigs.

Not only the cytotoxic activity itself, but also the interactions with other immune cells, enhanced the notion of a pro-inflammatory role for the eosinophil. It could be demonstrated that MBP induces histamine release by both mast cells and basophils [61]. Furthermore, EPO in combination with H_2O_2 and halides was shown to induce mast cell secretion [62].

In recent years, further evidence has suggested an involvement of the eosinophil in fungal, viral and bacterial defense. In 2008, Yoon et al. [63] described a concept for anti-fungal defense using *Alternaria alternata* as a disease model. The immune recognition of the fungus was dependent on its cell wall component β-glycan and mediated by CD11b – an integrin subunit and complement receptor on the eosinophil surface. The CD11b engagement led to release of the cytotoxic granule proteins onto the surface of the fungus, with the consequent destruction of that surface. As reported for helminthic killing, anti-fungal eosinophil-mediated immunity is thus achieved in a contact-dependent manner.

A viral cause for eosinophilia is not common [34]. In asthmatic patients and IL-5-transgenic mice, however, respiratory syncytial virus (RSV) infection led to an IL-5-dependent increase of eosinophils in the lung. Furthermore, the clearance of RSV

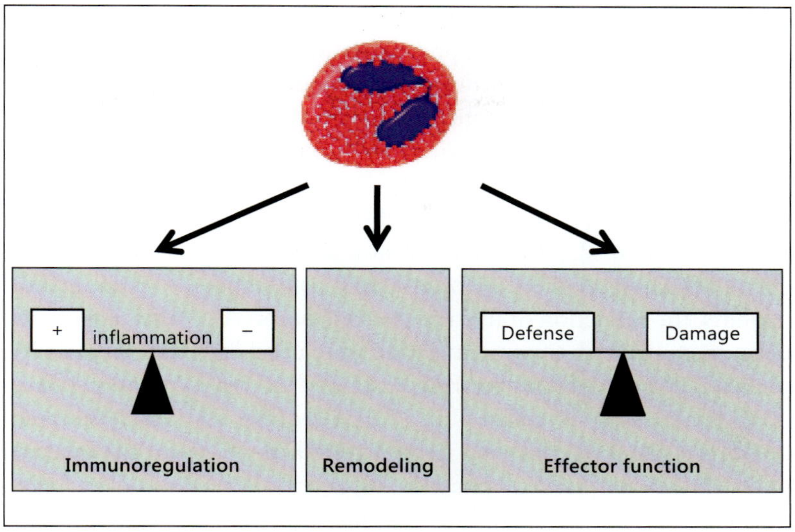

Fig. 4. The multiple functions of the eosinophil as conceived today.

was more efficient in IL-5-overexpressing transgenic mice than in wild-type mice, suggesting a beneficial role for eosinophils in RSV clearance. The mechanisms involved in eosinophil-mediated viral defense have been linked to their constitutive expression of Toll-like receptor 7, which recognizes single-stranded RNA. This finding was supported by a diminution of the RSV clearance upon knockout of MyD88, a protein acting downstream of Toll-like receptor 7 [64]. Furthermore, the RNase activities of eosinophil cationic protein and EDN have been associated with the eosinophil-mediated antiviral defense [65].

Bacterial infections are seldom associated with eosinophilia [34]. In vitro studies have, however, highlighted bacterial killing mediated by eosinophils. IL-5-transgenic mice demonstrated an improved clearance of intraperitoneal *Pseudomonas aeruginosa* while mice with a congenital deficiency of eosinophils showed an impaired clearance [66]. A fascinating mechanism of bacterial killing through eosinophils could be demonstrated by Yousefi et al. [67] in 2008. The LPS-induced catapult-like release of mitochondrial DNA from primed eosinophils was shown to form, together with granule proteins, extracellular net-like structures. These so-called eosinophil extracellular TRAPs trap and kill bacteria in vitro and in vivo.

The Immunoregulatory Role of Eosinophils

The identification of the production and secretion of pro- and anti-inflammatory cytokines and chemokines was indicative for an immunoregulatory role of eosinophils. At the beginning of the 1990s, eosinophil secretion of tumor growth factor (TGF)-α and expression of IL-3, IL-6, IL-8 and GM-CSF, as well as TGF-β, were all demonstrated. At sites of allergic stimulation, mRNA for IL-5 and GM-CSF could be detected in eosinophils, suggesting auto-/paracrine activity. In addition to PGE2 that had already been described previously, the secretion of further lipid mediators, such as PAF and LTC4, could be attributed to the eosinophil [67]. It was the investigation of lipid mediator secretion by eosinophils, other than following calcium ionophore treatment, that introduced the phenomenon of priming. A dramatic increase of LTC4 secretion was observed if eosinophils were pre-treated with IL-5 or IL-3 prior to incubation with fMLF, C5a or PAF compared to either one of these agents alone [68]. The plasticity of response by eosinophils and the capability to produce both pro- and anti-inflammatory cytokines has recently been shown in diseases of the skin that demonstrated, at least partially, different eosinophilic cytokine expression patterns [51, 69].

The Role of Eosinophils in Tissue Remodeling

The involvement of eosinophils in tissue remodeling was demonstrated in two mouse models, the Δdbl GATA and the IL-5-deficient models [70, 71]. A reduction of TGF-β expression was proposed as the underlying mechanism in the IL-5-deficient mouse model [71]. In the lungs of Δdbl GATA, however, Humbles et al. [70] could not show altered levels of TGF-β expression. In mild atopic asthmatic patients, the reduction of fibrosis markers observed upon mepolizumab treatment was accompanied by reduced TGF-β levels in the BAL fluid and TGF-β mRNA expression of eosinophils [72]. A reduction of fibrosis markers was also demonstrated in patients with eosinophilic esophagitis [48] and in allergen-challenged atopic skin [73] upon mepolizumab treatment.

Over time the different hypotheses for eosinophil function have brought us today to a view of the eosinophil as a multifunctional cell with effector and immunoregulatory roles, capable of being both a promoter of tissue damage and of remodeling (fig. 4).

Conclusions

The eosinophil has been the focus of many scientific disputes over more than a century. Nonetheless, the knowledge achieved concerning its development, regulation and function in disease has led to the development of diverse therapeutic approaches for the treatment of patients suffering from diseases associated with eosinophilia. The continuous investigations carried out over the years in eosinophil research and the corresponding increase in the understanding of the role of this cell in disease will allow further optimization of future therapeutic strategies.

References

1 Samter M: Eosinophils: the first 90 years; in Mahmoud AAF, Austen KF (eds): The Eosinophil in Health and Disease. New York, Grune and Stratton, 1980, pp 25–43.

2 Wharton-Jones T: The blood-corpuscle considered in its different phases of development in the animal series. Memoir I. Vertebrata. Philos Trans R Soc Lond 1846;136: 63–87.

3 Brewer DB: Max Schultze and the living, moving, phagocytosing leucocytes: 1865. Med Hist 1994;38:91–101.

4 Ehrlich P: Methodologische Beiträge zur Physiologie und Pathologie der verschiedenen Formen der Leukocyten. Z Klin Med 1880;1:553–560.

5 Brown TR: Studies on trichinosis, with especial reference to the increase of the eosinophilic cells in the blood and muscle, the origin of these cells and their diagnostic importance. J Exp Med 1898;3:315–347.

6 Biggart JH: The origin of the eosinophil granule. Ulster Med J 1933;2:47–52.

7 Ehrlich P: Ueber die specifischen Granulationen des Blutes. Arch Anat Physiol (Physiol Abt), 1879, pp 571–579.

8 Hirsch JG, Hirsch BI: Paul Ehrlich and the discovery of the eosinophil; in Mahmoud AAF, Austen KF (eds): The Eosinophil in Health and Disease. New York, Grune and Stratton, 1980, chapt 1, pp 3–23.

9 Rytömaa T: Organ distribution and histochemical properties of eosinophil granulocytes in rat. Acta Pathol Microbiol Scand 1960;50(suppl 140):1–118.

10 Tavassoli M: Eosinophil, eosinophilia, and eosinophilic disorders. Crit Rev Clin Lab Sci 1981;16:35–83.

11 Weller PF, Goetzl EJ: The human eosinophil. Am J Pathol 1980;100:791–820.

12 Fischkoff SA, Pollak A, Gleich GJ, Testa JR, Misawa S, Reber TJ: Eosinophilic differentiation of the human promyelocytic leukemia cell line, HL-60. J Exp Med 1984;160:179–196.

13 Vadas MA: Genetic control of eosinophilia in mice: gene(s) expressed in bone marrow-derived cells control high responsiveness. J Immunol 1982;128:691–695.

14 McNagny KM, Sieweke MH, Döderlein G, Graf T, Nerlov C: Regulation of eosinophil-specific gene expression by a c/EBP-Ets complex and GATA-1. EMBO J 1998;17: 3669–3680.

15 Yu C, Cantor AB, Yang H, Browne C, Wells RA, Fujiwara Y, Orkin SH: Targeted deletion of a high-affinity GATA-binding site in the GATA-1 promoter leads to selective loss of the eosinophil lineage in vivo. J Exp Med 2002;195:1387–1395.

16 Mahmoud AAF, Stone MK, Kellermeyer RW: Eosinophilopoietin: a circulating low molecular weight peptide-like substance which stimulates the production of eosinophils in mice. J Clin Invest 1977;60:675–682.

17 Basten A, Boyer MH, Beeson PB: Mechanism of eosinophilia. 1. Factors affecting the eosinophil response of rats to *Trichinella spiralis*. J Exp Med 1970;131:1271–1287.

18 Boyer MH, Basten A, Beeson PB: Mechanism of eosinophilia. 3. Suppression of eosinophilia by agents known to modify immune response. Blood 1970;36:458–469.

19 Basten A, Beeson PB: Mechanism of eosinophilia. 2. Role of the lymphocyte. J Exp Med 1970;131:1288–1305.

20 Dumonde DC, Wolstencroft RA, Panayi GS, Matthew M, Morley J, Howson WT: 'Lymphokines': non-antibody mediators of cellular immunity generated by lymphocyte activation. Nature 1969;224:38–42.

21 Sanderson CJ, O'Garra A, Warren DJ, Klaus GGB: Eosinophil differentiation factor also has B-cell growth factor activity: proposed name interleukin 4. Proc Natl Acad Sci USA 1986;83:437–440.

22 Azuma C, Tanabe T, Konishi M, Kinashi T, Noma T, Matsuda F, Yaoita Y, Takatsu K, Hammerström L, Smith CIE, Severinson E, Honjo T: Cloning of cDNA for human T-cell replacing factor (interleukin-5) and comparison with murine homologue. Nucleic Acids Res 1986;14:9149–9158.

23 Takatsu K, Tominaga A, Harada N, Mita S, Matsumoto M, Takahashi T, Kikuchi Y, Yamaguchi N: T cell-replacing factor (TRF)/interleukin 5 (IL-5): molecular and functional properties. Immunol Rev 1988;102: 107–135.

24 Yamaguchi Y, Hayashi Y, Sugama Y, Miura Y, Kasahara T, Kitamura S, Torisu M, Mita S, Tominaga A, Takatsu K, Suda T: Highly purified murine interleukin 5 (IL-5) stimulates eosinophil function and prolongs in vitro survival: IL-5 as an eosinophil chemotactic factor. J Exp Med 1988;167:1737–1742.

25 Lopez AF, Begley CG, Williamson DJ, Warren DJ, Vadas MA, Sanderson C: Murine eosinophil differentiation factor: an eosinophil-specific colony-stimulating factor with activity for human cells. J Exp Med 1986; 163:1085–1099.

26 Kinashi T, Harada N, Severinson E, Tanabe T, Sideras P, Konishi M, Azuma C, Tominaga A, Bergstedt-Lindqvist S, Takahashi M, Matsuda F, Yaoita Y, Takatsu K, Honjo T: Cloning of complementary DNA encoding T-cell replacing factor and identity with B-cell growth factor II. Nature 1986;324:70–73.

27 Mita S, Tominaga A, Hitoshi Y, Sakamoto K, Honjo T, Akagi M, Kikuchi Y, Yamaguchi N, Takatsu K: Characterization of high-affinity receptors for interleukin 5 on interleukin 5-dependent cell lines. Proc Natl Acad Sci USA 1989;86:2311–2315.

28 Takaki S, Tominaga A, Hitoshi Y, Mita S, Sonada E, Yamaguchi N, Takatsu K: Molecular cloning and expression of the murine interleukin-5 receptor. EMBO J 1990;9: 4367–4374.

29 Rolink AG, Melchers F, Palacios R: Monoclonal antibodies reactive with the mouse interleukin 5 receptor. J Exp Med 1989;169: 1693–1701.

30 Takaki S, Mita S, Kitamura T, Yonehara S, Yamaguchi N, Tominaga A, Miyajima A, Takatsu K: Identification of the second subunit of the murine interleukin-5 receptor: interleukin-3 receptor-like protein, AIC2B is a component of the high affinity interleukin-5 receptor. EMBO J 1991;10:2833–2838.

31 Dent LA, Strath M, Mellor AL, Sanderson CJ: Eosinophilia in transgenic mice expressing interleukin 5. J Exp Med 1990;172: 1425–1431.

32 Foster PS, Hogan SP, Ramsay AJ, Matthaei KI, Young IG: Interleukin 5 deficiency abolishes eosinophilia, airway hyperreactivity, and lung damage in a mouse asthma model. J Exp Med 1996;183:195–201.

33 Simon HU, Yousefi S, Schranz C, Schapowal A, Bachert C, Blaser K: Direct demonstration of delayed eosinophil apoptosis as a mechanism causing tissue eosinophilia. J Immunol 1997;158:3902–3908.

34 Simon D, Simon HU: Eosinophilic disorders. J Allergy Clin Immunol 2007;119: 1291-1300.

35 Hardy WR, Anderson RE: The hypereosinophilic syndromes. Ann Intern Med 1968;68: 1220–1229.

36 Chusid MJ, Dale DC, West BC, Wolff SM: The hypereosinophilic syndrome: analysis of fourteen cases with review of the literature. Medicine 1975;54:1–27.

37 Simon HU, Rothenberg ME, Bochner BS, Weller PF, Wardlaw AJ, Wechsler ME, Rosenwasser LJ, Roufosse F, Gleich GJ, Klion AD: Refining the definition of hypereosinophilic syndrome. J Allergy Clin Immunol 2010;126:45–49.

38 Simon HU, Plötz SG, Dummer R, Blaser K: Abnormal clones of T cells producing interleukin-5 in idiopathic eosinophilia. N Engl J Med 1999;341:1112–1120.

39 Cools J, DeAngelo DJ, Gotlib J, Stover EH, Legare RD, Cortes J, Kutok J, Clark J, Galinsky I, Griffin JD, Cross NCP, Tefferi A, Malone J, Alam R, Schrier SL, Schmid J, Rose M, Vandenberghe P, Verhoef G, Boogaerts M, Wlodarska I, Kantarjian H, Marynen P, Coutre SE, Stone R, Gilliland DG: A tyrosine kinase created by fusion of the PDGFRA and FIP1L1 genes as a therapeutic target of imatinib in idiopathic hypereosinophilic syndromes. N Engl J Med 2003;348:1201–1214.

40 Simon HU, Klion A: Therapeutic approaches to patients with hypereosinophilic syndromes. Semin Hematol 2012;49:160–170.

41 Rothenberg ME, Hogan SP: The eosinophil. Annu Rev Immunol 2006;24:147–174.

42 Plötz SG, Simon HU, Darsow U, Simon D, Vassina E, Yousefi S, Hein R, Smith T, Behrendt H, Ring J: Use of anti-interleukin-5 antibody in the hypereosinophilic syndrome with eosinophilic dermatitis. N Engl J Med 2003;349:2334–2339.

43 Leckie MJ, Ten Brinke A, Khan J, Diamant Z, O'Connor BJ, Walls CM, Mathur AK, Cowley HC, Chung KF, Djukanovic R, Hansel TT, Holgate ST, Sterk PJ, Barnes PJ: Effects of an interleukin-5 blocking monoclonal antibody on eosinophils, airway hyperresponsiveness, and the late asthmatic response. Lancet 2000;356:2144–2148.

44 Pavord ID, Korn S, Howarth P, Bleecker ER, Buhl R, Keene ON, Ortega H, Chanez P: Mepolizumab for severe eosinophilic asthma (DREAM): a multicentre, double-blind, placebo-controlled trial. Lancet 2012;380: 651–659.

45 Haldar P, Brightling CE, Hargadon B, Gupta S, Monteiro W, Sousa A, Marshall RP, Bradding P, Green RH, Wardlaw AJ, Pavord ID: Mepolizumab and exacerbations of refractory eosinophilic asthma. N Engl J Med 2009;360:973–984.

46 Nair P, Pizzichini MMM, Kjarsgaard M, Inman MD, Efthimiadis A, Pizzichini E, Hargreave FE, O'Bryne PM: Mepolizumab for prednisone-dependent asthma with sputum eosinophilia. N Engl J Med 2009;360: 985–993.

47 Flood-Page PT, Menzies-Gow AN, Kay AB, Robinson DS: Eosinophil's role remains uncertain as anti-interleukin-5 only partially depletes numbers in asthmatic airway. Am J Respir Crit Care Med 2003;167:199–204.

48 Straumann A, Conus S, Grzonka P, Kita H, Kephart G, Bussmann C, Beglinger C, Smith DA, Patel J, Byrne M, Simon HU: Anti-interleukin-5 antibody treatment (mepolizumab) in active eosinophilic oesophagitis: a randomized, placebo-controlled, double-blind trial. Gut 2010;59:21–30.

49 Archer GT, Hirsch JG: Isolation of granules from eosinophil leucocytes and study of their enzyme content. J Exp Med 1963;118: 227–286.

50 Hansel TT, De Vries IJ, Iff T, Rihs S, Wandzilak M, Betz S, Blaser K, Walker C: An improved immunomagnetic procedure for the isolation of highly purified human eosinophils. J Immunol Methods 1991;145:105–110.

51 Roth N, Städler S, Lemann M, Hösli S, Simon HU, Simon D: Distinct eosinophil cytokine expression patterns in skin diseases: the possible existence of functionally different eosinophil subpopulations. Allergy 2011;66:1477–1486.

52 Mahmoud AAF, Warren KS, Peters PA: A role for the eosinophil in acquired resistance to *Schistosoma mansoni* infection as determined by antieosinophil serum. J Exp Med 1975;142:805–813.

53 Glaubert AM, Butterworth AE, Sturrock RF, Houba V: The mechanism of antibody-dependent, eosinophil-mediated damage to schistosomula of *Schistosoma mansoni* in vitro: a study by phase-contrast and electron microscopy. J Cell Sci 1978;34:173–192.

54 Gleich GJ, Loegering DA, Maldonado JE: Identification of a major basic protein in guinea pig eosinophil granules. J Exp Med 1973;137:1459–1471.

55 Gleich GJ, Loegering DA, Adolphson CR: Eosinophils and brochial inflammation. Chest 1985;87:10S–13S.

56 Gleich GJ, Frigas E, Loegering DA, Wassom DL, Steinmuller D: Cytotoxic properties of the eosinophil major basic protein. J Immunol 1979;123:2925–2927.

57 Durack DT, Sumi SM, Klebanoff SJ: Neurotoxicity of human eosinophils. Proc Natl Acad Sci USA 1979;76:1443–1447.

58 Peterson CG, Venge P: Purification and characterization of a new cationic protein – eosinophil protein-X (EPX) – from granules of human eosinophils. Immunol 1983;50:19–26.

59 Olssen I, Venge P: Cationic proteins of human granulocytes. 2. Seperation of the cationic proteins of the granules of leukemic myeloid cells. Blood 1974;44:235–246.
60 Motojima S, Frigas E, Loegering DA, Gleich GJ: Toxicity of eosinophil cationic proteins for guinea pig tracheal epithelium in vitro. Am Rev Respir Dis 1989;139:801–805.
61 O'Donnell MC, Ackerman SJ, Gleich GJ, Thomas LJ: Activation of basophil and mast cell histamine release by eosinophil granule major basic protein. J Exp Med 1983;157: 1981–1991.
62 Henderson WR, Chi EY, Klebanoff SJ: Eosinophil peroxidase-induced mast cell secretion. J Exp Med 1980;152:265–279.
63 Yoon J, Ponikau JU, Lawrence C, Kita H: Innate anti-fungal immunity of human eosinophils mediated by a β2-integrin, CD11b. J Immunol 2008;181:2907–2915.
64 Stevens RL: Viral infections: beneficial role of eosinophils. Blood 2007;110:1406.
65 Adamko DJ, Yost BL, Gleich GJ, Fryer AD, Jacoby DB: Ovalbumin sensitization changes the inflammatory response to subsequent parainfluenza infection: eosinophils mediate airway hyperresponsiveness, M_2 muscarinic receptor dysfunction, and antiviral effects. J Exp Med 1999;190:1465–1477.
66 Linch SN, Kelly AM, Danielson ET, Pero R, Lee JJ, Gold JA: Mouse eosinophils possess potent antibacterial properties in vivo. Infect Immun 2009;77:4976–4982.
67 Yousefi S, Gold JA, Andina N, Lee JJ, Kelly AM, Kozlowski E, Schmid I, Straumann A, Reichenbach J, Gleich GJ, Simon HU: Catapult-like release of mitochondrial DNA by eosinophils contributes to antibacterial defense. Nat Med 2008;14:949–953.
68 Wardlaw AJ: Eosinphils in the 1990s: New perspectives on their role in health and disease. Postgrad Med J 1994;70:536–552.
69 Takafuji S, Bischoff SC, DeWeck AL, Dahinden CA: IL-3 and IL-5 prime normal human eosinophils to produce leukotriene C4 in response to soluble agonists. J Immunol 1991; 147:3855–3861.
70 Humbles AA, Lloyd CM, McMillan SJ, Friend DS, Xanthou G, McKenna EE, Ghiran S, Gerard NP, Yu C, Orkin SH, Gerard C: A critical role for eosinophils in allergic airways remodeling. Science 2004;305: 1776–1779.
71 Cho JY, Miller M, Baek KJ, Han JW, Nayar J, Lee SY, McElwain K, McElwain S, Friedman S, Broide DH: Inhibition of airway remodeling in IL-5-deficient mice. J Clin Invest 2004;113:551–560.
72 Flood-Page P, Menzies-Gow A, Phipps S, Ying S, Wangoo A, Ludwig MS, Barnes N, Robinson D, Kay AB: Anti-IL-5 treatment reduces deposition of ECM proteins in the bronchial subepithelial basement membrane of mild atopic asthmatics. J Clin Invest 2003;112:1029–1036.
73 Phipps S, Flood-Page P, Menzies-Gow A, Ong YE, Kay AB: Intravenous anti-IL-5 monocloncal antibody reduces eosinophils and tenascin deposition in allergen-challenged human atopic skin. J Invest Dermatol 2004;122:1406–1412.

Prof. Hans-Uwe Simon
Institute of Pharmacology, University of Bern
Friedbühlstrasse 49
CH–3010 Bern (Switzerland)
E-Mail hus@pki.unibe.ch

Bergmann K-C, Ring J (eds): History of Allergy. Chem Immunol Allergy. Basel, Karger, 2014, vol 100, pp 205–213
DOI: 10.1159/000358739

The Bradykinin-Forming Cascade: A Historical Perspective

Allen P. Kaplan

Department of Medicine, Medical University of South Carolina, Charleston, S.C., USA

Abstract

The formation of bradykinin in plasma requires interaction of three proteins, namely coagulation factor XII (Hageman factor), prekallikrein and high-molecular-weight kininogen (HK). Prekallikrein and HK circulate as a bimolecular complex. Initiation of the cascade upon binding to negatively charged surfaces (or macromolecules) is dependent on factor XII autoactivation, conversion of prekallikrein to kallikrein, and a feedback activation of factor XII by kallikrein. The latter reaction is extremely rapid relative to factor XII autoactivation. The kallikrein then digests HK to liberate bradykinin. The natural surface appears to be vascular endothelial cells which express binding proteins for factor XII and HK, and activation can proceed along the cell surface. Recent findings demonstrate that prekallikrein has enzymatic activity separate from that of kallikrein such that it can stoichiometrically bind and cleave HK to liberate bradykinin. It is normally prevented from doing so by the plasma C1 inhibitor. Release of heat shock protein 90 (HSP-90) from endothelial cells can convert prekallikrein to kallikrein (stoichiometrically) within the prekallikrein-HK complex, even in the absence of factor XII, and the prekallikrein-HK complex can autoactivate to generate kallikrein if phosphate is the buffering ion. The effects of phosphate ion and HSP-90 are additive. Thus, an active site appears to be induced in prekallikrein by binding to HK and any of the aforementioned reactions can generate kallikrein prior to factor XII activation by autoactivation of the HK-PK complex. This brief review highlights the major discoveries made over the past 50 years which have led to our current concepts regarding the constituents and mechanisms of activation of the plasma bradykinin-forming cascade.

The plasma pathway by which bradykinin is produced is known as 'contact activation' because the sequence of reactions leading to bradykinin production is initiated by interaction with negatively charged surfaces. Most are familiar with this phenomenon based on drawing blood into a glass test tube so that it clots. The negative surface charge of the silicate is the 'contact' that starts what is known as the intrinsic coagulation cascade with simultaneous formation of bradykinin. Three plasma proteins interact in plasma in order to produce bradykinin, namely factor XII (Hageman factor), prekallikrein and high-molecular-weight kininogen (HK). Although their interactions are quite complex, when taken together they can be considered to represent the intrinsic initiating step for blood coagulation [1]. Thus, all three proteins interact leading to optimal conversion of factor XII to factor XIIa with bradykinin as the by-product. Conversion of factor XI to factor XIa by factor XIIa represents the second step in this coagulation cascade, but factor XI has no role in bradykinin formation.

Factor XII

The discovery of plasma deficient in factor XII (Hageman factor deficiency) by Oscar Ratnoff is a good starting point historically [2] and, early on, Hageman factor was known to have functions in coagulation, fibrinolysis and bradykinin formation. The enzyme kallikrein was demonstrated as an activity based on its ability to cleave a kininogen to produce bradykinin. A seminal paper by Marion Webster [3] was one in which she attempted to isolate those factors in serum (or activated plasma) that were required to produce bradykinin by ion exchange chromatography. A γ-globulin fraction (i.e. IgG, primarily) possessed kallikrein activity but she also defined 4 other peaks of activity which on incubation with EDTA-plasma produced bradykinin, yet did not do so when incubated with a kininogen source. These peaks therefore represented enzymatic steps that precede kininogen cleavage by kallikrein – the distinction between HK and low-molecular-weight kininogen (LK) was not yet evident – their relationship to factor XII was not known, and prekallikrein was not a defined entity. My own work on the bradykinin-forming cascade began with an attempt to identify all of these peaks of activity. The result was that all 4 represented differing forms of activated factor XII; the largest is now known as factor XIIa and the smallest, and only stable form, a 'fragment', is factor XIIf of about 30 kDa [4]. Fractionation of inactivated plasma revealed that incubation of the initial γ-globulin peak obtained on ion exchange chromatography with factor XIIa or factor XIIf generated kallikrein activity and, therefore, contained a kallikrein precursor designated 'prekallikrein'.

Unactivated factor XII was purified by Cochrane and Wuepper [5] subsequent to the purification and characterization of the activated forms [6]. There was controversy regarding the activation mechanism because Revak et al. [7] proposed that factor XIIa and factor XIIf represented two differing pathways for factor XII activation; the formation of factor XIIa required cleavage within a key disulfide bridge such that reduction yielded a heavy chain of 50 kDa and a light chain of 30 kDa, while formation of factor XIIf was a product of cleavage external to the disulfide bond. These forms of activated factor XII were renamed α-factor XIIa and β-factor XIIa [7], and represent terminology still used by some. However, the original mechanism [6] required formation of factor XIIa first (i.e. first cleavage within the disulfide bridge as an absolute requirement for an active enzyme to result) while factor XIIf represented a later cleavage product of factor XIIa. This proved to be correct once careful kinetics and bond cleavages were established [8]. The term factor XIIa is consistent with terminology for a coagulation factor (e.g. factor XIIa, IXa, VIIa, etc.) while factor XIIf does not (it retains only 4% of the coagulant activity of factor XIIa) [6], yet factor XIIf activates prekallikrein readily (fig. 1) until it is inactivated by C1 inhibitor (INH).

Cleavage of factor XII was shown to be a requisite for activation, which is facilitated when it is bound to negatively charged surfaces or macromolecules [9]; thus, the 'contact activation' surface renders the factor XIIa substrate. A prior idea that a conformational change occurs upon factor XII binding to surfaces that leads to active site expression was therefore disproved. Yet, incubation of purified factor XII with a synthetic substrate that turns yellow upon factor XII activation revealed seemingly spontaneous activation of factor XII (fig. 2). When the product of the reaction was examined, it was completely cleaved. The explanation turned out to be due to autoactivation [10] in which trace amounts of factor XIIa present in the factor XII preparation (less than 0.01%, i.e. less than 1 molecule in 10,000) is sufficient to ac-

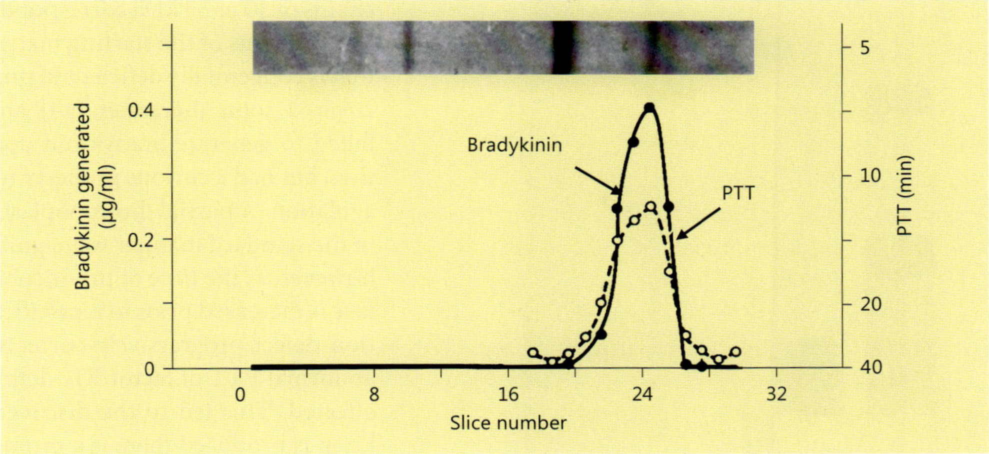

Fig. 1. Factor XIIf has bradykinin-forming activity and retains clotting activity. Factor XIIf was purified from plasma by ion exchange chromatography and gel electrophoresis. A concentrate of bradykinin-forming activity was subjected to SDS gel electrophoresis. The SDS gel was sliced into 32 sections; each section was sliced, solubilized and assayed for bradykinin formation as well as the ability to correct the clotting abnormality of factor XII-deficient plasma (PTT). Slices 20–26 possessed both active activities with a peak at slice 25 in a prealbumin region of the SDS gel containing two closely paced bands.

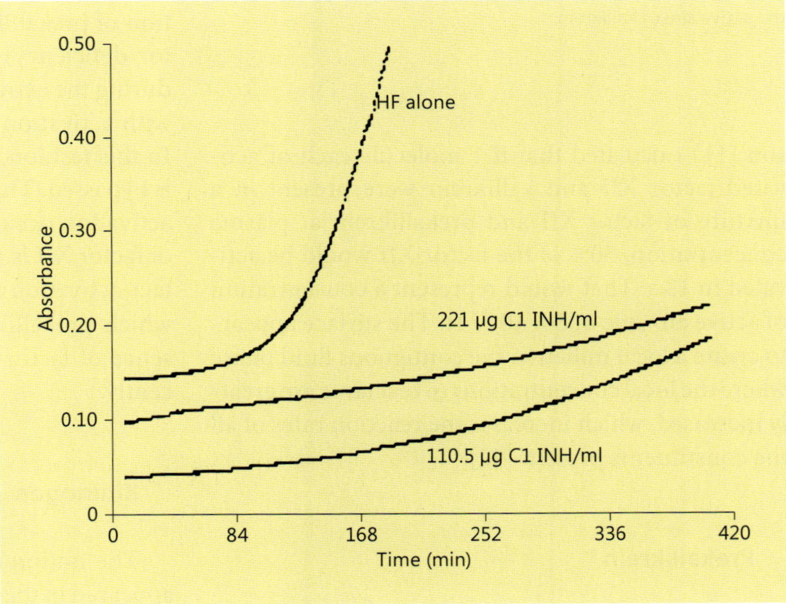

Fig. 2. Autoactivation of factor XII (HF) as assessed by cleavage of Pro-Phe-Arg *p*-nitroanidide to liberate *p*-nitrophenol. OD at 250 nm is shown. A concave upward increasing curve is produced; however, a lag time of close to 1 h (60 min) is seen. Inhibition of the curvature (autoactivation) by a half normal level of C1 INH (110.5 µg/ml) and a normal C1 INH (221 µg/ml) is shown.

count for the result. Stated another way, factor XIIa activates surface-bound factor XII to produce more factor XIIa and then factor XIIf. The reaction rate is very slow initially, then continuously increases since the concentration of enzyme is not constant (as it is in usual enzymes/substrate reactions) but instead is continuously increasing. The source of this putative trace factor XIIa in plasma is unknown and is far below our abilities to measure, although some possibilities are discussed below. Tankersley and Finlay-

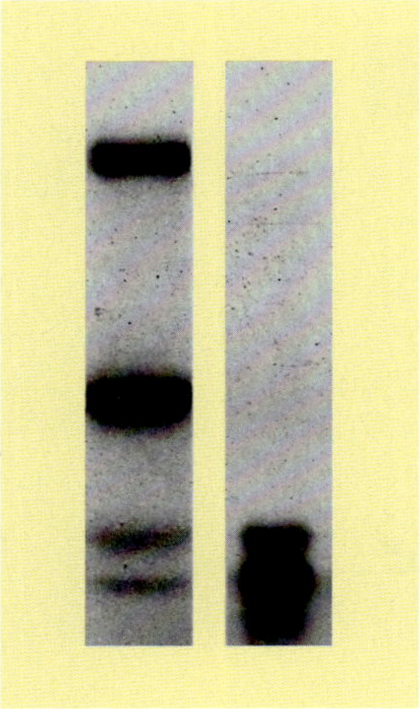

Fig. 3. Prekallikrein conversion of kallikrein. Reduced SDS gel electrophoresis (left gel) followed by radioautography of H^3-prekallikrein (top band, 82–84 kDa) and after conversion of approximately 50% of the prekallikrein to kallikrein by incubation with factor XIIf. The heavy kallikrein chain is at the middle of the gel (50 kDa) and two light chains at 32 and 34 kDa are seen below. Further incubation with D^4-DFP followed by a C^{14} radioautogram (right gel) reveals the incorporation of DFP into the light chains, which have the active site of kallikrein.

son [11] calculated that if 1 molecule each of activated factor XII and kallikrein were present in a mixture of factor XII and prekallikrein at plasma concentration, 50% of the factor XII would be activated in 13 s. That would represent a concentration of active enzyme of 5×10^{-13} M. The surface appears to create a local milieu in the contiguous fluid phase where the local concentrations of reactants are greatly increased, which increases the reaction rates of all the constituents present [12].

Prekallikrein

Prekallikrein was purified from 4 liters of human plasma [13] and was demonstrated to have 2 bands on SDS gel electrophoresis that differ in carbohydrate contact, but are otherwise functionally identical, and are present in everyone. Conversion to kallikrein by factor XIIa or factor XIIf occurred by cleavage within a critical disulfide bound such that a heavy chain of 50 kDa is disulfide linked to light chains of 30 or 33 kDa corresponding to the two molecular forms of the starting material (fig. 3). Plasma that is congenitally deficient in prekallikrein was discovered soon thereafter [14] and, as anticipated, failed to generate bradykinin upon contact activation, but had a curious property regarding blood coagulation. A partial thromboplastin time performed in the standard manner was significantly prolonged; however, as the time of pre-incubation with the surface is increased prior to recalcification, the coagulation defect progressively corrects. By contrast, the abnormal PTT of factor XII-deficient plasma is unaffected. This led to the discovery that once kallikrein is produced there is a prominent feedback activation of factor XII to factor XIIa and factor XIIf [15, 16], which dramatically increases the rate of contact activation. In this fashion, factor XIIa (produced by autoactivation of factor XII) converts prekallikrein to kallikrein, and kallikrein rapidly activates factor XII. Quantitatively, the major factor XII activator is therefore kallikrein. The autocorrection of prekallikrein-deficient plasma (Fletcher factor deficiency) is due to factor XII autoactivation during the extra time of incubation with the surface, with activation of factor XI prior to recalcification. In this fashion, the need for the kallikrein feedback is bypassed. This result also confirms that factor XII activation occurs first and that kallikrein activation of factor XII is not an absolute requirement for contact activation to proceed. An alternative route by which prekallikrein might be activated in the absence of factor XII did not seem possible until recently.

Kininogen

The notion of two kininogens, i.e. HK and LK, appeared in the late 1960s [17]. Their distinction was based not only on size difference, but kinetic analysis also indicated that there are kininogens (the number was actually not clear) that are readily cleaved by plasma kallikrein (with K_m and V_{max} consistent with that) and kininogens that are more readily cleaved by tissue kallikrein [18] than plasma kallikrein. Questions were then raised as to whether the lower-molecular-weight form(s) might be a cleavage product of the higher, or the higher an aggregate of the lower. The discovery of plasma deficient in one or more kininogens was extremely helpful in sorting out the possibilities. Flaujeac-deficient plasma [19] possessed LK, but no HK. It was almost as abnormal as factor XII-deficient plasma, i.e. contact activation did not produce bradykinin and there were marked abnormalities of intrinsic coagulation and fibrinolysis. Williams plasma [20], discovered at the same time, had the same functional abnormalities but no kininogen at all. At that time we collaborated with Dr. Jack Pierce to reconstitute this plasma with HK and LK that he was able to separate by ion exchange chromatography. Each had a multiplicity of molecular forms. However, some were readily cleaved kinetically by plasma kallikrein (HK) and some were relatively resistant to cleavage (LK). When we reconstituted Williams plasma with any fraction designated HK, all abnormalities were corrected, while LK fractions had no effect. Thus, two kininogens seemed more likely than one being derived from the other, and HK appeared to have a special role in all factor XII-dependent processes.

This led to further studies of the structure of HK and its interactions with prekallikrein. A key discovery was that prekallikrein and HK [21] circulate as a biomolecular complex (HK and factor XI also circulate as a bimolecular complex) and, at plasma equilibrium conditions, about 75–80% of prekallikrein circulates bound. Subsequent structural studies of HK demonstrated that cleavage by plasma kallikrein to release bradykinin results in the formation of kinin-free HK in which a heavy chain of 62 kDa is disulfide linked to a light chain of 56 kDa. The light chain is then further degraded to 42 kDa [22]. Employing immunologic methods with antibodies to the heavy and light chains of HK, we could demonstrate that HK and LK shared heavy chains and that the light chains of each are completely different [22]. Once protein sequencing as well as c-DNA and genomic cloning of HK and LK were accomplished [23–25], it became clear that they are derived by alternative splicing which begins 9 amino acids beyond the bradykinin sequence, with separate exons for their respective light chains. As anticipated, the portion of HK responsible for all the HK kinetic effects pertaining to contact activation are functions of the light chain (domains 5 and 6 of HK) [26] and domain 5 binds to initiating surfaces while domain 6 binds either prekallikrein or factor XI (but not both simultaneously; fig. 4). HK is present in sufficient molar excess such that 95% of factor XI circulated bound while, as noted above, for prekallikrein it is 75–80%. LK has no role in contact activation while tissue kallikrein does not bind to HK.

Binding to Endothelial Cells

Although many substances were known to serve as initiating surfaces for contact activation (glass test tubes, glass beads, endotoxin, uric acid and pyrophosphate crystals), the nature of any 'physiologic' surface remained an enigma for quite some time. In 1979, a series of papers appeared indicating that HK binds to endothelial cells and platelets, and that such binding is zinc dependent [27]. This led to a search for binding proteins on the surface of endothelial cells. One approach was to prepare an affinity column with HK, solubilize endothelial cell membranes in zinc-containing buffers, allow interaction with the HK column, elute the binding protein(s), and identify them by amino acid sequencing and/or immunologic methods. The first such protein obtained was gC1qR, a receptor for the globular heads of the first component of complement. This was first isolated and reported by Herwald et al. [28] and Joseph et al. [29]. The latter authors also noted zinc-dependent binding of factor XII to gC1qR [29] and that factor XII and HK could compete for binding, indicating that they interacted with the same or similar binding proteins, and with comparable affinities. Thus, if either protein was bound to the cell, it could be completely displaced by a large molar excess of the other. The cell surface-binding domains of HK included domain 3 (on the C-terminal portion of the heavy chain) and domain 5 of the light chain; yet interaction with gC1qR was dependent on the light chain (i.e. domain 5), and prekallikrein could be brought to the cell surface by virtue of its binding to domain 6. In fact, a separate binding site for prekallikrein has not been found. However, a second cell surface-binding protein for HK was suspected, since a zinc-dependent binding site at domain 3 could be

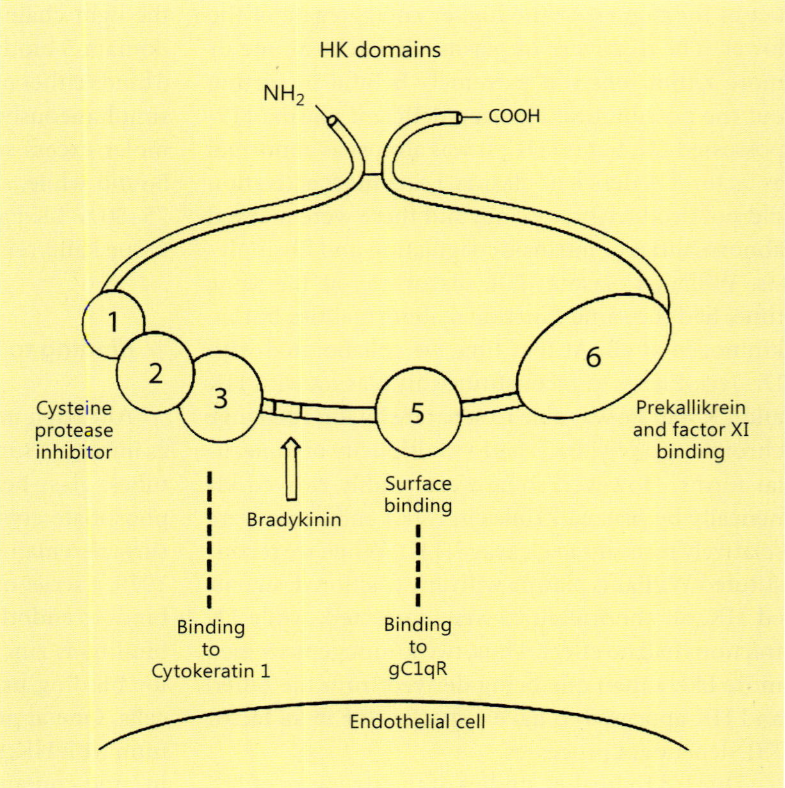

Fig. 4. Domain structure of HK. Domains 1–3 are within the heavy chain while domains 5 and 6 are part of the light chain. Domains 2 and 3 possess cysteine protease inhibitory activity and can, for example, inactivate pain. Domain 5 contains the histidine-rich region which binds to negatively charged surfaces (as does factor XII) and domain 6 has the overlapping binding sites for prekallikrein and factor XII. Binding to endothelial cells is a function of both domains 3 and 5, which bind to cytokeratin 1 and gC1qR, respectively.

defined. This was first identified by Hasan et al. [30] to be cytokeratin 1. Since our HK affinity column led to isolation of gC1qR, we prepared an affinity column to which the heavy chain of HK was bound, and then isolated cytokeratin 1 from a solubilized endothelial cell membrane preparation. Using antisera to gC1qR and cytokeratin 1, we could demonstrate incremental inhibition of HK binding to endothelial cells. Factor XII was shown to interact with both cytokeratin 1 and gC1qR; however, the binding to gC1qR is far easier to demonstrate. These results did not explain how factor XII might competitively remove all bound HK molecules, particularly if some molecules of HK were bound to cytokeratin 1 or alternatively, if HK were simultaneously bound to cytokeratin 1 and gC1qR (i.e. a 'two-hit binding') with heavy chain domain 3 bound to cytokeratin 1 and light chain domain 5 bound to gC1qR.

Soon thereafter, a third binding molecule, namely u-PAR (urokinase plasminogen activator receptor), was found to bind HK. However, the affinity for cleaved, kinin-free HK was found to be much greater than that for native HK. This is consistent with the fact that we could not isolate u-PAR by affinity chromatography using HK as the ligand. However, binding of factor XII to u-PAR could be readily demonstrated. At this point, three plasma entities (HK-heavy chain, HK-light chain and factor XII) could bind to 3 cell membrane proteins (gC1qR, cytokeratin 1 and u-PAR) and the possibility that all 3 cell membrane proteins might exist in a trimolecular complex was considered. It was realized that this was not the case once interactions among these proteins were studied. Joseph et al. [31] demonstrated that cytokeratin 1 could bind to either u-PAR or gC1qR, but u-PAR and gC1qR would not bind to each other. Then, when antisera were used to isolate the proteins from solubilized cell membranes, antibody to gC1qR led to the isolation of a complex of gC1qR and cytokeratin 1 with no u-PAR evident, while an antibody

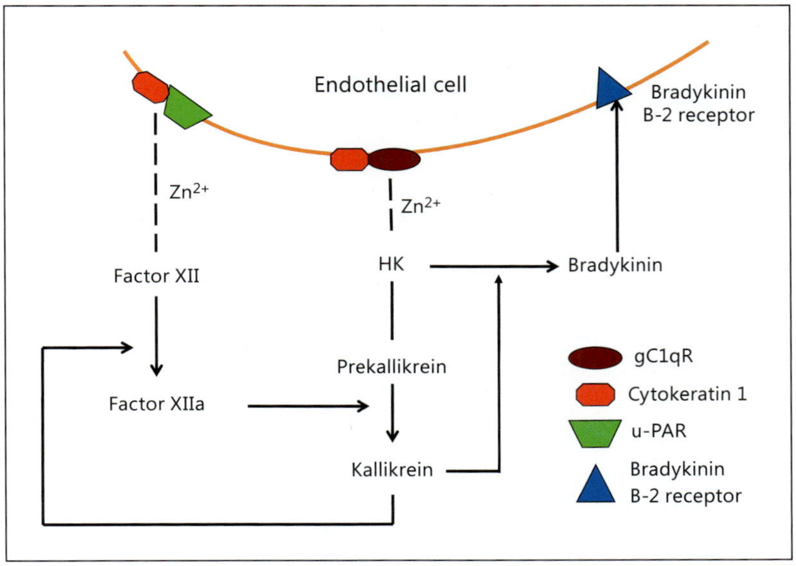

Fig. 5. Activation of the bradykinin-forming cascade along the surface of vascular endothelial cells. Zinc-dependent binding of factor XII and HK is shown and the predominant surface binding moieties are indicated.

to cytokeratin 1 led to isolation of both u-PAR and gC1qR. It became clear that these proteins exist in the cell membrane as two bimolecular complexes: gC1qR-cytokeratin 1 and u-PAR-cytokeratin 1 [31]. The latter complex has been confirmed to be expressed along the surface of endothelial cells by immune electron microscopy [32]. Furthermore, gC1qR is present in excess; thus, molecules of HK or factor XII could be found bound to three different cell surface binding sites, namely free gC1qR or the complexes of gC1qR-cytokeratin 1 or u-PAR-cytokeratin 1. Factor XII and HK would compete equally for gC1qR sites, while factor XII would preferentially bind to u-PAR cytokeratin 1 and HK would preferentially bind to gC1qR-cytokeratin 1. The actual distribution of HK or factor XII binding to each of these cell membrane constituents at plasma concentration of each protein is not known (fig. 5).

Activation along the cell surface might localize bradykinin formation to a particular site; however, perturbation of endothelial cells to initiate activation in the manner of a 'surface' has not yet been demonstrated. It is of interest, however, that binding of factor XII to gC1qR can lead to slow factor XII autoactivation as is seen with more traditional initiating surfaces, while binding to cytokeratin 1 does not, and binding to u-PAR has not been tested. However, incubation of endothelial cells with human plasma leads to conversion of prekallikrein to kallikrein, while plasma deficient in factor XII, prekallikrein or HK does not activate (within 1 h), indicating a requirement for all the constituents needed for contact activation. Yet further incubation for many hours leads to the activation of the factor XII-deficient plasma, but not the plasma deficient in prekallikrein or HK. When this was tested by Schmaier et al. [27] utilizing purified proteins bound to endothelial cells, they too found activation of prekallikrein in the absence of factor XII, presumably by some endothelial cell constituent. They questioned whether factor XII can autoactivate on endothelial cell surfaces at all. However, our own experiments, which were described above, suggest otherwise. Either way, the presence of a factor XII-independent pathway for kallikrein production was clearly evident.

When the endothelial cell factor was isolated by each group, we purified heat shock protein 90 (HSP-90) [33], which activates the complex of prekallikrein-HK in a stoichiometric reaction that requires zinc ion, while Shariat-Madar et al. [34] isolated a prolylcarboxypeptidase that may do the same thing. It is important to note that HSP-90, and probably prolylcarboxypeptidase, are not prekallikrein activa-

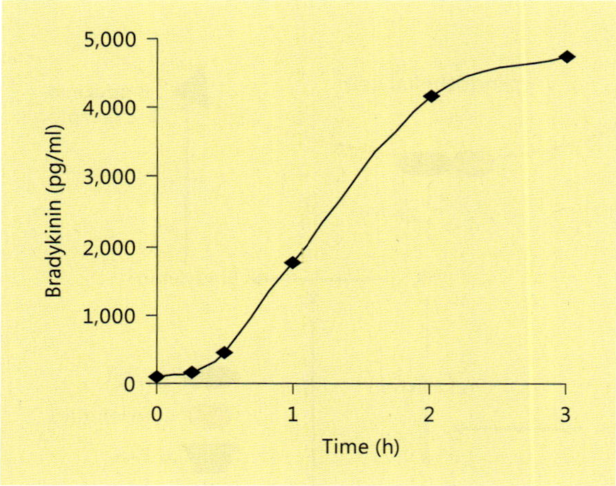

Fig. 6. Prekallikrein is incubated with an equimolar quantity of HK and a time course of bradykinin generation is shown. The HK is completely cleaved at the end of the experiment while prekallikrein reveals no conversion to kallikrein. The reaction is inhibited completely by corn trypsin inhibitor, which has no effect on plasma kallikrein.

tors as factor XIIa or factor XIIf are, and require prekallikrein bound to HK as a complex. These observations do suggest the possibility of initiating the cascade by formation of kallikrein first, followed by activation of factor XII. The kinetics would then switch from stoichiometric, which is relatively inefficient for bradykinin formation, to classical Michaelis Menton kinetics, with a burst of activity that is factor XII-dependent.

A Surprise: Prekallikrein Is an Enzyme

During studies of HSP-90-dependent conversion of prekallikrein, one control was to leave out the HSP-90 and incubate the prekallikrein-HK complex in buffer. No conversion to kallikrein was noted, although cleavage of HK to release bradykinin was repeatedly observed (fig. 6). The formation of bradykinin was directly proportional to the addition of prekallikrein to excess HK with a maximum at a 1:1 molar ratio, indicating stoichiometric cleavage of HK [35]. Corn trypsin inhibitor, a known inhibitor of factor XIIa and factor XIIf, inhibited HK cleavage, yet did not inhibit plasma kallikrein. This allowed the distinction of the active site within prekallikrein from the active site of kallikrein. This reaction, in which prekallikrein cleaves HK, is normally inhibited by C1 INH (which is relevant to a discussion about hereditary angioedema). The addition of HSP-90 in a zinc-containing buffer leads to conversion of prekallikrein to kallikrein. Since HSP-90 has no known proteolytic activity, we speculate that prekallikrein can autoactivate when bound to HK plus HSP-90.

It should be noted that zinc is an absolute requirement for binding of factor XII and HK to the endothelial cell surface, as well as for the interaction of HSP-90 with the prekallikrein HK complex. It is not necessary for prekallikrein cleavage of HK. Contact activation (factor XII plus prekallikrein, plus HK) has no ion requirement but the kinetics of activation are increased by the presence of zinc ion and phosphate ion, both of which are present in plasma.

Concluding Remarks

Key questions that remain regarding the plasma bradykinin-forming pathway all have to do with issues regarding the molecular mechanisms by which the cascade is activated in vivo, and in bradykinin-mediated diseases in particular. Can small amounts of factor XIIa be produced in vivo by virtue of its binding to endothelial cells? Do we always have trace amounts of kallikrein present because the prekallikrein-HK complex can autoactivate in a phosphate-containing milieu even in the presence of C1 INH? Perhaps endothelial cell activation can release HSP-90 to increase the local conversion of prekallikrein to kallikrein such that kallikrein activation of factor XII becomes kinetically favored. Although factor XII autoactivation is a relatively slow process, a mixture of factor XII and prekallikrein activates rapidly even in the absence of an initiating surface. Is this due to trace amounts of each type of active enzyme present? Since this can occur in the absence of HK [16], one cannot invoke the enzymatic site within prekallikrein as a possible initiator, and a firm complex between factor XII and prekallikrein has never been demonstrated. These issues are of theoretical interest and the answers may be critical to understanding bradykinin-mediated diseases such as hereditary angioedema.

References

1 Kaplan AP, Joseph K, Silverberg M: Pathways for bradykinin formation and inflammatory disease. J Allergy Clin Immunol 2002;109:195–209.

2 Ratnoff O, Colopy J: A familial hemorrhagic trait associated with a deficiency of a clot-promoting fraction of plasma. J Clin Invest 1955;34:602–612.

3 Webster M: Human plasma kallikrein, its activation and pathological role. Fed Proc 1968;27:84–89

4 Kaplan AP, Austen KF: A pre-albumin activator of prekallikrein. J Immunol 1970;105:802–811.

5 Cochrane C, Wuepper K: The first component of the kinin-forming system in human and rabbit plasma: its relationship to clotting factor XII (Hageman factor). J Exp Med 1971;134:986–1004.

6 Kaplan AP, Austen KF: A prealbumin activator of prekallikrein. 2. Derivation of activators of prekallikrein from active Hageman factor by digestion with plasmin. J Exp Med 1971;133:696–712.

7 Revak S, Cochrane C, Bouma B, et al: Surface and fluid phase activities of two forms of activated Hageman factor produced during contact activation of plasma. J Exp Med 1978;147:719–729.

8 Dunn JT, Kaplan AP: Formation and structure of human Hageman factor fragments. J Clin Invest 1982;70:627–631.

9 Griffin JH: Role of surface in surface-dependent activation of Hageman factor (blood coagulation factor XII). Proc Natl Acad Sci USA 1978;75:1998–2002.

10 Silverberg M, Dunn J, Garen L, et al: Autoactivation of human Hageman factor: demonstration utilizing a synthetic substrate. J Biol Chem 1980;255:7281–7286.

11 Tankersley DL, Finlayson JS: Kinetics of activation and autoactivation of human factor XII. Biochemistry 1984;23:273–279.

12 Griffin JH, Cochrane CG: Mechanisms for the involvement of high molecular weight kininogen in surface-dependent reactions of Hageman factor. Proc Natl Acad Sci USA 1976;73:2554–2558.

13 Mandle RJ, Kaplan A: Hageman factor substrates: human plasma prekallikrein: mechanism of activation by Hageman factor and participation in Hageman factor-dependent fibrinolysis. J Biol Chem 1977;252:6097–6104.

14 Wuepper KD: Prekallikrein deficiency in man. J Exp Med 1973;138:1345–1355.

15 Cochrane CG, Revak SD, Wuepper KD: Activation of Hageman factor in solid and fluid phases: a critical role of kallikrein. J Exp Med 1973;138:1564–1583.

16 Meier H, Pierce J, Colman R, et al: Activation and function of human Hageman factor: the role of high molecular weight kininogen and prekallikrein. J Clin Invest 1977;60:18–31.

17 Jacobson S, Kritz M: Some data on two purified kininogens from human plasma. Br J Pharmacol 1967;29:25–36.

18 Pierce J: Structural features of plasma kinins and kininogens. Fed Proc 1968;27:52–57.

19 Wuepper KD, Miller DR, Lacombe MJ: Flaujeac trait: deficiency of human plasma kininogen. J Clin Invest 1975;56:1663–1672.

20 Colman RW, Bagdasarian A, Talamo RC, et al: Williams trait: human kininogen deficiency with diminished levels of plasminogen proactivator and prekallikrein associated with abnormalities of the Hageman factor-dependent pathways. J Clin Invest 1975;56:1650–1662.

21 Mandle R, Colman R, Kaplan A: Identification of prekallikrein and high-molecular-weight kininogen as a complex in human plasma. Proc Natl Acad Sci USA 1976;73:4179–4183.

22 Thompson RE, Mandle R Jr, Kaplan AP: Characterization of human high molecular weight kininogen: procoagulant activity associated with the light chain of kinin-free high molecular weight kininogen. J Exp Med 1978;147:488–499.

23 Kitamura N, Kitagawa H, Fukushima D, et al: Structural organization of the human kininogen gene and a model for its evolution. J Biol Chem 1985;260:8610–8617.

24 Kellermann J, Lottspeich F, Henschen A, et al: Completion of the primary structure of human high-molecular-mass kininogen: the amino acid sequence of the entire heavy chain and evidence for its evolution by gene triplication. Eur J Biochem 1986;154:471–478.

25 Takagaki Y, Kitamura N, Nakanishi S: Cloning and sequence analysis of cDNAs for human high molecular weight and low molecular weight prekininogens: primary structures of two human prekininogens. J Biol Chem 1985;260:8601–8609.

26 Thompson RE, Mandle R Jr, Kaplan AP: Studies of binding of prekallikrein and factor XI to high molecular weight kininogen and its light chain. Proc Natl Acad Sci USA 1979;76:4862–4866.

27 Schmaier AH, Kuo A, Lundberg D, et al: The expression of high molecular weight kininogen on human umbilical vein endothelial cells. J Biol Chem 1988;263:16327–16333.

28 Herwald H, Dedio J, Kellner R, et al: Isolation and characterization of the kininogen-binding protein p33 from endothelial cells: identity with the gC1q receptor. J Biol Chem 1996;271:13040–13047.

29 Joseph K, Ghebrehiwet B, Peerschke EI, et al: Identification of the zinc-dependent endothelial cell binding protein for high molecular weight kininogen and factor XII: identity with the receptor that binds to the globular 'heads' of C1q (gC1q-R). Proc Natl Acad Sci USA 1996;93:8552–8557.

30 Hasan AA, Zisman T, Schmaier AH: Identification of cytokeratin 1 as a binding protein and presentation receptor for kininogens on endothelial cells. Proc Natl Acad Sci USA 1998;95:3615–3620.

31 Joseph K, Tholanikunnel B, Ghebrehiwet B, et al: Interaction of high molecular weight kininogen biding proteins on endothelial cells. Thromb Haemost 2004;91:61–70.

32 Mahdi F, Shariat-Madar Z, Todd RF 3rd, et al: Expression and colocalization of cytokeratin 1 and urokinase plasminogen activator receptor on endothelial cells. Blood 2001;97:2342–2350.

33 Joseph K, Tholanikunnel B, Kaplan A: Heat shock protein 90 catalyzes activation of the prekallikrein-kininogen complex in the absence of factor XII. Proc Natl Acad Sci USA 2002;99:896–900.

34 Shariat-Madar Z, Mahdi F, Schmaier A: Identification and characterization of prolylcarboxypeptidase as an endothelial cell prekallikrein activator. J Biol Chem 2002;277:17962–17969.

35 Joseph K, Tholanikunnel B, Kaplan A: Factor XII-independent cleavage of high molecular weight kininogen by prekallikrein and inhibition by C1 inhibitor. J Allergy Clin Immunol 2009;124:143–149.

Dr. Allen P. Kaplan
Department of Medicine
Medical University of South Carolina
171 Ashley Avenue
Charleston, SC 29425–2220 (USA)
E-Mail kaplana@musc.edu

3

Bergmann K-C, Ring J (eds): History of Allergy. Chem Immunol Allergy. Basel, Karger, 2014, vol 100, pp 214–226
DOI: 10.1159/000358740

Histamine Receptors and Antihistamines: From Discovery to Clinical Applications

Mauro Cataldi[a] · Francesco Borriello[b] · Francescopaolo Granata[b] · Lucio Annunziato[a] · Gianni Marone[b]

[a]Department of Neuroscience, Reproductive and Odontostomatologic Sciences, and [b]Department of Translational Medical Sciences and Center for Basic and Clinical Immunology Research (CISI), School of Medicine, University of Naples Federico II, Naples, Italy

Abstract

The synthesis and the identification of histamine marked a milestone in both pharmacological and immunological research. Since Sir Henry Dale and Patrick Laidlaw described some of its physiological effects in vivo in 1910, histamine has been shown to play a key role in the control of gastric acid secretion and in allergic disorders. Using selective agonists and antagonists, as well as molecular biology tools, four histamine receptors (H_1R, H_2R, H_3R and H_4R) have been identified. The Nobel Prize in Physiology and Medicine was awarded to Daniel Bovet in 1957 for the discovery of antihistamines (anti-H_1R) and to Sir James Black in 1988 for the identification of anti-H_2R antagonists. Anti-H_1R and anti-H_2R histamine receptor antagonists have revolutionized the treatment of certain allergic disorders and gastric acid-related conditions, respectively. More recently, anti-H_3R antagonists have entered early-phase clinical trials for possible application in obesity and a variety of neurologic disorders. The preferential expression of H_4R by several immune cells and its involvement in the development of allergic inflammation provide the rationale for the use of anti-H_4R antagonists in allergic and in other immune-related disorders.

The discovery and characterization of histamine, its receptors and blocking drugs is one of the most fascinating chapters of the history of medicine. Pharmacologists, medicinal chemists, molecular biologists and clinical immunologists all contributed to the synthesis and clinical application of some of the most successful and widely used drugs ever. Outstanding scientists worked in this field and two Nobel Prizes have been awarded for the discovery of histamine H_1 (Daniel Bovet in 1957) and H_2 (Sir James Black in 1988) receptor (H_1R and H_2R) antagonists. Although histamine was synthesized and characterized at the beginning of the last century, new knowledge of this mediator and its pharmacological properties continue to accumulate day by day. In the present chapter, we will review this extraordinary story with a special emphasis on its implications in allergy and clinical immunology.

The Discovery of Histamine

In 1907, Windaus and Vogt [1] chemically synthesized and, in 1910, Ackermann [2] isolated histamine as a metabolite of bacterial histidine fermentation. Henry Dale, a young pharmacologist at Sir Wellcome's research laboratories in London, was working on ergot fungi extracts that were used for the treatment of postpartum bleeding. Dale's mission was to identify the active ingredient(s) responsible for this activity [3]. Dale had the intuition that a novel substance could have a much higher contractant activity on the uterus than all those identified so far. Watching a demonstration of the new in vitro assay for uterus contraction developed by Kehrer, a German obstetrician, he realized that the so-called 'ergotinum dialysatum' of Wernich was much more potent than ergot itself. With the help of the chemist George Barger, Dale isolated a new base from ergotinum dialysatum that could replicate the effect of the dialysatum on a cat uterus [4, 5].

In 1910, Dale and Laidlaw reported the first physiological characterization of β-imidazolyl ethylamine, the chemical formula of histamine [6]. This work remains a milestone in pharmacology for its exhaustive experimental approach and for the tremendous impact it had on future research. They demonstrated that this molecule caused vasodilation, the contraction of smooth muscles in the airways, uterus and the intestine, stimulated heart rate and contractility, and induced a shock-like syndrome when injected into animals.

During the following decade, the effects of histamine administration were intensively investigated. In 1920, Popielski [7] reported that histamine also affects the activity of the stomach by potently stimulating hydrochloric acid secretion in the dog. In 1924, Lewis and Grant [8] described the classic 'triple response' elicited by the subcutaneous injection of histamine consisting of a red spot due to vasodilatation, a wheal which was the consequence of increased permeability and flare due to an axon reflex.

During the first 20 years after the synthesis of histamine, it was unclear whether this mediator could have any physiological role. In 1927, C.H. Best et al. [9] isolated crystalline histamine from liver and lungs, providing formal evidence that histamine is physiologically present in the body. Later, W. Feldberg and coworkers [10–12] provided compelling evidence that histamine is a mediator of experimental anaphylaxis. In 1952, J.F. Riley and G.B. West [13, 14] demonstrated that mast cells are the predominant cellular source of histamine. Subsequently, basophil leukocytes were identified as the main source of histamine among blood cells [15].

The Synthesis of the First Antihistamines and the Identification of H_1R

In 1937, while working in the laboratory of Ernest Fourneau at the Institut Pasteur in Paris, Daniel Bovet started a research program aiming to identify new drugs that could block the actions of histamine. Bovet tested several compounds that were part of the large collection of molecules previously synthesized by Fourneau [16]. He described two benzodioxanes, compound 883 F and compound 933 F, which were slightly effective in preventing histamine shock in guinea pig [17–19]. Based on these results, twenty congeners of these compounds were synthesized leading, in 1937, to the identification of the first potent histamine antagonists, thymoxyethyldiethylamine (929 F) [20] and N,N'-diethyl-N'-phenyl-N'-ethylethylenediamine (1571 F) [21]. Unfortunately, these compounds proved to be too toxic for clinical development. More effective and better-tolerated compounds were soon developed by chemical modification of their structure. Bernard Halpern [22] first used N'-dimethylethylenediamine clinically, which matched the requirements of safety and efficacy for clinical development in humans. It has been marketed since 1942 by Rhone-Poulenc under the brand name of Antergan. This compound was soon replaced by its derivative, mepyramine, which was marketed under the brand name of Neo-Antergan and for years represented the gold standard of histamine H_1R antagonists.

The Identification of H_2R and the Synthesis of the First H_2 Blockers

In the late 1940s, it became clear that some of the actions of histamine were refractory to inhibition by classical antihistamines. In particular, mepyramine did not block the effects of histamine on heart rate and on gastric hydrochloric acid secretion [23, 24]. In 1948, Folkow et al. [25] first suggested that two different classes of histamine receptors should exist because the antihistamine blocker Benadryl could block the vasodilator effect of low, but not of high concentrations of histamine. A limitation of those studies was the absence of a mathematical model to analyze the interactions between increasing concentrations of agonists (e.g. histamine) and antagonists (e.g. antihistamines). In 1947, Hans Schild [26] described a mathematical method for the evaluation of drug antagonism (the pA2 value). In particular, he evaluated the effects of two antihistamines (Neo-Antergan and Benadryl) on histamine-induced ileum contraction. By applying the pA2 method, Ash and Schild [27] showed that H_1R antagonized by meperidine and diphenhydramine mediate the effects of histamine on intestinal and uterine tone. Whilst not specifically stated in their 1966 paper, the results implied that other receptor(s) could be responsible for the histamine effects insensitive to classical antihistamines.

The discovery of histamine H_2R is linked to the name of the Nobel Laureate Sir James Black [28]. He hypothesized that anti-H_2 drugs should be more similar to histamine because anti-H_1 compounds were significantly different to histamine. Therefore, the idea behind the project was to modify the molecule of histamine. This approach led to the identification of burimamide that blocked histamine effects on both the beating guinea pig atrium and the rat gastric acid secretion [29]. These findings, communicated in a classical paper in *Nature* in 1972 [29], provided the first pharmacological demonstration of H_2R distinct from H_1R. After burimamide, several other H_2R antagonists were developed that revolutionized the treatment of peptic ulcer [28, 30, 31].

Evidence that histamine acting through H_2R induces both a G_s-dependent increase in intracellular cAMP concentrations and a G_q-dependent increase in $[Ca^{2+}]_i$ was obtained in different tissue and cell preparations, including gastric mucosal cells, vascular smooth muscle cells, brain slices and adipocytes [32]. In 1973, Lichtenstein and Gillespie [33] reported that H_2R are functionally present on human basophils. Subsequently, H_2R were found on rodent mast cells [34], human eosinophils [35, 36] and human neutrophils [37].

Histamine in the Brain

When Antergan entered clinical use, it was reported that it induced marked sedation. It soon became clear that this characteristic was typical of the entire class of the first generation of anti-H_1 drugs. In 1943, Kwiatkowski found small amounts of histamine in different brain regions. With the development of antibodies directed against histidine decarboxylase, different groups mapped histaminergic neurons and their projections in the brain [38–41]. Histaminergic neurons are localized in the tuberomammillary nucleus of the hypothalamus, project to all major areas of the brain, and are involved in several functions including the regulation of sleep/wakefulness, feeding and memory processes. The presence of histaminergic neurons and H_1R in the brain underlies the sedative effects of the classical H_1 antagonists. There are also H_2R in the brain, but their functions are more limited compared to H_1R and H_3R [42].

In 1983, Jean-Charles Schwartz and colleagues [43] reported that histamine does inhibit its own release in the isolated rat brain cortex. This histamine inhibitory activity was mimicked with an higher potency by N^α- and N^α,N^α-methylhistamine, two compounds weakly effective on H_1R and H_2R; in addition, H_1R or H_2R agonists, as well as H_1R antagonists, were ineffective [43]. Conversely, several H_2 blockers, like burimamide, and the H_2R partial agonist impromidine, antagonized histamine release autoinhibition [43]. These effects were observed at concentrations much higher than those required to block H_2R. Importantly, Schild plot analysis demonstrated that these effects could not be explained as an action on H_2R [43]. Based on these findings it was proposed that an H_3R could exist in the brain. The same group reported the synthesis of selective ligands for H_3R, including the agonist (R)-α-methylhistamine and the antagonist thioperamide [44]. Using selective H_3R agonists and antagonists it was shown that signal transduction by the H_3R is mediated by pertussis toxin-sensitive G_i/G_o proteins leading to a decrease in intracellular cAMP concentrations [45, 46] and to a decrease in extracellular Ca^{2+} influx in neurons [47].

The group of Manfred Göthert showed that H_3R also inhibit the release of other neurotransmitters, including noradrenaline and serotonin [48–52]. Thus, histamine H_3R modulate neurotransmitter release acting as presynaptic autoreceptors or heteroreceptors.

There is compelling evidence that H_3R could be involved in several neurological diseases like sleep-wake disorders, Alzheimer's disease and cognitive disorders, as well as in obesity [53]. Several H_3R agonists and inverse agonists/antagonists have been synthesized and some of these compounds are now being tested for therapeutic use in neurological disorders and obesity [53, 54].

Cloning of H_1R, H_2R and H_3R, and Generation of Histamine Receptor Knockout Mice

Molecular biology entered the field of histamine pharmacology in the 1990s with the cloning of histamine receptors and the generation of histamine receptor knockout mice. In 1991, Gantz et al. [55] cloned the canine H_2R gene. Molecular biologists in different laboratories were rapidly successful in cloning the H_2R gene from other species, including human [56], rat [57] and guinea pig [58]. Once the H_2R cDNAs were cloned, detailed studies on the tissue distribution of these receptors became possible, confirming and extending previous functional data showing that these receptors are highly expressed in a variety of tissues and immune cells [59–61].

Cloned H_2R were heterologously expressed for signal transduction and structure-activity studies. The group of Henk Timmerman [62] demonstrated that recombinant rat H_2R heterologously expressed in CHO cells have a spontaneous activity that can be inhibited by H_2 antagonists. This observation was made when the allosteric theory of receptor activity was rapidly becoming popular after the seminal work on mutant adrenergic receptors by Robert Lefkowitz et al. [63]. Following the publication of Timmerman's paper, H_2 antagonists became the paradigmatic example of inverse agonists in pharmacology. It should be noted that, similar to the Schild plot analysis, another fundamental concept in pharmacology found a relevant application in histamine research.

In 2000, Kobayashi et al. [64] generated H_2R knockout mice. Homozygous mutant mice were phenotypically normal and, unexpectedly, showed normal basal gastric pH. A marked hypertrophy of gastric mucosa and high circulating levels of gastrin were found in these mice, suggesting that when the histamine-dependent major regulatory system of hydrochloric acid secretion is genetically destroyed, compensatory mechanisms are activated to maintain normal gastric secretion. Interestingly, these mice showed a dysregulated T lymphocyte activity. H_2R knockout mice display upregulation of both Th1 and Th2 cytokines and decreased OVA-specific IgE production compared with wild-type and H_1R knockout mice [65].

H_2R gene expression increased in human interleukin (IL)-4+ T cells upon bee venom exposure of non-allergic beekeepers [66] and in basophils during the first hours of ultra-rush venom immunotherapy [67]. H_2R upregulation was responsible for the inhibition of IL-4 and the stimulation of IL-10 secretion by IL-4+ T cells [66] as well as the inhibition of histamine release and cytokine secretion from basophils [33, 67]. In addition, activation of H_2R inhibits histamine release from rodent mast cells [34], neutrophil activation [37], eosinophil chemotaxis [35] and degranulation [36], γδ T cell-mediated cytotoxicity [68], and reduces the inflammatory response of dendritic cells (DCs) to microbial ligands [69, 70].

Owing to the inhibitory effect exerted on several immune cells, H_2R may play a role in the development of allergy and possibly other immune-mediated disorders. Interestingly, the use of histamine dihydrochloride (a salt of histamine) in conjunction with low-dose IL-2 has been proposed as a relapse-preventive immunotherapy for patients with acute myeloid leukemia [71, 72]. It is thought that myeloid cell-derived reactive oxygen species inhibit natural killer (NK) cell-mediated killing of human acute myeloid leukemia blasts. Histamine via H_2R protects NK cells from myeloid cell-dependent inactivation, probably through inhibition of reactive oxygen species production [73].

In 1991, Yamashita et al. [74] cloned the H_1R gene. Thanks to H_1R cDNA cloning, the tissue distribution of these receptors could be studied by Northern blot analysis. The expression of H_1R was found to be high in the lung and small intestine, moderate in the adrenal medulla and uterus, and low in the cerebral cortex and spleen [74]. The H_1R was later cloned in other species including mouse [75], rat [76] and human [77]. Heterologously expressed H_1R triggered the activation of phospholipase C, the accumulation of IP_3 and an increase in $[Ca^{2+}]_i$ via G_q proteins [78, 79].

Studies on recombinant H_1R also helped to clarify the apparent paradox of the increase in intracellular cAMP concentration blocked by H_1 blockers that had been reported since the end of the 1970s in different native preparations [80, 81]. Working on heterologously expressed human H_1R in CHO cells, Maruko et al. [82] demonstrated that adenylate cyclase is indirectly activated upon H_1R activation via $G_{\beta\gamma}$ subunits released from G_q proteins.

In 1996, Inoue et al. [75] produced knockout mice for the H_1R. The study of these animals confirmed and extended previous knowledge on the physiological roles of H_1-mediated histamine effects. H_1R knockout mice have an impairment in locomotor activity and exploratory behavior, and a decrease in aggression and anxiety [83]. The study of the behavioral effect of H_1R raised great interest because of its possible implications in the pharmacological activity of antipsychotic drugs, a class of compounds also acting on H_1R [84]. In addition, studies performed on these knockout mice provided evidence that histamine via H_1R could be involved in the neurotensin anorexic effect [85]. H_1R knockout mice also showed a significant impairment in nociception and an enhancement in the sensitivity to the analgesic effect of morphine, confirming the role of these receptors in pain perception [83, 86, 87].

H_1R knockout mice showed lower percentages of IFN-γ-producing T cells and produced more OVA-specific IgG1 and IgE compared with wild-type mice [65]. Interestingly, although allergen-stimulated T cells from H_1R knockout mice exhibited an enhanced production of Th2 cytokines, allergen-challenged H_1R knockout mice showed reduced lung Th2 cytokines associated with lower airway inflammation, goblet cell metaplasia and airway hyperresponsiveness. These conflicting results can be explained, at least in part, considering that histamine promotes T cell chemotaxis. Thus, defective T cell trafficking could be responsible for reduced lung inflammation in allergen-challenged H_1R knockout mice [88].

The effects of histamine acting via H_1R on the immune system extend well beyond those described for T cells. Human lung macrophages (HLM), monocyte-derived macrophages (MDM) and monocyte-derived DCs express higher levels of H_1R compared with precursor monocytes. Histamine induces the release of pro-inflammatory mediators (β-glucuronidase, IL-8 and IL-6) by MDM and HLM through the activation of H_1R [89–91].

Interestingly, gene variability of the H_1R can influence the risk of developing specific disorders. *Bphs*, one of the first non-major histocompatibility complex-linked genes associated with the susceptibility of murine models to autoimmune diseases, was identified with the H_1R [92]. In addition, polymorphisms of the H_1R were associated with the risk of developing Parkinson's disease [93].

Despite the intense efforts of several laboratories, H_3R cloning proved a formidable task. It was not until 1999 that Lovenberg et al. [94] attained this important result by a reverse approach. They were working at R.W. Johnson Pharmaceutical Research Institute on the identification of orphan GPCR. Among the almost 30 different orphan receptors they identified GPCR97, which was highly expressed in the brain and showed a significant structural homology with several members of the biogenic amine receptor superfamily. When heterologously expressed in different cell lines this receptor conferred a high responsiveness to the inhibitory action of histamine on adenylate cyclase activity, thus behaving as a new histamine receptor: it was dubbed the H_3R [94, 95]. Recombinant H_3R showed a pharmacological profile indistinguishable from H_3R [94]. Importantly, as observed for H_2R, H_3R also showed a relevant constitutive activity in heterologous expression systems [96, 97]. Evidence that these receptors are also constitutively activated in native preparations was reported, suggesting that they could also regulate neurotransmitter release in the absence of histamine [98].

Different isoforms of the H_3R were identified both in humans [99] and in rodents [95, 100]. Evidence was reported for isoform-specific differences in signal transduction as some isoforms, but not all, activated the MAPK cascade and caused arachidonic acid release [95, 100]. Once the H_3 gene was cloned, the tissue distribution of this receptor was explored by RT-PCR and in situ hybridization. These studies confirmed its preferential localization in the brain with minor expression in other tissues, including stomach, intestine, skin and thymus [100, 101].

In 2002, Toyota et al. [102] reported the generation of H_3R knockout mice. Unexpectedly, these mice showed a decrease in locomotor activity, wheel-running behavior and body temperature, which was interpreted as the consequence of compensatory mechanisms, such as H_1R downregulation, triggered by the increased availability of histamine in the synapse. Similarly, a mild obesity [103] and a reduction in anxiety [104] were reported in these mice.

Identification and Cloning of H_4R

At the end of 2000, both Oda et al. [105] and Nakamura et al. [106] reported the cloning of a new histamine receptor that they designated H_4R. This result was attained by screening the human genome database for sequences similar to that of H_3R. The newly cloned receptor showed a very limited homology with all the known histamine receptors (approximately 31% with H_3R and only 23% and 22% with H_1R and H_2R, respectively). The existence of similar receptors was confirmed in other animal species, including mouse, rat, monkey, pig and guinea pig [107–109]. With the discovery of the H_4R gene, the pharmacology of these receptors could be accurately defined in heterologous expression systems. It was established that whereas the pharmacological profile of H_4R is different from that of H_1R and H_2R, some overlap does exist with H_3R. Specifically, thioperamide acts as an inverse agonist both on H_3R and on H_4R and (R)-α-methylhistamine, immepip and imetit activate both these classes of receptors [110]. Conversely, clobenpropit and burimamide block H_3R and activate H_4R [111]. These initial pharmacological data showed that no available drug could distinguish between H_4R and H_3R, and prompted the development of selective H_4R-acting drugs. To this aim, Jablonowski et al. [110], working at the Johnson & Johnson pharmaceutical research laboratories, started a high-throughput screening program to identify in the company compound collection new molecules acting on recombinant H_4R. This effort led to the identification of several indolylpiperazine whose SAR analysis provided useful information needed for the synthesis of the first selective H_4R blocker, compound JNJ 7777120 [110, 112].

H_4R is preferentially expressed on immune cells, namely eosinophils [113, 114], basophils [115], mast cells [112, 116, 117], NK cells, DCs, monocytes [118] and T cells [68, 119–122]. The activation of this receptor is emerging as an important mechanism for the modulation of chemotaxis as well as several other functions of these cells [59].

Hofstra et al. [117] demonstrated that H_4R modulates mast cell chemotaxis by a $G_{i/o}$-dependent PTX-sensitive mechanism. Mast cells from wild-type and H_3R-deleted mice migrated in response to histamine, while mast cells from the H_4R-deleted mice did not. Conversely, no role for H_4R could be demonstrated in IgE-dependent mast cell degranulation [117]. Compound JNJ 7777120 prevented histamine-induced $[Ca^{2+}]_i$ increase as well as mast cell chemotaxis and submucosal mast cell accumulation in the trachea of mice after histamine inhalation [112]. By using siRNAs directed against H_4R, Godot et al. [116] showed that histamine acting through H_4R enhanced CXCL12-induced chemotaxis of mast cell precursors, but not mature mast cells. A role for H_4R was also demonstrated in the modulation of eosinophil chemotaxis [113, 114]. Recently, it was shown in a mouse model of allergic rhinitis that histamine released from mast cells recruits H_4R-expressing basophils to the nasal cavity, an event that

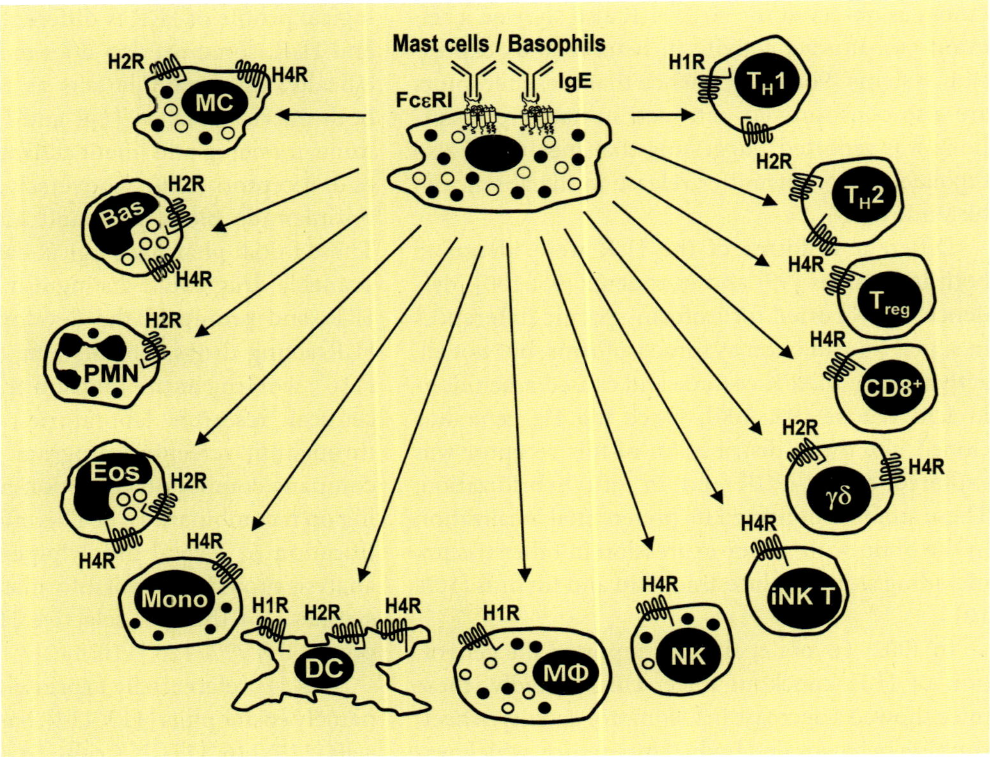

Fig. 1. Schematic representation of the expression of histamine receptors in inflammatory and immune cells. Histamine, contained in human mast cells (MC; ~3 pg/cell) and basophils (Bas; ~1 pg/cell), can be released by immunologic and non-immunologic stimuli. Histamine via H_4R induces the chemotaxis of several immune cells, namely mast cell precursors, basophils, eosinophils (Eos), monocytes (Mono), DCs, IL-2-activated NK cells, γδ T cells and regulatory T cells (Treg). Moreover, H_4R activation induces IL-16 and IL-31 secretion by CD8 T cells and Th2 lymphocytes, respectively, and enhances cytokine secretion from invariant NK T (iNKT) cells. H_2R exerts mainly an inhibitory effect on immune cells. H_2R activation inhibits human basophil degranulation and cytokine secretion, histamine release from rodent mast cells, neutrophil activation, eosinophil chemotaxis and degranulation, γδ T cell-mediated cytotoxicity, and reduces the pro-inflammatory response of DCs to microbial ligands. H_2R negatively regulates both Th1 and Th2 lymphocytes. In addition, H_2R gene expression increases in human IL-4+ T cells upon bee venom exposure in non-allergic beekeepers and its activation inhibits IL-4 and stimulates IL-10 secretion. Histamine enhances Th1 responses by triggering the H_1R. HLM, MDM and monocyte-derived DCs express higher levels of H_1R compared with precursor monocytes. Histamine induces the release of pro-inflammatory mediators (β-glucuronidase, IL-8 and IL-6) by HLM and MDM through the activation of H_1R.

was required for the development of early- or late-phase nasal responses following allergen challenge [115].

A role in the control of lymphocyte activity was also proposed based on the evidence that H_4R blockers prevent histamine-induced IL-16 release by human CD8 T cells [119]. This could be of particular importance because IL-16 induces the chemotaxis of several immune cells (CD4 T lymphocytes, eosinophils and DCs) [123–125] and has been found in the bronchoalveolar fluid of allergen- or histamine-challenged asthmatics [126–128]. In addition, this cytokine is highly expressed by eosinophils and mast cells [129] in the bronchial mucosa of atopic asthmatics [130]. H_4R is also expressed by CD4 T cells and intratracheal administration of an H_4R agonist-mitigated airway inflammation in a murine model of allergic asthma. This anti-inflammatory effect was associated with an increase in IL-10 and IFN-γ, and a decrease in IL-13 in the bronchoalveolar lavage fluid as well as the recruitment of FoxP3+ T cells. In vitro data confirmed that, among T lymphocytes, a specific H_4R agonist preferentially induces the chemotaxis of CD4+CD25+FoxP3+ cells [122].

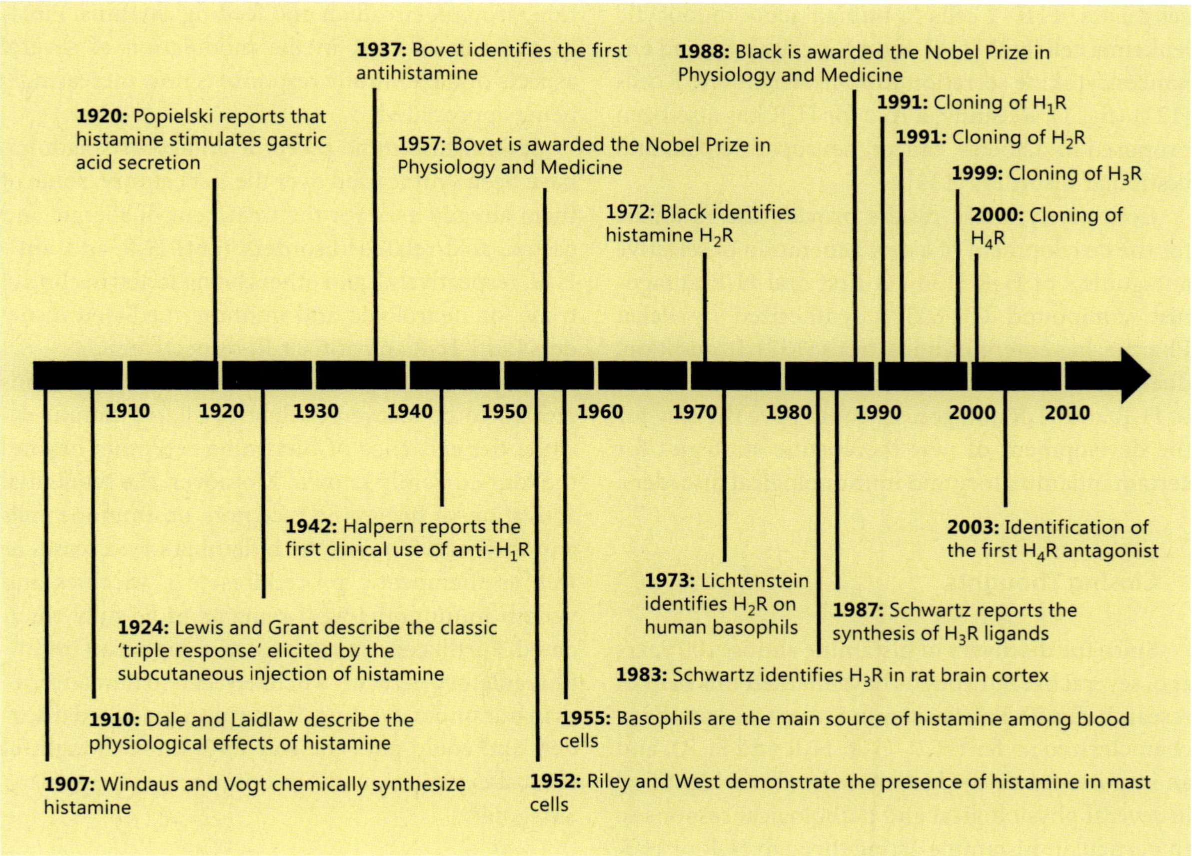

Fig. 2. A timeline of the major breakthroughs in histamine research.

Although the latter study suggests that H_4 receptor activation protects from allergic airway inflammation, it should be noted that H_4R agonists were administered intratracheally and before antigen challenge. In addition, possible discrepancies between human and mouse cells should be taken into account. For example, conversely to what has been observed in mice, H_4R is highly expressed by Th2 cells or CD4 T cells stimulated with IL-4. Moreover, polyclonally activated peripheral blood mononuclear cells or Th2 cells stimulated with H_4R agonists upregulated IL-31 mRNA, a cytokine involved in skin allergic inflammation and the induction of pruritus. Specific H_4 agonists have been shown to induce itch, whereas pretreatment with H_4R antagonists reduced the itch response to either H_4 agonists or histamine. Interestingly, the effects of H_4R antagonists on pruritus are enhanced by the concurrent blockade of H_1R [131–133]. Thus, H_4R might contribute to skin allergic inflammation by activating Th2 cells and inducing pruritus via IL-31 [120].

In summary, although the balance between pro-inflammatory and anti-inflammatory effects of H_4R needs to be fully elucidated and requires further investigation, these findings suggest that H_4R could play a role in allergic inflammation and could, therefore, be a potential target for drug intervention.

H_4R has also been involved in the pathogenesis of non-allergic disorders. H_4R blockade decreased neutrophil accumulation in experimental models of peritonitis [112] and pleurisy [134]. Moreover, H_4R activation induces chemotaxis of IL-2-activated NK cells, DCs, THP-1 cells (a human acute monocytic leukemia cell line) [118] and γδ T cells [68], and enhances cytokine secretion from invariant NK T cells [121] (fig. 1). Recently, a role for H_4R has also been proposed in diabetes, cancer, neuropathic pain and vestibular disorders [135].

Collectively, these results provide the rationale for the development of a new generation of selective antagonists of H_4R [136]. A first oral H_4R antagonist, compound UR-63325 synthesized by Palau Pharma, has entered clinical trials [137]. In addition, dual H_1R/H_4R antagonists and/or the combination of H_1R and H_4R antagonists could pave the way for the development of new therapeutic strategies for certain inflammatory and immunological disorders.

Closing Thoughts

Since the discovery of histamine almost 100 years ago, several breakthroughs have marked this field of research (fig. 2). Four histamine receptors have been characterized so far (H_1R, H_2R, H_3R and H_4R), and an important role for histamine has been identified in several physiological and pathological responses. In particular, histamine acting through H_1R or H_2R plays a fundamental role in the development of allergic disorders and in the regulation of gastric acid secretion, respectively. Although all histamine receptors are expressed in the brain, the preferential expression of H_3R in the central nervous system underlies its pivotal role in the regulation of basic homeostatic and higher functions, including cognition, arousal, circadian and feeding rhythms. Finally, the role of H_4R in the modulation of several aspects of the immune response is now increasingly being appreciated.

Several histamine receptor antagonists/agonists have been synthesized over the last century, some of them already used for the treatment of allergic and gastric acid-related disorders (anti-H_1R and anti-H_2R, respectively), and others being tested in clinical trials for neurologic and immune-mediated disorders (anti-H_3R and anti-H_4R, respectively).

Despite these great advances, several questions remain to be answered. First of all, we cannot exclude the existence of histamine receptors beyond the four currently known. Moreover, the sequential activation of histamine receptors on immune cells and their roles in chronic inflammatory diseases as well as therapeutic procedures (e.g. vaccines and venom immunotherapy) remains to be fully elucidated. Further examination of this important immunoregulatory network will likely lead to new advances in our understanding of immune-mediated disorders and could pave the way for a more thoughtful clinical exploitation of histamine receptor agonists/antagonists.

Acknowledgements

This work was supported in part by grants from the Ministero dell'Istruzione, Università e Ricerca (MIUR), the Istituto Superiore di Sanità AIDS project 'Role of Basophils in HIV-1 Infection', the Regione Campania 'CISI-Lab Project', CRÈME Project and TIMING Project.

References

1 Windaus A, Vogt W: Synthese des Imidazolyl-äthylamins. Ber Dtsch Chem Ges 1907;40:3691–3695.
2 Ackermann D: Über den bakteriellen Abbau des Histidins. Zeitschr Physiol Chem 1910;65;504–510.
3 Barger G, Dale HH: Ergotoxine and some other constituents of ergot. Biochem J 1907; 2:240–299.
4 Barger G, Dale HH: The presence in ergot and physiological activity of β-imidazolylethylamine. J Physiol 1910;Supp 40:xxxviii–xl.
5 Barger G, Dale HH: Chemical structure and sympathomimetic action of amines. J Physiol 1910;41:19–59.
6 Dale HH, Laidlaw PP: The physiological action of β-iminazolylethylamine. J Physiol 1910;41:318–344.
7 Popielski L: β-Imidazolyläthylamin und die Organextrakte Erster Teil: β-Imidazolyläthylamin als mächtiger Erreger der Magendrüsen. Pfluegers Arch 1920;178:214–236.
8 Lewis T, Grant RT: Vascular reactions of the skin to injury. 11. The liberation of histamine-like substance in the injured skin, the underlying cause of factitious urticaria and of wheals produced by burning; and observations upon the nervous control of certain skin reactions. Heart 1924;11:209–265.
9 Best CH, Dale HH, Dudley HW, Thorpe WV: The nature of the vaso-dilator constituents of certain tissue extracts. J Physiol 1927;62:397–417.

10 Feldberg W, O'Connor WJ: The liberation of histamine from the perfused lung by peptone. J Physiol 1937;90:288–295.
11 Feldberg W, Keogh EV: Liberation of histamine from the perfused lung by staphylococcal toxin. J Physiol 1937;90:280–287.
12 Feldberg W, Kellaway CH: Liberation of histamine from the perfused lung by snake venoms. J Physiol 1937;90:257–279.
13 Riley JF, West GB: The presence of histamine in tissue mast cells. J Physiol 1953; 120:528–537.
14 Riley JF, West GB: Histamine in tissue mast cells. J Physiol 1952;117:72P–73P.
15 Graham HT, Lowry OH, Wheelwright F, Lenz MA, Parish HH Jr: Distribution of histamine among leukocytes and platelets. Blood 1955;10:467–481.
16 Fourneau E, Maderni P, de Lestrange Y: Bases hétérocycliques provenant des coumaranes et du phényldioxane. J Pharm Chim 1933;18:185–191.
17 Fourneau E, Bovet D: Recherches sur l'action sympathicolytique d'un nouveau dérivé du dioxane. Arch Int Pharmacodyn 1933;46:178–191.
18 Fourneau E, Bovet D: Recherches sur l'action sympatholytique de nouveaux dérivés du dioxane. CR Soc Biol Paris 1933;113: 388–390.
19 Ungar G, Parrot JL, Bovet D: Inhibition des effets de l'histamine sur l'intestin isolé du cobaye par quelques substances sympathicomimetiques et sympathicolitiques. CR Soc Biol Paris 1937;124:445–446.
20 Bovet D, Staub AM: Action protectrice des éthers phénoliques au cours de l'intoxication histaminique. CR Soc Biol Paris 1937;124: 547–549.
21 Staub AM: Recherches sur quelque bases synthetique antagonistes de l'histamine. Ann Inst Pasteur 1939;63:400–436.
22 Halpern BN: Etude expérimentale des antihistaminiques de synthèse: essais de chimiothérapie des états allergiques. J Med Lyon 1942;23:409.
23 Ashford CA, Heller H, Smart GA: The action of histamine on hydrochloric acid and pepsin secretion in man. Br J Pharmacol Chemother 1949;4:153–161.
24 Parsons ME, Ganellin CR: Histamine and its receptors. Br J Pharmacol 2006;147(suppl 1):S127.
25 Folkow B, Haeger K, Kahlson G: Observations on reactive hyperaemia as related to histamine on drugs antagonising vasodilatation induced by histamine and the vasodilator properties of adenosine triphosphate. Acta Physiol Scand 1948;15:264–278.
26 Schild HO: pA, a new scale for the measurement of drug antagonism. Br J Pharmacol Chemother 1947;2:189–206.
27 Ash AS, Schild HO: Receptors mediating some actions of histamine. Br J Pharmacol Chemother 1966;27:427–439.
28 Ganellin CR: Personal reflections on Sir James Black (1924–2010) and histamine. Inflamm Res 2011;60:103–110.
29 Black JW, Duncan WA, Durant CJ, Ganellin CR, Parsons EM: Definition and antagonism of histamine H_2-receptors. Nature 1972;236:385–390.
30 Jensen KG, Rune S, Wulff HR: Cimetidine and gastric ulcer healing. Br Med J 1977;2: 1479.
31 Bradshaw J, Brittain RT, Clitherow JW, Daly MJ, Jack D, Price BJ, Stables R: Ranitidine (AH 19065): a new potent, selective histamine H_2-receptor antagonist [proceedings]. Br J Pharmacol 1979;66:464P.
32 Del Valle J, Gantz I: Novel insights into histamine H_2 receptor biology. Am J Physiol 1997;273:G987–G996.
33 Lichtenstein LM, Gillespie E: Inhibition of histamine release by histamine controlled by H_2 receptor. Nature 1973;244:287–288.
34 Masini E, Blandina P, Brunelleschi S, Mannaioni PF: Evidence for H_2-receptor-mediated inhibition of histamine release from isolated rat mast cells. Agents Actions 1982; 12:85–88.
35 Clark RA, Gallin JI, Kaplan AP: The selective eosinophil chemotactic activity of histamine. J Exp Med 1975;142:1462–1476.
36 Ezeamuzie CI, Philips E: Histamine H_2 receptors mediate the inhibitory effect of histamine on human eosinophil degranulation. Br J Pharmacol 2000;131:482–488.
37 Burde R, Seifert R, Buschauer A, Schultz G: Histamine inhibits activation of human neutrophils and HL-60 leukemic cells via H_2-receptors. Naunyn Schmiedebergs Arch Pharmacol 1989;340:671–678.
38 Panula P, Yang HY, Costa E: Histamine-containing neurons in the rat hypothalamus. Proc Natl Acad Sci USA 1984;81: 2572–2576.
39 Steinbusch HW, Sauren Y, Groenewegen H, Watanabe T, Mulder AH: Histaminergic projections from the premammillary and posterior hypothalamic region to the caudate-putamen complex in the rat. Brain Res 1986;368:389–393.
40 Watanabe T, Taguchi Y, Hayashi H, Tanaka J, Shiosaka S, Tohyama M, Kubota H, Terano Y, Wada H: Evidence for the presence of a histaminergic neuron system in the rat brain: an immunohistochemical analysis. Neurosci Lett 1983;39:249–254.
41 Watanabe T, Taguchi Y, Shiosaka S, Tanaka J, Kubota H, Terano Y, Tohyama M, Wada H: Distribution of the histaminergic neuron system in the central nervous system of rats; a fluorescent immunohistochemical analysis with histidine decarboxylase as a marker. Brain Res 1984;295:13–25.
42 Passani MB, Blandina P: Histamine receptors in the CNS as targets for therapeutic intervention. Trends Pharmacol Sci 2011;32: 242–249.
43 Arrang JM, Garbarg M, Schwartz JC: Autoinhibition of brain histamine release mediated by a novel class (H_3) of histamine receptor. Nature 1983;302:832–837.
44 Arrang JM, Garbarg M, Lancelot JC, Lecomte JM, Pollard H, Robba M, Schunack W, Schwartz JC: Highly potent and selective ligands for histamine H_3-receptors. Nature 1987;327:117–123.
45 Clark EA, Hill SJ: Sensitivity of histamine H_3 receptor agonist-stimulated [^{35}S]GTPγ[S] binding to pertussis toxin. Eur J Pharmacol 1996;296:223–225.
46 Clark MA, Korte A, Egan RW: Guanine nucleotides and pertussis toxin reduce the affinity of histamine H_3 receptors on AtT-20 cells. Agents Actions 1993;40:129–134.
47 Blandizzi C, Colucci R, Tognetti M, De Paolis B, Del Tacca M: H_3 receptor-mediated inhibition of intestinal acetylcholine release: pharmacological characterization of signal transduction pathways. Naunyn Schmiedebergs Arch Pharmacol 2001;363: 193–202.
48 Fink K, Schlicker E, Neise A, Gothert M: Involvement of presynaptic H_3 receptors in the inhibitory effect of histamine on serotonin release in the rat brain cortex. Naunyn Schmiedebergs Arch Pharmacol 1990;342: 513–519.
49 Schlicker E, Behling A, Lummen G, Gothert M: Histamine H_{3A} receptor-mediated inhibition of noradrenaline release in the mouse brain cortex. Naunyn Schmiedebergs Arch Pharmacol 1992;345:489–493.
50 Schlicker E, Betz R, Gothert M: Histamine H_3 receptor-mediated inhibition of serotonin release in the rat brain cortex. Naunyn Schmiedebergs Arch Pharmacol 1988;337: 588–590.
51 Schlicker E, Fink K, Hinterthaner M, Gothert M: Inhibition of noradrenaline release in the rat brain cortex via presynaptic H_3 receptors. Naunyn Schmiedebergs Arch Pharmacol 1989;340:633–638.
52 Schlicker E, Malinowska B, Kathmann M, Gothert M: Modulation of neurotransmitter release via histamine H_3 heteroreceptors. Fundam Clin Pharmacol 1994;8:128–137.
53 Leurs R, Bakker RA, Timmerman H, de Esch IJ: The histamine H_3 receptor: from gene cloning to H_3 receptor drugs. Nat Rev Drug Discov 2005;4:107–120.
54 Sander K, Kottke T, Stark H: Histamine H_3 receptor antagonists go to clinics. Biol Pharm Bull 2008;31:2163–2181.

55 Gantz I, Schaffer M, DelValle J, Logsdon C, Campbell V, Uhler M, Yamada T: Molecular cloning of a gene encoding the histamine H_2 receptor. Proc Natl Acad Sci USA 1991;88: 429–433.
56 Gantz I, Munzert G, Tashiro T, Schaffer M, Wang L, DelValle J, Yamada T: Molecular cloning of the human histamine H_2 receptor. Biochem Biophys Res Commun 1991; 178:1386–1392.
57 Ruat M, Traiffort E, Arrang JM, Leurs R, Schwartz JC: Cloning and tissue expression of a rat histamine H_2-receptor gene. Biochem Biophys Res Commun 1991;179: 1470–1478.
58 Traiffort E, Vizuete ML, Tardivel-Lacombe J, Souil E, Schwartz JC, Ruat M: The guinea pig histamine H_2 receptor: gene cloning, tissue expression and chromosomal localization of its human counterpart. Biochem Biophys Res Commun 1995;211:570–577.
59 Ferstl R, Akdis CA, O'Mahony L: Histamine regulation of innate and adaptive immunity. Front Biosci 2012;17:40–53.
60 Honrubia MA, Vilaro MT, Palacios JM, Mengod G: Distribution of the histamine H_2 receptor in monkey brain and its mRNA localization in monkey and human brain. Synapse 2000;38:343–354.
61 Matsuda N, Jesmin S, Takahashi Y, Hatta E, Kobayashi M, Matsuyama K, Kawakami N, Sakuma I, Gando S, Fukui H, Hattori Y, Levi R: Histamine H_1 and H_2 receptor gene and protein levels are differentially expressed in the hearts of rodents and humans. J Pharmacol Exp Ther 2004;309:786–795.
62 Smit MJ, Leurs R, Alewijnse AE, Blauw J, Van Nieuw Amerongen GP, Van De Vrede Y, Roovers E, Timmerman H: Inverse agonism of histamine H_2 antagonist accounts for upregulation of spontaneously active histamine H_2 receptors. Proc Natl Acad Sci USA 1996;93:6802–6807.
63 Lefkowitz RJ, Cotecchia S, Samama P, Costa T: Constitutive activity of receptors coupled to guanine nucleotide regulatory proteins. Trends Pharmacol Sci 1993;14:303–307.
64 Kobayashi T, Tonai S, Ishihara Y, Koga R, Okabe S, Watanabe T: Abnormal functional and morphological regulation of the gastric mucosa in histamine H_2 receptor-deficient mice. J Clin Invest 2000;105:1741–1749.
65 Jutel M, Watanabe T, Klunker S, Akdis M, Thomet OA, Malolepszy J, Zak-Nejmark T, Koga R, Kobayashi T, Blaser K, Akdis CA: Histamine regulates T-cell and antibody responses by differential expression of H_1 and H_2 receptors. Nature 2001;413:420–425.
66 Meiler F, Zumkehr J, Klunker S, Ruckert B, Akdis CA, Akdis M: In vivo switch to IL-10-secreting T regulatory cells in high dose allergen exposure. J Exp Med 2008;205:2887–2898.
67 Novak N, Mete N, Bussmann C, Maintz L, Bieber T, Akdis M, Zumkehr J, Jutel M, Akdis C: Early suppression of basophil activation during allergen-specific immunotherapy by histamine receptor 2. J Allergy Clin Immunol 2012;130:1153–1158.
68 Truta-Feles K, Lagadari M, Lehmann K, Berod L, Cubillos S, Piehler S, Herouy Y, Barz D, Kamradt T, Maghazachi A, Norgauer J: Histamine modulates γδ-T lymphocyte migration and cytotoxicity, via Gi and Gs protein-coupled signalling pathways. Br J Pharmacol 2010;161:1291–1300.
69 Frei R, Ferstl R, Konieczna P, Ziegler M, Simon T, Rugeles TM, Mailand S, Watanabe T, Lauener R, Akdis CA, O'Mahony L: Histamine receptor 2 modifies dendritic cell responses to microbial ligands. J Allergy Clin Immunol 2013;132:194–204.
70 Mazzoni A, Leifer CA, Mullen GE, Kennedy MN, Klinman DM, Segal DM: Cutting edge: histamine inhibits IFN-α release from plasmacytoid dendritic cells. J Immunol 2003; 170:2269–2273.
71 Thoren FB, Romero AI, Brune M, Hellstrand K: Histamine dihydrochloride and low-dose interleukin-2 as post-consolidation immunotherapy in acute myeloid leukemia. Expert Opin Biol Ther 2009;9: 1217–1223.
72 Brune M, Castaigne S, Catalano J, Gehlsen K, Ho AD, Hofmann WK, Hogge DE, Nilsson B, Or R, Romero AI, Rowe JM, Simonsson B, Spearing R, Stadtmauer EA, Szer J, Wallhult E, Hellstrand K: Improved leukemia-free survival after postconsolidation immunotherapy with histamine dihydrochloride and interleukin-2 in acute myeloid leukemia: results of a randomized phase 3 trial. Blood 2006;108:88–96.
73 Brune M, Hansson M, Mellqvist UH, Hermodsson S, Hellstrand K: NK cell-mediated killing of AML blasts: role of histamine, monocytes and reactive oxygen metabolites. Eur J Haematol 1996;57:312–319.
74 Yamashita M, Fukui H, Sugama K, Horio Y, Ito S, Mizuguchi H, Wada H: Expression cloning of a cDNA encoding the bovine histamine H_1 receptor. Proc Natl Acad Sci USA 1991;88:11515–11519.
75 Inoue I, Taniuchi I, Kitamura D, Jenkins NA, Gilbert DJ, Copeland NG, Watanabe T: Characteristics of the mouse genomic histamine H_1 receptor gene. Genomics 1996;36: 178–181.
76 Fujimoto K, Horio Y, Sugama K, Ito S, Liu YQ, Fukui H: Genomic cloning of the rat histamine H_1 receptor. Biochem Biophys Res Commun 1993;190:294–301.
77 Fukui H, Fujimoto K, Mizuguchi H, Sakamoto K, Horio Y, Takai S, Yamada K, Ito S: Molecular cloning of the human histamine H_1 receptor gene. Biochem Biophys Res Commun 1994;201:894–901.
78 De Backer MD, Gommeren W, Moereels H, Nobels G, Van Gompel P, Leysen JE, Luyten WH: Genomic cloning, heterologous expression and pharmacological characterization of a human histamine H_1 receptor. Biochem Biophys Res Commun 1993;197: 1601–1608.
79 Booth RG, Moniri NH, Bakker RA, Choksi NY, Nix WB, Timmerman H, Leurs R: A novel phenylaminotetralin radioligand reveals a subpopulation of histamine H_1 receptors. J Pharmacol Exp Ther 2002;302: 328–336.
80 Dismukes RK, Daly JW: Adaptive responses of brain cyclic AMP-generating systems to alterations in synaptic input. J Cyclic Nucleotide Res 1976;2:321–336.
81 Marley PD, Thomson KA, Jachno K, Johnston MJ: Histamine-induced increases in cyclic AMP levels in bovine adrenal medullary cells. Br J Pharmacol 1991;104:839–846.
82 Maruko T, Nakahara T, Sakamoto K, Saito M, Sugimoto N, Takuwa Y, Ishii K: Involvement of the βγ subunits of G proteins in the cAMP response induced by stimulation of the histamine H_1 receptor. Naunyn Schmiedebergs Arch Pharmacol 2005;372:153–159.
83 Yanai K, Son LZ, Endou M, Sakurai E, Nakagawasai O, Tadano T, Kisara K, Inoue I, Watanabe T: Behavioural characterization and amounts of brain monoamines and their metabolites in mice lacking histamine H_1 receptors. Neuroscience 1998;87:479–487.
84 Dai H, Okuda T, Sakurai E, Kuramasu A, Kato M, Jia F, Xu AJ, Iinuma K, Sato I, Yanai K: Blockage of histamine H_1 receptor attenuates social isolation-induced disruption of prepulse inhibition: a study in H_1 receptor gene knockout mice. Psychopharmacology (Berl) 2005;183:285–293.
85 Ohinata K, Shimano T, Yamauchi R, Sakurada S, Yanai K, Yoshikawa M: The anorectic effect of neurotensin is mediated via a histamine H_1 receptor in mice. Peptides 2004;25:2135–2138.
86 Mobarakeh JI, Sakurada S, Katsuyama S, Kutsuwa M, Kuramasu A, Lin ZY, Watanabe T, Hashimoto Y, Yanai K: Role of histamine H_1 receptor in pain perception: a study of the receptor gene knockout mice. Eur J Pharmacol 2000;391:81–89.
87 Mobarakeh JI, Sakurada S, Hayashi T, Orito T, Okuyama K, Sakurada T, Kuramasu A, Watanabe T, Yanai K: Enhanced antinociception by intrathecally-administered morphine in histamine H_1 receptor gene knockout mice. Neuropharmacology 2002;42: 1079–1088.

88 Bryce PJ, Mathias CB, Harrison KL, Watanabe T, Geha RS, Oettgen HC: The H1 histamine receptor regulates allergic lung responses. J Clin Invest 2006;116:1624–1632.
89 Triggiani M, Petraroli A, Loffredo S, Frattini A, Granata F, Morabito P, Staiano RI, Secondo A, Annunziato L, Marone G: Differentiation of monocytes into macrophages induces the upregulation of histamine H_1 receptor. J Allergy Clin Immunol 2007;119:472–481.
90 Marone G, Gentile M, Petraroli A, De Rosa N, Triggiani M: Histamine-induced activation of human lung macrophages. Int Arch Allergy Immunol 2001;124:249–252.
91 Triggiani M, Gentile M, Secondo A, Granata F, Oriente A, Taglialatela M, Annunziato L, Marone G: Histamine induces exocytosis and IL-6 production from human lung macrophages through interaction with H_1 receptors. J Immunol 2001;166:4083–4091.
92 Ma RZ, Gao J, Meeker ND, Fillmore PD, Tung KS, Watanabe T, Zachary JF, Offner H, Blankenhorn EP, Teuscher C: Identification of Bphs, an autoimmune disease locus, as histamine receptor H_1. Science 2002;297:620–623.
93 Garcia-Martin E, Ayuso P, Luengo A, Martinez C, Agundez JA: Genetic variability of histamine receptors in patients with Parkinson's disease. BMC Med Genet 2008;9:15.
94 Lovenberg TW, Roland BL, Wilson SJ, Jiang X, Pyati J, Huvar A, Jackson MR, Erlander MG: Cloning and functional expression of the human histamine H_3 receptor. Mol Pharmacol 1999;55:1101–1107.
95 Drutel G, Peitsaro N, Karlstedt K, Wieland K, Smit MJ, Timmerman H, Panula P, Leurs R: Identification of rat H_3 receptor isoforms with different brain expression and signaling properties. Mol Pharmacol 2001;59:1–8.
96 Wieland K, Bongers G, Yamamoto Y, Hashimoto T, Yamatodani A, Menge WM, Timmerman H, Lovenberg TW, Leurs R: Constitutive activity of histamine H_3 receptors stably expressed in SK-N-MC cells: display of agonism and inverse agonism by H_3 antagonists. J Pharmacol Exp Ther 2001;299:908–914.
97 Rouleau A, Ligneau X, Tardivel-Lacombe J, Morisset S, Gbahou F, Schwartz JC, Arrang JM: Histamine H_3-receptor-mediated [^{35}S] GTP gamma[S] binding: evidence for constitutive activity of the recombinant and native rat and human H_3 receptors. Br J Pharmacol 2002;135:383–392.
98 Morisset S, Rouleau A, Ligneau X, Gbahou F, Tardivel-Lacombe J, Stark H, Schunack W, Ganellin CR, Schwartz JC, Arrang JM: High constitutive activity of native H_3 receptors regulates histamine neurons in brain. Nature 2000;408:860–864.
99 Coge F, Guenin SP, Audinot V, Renouard-Try A, Beauverger P, Macia C, Ouvry C, Nagel N, Rique H, Boutin JA, Galizzi JP: Genomic organization and characterization of splice variants of the human histamine H_3 receptor. Biochem J 2001;355:279–288.
100 Morisset S, Sasse A, Gbahou F, Heron A, Ligneau X, Tardivel-Lacombe J, Schwartz JC, Arrang JM: The rat H_3 receptor: gene organization and multiple isoforms. Biochem Biophys Res Commun 2001;280:75–80.
101 Heron A, Rouleau A, Cochois V, Pillot C, Schwartz JC, Arrang JM: Expression analysis of the histamine H_3 receptor in developing rat tissues. Mech Dev 2001;105:167–173.
102 Toyota H, Dugovic C, Koehl M, Laposky AD, Weber C, Ngo K, Wu Y, Lee DH, Yanai K, Sakurai E, Watanabe T, Liu C, Chen J, Barbier AJ, Turek FW, Fung-Leung WP, Lovenberg TW: Behavioral characterization of mice lacking histamine H_3 receptors. Mol Pharmacol 2002;62:389–397.
103 Takahashi K, Suwa H, Ishikawa T, Kotani H: Targeted disruption of H_3 receptors results in changes in brain histamine tone leading to an obese phenotype. J Clin Invest 2002;110:1791–1799.
104 Rizk A, Curley J, Robertson J, Raber J: Anxiety and cognition in histamine H_3 receptor$^{-/-}$ mice. Eur J Neurosci 2004;19:1992–1296.
105 Oda T, Morikawa N, Saito Y, Masuho Y, Matsumoto S: Molecular cloning and characterization of a novel type of histamine receptor preferentially expressed in leukocytes. J Biol Chem 2000;275:36781–36786.
106 Nakamura T, Itadani H, Hidaka Y, Ohta M, Tanaka K: Molecular cloning and characterization of a new human histamine receptor, HH_4R. Biochem Biophys Res Commun 2000;279:615–620.
107 Liu C, Wilson SJ, Kuei C, Lovenberg TW: Comparison of human, mouse, rat, and guinea pig histamine H_4 receptors reveals substantial pharmacological species variation. J Pharmacol Exp Ther 2001;299:121–130.
108 Oda T, Matsumoto S, Masuho Y, Takasaki J, Matsumoto M, Kamohara M, Saito T, Ohishi T, Soga T, Hiyama H, Matsushime H, Furuichi K: cDNA cloning and characterization of porcine histamine H_4 receptor. Biochim Biophys Acta 2002;1575:135–138.
109 Oda T, Matsumoto S, Matsumoto M, Takasaki J, Kamohara M, Soga T, Hiyama H, Kobori M, Katoh M: Molecular cloning of monkey histamine H_4 receptor. J Pharmacol Sci 2005;98:319–322.
110 Jablonowski JA, Grice CA, Chai W, Dvorak CA, Venable JD, Kwok AK, Ly KS, Wei J, Baker SM, Desai PJ, Jiang W, Wilson SJ, Thurmond RL, Karlsson L, Edwards JP, Lovenberg TW, Carruthers NI: The first potent and selective non-imidazole human histamine H_4 receptor antagonists. J Med Chem 2003;46:3957–3960.
111 Lim HD, van Rijn RM, Ling P, Bakker RA, Thurmond RL, Leurs R: Evaluation of histamine H_1-, H_2-, and H_3-receptor ligands at the human histamine H_4 receptor: identification of 4-methylhistamine as the first potent and selective H_4 receptor agonist. J Pharmacol Exp Ther 2005;314:1310–1321.
112 Thurmond RL, Desai PJ, Dunford PJ, Fung-Leung WP, Hofstra CL, Jiang W, Nguyen S, Riley JP, Sun S, Williams KN, Edwards JP, Karlsson L: A potent and selective histamine H_4 receptor antagonist with anti-inflammatory properties. J Pharmacol Exp Ther 2004;309:404–413.
113 Buckland KF, Williams TJ, Conroy DM: Histamine induces cytoskeletal changes in human eosinophils via the H_4 receptor. Br J Pharmacol 2003;140:1117–1127.
114 O'Reilly M, Alpert R, Jenkinson S, Gladue RP, Foo S, Trim S, Peter B, Trevethick M, Fidock M: Identification of a histamine H_4 receptor on human eosinophils – role in eosinophil chemotaxis. J Recept Signal Transduct Res 2002;22:431.
115 Shiraishi Y, Jia Y, Domenico J, Joetham A, Karasuyama H, Takeda K, Gelfand EW: Sequential engagement of FcεRI on mast cells and basophil histamine H_4 receptor and FcεRI in allergic rhinitis. J Immunol 2013;190:539–548.
116 Godot V, Arock M, Garcia G, Capel F, Flys C, Dy M, Emilie D, Humbert M: H_4 histamine receptor mediates optimal migration of mast cell precursors to CXCL12. J Allergy Clin Immunol 2007;120:827–834.
117 Hofstra CL, Desai PJ, Thurmond RL, Fung-Leung WP: Histamine H_4 receptor mediates chemotaxis and calcium mobilization of mast cells. J Pharmacol Exp Ther 2003;305:1212–1221.
118 Damaj BB, Becerra CB, Esber HJ, Wen Y, Maghazachi AA: Functional expression of H_4 histamine receptor in human natural killer cells, monocytes, and dendritic cells. J Immunol 2007;179:7907–7915.
119 Gantner F, Sakai K, Tusche MW, Cruikshank WW, Center DM, Bacon KB: Histamine H_4 and H_2 receptors control histamine-induced interleukin-16 release from human $CD8^+$ T cells. J Pharmacol Exp Ther 2002;303:300–307.
120 Gutzmer R, Mommert S, Gschwandtner M, Zwingmann K, Stark H, Werfel T: The histamine H_4 receptor is functionally expressed on TH2 cells. J Allergy Clin Immunol 2009;123:619–625.

3

121 Leite-de-Moraes MC, Diem S, Michel ML, Ohtsu H, Thurmond RL, Schneider E, Dy M: Cutting edge: histamine receptor H_4 activation positively regulates in vivo IL-4 and IFN-γ production by invariant NKT cells. J Immunol 2009;182:1233–1236.
122 Morgan RK, McAllister B, Cross L, Green DS, Kornfeld H, Center DM, Cruikshank WW: Histamine 4 receptor activation induces recruitment of FoxP3+ T cells and inhibits allergic asthma in a murine model. J Immunol 2007;178:8081–8089.
123 Center DM, Cruikshank W: Modulation of lymphocyte migration by human lymphokines. 1. Identification and characterization of chemoattractant activity for lymphocytes from mitogen-stimulated mononuclear cells. J Immunol 1982;128:2563–2568.
124 Kaser A, Dunzendorfer S, Offner FA, Ryan T, Schwabegger A, Cruikshank WW, Wiedermann CJ, Tilg H: A role for IL-16 in the cross-talk between dendritic cells and T cells. J Immunol 1999;163:3232–3238.
125 Rand TH, Cruikshank WW, Center DM, Weller PF: CD4-mediated stimulation of human eosinophils: lymphocyte chemoattractant factor and other CD4-binding ligands elicit eosinophil migration. J Exp Med 1991;173:1521–1528.
126 Lim KG, Wan HC, Resnick M, Wong DT, Cruikshank WW, Kornfeld H, Center DM, Weller PF: Human eosinophils release the lymphocyte and eosinophil active cytokines, RANTES and lymphocyte chemoattractant factor. Int Arch Allergy Immunol 1995;107:342.
127 Mashikian MV, Tarpy RE, Saukkonen JJ, Lim KG, Fine GD, Cruikshank WW, Center DM: Identification of IL-16 as the lymphocyte chemotactic activity in the bronchoalveolar lavage fluid of histamine-challenged asthmatic patients. J Allergy Clin Immunol 1998;101:786–792.
128 Krug N, Cruikshank WW, Tschernig T, Erpenbeck VJ, Balke K, Hohlfeld JM, Center DM, Fabel H: Interleukin 16 and T-cell chemoattractant activity in bronchoalveolar lavage 24 h after allergen challenge in asthma. Am J Respir Crit Care Med 2000;162:105–111.
129 Laberge S, Pinsonneault S, Ernst P, Olivenstein R, Ghaffar O, Center DM, Hamid Q: Phenotype of IL-16-producing cells in bronchial mucosa: evidence for the human eosinophil and mast cell as cellular sources of IL-16 in asthma. Int Arch Allergy Immunol 1999;119:120–125.
130 Laberge S, Ernst P, Ghaffar O, Cruikshank WW, Kornfeld H, Center DM, Hamid Q: Increased expression of interleukin-16 in bronchial mucosa of subjects with atopic asthma. Am J Respir Cell Mol Biol 1997;17:193–202.
131 Dunford PJ, Williams KN, Desai PJ, Karlsson L, McQueen D, Thurmond RL: Histamine H_4 receptor antagonists are superior to traditional antihistamines in the attenuation of experimental pruritus. J Allergy Clin Immunol 2007;119:176–183.
132 Marson CM: Targeting the histamine H_4 receptor. Chem Rev 2011;111:7121–7156.
133 Yamaura K, Oda M, Suwa E, Suzuki M, Sato H, Ueno K: Expression of histamine H_4 receptor in human epidermal tissues and attenuation of experimental pruritus using H_4 receptor antagonist. J Toxicol Sci 2009;34:427–431.
134 Takeshita K, Sakai K, Bacon KB, Gantner F: Critical role of histamine H_4 receptor in leukotriene B_4 production and mast cell-dependent neutrophil recruitment induced by zymosan in vivo. J Pharmacol Exp Ther 2003;307:1072–1078.
135 Kiss R, Keseru GM: Histamine H_4 receptor ligands and their potential therapeutic applications: an update. Expert Opin Ther Pat 2012;22:205–221.
136 Thurmond RL, Gelfand EW, Dunford PJ: The role of histamine H_1 and H_4 receptors in allergic inflammation: the search for new antihistamines. Nat Rev Drug Discov 2008;7:41–53.
137 Salcedo C, Pontes C, Merlos M: Is the H_4 receptor a new drug target for allergies and asthma? Front Biosci (Elite Ed) 2013;5:178–187.

Prof. Gianni Marone
Department of Translational Medical Sciences and
Center for Basic and Clinical Immunology Research (CISI)
Division of Clinical Immunology and Allergy
University of Naples Federico II, via S. Pansini 5
IT–80131 Naples (Italy)
E-Mail marone@unina.it

4 Detection of Environmental Influences and Allergens

Bergmann K-C, Ring J (eds): History of Allergy. Chem Immunol Allergy. Basel, Karger, 2014, vol 100, pp 228–233
DOI: 10.1159/000358743

Pollen and Pollinosis

Matt Smith[a] · Uwe Berger[a] · Heidrun Behrendt[b] · Karl-Christian Bergmann[c]

[a]Research Unit Aerobiology and Pollen Information, Department of Oto-Rhino-Laryngology, Medical University of Vienna, Vienna, Austria; [b]ZAUM – Center of Allergy and Environment, Helmholtz Zentrum München/Technical University of Munich, Munich, and [c]Allergy Centre Charité, Universitätsmedizin, Berlin, Germany

Abstract

Pollen grains only represent a small fraction of the total amount of the viable biological particles present in the air, but pollen are the most important aeroallergens in the outdoor environment. The analysis of pollen has traditionally been carried out by microscopy, which can be traced back to the 17th century. Modern advances in molecular analysis could improve information for allergy sufferers and health care professionals. Pollen allergy (pollinosis) was first described in the 19th century. The prevalence of respiratory diseases increased dramatically during the latter part of the 20th century and millions of individuals are now affected. A number of scientists devised equipment to examine airborne biological particles during the 19th century, but aerobiological monitoring only became standardized during the 20th century. Airborne pollen are routinely monitored in many parts of the world, such as North America and Europe, and the first limited network has also been created for monitoring airborne allergen concentrations. Monitoring of the environment is often based on a combination of measurements and model results. Source-based models can increase our knowledge of airborne pollen because they can explain situations and processes that are almost impossible to understand using observations alone.

Pollen grains only represent a small fraction of the total amount of the viable biological particles present in the air [1]. However, pollen are the most important aeroallergens in the outdoor environment. They are the male gametophyte of seed plants (spermatopsids), of which there are two categories: the gymnosperms (from the Greek 'naked seed') and the more advanced angiosperms (from the Greek 'seed vessel'). The latter first became abundant during the Cretaceous period about 100 million years ago. The seed protects the embryo from unfavorable growing conditions and facilitates the distribution of the embryo away from the parent plant. This makes spermatopsids the most successful terrestrial plants as they are able to colonize and adapt to a wide range of different habitats [2].

Pollen grains produce the male gametes and transfer them to the female gametes during sexual reproduction [3]. This transfer is carried out by insects (entomophily) in the majority of species, but pollinators may also be other animals such as birds or bats (zoophily). Wind pollination (anemophily) only occurs in about 10% of over 250,000 pollen-producing species [1], but this fertilization process is the most important in terms of allergy.

Anemophily is generally considered to be a secondary adaptation from entomophilous plants [3]. Wind-pollinated plants have reduced the normal means of attracting animal visitors, such as through nectar, color or scent, and instead produce enormous quantities of pollen to compensate for the fact that many grains do not reach their targets. These pollen grains are often dry, smooth and relatively small (approx. 20–60 μm), and can easily become airborne [1, 3]. However, there are exceptions. For instance, wind-pollinated plants can produce pollen grains that have a sculptured exine (e.g. *Ambrosia*) or are large and have features like air sacs that lower the pollen grain's density so that it can be transported in the in air (e.g. Pinaceae pollen can be >80 μm in diameter) [3].

The pollen grains are the carriers of the antigenic material responsible for allergic diseases. The most important allergens are proteins or polypeptides, although polysaccharides, glycoproteins and lipoproteins can also act as allergens [3]. Pollen-derived allergens are also released with pollen granules, starch grains and other, non-protein substances. Lipids are a major part of the pollen exine and exudate, such as the so-called pollen-associated lipid mediators, PALMs, which help the pollen tube to penetrate the stigma and are essential in the plant fertilization process [4].

Analysis of Airborne Pollen and Pollen Allergens

Pollen grains can be classified and identified on the basis of their morphology, such as shape, size, number and characteristics of the apertures, and the structure of the outer surface of the exine (fig. 1a, b) [1]. The analysis of pollen has traditionally been carried out by microscopy, e.g. light microscopy or scanning electron microscopy.

The use of microscopy can be traced back to the natural philosophers of the 17th century. Perhaps the single greatest experimental scientist from this time was Robert Hooke (1635–1703). Hooke was fascinated by microscopy; he invented the first practical compound microscope and founded microscopic biology with his pioneering work *Micrographia* (1665). Hooke's publication contained accurate microscopic observations and detailed drawings, and when describing the angular spaces he saw in a thin section of cork he coined the term 'cell' because they reminded him of the cells of a monastery [5, 6].

A contemporary of Hooke's was Anton van Leeuwenhoek (1632–1723), a Dutch tradesman and scientist from Delft in the Netherlands who investigated the natural world using microscopes he built himself. Between 1673 and 1683, he first described organisms such as bacteria and protozoa, as well as some yeasts and molds. The instruments used by van Leeuwenhoek were single biconvex lenses, with magnification in the range of ×50–200, which were mounted between two metal plates. The object to be examined was raised or lowered and rotated on its axis by a coarse-threaded screw. The eye would almost need to be in contact with the glass due to the short (approx. 1 mm) focal lengths of the lens [6, 7].

The Italian Marcello Malpighi (1628–1694; fig. 2) was a microscopist who is credited as being the first to see capillaries as well as a founder of embryology, comparative anatomy, histology and plant anatomy. Malpighi and his contemporary and cofounder of plant anatomy, the English scientist Nehemiah Grew (1641–1712; fig. 3), carried out systematic studies on the microscopic structure of plants. Malpighi published *Anatome Plantarum* in two parts in 1675 and in 1679 [8]. Grew presented his work entitled *The Anatomy of Plants* in 1682 (fig. 4), which includes the first known description of pollen (fig. 5) [6].

Many of the pollen grains collected from the air can be identified to the level of genus (e.g. *Betula*) but some can only be recognized as belonging to a certain family (e.g. Poaceae) and others can simply be described as a 'type' (e.g. Taxaceae/Cupressaceae type). At present, relatively few pollen grains found

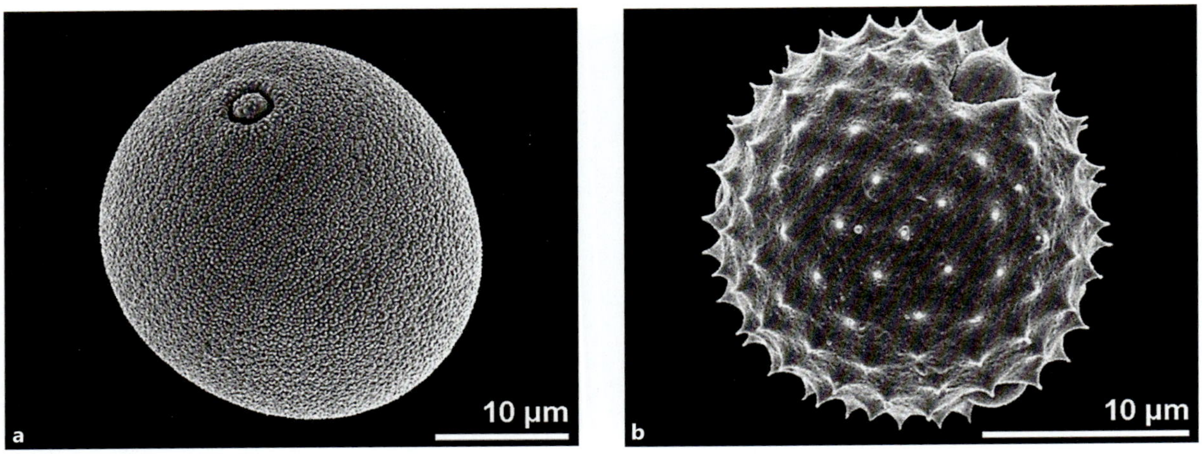

Fig. 1. Pollen grains of *Dactylis glomerata* (Poaceae family; **a**) and *Ambrosia artemisiifolia* (Asteraceae family; **b**). Note the different characteristics that can be used for identification. For example, *D. glomerata* is a medium-sized (26–50 µm) grain with a smooth exine (outer layer of the wall of the pollen grain) and a single pore (monoporate) with an annulus and operculum. In contrast, *A. artemisiifolia* is a small (10–25 µm) grain, covered in short spines and has three furrows with pores inside (tricolporate).

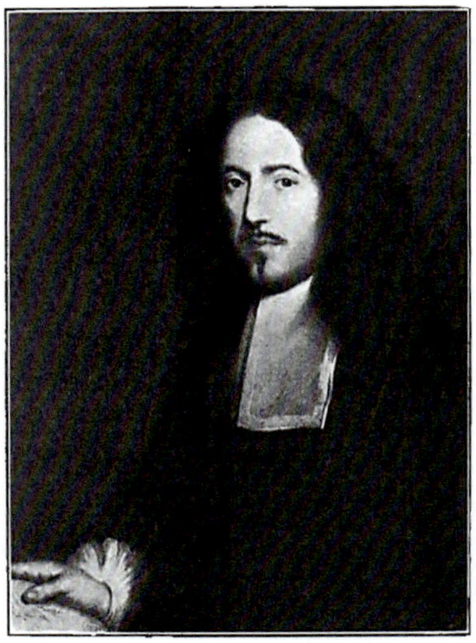
2

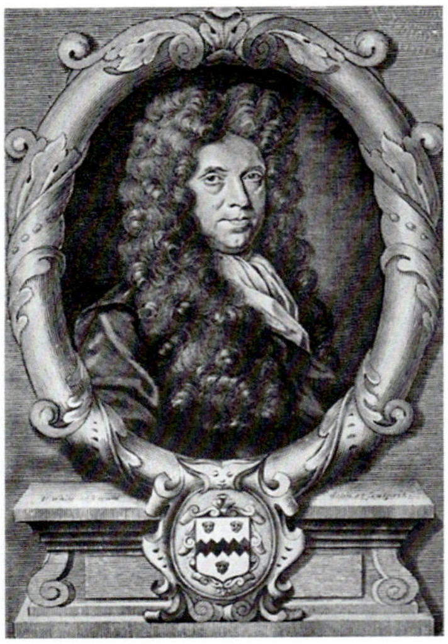
3

Fig. 2. Marcello Malpighi (1628–1694), by A.M. Tobar.
Fig. 3. Nehemiah Grew (1641–1712).

in air samples can be identified to the species level (e.g. *Urtica membranacea*). In 1869, the Swiss chemist Friedrich Miescher (1844–1895) identified what he termed 'nuclein' inside the nuclei of human white blood cells. The term nuclein was eventually to become known as deoxyribonucleic acid, or DNA [9]. DNA sequencing has now advanced understanding about plant phylogeny and could be used to identify pollen grains to the species level [10].

The amount of allergen contained in pollen has also been shown to vary spatially and temporally [11], and so monitoring airborne allergen concentrations in ambient air might be required if the aim is to provide information related to pollen allergy. A number of pollen allergens have been identified, isolated and characterized by different workers, such as David Marsh and coworkers who examined the perennial ryegrass group during the 1960s and 1970s [12]. In addition, laboratories around the world can

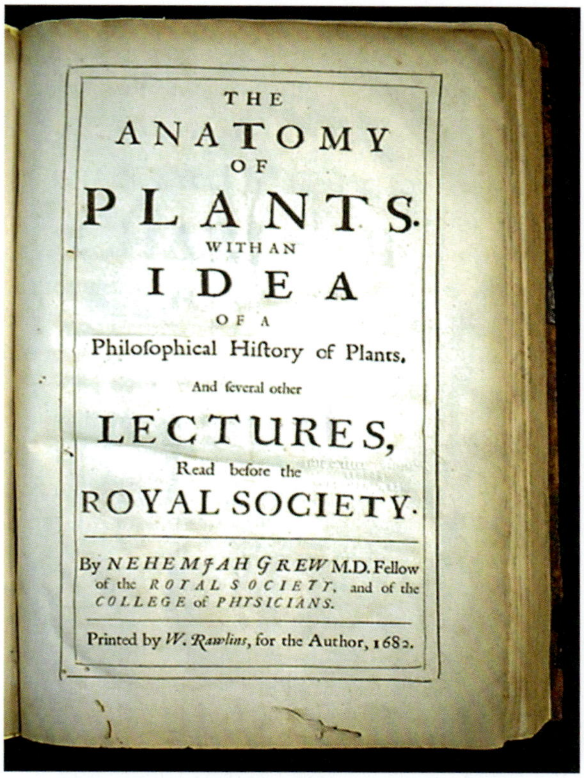

THE
ANATOMY
OF
PLANTS.
WITH AN
IDEA
OF A
Philoſophical Hiſtory of Plants.
And ſeveral other
LECTURES,
Read before the
ROYAL SOCIETY.

By NEHEMJAH GREW M.D. Fellow of the ROYAL SOCIETY, and of the COLLEGE of PHYSICIANS.

Printed by W. Rawlins, for the Author, 1682.

Fig. 4. *The Anatomy of Plants*, by N. Grew.

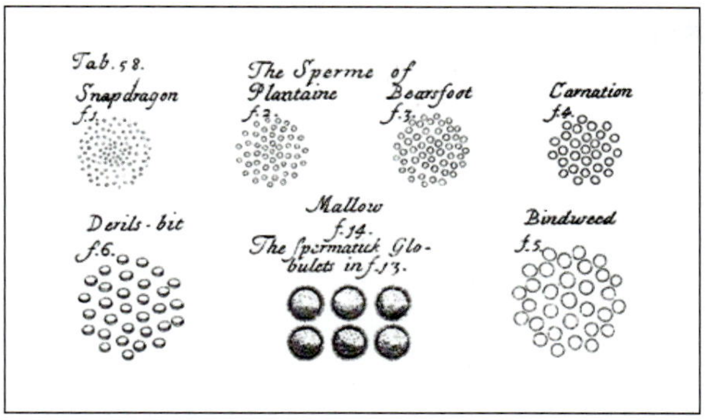

Fig. 5. The first pictures of pollen made by N. Grew.

now carry out immunoassays following the invention of the enzyme immunoassay, EIA, and enzyme-linked immunosorbent assay, ELISA, which were developed independently and simultaneously by two different research groups in 1971: Peter Perlmann and Eva Engvall at Stockholm University in Sweden, and Anton Schuurs and Bauke van Weemen in the Netherlands [13].

First Descriptions of the Disease

Pollen allergy (pollinosis) was first described at the beginning of the 19th century [14]. The prevalence of allergic respiratory diseases, such as asthma and allergic rhinitis, increased dramatically during the latter part of the 20th century [15] and millions of individuals are now affected. The first clinical description of the disease is accredited to John Bostock (1773–1846), who was a physician at Guy's Hospital in London. Bostock presented his 'Case of a periodical affection of the eyes and chest' to the Royal Society of Medicine on March 16, 1819 [14]. He described 'an unusual train of symptoms' that made their appearance at the beginning or middle of June in every year with a greater or lesser degree of violence. These were symptoms that he experienced himself: eyes that became inflamed, irritation of the nose, sneezing, tightness of the chest, difficulty in breathing and languor [14, 16].

Bostock later used the term 'catarrhus aestivus', or summer catarrh, to describe the malaise, but he failed to find a causal explanation [14]. This was left to John Elliotson (1791–1868). In a clinical lecture delivered at St. Thomas's Hospital on March 31, 1831, Elliotson attributed the symptoms of hay fever to the 'emanation from the flower of the grass'. In the same lecture, Elliotson also refuted Brostock's claim that the disease was confined to the higher ranks of society and argued that the prevalence of the disease was underestimated in the 'lower orders' because poorer people did not seek to visit physicians but instead had their symptoms treated in dispensaries [16, 17].

In 1873, Charles H. Blackley [18] was the first person to demonstrate the 'nature and modus operandi' of hay fever through a 'systematic course of experiments' that he carried out on himself and presented in his seminal publication *Experimental Researches on the Causes and Nature of Catarrhus Aestivus* [18]. Interestingly, the first allergies of *Ambrosia* pollen, which belongs to the Asteraceae family, were described as 'autumnal cattarrh' by Dr. W.M.

4

Wyman (1812–1903) in the USA at about the same time that Blackley was discovering the role of grass pollen in hay fever in England [19].

Blackley's experiments were notable for their methodical approach to evaluating and rejecting other possible causes of hay fever, but his work was not universally and immediately accepted by his peers. In 1903, William P. Dunbar confirmed Blackley's theories about the causal role of pollen [16] and, in 1906, Alfred Wolff-Eisner recognized that it was the proteins in pollen that provoked symptoms in his work concerned with the nature of hay fever and its treatment [20]. Allergy to pollen is now confirmed as being an immunoglobulin E-mediated allergy [1], although our general understanding of the mechanisms of pollen-induced allergy is still to be improved by work into substances such as PALMs [4].

Monitoring and Monitoring Networks

In his publication, Blackley [18] also described novel apparatus that he used for collecting, measuring and following day-to-day and seasonal variations in airborne pollen [16]. These studies allowed him to identify environmental factors that influence the amount of pollen in the atmosphere, such as rainfall, which he described as being able to 'completely clear the air of pollen'. Similar work is still carried out today by operators of pollen-monitoring sites who strive to understand and predict atmospheric concentrations of allergenic pollen [21].

Blackley was not the only investigator during the 19th century who was examining the air flora; a number of other scientists were also developing equipment to conduct aerobiological investigations. Some of the most well-known include the aeroscope invented by Pouchet (1859) and the aeroconiscopes of Maddox (1870) and Cunningham (1873). Pierre Miquel (1850–1922) worked at the Observatoire Montsouris in Paris for more than a quarter of a century and was the first to make a long-term survey of the microbial content of the atmosphere by volumetric methods using a modified aeroscope [6, 22, 23].

The first attempts to standardize aerobiological monitoring came during the 20th century. The gravimetric Durham sampler [24] was adopted by the Pollen and Mold Committee of the American Academy of Allergy. It is easy to use, inexpensive and requires no moving parts or electric power. The main disadvantages are that the volume of air sampled is unknown and so concentrations and efficiency cannot be calculated [25].

The volumetric spore trap was designed by Jim Hirst [26] in 1952. The Hirst-type trap is a sampler with a suction pump that was the forerunner of the modern Burkard (http://www.burkard.co.uk/ and http://www.burkardscientific.co.uk/) and Lanzoni (http://www.lanzoni.it/home.html) traps. Hirst-type volumetric samplers are still operated by the majority of monitoring centers throughout the world [6]. However, rotating impaction samplers are also used, the first of which was the rotorod designed by W.A. Perkins in 1957 [25].

Airborne pollen are monitored in North America by the National Allergy Bureau, which is certified by the American Academy of Allergy, Asthma and Immunology (AAAAI). In Europe, pollen data from participating sites are sent to the European Aeroallergen Network (EAN) database, which was established in the late 1980s [1] and is administered by the Medical University of Vienna. In addition to pollen monitoring, the EU-funded project Health Impacts of Airborne Allergen Information Network (HIALINE; http://www.hialine.com/) created the first limited network for monitoring airborne allergen concentrations.

Today, monitoring of the environment is often based on a combination of measurements and model results. Source-based forecast models include emission source data, a description of emission variation, and an atmospheric transport model system. Such models can improve understanding of pollen levels as they explain situations and processes that are almost impossible to understand using observations alone [21].

Acknowledgements

The authors would like to thank the Society for the Promotion of Palynological Research in Austria (http://www.paldat.org/) for the use of the figures, and particularly Martina Weber and Ursula Schachner for their help and support.

References

1 Rantio Lehtimaki A: Aerobiology of pollen and pollen antigens; in Cox CS, Wathes CM (eds): Bioaerosols Handbook. Florida, CRC Press, 1995, pp 387–406.
2 Zeiger T: Plant Physiology. Sunderland, Sinauer Associates, 1998.
3 Emberlin J: Aerobiology; in Busse WW, Holgate ST (eds): Asthma and Rhinitis. Hoboken, Blackwell Science, 2000, vol 2, pp 1083–1105.
4 Gilles S, Mariani V, Bryce M, Mueller M, Ring J, Behrendt H, Jakob T, Traidl-Hoffmann C: Pollen allergens do not come alone: pollen associated lipid mediators (PALMS) shift the human immune systems towards a TH2-dominated response. Allergy Asthma Clin Immunol 2009;5:3.
5 Gale Biography in Context: Robert Hooke. Gale Document Number: GALE K1631003108.
6 Scheifinger H, Belmonte J, Buters J, Celenk S, Damialis A, Dechamp C, García-Mozo H, Gehrig R, Grewling L, Halley JM, Hogda K-A, Jäger S, Karatzas K, Karlsen S-R, Koch E, Pauling A, Peel R, Sikoparija B, Smith M, Galán-Soldevilla C, Thibaudon M, Vokou D, Weger LA: Monitoring, modelling and forecasting of the pollen season; in Sofiev M, Bergmann K-C (eds): Allergenic Pollen. Dordrecht, Springer, 2013, pp 71–126.
7 Gale Biography in Context: Leeuwenhoek, Anton van (1632–1723). Gale Document Number: GALE A148472101
8 Gale Biography in Context: Malpighi, Marcello (1628–1694). Gale Document Number: GALE A148478013.
9 Pray L: Discovery of DNA structure and function: Watson and crick. Nat Ed 2008;1: 100.
10 Kraaijeveld K, Ventayol-Garcia M, van Schadewijk A, van der Steen L, Hiemstra P, den Dunnen J, De Weger LA: Efficient characterization and quantification of airborne pollen using DNA sequencing: a progress report. Allergol Immunol 2012;9:187.
11 Buters JTM, Kasche A, Weichenmeier I, Schober W, Klaus S, Traidl-Hoffmann C, Menzel A, Huss-Marp J, Krämer U, Behrendt H: Year-to-year variation in release of bet v 1 allergen from birch pollen: evidence for geographical differences between west and south Germany. Int Arch Allergy Immunol 2008;145:122–130.
12 Esch RE: Grass pollen allergens; in Lockey RF, Bukantz SC, Bousqet J (eds): Allergens and Allergen Immunotherapy. New York, Marcel Dekker, 2004.
13 Lequin RM: Enzyme immunoassay (EIA)/enzyme-linked immunosorbent assay (ELISA). Clin Chem 2005;51:2415–2418.
14 Bostock J: Case of a periodical affection of the eyes and chest. Med Chir Trans 1819;10: 161–165.
15 D'Amato G, Cecchi L: Effects of climate change on environmental factors in respiratory allergic diseases. Clin Exp Allergy 2008; 38:1264–1274.
16 Jackson M: Allergy: The History of a Modern Malady. London, Reaktion, 2007.
17 Elliotson J: St. Thomas's hospital: clinical lecture delivered by Dr. Elliotson, 18 June 1831. Lancet 1831;16:366–376.
18 Blackley CH: Experimental Researches on the Causes and Nature of Catarrhus Aestivus (Hay-Fever or Hay-Asthma). Oxford, Oxford Historical Books, 1873.
19 Wyman M: Autumnal catarrh. Boston Med Surg J 1875;93:209–212.
20 Ring J, Gutermuth J: 100 years of hyposensitization: history of allergen-specific immunotherapy (ASIT). Allergy 2011;66:713–724.
21 Smith M, Skjøth CA, Jäger S, Berger UE: Modelling and forecasting: methods in aerobiology. Allergol Immunol 2012;9:75–79.
22 Erdtman G: An Introduction to Pollen Analysis. Waltham, Chronica Botanica, 1943.
23 Gregory PH: The Microbiology of the Atmosphere. London, Leonard Hill, 1961.
24 Durham OC: The volumetric incidence of atmospheric allergens; a proposed standard method of gravity sampling, counting, and volumetric interpolation of results. J Allergy 1946;17:79–86.
25 Ogden EC, Raynor GS, Hayes JV, Lewis DM, Haines JH: Manual for Sampling Airborne Pollen. New York, Hafner Press, 1976.
26 Hirst JM: An automatic volumetric spore trap. Ann Appl Biol 1952;39:257–265.

Dr. Matt Smith
Forschungsgruppe Aerobiologie und Polleninformation
HNO Klinik, Medizinische Universität Wien
Währinger Gürtel 18–20
AT–1090 Wien (Austria)
E-Mail aeromattsmith@gmail.com

Bergmann K-C, Ring J (eds): History of Allergy. Chem Immunol Allergy. Basel, Karger, 2014, vol 100, pp 234–242
DOI: 10.1159/000358860

Mites and Allergy

Enrique Fernández-Caldas[a, b] · Leonardo Puerta[c] · Luis Caraballo[c]

[a]Inmunotek SL, Madrid, Spain; [b]Division of Allergy and Immunology, College of Medicine, University of South Florida, Tampa, Fla., USA; [c]Institute for Immunological Research, University of Cartagena, Cartagena, Colombia

Abstract

Allergic diseases triggered by mite allergens include allergic rhinoconjunctivitis, asthma, atopic dermatitis and other skin diseases. Since the early discovery of the allergenic role of mites of the genus *Dermatophagoides* in the mid 1960s, numerous species have been described as the source of allergens capable of sensitizing and inducing allergic symptoms in sensitized and genetically predisposed individuals. The main sources of allergens in house dust worldwide are the fecal pellets of the mite species *D. pteronyssinus*, *D. farinae*, *Euroglyphus maynei* and the storage mites *Blomia tropicalis*, *Lepidoglyphus destructor* and *Tyropahgus putrescentiae*. Group 1 and 2 allergens are major house dust mite allergens. The main allergens in storage mites include fatty acid-binding proteins, tropomyosin and paramyosin homologues, apolipophorin-like proteins, α-tubulins and others, such as group 2, 5 and 7 allergens. Cross-reactivity is an important and common immunological feature among mites. Currently, purified native or recombinant allergens, epitope mapping, proteomic approaches and T cell proliferation techniques are being used to assess cross-reactivity. Mites contain potent enzymes capable of degrading a wide range of substrates. Most mite allergens are enzymes. Advances in genomics and molecular biology will improve our ability to understand the genetics of specific IgE responses to mites. Mite allergen avoidance and immunotherapy are the only two allergen-specific ways to treat mite-induced respiratory and cutaneous diseases.

In 1922, Giocomo R. Ancona (1886–1976) studied 21 mill workers suffering from asthma and realized that the disease was induced by the grain mite, *Pediculoides ventricosus* [1]. It was novel to establish mites as a possible trigger of asthma and identified a potentially important new source of allergens. Later on, the scientist and physician Willem Storm van Leeuwen (1882–1933; fig. 1) became interested in 'house-dust asthma', inspired by publications in the USA. Cooke [2] suggested in 1922 that a specific allergen could be responsible for the allergenicity of house dust. One of the main problems associated

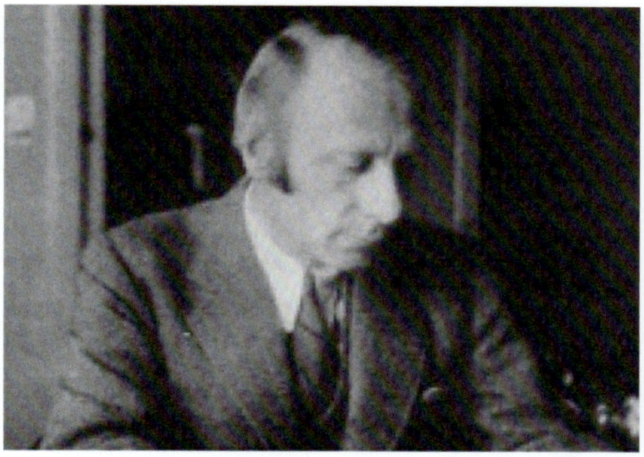

Fig. 1. Willem Storm van Leeuwen.

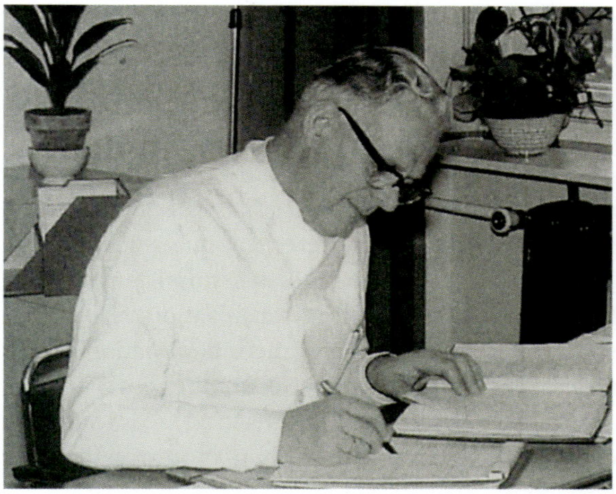

Fig. 2. Reindert Voorhorst.

with house dust was that skin tests with other allergen extracts often remained negative, but provocations with the dust induced asthma attacks. Storm van Leeuwen indicated that 'intradermal skin reactions may serve to diagnose the allergic state, but not to make a specific diagnosis. ... Doubtless cases of allergy exist which give negative skin tests ... with an extract of the allergen which causes the attacks' [3]. In 1923, Storm van Leeuwen conducted a very special experiment. He went with three asthmatic individuals from the Netherlands to the high mountain area near St. Moritz in Switzerland. Within a few days the asthmatic patients were free of asthma symptoms. However, when the patients inhaled house dust contained in a box and sampled from their flats, they also had exacerbations of their asthma in St. Moritz [4].

It had already been known for many years that asthmatic patients had fewer symptoms in high mountain areas, but now an explanation for the reason had been provided. In 1931, Peipers [5] suggested the presence of numerous allergens in house dust. However, it was not until 1964 that the Dutch group comprised of R. Voorhorst (fig. 2) and the married couple F.T. Spieksma and M.I. Spieksma-Boezeman (fig. 3) demonstrated the presence of house dust mites in dust samples collected in flats in Juliana Street in Leiden, the Netherlands (fig. 4). Mrs. Spieksma-Boezeman was able to demonstrate that mites are the main allergen source in house dust [6]. She also established that there were clearly more mites in the dust from a damp house and that the allergen content was also higher. One of the first appreciations of the new idea of mites as the origin of the house dust allergen came from Jack Pepys [7], as well as from other groups that published confirmative reports [8]. Simultaneously, the Japanese biologist Shiro Oshima, trying to identify parasites causing skin afflictions in schoolchildren in Yokohama, reported the finding of *Dermatophagoides* species in 'tatami' floor coverings [9]. Contact with Japanese colleagues resulted in the first confirming report from countries outside of Europe [10]. Many other scientists and physicians collaborated in the discovery and establishment of house dust mites as one of the most important sources of allergens in house dust worldwide, and we extend our most sincere recognition to them all.

Since the early demonstration that dust mites were the origin of the allergenicity of house dust, numerous mite species have been described as the source of allergens capable of sensitizing and inducing allergic symptoms in sensitized and genetically predisposed individuals [11]. The overall treatment of these mite-allergic patients focuses primarily on education, the reduction of allergen exposure, pharmacotherapy to reduce allergic inflammation and bronchoconstriction, and immunotherapy. Patients who are exposed to large quantities of mite allergens may experience a

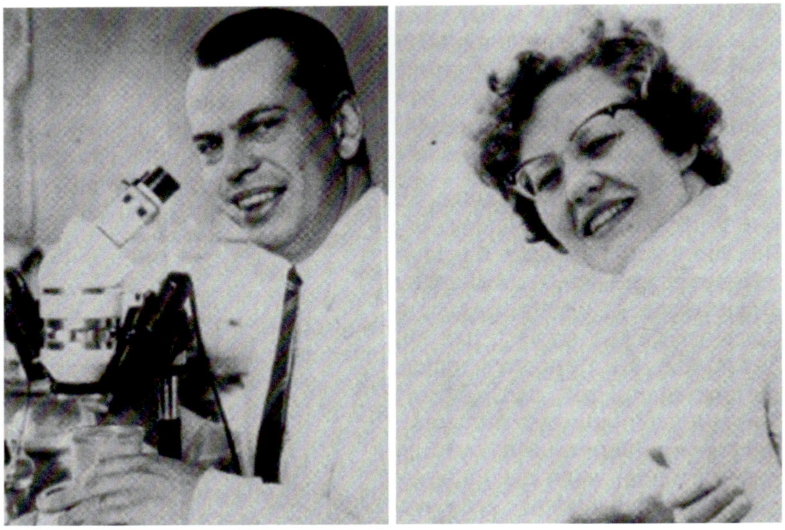

Fig. 3. Family Spieksma: Frits T.M. Spieksma and Marise Spieksma-Boezeman.

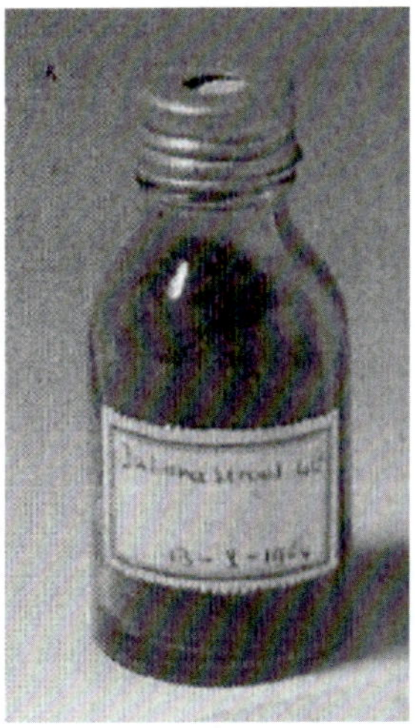

Fig. 4. Bottle with a dust sample collected in 1964 in which mites were detected by Spieksma-Boezeman and Spieksma. The content of the little bottle is a small portion from a mixture of two 5-gram samples of floor dust collected with a vacuum cleaner from the ground floor of a small house in Leiden on October 13, 1964. It was part of a sampling series from three houses with different grades of dampness. The address was Julianastraat 48 and it was the dampest of the three. Samples were taken every 3 weeks. The house does not exist anymore – it was demolished because of poor quality. From the two original 5-gram samples, mites were isolated and counted as described in two published articles [50, 51] and in a personal communication from Frits Spieksma to K.C. Bergmann. Approximately 1,600 mites of the genus *Dermatophagoides*, almost exclusively *D. pteronyssinus*, were identified in the sample.

progressive deterioration in $PD_{20}FEV_1$. This fact is consistent with a chronic inflammatory and remodeling process of the lungs, as has been suggested for several animal models, including rhesus monkeys, sheep and mice [12]. There is ample evidence that continuous exposure to mites is an important risk factor for the development of sensitization, allergic respiratory diseases and chronic inflammation of the lungs. Sensitization to house dust mites is a major independent risk factor for asthma in all areas where the climate is conducive to mite population growth. It has been demonstrated that there is a significant dose-response relationship between exposure to mite allergens and subsequent sensitization. Exposure to house dust mite antigen can induce airway epithelial shedding even in subjects with low eosinophil airway infiltration, thus supporting the idea that epithelial damage in asthmatics sensitized to *Dermatophagoides* may be due to the proteolytic activity of the mite allergens [13].

The most studied species belong to the family Pyroglyphidae, especially *D. pteronyssinus*, *D. farinae* and *Euroglyphus maynei*, and are called house dust mites. House dust mites are commonly present in human dwellings and are especially abundant in mattresses, sofas, carpets and blankets. Numerous mite allergens have been purified, sequenced and cloned. An important group of mites, referred to as 'storage mites', mainly comprises members of the Acaridae and Glycyphagidae families that live in stored food and grains. All mite species present in the home environment and capable of inducing immunoglobulin (Ig) E-mediated sensitization are called 'domestic mites' [14]. Approximately 150 storage mite species are known [15], and approximately 20 can be considered to be important from an economic and sanitary perspective [16]. The most studied species are *Blomia tropicalis*, due to its abundance in tropical and subtropical regions of the world [17], and *Lepidoglyphus destructor*, because of its frequent presence in barns. Storage mite species can be present in kitchen floor dust, cupboards and pantries. In humid homes, storage mites can also be found in mattress dust. They can be an important plague with economical consequences and cause occupational respiratory allergies in farmers and other occupationally exposed individuals. The most important genera are *Lepidoglyphus* (family Glycyphagidae), *Glycyphagus* (family Glycyphagidae), *Acarus* (family Acaridae), *Tyrophagus* (family Acaridae), *Aleuroglyphus* (family Acaridae), *Suidasia* (family Suidasidae), *Chortoglyphus* (family Chortoglyphidae) and *Cheyletus* (family Cheyletidae).

Allergens from House Dust Mites

Mite allergens are present in mite bodies, secretion and excretion. Fecal particles contain the greatest proportion of mite allergen [18]. Mite allergens can be detected in many areas of the home, including beds, carpets, upholstered furniture and clothing. Leather-covered couches, wooden furniture and bare floors contain fewer. Beds are the perfect habitat for mites since they provide the ideal temperature, food and moisture for their proliferation, and the allergens they produce accumulate deep inside mattresses and pillows, especially when they are old. Information on the distribution of house dust mites provides valuable information with which to design environmental control strategies. They can also be detected in the air; studies using volumetric samples equipped with sizing devices have shown that mite allergens remain airborne for a short period of time. Allergenic activity has been detected in particles smaller than 1 μm and in particles larger than 10 μm. It has been suggested that mite fecal pellets may occasionally enter the lung and cause inflammation and bronchoconstriction [19].

Most of the isolated allergens have been placed in groups based on their chronological characterization and/or homology with previously purified allergens. Purified allergens are named according to the first three letters of the genus, the first letter of the species and a number indicating the group in which they are placed. Thus, the first identified allergen of *D. pteronyssinus* was named Der p 1 and belongs to group 1. When several isoforms exist they have to be reflected in the denomination, e.g. Der p 1.0101 and Der p 1.0201. The best-studied groups are group 1 (Der p 1 and Der f 1) and group 2 (Der p 2 and Der f 2). They are considered major allergens based on the frequency of patients sensitized and the amount of specific IgE. In Europe, more than 95% of mite-allergic patients are sensitized to Der p 1 and Der p 2. Der p 1 is a glycoprotein with sequence homology and thiol protease functions similar to the enzymes papain, actinidin, bromelain and cathepsins B and H [20]. Der p 1 may upregulate the IgE synthesis by cleaving the low-affinity IgE receptor (CD23) from the surface of human B cell lymphocytes [21]. Der p 1 may also cleave the α-subunit of the interleukin (IL)-2 receptor (IL-2R or CD25) from the surface of human peripheral blood T cells and, as a result, these cells show markedly diminished proliferation and interferon-γ secretion, which consequently bias the immune response towards Th2 cells. It has been shown that the cysteine protease activity of Der p 1 seems to selectively enhance the IgE response and that the proteolytic activity of Der p 1 conditions T cells to produce more IL-4 and less interferon-γ [22, 23]. The enzymatic activity for Der p 1 and other mite allergens may also contribute to their immunogenicity by increasing mucosal permeability. Der p 1 and Der f 1 also cleave SP-A and SP-D lung collectins which have protective roles in allergy. The cleavage and consequent inactivation of SP-A and SP-D may be a novel mechanism to account for the potent allergenicity of Der p 1 and Der f 1 [24]. Due to its high prevalence in house dust and worldwide distribution, the group 1 allergen is used as a standard to

Table 1. Biological function, molecular weight (MW) and prevalence of specific IgE binding of several mite allergens [adapted from 50]

Group	Biological function	MW, kDa	Mite species	IgE binding, %
1	Cysteine protease	25	Dp, Df, Dm, Ds, Em, Bt, As, Ao, Sm, Tp	70–100
2	Niemann-pick type C2 protein Recognition and binding of lipids; similar to MD-2	14	Dp, Df, Dm, Ds, Em, Ld, Gd, Bt, As, Ao, Sm, Tp	80–100
3	Trypsin	28–30	Dp, Df, Dm, Ds, Em, Gd, Bt, As, Ao, Sm, Tp	16–100
4	α-Amylase	57	Dp, Df, Em, Bt, As, Sm, Tp	25–46
5	Unknown	15	Dp, Df, Ds, Ld, Gd, Bt, Ao, Sm, Tp	50–70
6	Chymotrypsin	25	Dp, Df, Ds, Bt, Ao, Sm	40
7	Lipid-binding protein; similar to proteins in the TLR pathway	22–31	Dp, Df, Ld, Gd, Bt, As, Ao, Sm, Tp	50
8	Glutathione-S-transferase	26	Dp, Df, Ld, Gd, Bt, As, Ao, Sm	40
9	Collagenolytic serine protease	30	Dp, Df, Dm, Bt, Ao, Sm	90
10	Tropomyosin	33–37	Dp, Df, Ld, Gd, Bt, As, Ao, Sm, Tp, Ca	50–95
11	Paramyosin	92–110	Dp, Df, Dm, Bt	80
12	Unknown	14	Bt	50
13	Fatty acid-binding proteins	14–15	Dp, Df, Ld, Gd, Bt, As, Ao, Sm, Tp	10–23
14	Lipid-binding apolipophorin	177	Dp, Df, Dm, Em, Bt	90
15	Chitinase	98–109	Dp, Df, Dm, Bt	70
16	Gelsolin-like protein/villin	53	Df	35
17	EF-hand calcium-binding protein	53	Df	35
18	60-kDa chitinase	60	Dp, Df	50–60
19	Antimicrobial peptide	7.2	Bt	10
20	Arginine kinase	40	Dp, Df, Ao	?
21	Unknown	13.2	Dp, Bt	?
22	Unknown	14	Dp, Df, Ao, As, Tp	?
23	Homology to peritrophin-A domain	14	Dp	74
24	Troponin C	18	Tp	10.6

Ao = *A. ovatus;* As = *A. siro;* Bt = *B. tropicalis;* Ca = *C. arcuatus;* Df = *D. farinae;* Dm = *D. microceras;* Dp = *D. pteronyssinus;* Em = *E. mayne;* Gd = *G. domesticus;* Ld = *L. destructor;* Tp = *T. putrescentiae;* Sm = *S. medanensis.*

estimate environmental exposure to *Dermatophagoides* spp. in the indoor environment.

Der p 2 and Der f 2 are heat- and pH-stable proteins of 14 kDa [25, 26]. These allergens have 88% sequence similarity. In their native stage and expressed as a fusion protein, both have an 83% frequency of specific IgE recognition [27]. Crystallographic studies suggest that Der p 2 is a lipid-binding protein [28]. Der f 2 binds lipopolysaccharide (LPS) in a manner similar to the binding by MD-2. The hydrophobic LPS-binding residues are similar in all of the group 2 allergen sequences [29]. Considering that MD-2 loads LPS onto Toll-like receptor (TLR) 4, it has been suggested that group 2 allergenicity might be enhanced by a similar interaction. It has been demonstrated that rDer p 2 could act directly on airway smooth muscle cells activating the TLR2 signaling pathway, but not on TLR4. A list containing the most relevant and characterized mite allergens is shown in table 1.

Allergens from Storage Mites

Several storage mite allergens have been purified, cloned and sequenced [30]. Some of these allergens can be considered as pan allergens and are present in *B. tropicalis*, *L. destructor*, *G. domesticus*, *T. putres-*

Table 2. Main families and species of storage mites that have been described as allergenic

Family	Species
Glycyphagidae	*Glycyphagus domesticus*
	Glycyphagus privatus
	Gohieria fusca
	Lepidoglyphus destructor
Echimyopodidae	*Blomia tropicalis*
	Blomia kulagini
	Blomia tjibodas
Chortoglyphidae	*Chortoglyphus arcuatus*
Ebertiidae	*Suidasia medanensis*
Acaridae	*Tyrophagus putrescentiae*
	Tyrophagus longior
	Acarus siro
	Acarus farris
	Thyreophagus entomophagus
	Aleuroglyphus ovatus
Cheyletidae	*Cheyletus eruditus*
	Cheyletus tenuipilis
	Cheyletus malaccensis

Table 3. Other mite families and species of allergenic mites, excluding house dust and storage mites

	Family	Species
Parasites of plants	Tetranychidae	*Tetranychus urticae*
		Panonychus ulmi
		Panonychus citri
	Tydeidae	*Pronematus davisi*
Predator	Phytoseiidae	*Amblyseius cucumeris*
		Phytoseiulus persimilis
	Hypoaspidae	*Hypoaspis miles*
	Hemisarcoptidae	*Hemisarcoptes cooremani*
Parasites of animals	Varroaidae	*Varroa* spp.
	Sarcoptidae	*Sarcoptes scabiei*
	Analgidae	*Diplaegidia columbae*
	Ixodidae	*Ixodes pacificus*
		Ixodes holociclus
		Ixodes ricinus
		Riphicephalus spp.
	Argasidae	*Argas reflexus*

centiae, *A. siro*, *A. ovatus*, *S. medanensis* and *Thyreophagus entomophagus*. Table 2 shows a list of the main families and species of storage mites that have been described as allergenic [31]. Some of these allergens have shown sequence homology and biological function similar to those previously described in *Dermatophagoides* spp. (see table 1). The main allergens described in storage mites include fatty acid-binding proteins, tropomyosin and paramyosin homologues, apolipophorin-like proteins, α-tubulins and others, such as group 2, 5 and 7 allergens. A list of other mite families and species of allergenic mites, excluding house dust and storage mites, is shown in table 3.

Cross-Reactivity of Mite Allergens

Cross-reactivity is a common feature among mite allergens, especially in those from taxonomically related species. Cross-reactivity may also be the cause of mite polysensitization, which is observed in some mite-allergic individuals. Cross-reactivity among group 2 allergens from storage mites, *L. destructor*, *T. putrescentiae* and *G. domesticus* is high, whereas there is only limited cross-inhibition between Der p 2 and the non-pyroglyphid mite allergens. This lack of cross-reactivity between Der p 2 and the group 2 of storage mites is a result of the multiple amino acid substitutions across the surface [32]. Other studies have shown limited cross-reactivity between *D. pteronyssinus*, *L. destructor* and *T. putrescentiae* [33, 34], but others have reported a greater cross-reactivity between *Dermatophagoides* and *T. putresentiae* [35]. A low degree of cross-reactivity between *D. pteronyssinus*, *A. siro* and *T. putrescentiae* was described in one study, whereas cross-reactivity between *L. destructor* and *A. siro* was high [36]. Individuals allergic to the *Dermatophagoides* spp. may experience allergic symptoms after eating crustaceans and mollusks. Der f 10 and Der p 10, proteins with homology to tropomyosin from various animals, are involved in the cross-reactivity among *Dermatophagoides* spp., mollusks and crustaceans. The 36-kDa cross-reactive tropomyosin present in mites, various insects (chironomids, mosquitoes and cockroaches) and shrimp [37] is responsible for cross-reactivity among different arthropods [38]. Immunochemical studies have demonstrated that allergens from snails, crustaceans, cockroaches and chironomids cross-react with house dust mite allergens. However, house dust mites are usually the primary source of sensitizing allergens.

Tropomyosin is also involved in the cross-reactivity between mites and parasites. A high degree of cross-reactivity between extracts of house dust mites and *Ascaris* has been demonstrated. Several allergens are implicated, such as tropomyosin and glutathione-S-tranferases [39]. *A. lumbricoides* tropomyosin (Asc l 3) is an allergen cross-reactive with mite tropomyosins. IgE reactivity to this allergen is very frequent in both asthmatic and normal subjects sensitized to *Ascaris* [40]. Filarial and mite tropomyosins are similar, with a 72% identity at the amino acid level and overlapping predicted 3D structures. Filarial infection induces strong cross-reactive anti-tropomyosin antibody responses that may affect sensitization and regulation of allergic reactivity.

Effect of Parasitic Infections on Mite Allergy

The association of allergy with helminthiases was perceived before the discovery of IgE. However, being able to detect blood levels of this antibody allowed the discovery of the first shared phenotype between ascariasis and asthma: high total IgE levels. This raised the idea that the allergic and anti-parasitic immune responses were similar and, in addition, helminth infections could increase the symptoms of allergy. However, later studies have shown a low prevalence of both allergy and positivity of skin tests (including mites) in areas of great endemicity of helminth infections, suggesting that chronic and high-parasite-load infections induce immunosuppression, an aspect that has been widely documented in recent years although the mechanisms are not fully elucidated [41, 42]. Similarly, in regions with low endemicity where helminth infections are mild-to-moderate and deworming programs are permanent, it has been shown that allergic diseases such as asthma are more common. This is an important historical point since it involves the manifestations of allergy in almost half of the world's population, among which hygiene conditions are improving progressively, the severity of parasitic infections is diminishing and the prevalence of allergies is increasing, especially in urban settings [43]. An important advancement has been made with the description of cross-reactivity between mites and *Ascaris* allergens [39]. Several scenarios should be considered to explain the immunological interaction between mites and parasites. First, there are many chances of early life exposure to allergens from mites and antigens and *A. lumbricoides*. This has been observed in children from tropical regions [44, 45]. Second, parasitized preschool and school-aged children in underdeveloped tropical countries receive regular anti-helminth drug therapy during mass deworming programs. Since the fundamental socio-economic causes of the infections are not eliminated, children become re-infected several times and this sort of modified secondary immune response may be boosters of the IgE reactivity against cross-reactive allergens from other sources (e.g. mites). Third, mite allergen exposure is perennial and very intense in the tropics; therefore, in the *Ascaris*-infected population (current or past) susceptible to asthma, this may be another cause of the increasing IgE responses to cross-reactive allergens. To better study the effects of the immune responses to *Ascaris* on allergy, it is important to identify the molecules that induce allergy symptoms, those that generate a protective IgE immune response and those that promote both effects. A systematic approach to identify the antigens and allergens of *A. lumbricoides*, inducing immune responses in humans, is needed.

Environmental Control

The methods recommended for reducing exposure to house dust mite allergens have not changed much over the last 30 years. The implementation of these methods has provided inconsistent clinical benefit [46], especially in longitudinal prevention studies. However, studies using very strict measures have produced positive results. Evidence that mite allergy is more common in certain countries suggests that there are critical environmental factors which influence the prevalence, incidence and severity of mite-allergic asthma. The main question remains of whether we are able to control or influence these conditions. It is well established that ambient humidity and temperature are important factors for the development of mite allergy. Other factors, such as exposure to irritants, adjuvants or substances interacting directly with the innate immune system, remain less clear. The role of allergen exposure in the etiology of allergic sensitization and asthma is very complex [47]. Allergen avoidance is a successful treatment for occupational asthma in many settings and, as such, it should be considered for other occupational or environmental diseases. Although many strategies may reduce allergen levels, its effect in reducing inflammation is not so obvious. Removal of carpets, changing old mite-infested mattresses, pillows and sofas, and improving ventilation are all changes that make sense, but in some cases are not enough to produce a clinical benefit. It is also evident that a successful strategy would be attacking the mite reservoirs with a combination of methods – just one action alone is not enough. Controlling exposure to mite aeroallergens and adjuvant factors seems mandatory.

Mite Immunotherapy

Sensitivity and exposure to high levels of mite allergens is an important risk factor for developing and maintaining bronchial hyperreactivity [48]. However, in light of publications that have shown pessimistic results using environmental control measures, immunotherapy with mite extracts has emerged as a solid treatment of mite-induced allergic respiratory diseases. Numerous studies have shown the efficacy of mite sublingual and subcutaneous immunotherapy [12]. The future treatment of mite-induced allergies will not be changed much, although it will be based on a more accurate diagnosis and better immunotherapy treatments. The need to improve the quality of current allergen extracts for diagnosis and treatment is clear [49].

References

1 Ancona A: Asma bronchiale anafilattico. 2. Asma epidemic da pediculosis ventricosus. Sperimentale 1922;6:270.

2 Cooke RA: Studies in specific hypersensitiveness. 4. New etiologic factors in bronchial asthma. J Immunol 1922;7:147.

3 Storm van Leeuwen W: Allergic Diseases: Diagnosis and Treatment of Bronchial Asthma, Hay Fever and Other Allergic Diseases. Philadelphia, Lippincott, 1925, pp 41, 43.

4 Storm van Leeuwen W: Bronchial asthma in relation to climate. Proc R Soc Med 1924;17:19–26.

5 Peipers A: Über die Frage der Identität des Hausstauballergens. Z Immun Forsch 1931; 71:359.

6 Voorhosrt R, Spieksma-Boezeman MI, Spieksma FT: Is a mite (*Dermatophagoides* spp) the producer of the house-dust mite allergen? Allerg Asthma (Leipz) 1964; 10:329–334.

7 Pepys J, Chan M, Hargreave FE: Mites and house-dust allergy. Lancet 1968;i:1270–1272.

8 Brown HM, Filer JL: Role of mites in allergy to house dust. Br Med J 1968;3:646–647.

9 Oshima S: Observations of floor mites collected in Yokohama. 1. On the mites found in several schools in summer. Jap J San Zool 1964;15:233–244.

10 Miyamoto T, Oshima S, Ishizaki T, Sato S: Allergenic identity between the common floor mite *(Dermatophagoides farinae)* and house dust as a causative antigen in bronchial asthma. J Allergy 1968;42:14–28.

11 Voorhosrt R, Spieksma FTM, Varekamp H: House Dust Atopy and the House Dust Mite *Dermatophagoides pteronyssinus* (Troueessart, 1897). Leiden, Stafleu's Scientific, 1969.

12 Fernández-Caldas E, Iraola V, Boquete M, Nieto A, Casanovas M: Mite immunotherapy. Curr Allergy Asthma Rep 2006;6:413–419.

13 Piacentini GL, Vicentini L, Mazzi P, Chilosi M, Martinati L, Boner AL: Mite-antigen avoidance can reduce bronchial epithelial shedding in allergic asthmatic children. Clin Exp Allergy 1998;28:561–567.

14 Platts-Mills TA, Vervloet D, Thomas WR, et al: Indoor allergens and asthma: report of the Third International Workshop. J Allergy Clin Immunol 1997;100:S2–S24.

15 Smiley RL: The ordinal and subordinal names of mites with a list of mite pests of stored food products. Proc Int Work Conf Stored Prod Entomol 1983;3:37–43.

16 Fernández-Caldas E: Mite species of allergologic importance in Europe. Allergy 1997; 52:383–387.

17 Fernández-Caldas E, Lockey RF: *Blomia tropicalis*, a mite whose time has come. Allergy 2004;59:1161–1164.

18 Tovey ER, Chapman MD, Platts-Mills TAE: Mite feces are a major source of house dust allergens. Nature 1982;289:592–593.

19 Fergusson P, Broide DH: Environmental and bronchoalveolar lavage *Dermatophagoides pteronyssinus* antigen levels in tropic asthmatics. Am J Respir Crit Care Med 1995;151:71–74.

20 Chua KY, Stewart GA, Thomas WR, Simpson RJ, Dilworth RJ, Plozza TM, Turner KJ: Sequence analysis of cDNA coding for a major house dust mite allergen, Der p 1 homology with cysteine proteases. J Exp Med 1988;167:175–182.

21 Hewitt CRA, Brown AP, Hart BJ, et al: A major house dust mite allergen disrupts the immunoglobulin E network by selectively clearing CD23: innate protection by antiproteases. J Exp Med 1995;182:1537–1544.

22 Gough L, Sewell HF, Shakib F: The proteolytic activity of the major dust mite allergen Der p 1 enhances the IgE antibody response to a bystander antigen. Clin Exp Allergy 2001;31:1594–1598.

23 Ghaemmaghami AM, Robins A, Gough L, Sewell HF, Shakib F: Human T cell subset commitment determined by the intrinsic property of antigen: the proteolytic activity of the major mite allergen Der p 1 conditions T cells to produce more IL-4 and less IFN-γ. Eur J Immunol 2001;31:1211–1216.

24 Deb R, Shakib F, Reid K, Clark H: Major house dust mite allergens Der p 1 and Der f 1 degrade and inactivate lung surfactant proteins-A and -D. J Biol Chem 2007;282: 36808–36819.

25 Ovsyannikova IG, Vailes LD, Li Y, Heymann PW, Chapman MD: Monoclonal antibodies to group II *Dermatophagoides* spp allergens: murine immune response, epitope analysis, and development of a two-site ELISA. J Allergy Clin Immunol 1994;94: 537–546.

26 Lombardero M, Heymann PW, Platts-Mills TA, Fox JW, Chapman MD: Conformational stability of B cell epitopes on group I and group II *Dermatophagoides* spp allergens: effect of thermal and chemical denaturation on the binding of murine IgG and human IgE antibodies. J Immunol 1990;144:1353–1360.

27 Chua KY, Doyle CR, Simpson RJ, Turner KJ, Stewart GA, Thomas WR: Isolation of cDNA coding for the major mite allergen Der p 2 by IgE plaque immunoassay. Int Arch Allergy Appl Immunol 1990;91:118–123.

28 Derewenda U, Li J, Derewenda Z, Dauter Z, Mueller GA, Rule GS, Benjamin DC: The crystal structure of a major dust mite allergen Der p 2, and its biological implications. J Mol Biol 2002;318:189–197.

29 Ichikawa S, Takai T, Yashiki T, Takahashi S, Okumura K, Ogawa H, Kohda D, Hatanaka H: Lipopolysaccharide binding of the mite allergen Der f 2. Genes Cells 2009;14:1055–1065.

30 Fernández-Caldas E, Iraola V, Carnés J: Molecular and biochemical properties of storage mites (except *Blomia* species). Protein Pept Lett 2007;14:954–959.

31 Fernández-Caldas E, Iraola Calvo V: Mite allergens. Curr Allergy Asthma Rep 2005;5: 402–410.

32 Smith AM, Benjamin DC, Hozic N, Derewenda U, Smith WA, Thomas WR, Gafvelin G, van Hage-Hamsten M, Chapman MD: The molecular basis of antigenic cross-reactivity between the group 2 mite allergens. J Allergy Clin Immunol 2001;107: 977–984.

33 Luczynska CM, Griffin P, Davies RJ, Topping MD: Prevalence of specific IgE to storage mites *(A. siro, L. destructor* and *T. longior)* in an urban population and crossreactivity with the house dust mite *(D. pteronyssinus)*. Clin Exp Allergy 1990;20: 403–406.

34 van Hage-Hamsten M, Johansson SG, Johansson E, Wiren A: Lack of allergenic cross-reactivity between storage mites and *Dermatophagoides pteronyssinus*. Clin Allergy 1987;17:23–31.

35 Park JW, Ko SH, Yong TS, Ree HI, Jeoung BJ, Hong CS: Cross-reactivity of Tyrphagus putrescentiae with *Dermatophagoides farinae* and *Dermatophagoides pteronyssinus* in urban areas. Ann Allergy Asthma Immunol 1999;83:533–539.

36 Johansson E, Johansson SG, Van Hage-Hamsten M: Allergenic characterization of *Acarus siro* and *Tyrophagus putrescentiae* and their crossreactivity with *Lepidoglyphus destructor* and *Dermatophagoides pteronyssinus*. Clin Exp Allergy 1994;24: 743–751.

37 Witteman AM, Akkerdaas JH, van Leeuwen J, van der Zee JS, Aalberse RC: Identification of a cross-reactive allergen (presumably tropomyosin) in shrimp, mite and insects. Int Arch Allergy Immunol 1994;105:56–61.

38 van Ree R, Antonicelli L, Akkerdaas JH, Pajno GB, Barberio G, Corbetta L, Ferro G, Zambito M, Garritani MS, Aalberse RC, Bonifazi F: Asthma after consumption of snails in house-dust-mite-allergic patients: a case of IgE cross-reactivity. Allergy 1996; 51:387–393.

39 Acevedo N, Sánchez J, Erler A, Mercado D, Briza P, Kennedy M, Fernandez A, Gutierrez M, Chua KY, Cheong N, Jiménez S, Puerta L, Caraballo L: IgE cross-reactivity between *Ascaris* and domestic mite allergens: the role of tropomyosin and the nematode polyprotein ABA-1. Allergy 2009;64: 1635–1643.

40 Acevedo N, Erler A, Briza P, Puccio F, Ferreira F, Caraballo L: Allergenicity of *Ascaris lumbricoides* tropomyosin and IgE sensitization among asthmatic patients in a tropical environment. Int Arch Allergy Immunol 2011;154:195–206.

41 Cooper PJ: Interactions between helminth parasites and allergy. Curr Opin Allergy Clin Immunol 2009;9:29–37.

42 Maizels RM: Parasite immunomodulation and polymorphisms of the immune system. J Biol 2009;8:62.

43 Caraballo L, Acevedo N: New allergens of relevance in tropical regions: the impact of *Ascaris lumbricoides* infections. WAO J 2011;4:77–84.

44 Hagel I, Cabrera M, Hurtado MA, Sanchez P, Puccio F, Di Prisco MC, Palenque M: Infection by *Ascaris lumbricoides* and bronchial hyper reactivity: an outstanding association in Venezuelan school children from endemic areas. Acta Trop 2007;103:231–241.

45 López N, de Barros-Mazon S, Vilela MM, Condino Neto A, Ribeiro JD: Are immunoglobulin E levels associated with early wheezing? A prospective study in Brazilian infants. Eur Respir J 2002;20:640–645.

46 Tovey E, Ferro A: Time for new methods for avoidance of house dust mite and other allergens. Curr Allergy Asthma Rep 2012;12: 465–477.

47 Tovey ER, Marks GB: It's time to rethink mite allergen avoidance. J Allergy Clin Immunol 2011;128:723–727.

48 Sears MR, Greene JM, Willan AR, et al: A longitudinal, population-based, cohort study of childhood asthma followed to adulthood. N Engl J Med 2003;349:1414–1422.

49 Chen KW, Blatt K, Thomas WR, Swoboda I, Valent P, Valenta R, Vrtala S: Hypoallergenic Der p 1/Der p 2 combination vaccines for immunotherapy of house dust mite allergy. J Allergy Clin Immunol 2012;130:435–443.

50 Spieksma FTM, Spieksma-Boezeman MIA: The mite fauna of house dust with particular reference to the house-dust mite *Dermatophagoides pteronyssinus* (Trouessart, 1897). Acarologia 1967;9:226–241.

51 Voorhorst R, Spieksma FTM, Varekamp H, Leupen MJ, Lyklema A W: The house-dust mite *(Dermatophagoides pteronyssinus)* and the allergens it produces: identity with the house-dust allergen. J Allergy 1967;39: 325–339.

Dr. Enrique Fernández-Caldas
Inmunotek SL
Calle Punto Mobi, 5
ES–28805 Alcalá de Henares, Madrid (Spain)
E-Mail efcaldas@inmunotek.com

Bergmann K-C, Ring J (eds): History of Allergy. Chem Immunol Allergy. Basel, Karger, 2014, vol 100, pp 243–247
DOI: 10.1159/000358862

Mammalian Airborne Allergens

Rob C. Aalberse

Sanquin Blood Supply Foundation and Academic Medical Centre, Amsterdam, The Netherlands

Abstract

Historically, horse dandruff was a favorite allergen source material. Today, however, allergic symptoms due to airborne mammalian allergens are mostly a result of indoor exposure, be it at home, at work or even at school. The relevance of mammalian allergens in relation to the allergenic activity of house dust extract is briefly discussed in the historical context of two other proposed sources of house dust allergenic activity: mites and Maillard-type lysine-sugar conjugates. Mammalian proteins involved in allergic reactions to airborne dust are largely found in only 2 protein families: lipocalins and secretoglobins (Fel d 1-like proteins), with a relatively minor contribution of serum albumins, cystatins and latherins. Both the lipocalin and the secretoglobin family are very complex. In some instances this results in a blurred separation between important and less important allergenic family members. The past 50 years have provided us with much detailed information on the genomic organization and protein structure of many of these allergens. However, the complex family relations, combined with the wide range of post-translational enzymatic and non-enzymatic modifications, make a proper qualitative and quantitative description of the important mammalian indoor airborne allergens still a significant proteomic challenge.

For quite some time horse allergen was a favorite study object, partially due to the easy availability of large quantities of horse dandruff. Horse serum albumin was implicated from the start in allergic reactions as it was available for testing via the simple fractionation of plasma proteins into albumin and globulins. However, with the advent of more sophisticated biochemical fractionation procedures, pioneered in the allergen field by Dennis Stanworth in Birmingham, UK, it became clear that the major allergenic activity was not plasma derived. In 1957, he described a glycoprotein with a molecular weight of 34 kDa (calculated from the osmotic pressure of the protein solution) [1]. This description fits remarkably well with our current view on Equ c 1, a dimeric, glycosylated lipocalin.

Mammalian Allergens and the Identification of 'the House Dust Allergen'

A close proximity to the offending animal was an obvious reason to causally relate substances from the animal to the allergic symptoms of the patient. It took some time before it was widely accepted that mammalian allergens were an important source of indoor allergens and contributed substantially to the allergenicity of house dust extract, even when no mammalian pets were present. At least 3 issues contributed to this delay in acceptance. Firstly, the skin test reactivity of an extract prepared from dust collected from locations without pets was not obviously lower than that of regular house dust extracts. Secondly, the enthusiasm following the identification of house dust mites by Voorhorst et al. [2] as an important new source of indoor allergens led many allergists to conclude that all indoor allergies were due to these mites [see also Fernández-Caldas et al., this vol., pp. 234–242]. However, sceptics who were not convinced by the importance of mites were often attracted by a radically different explanation: products of the Maillard reaction as the universal allergenic structures.

The Postulated Role of Maillard Reaction Products

In 1966, Bleumink and Berrens [3] hit the pages of *Nature* with reports of their experiments with lactoglobulin. They showed that the skin test activity of lactoglobulin was increased by the incubation of the protein with some simple sugars under conditions that were favorable for the Maillard reaction. This non-enzymatic reaction between the sugar and lysines in proteins had been thoroughly studied by food chemists because it caused changes in the color (browning) and taste of foods. This observation, combined with the brownish color of many allergen extracts (and also of the few 'purified' allergens that were available at the time), led Berrens to the hypothesis that allergenicity was due to these lysine-sugar products. Differences in allergenicity were assumed to be due to quantitative and qualitative differences in the condensation products. According to this hypothesis extracts of animal dander were not essentially different from other allergens (including house dust extracts) – it was all a single type of reactivity. The type of carrier protein was considered to be of little relevance. The public debates between Voorhorst and Berrens on the merits of mites and lysine sugars, respectively, were highly memorable.

When radioallergosorbent test (RAST) and RAST inhibition studies showed that immunoglobulin (Ig) E binding to house dust extract was predominantly due to components in mite extracts, but also that the content of cat allergen was sufficient to contribute at least as much to IgE binding to house dust from sera selected to be mite negative and cat positive [4, 5], neither Voorhorst nor Berrens were willing to accept these results. Both felt that these results just showed that IgE had nothing to do with atopic allergy as they knew it. It took the extraordinary explosion of biochemical technologies to fully settle this debate. It was only after the second international workshop on indoor allergens [6] that the ubiquitous indoor presence of cat allergens, even in the absence of cats, became generally accepted.

Developments in Technologies for the Characterization of Allergens

Until IgE-based techniques became available, allergenicity measurements depended on titrated skin tests. Even if finding volunteers for testing allergenic fractions was easier at that time (before 1970), a biochemist's task was difficult: the high sensitivity of the skin test was not really an advantage, whereas the poor precision was a major obstacle for allergen characterization. With the advent IgE came RAST and RAST inhibition [7]. IgE-based electrophoretic procedures such as crossed radioimmunoelectrophoresis, CRIE [8] and immunoblotting [9] proved to be powerful analytical tools.

Monoclonal antibodies to mammalian allergens such as Fel d 1 became available in the mid-1980s as anti-Fel d 1 [10]. These monoclonal antibodies have proven to be extremely valuable both for analytical as well as preparative purposes.

The most important technical development was undoubtedly the cloning and expression of allergens via recombinant DNA technology. Whereas screening of phage libraries was very successful for mites and pollen allergens, this approach did not work as well with the mammalian allergens. The first mammalian allergens were cloned using an alternative strategy: fragments of the purified allergen were chemically sequenced and subsequently this amino acid sequence information was used to devise DNA probes suitable for PCR amplification of cDNA. Using the pure allergens, high-resolution structural information from X-ray crystallography allowed a detailed view of these allergens. Early examples were lipocalin allergens from rat and mouse in 1992 [11]. The 3D structure of the secretoglobin allergen Fel d 1 was initially problematic, but was soon corrected by the same authors [12].

These technological developments have solved many of the uncertainties in the allergen field. This may have generated the idea that understanding mammalian allergens is basically simple – lipocalins, secretoglobins and serum albumins, and possibly also cystatins [13] and latherins [14, 15] – if you know these few protein families, you may think you know it (almost) all. However, having now much more precise information than we may have wished for, we are facing new questions, some of which were quite unexpected.

Persistent Contaminants and Mind-Boggling Complexities

Considering the life cycle of airborne allergens, it should not come as a surprise that the allergen at its final allergological destination (an antigen-presenting cell, a B cell or a mast cell) is not a textbook-type protein anymore [16]. Instead, it has been exposed to enzymatic and non-enzymatic attacks, possibly including exposure to aggressive atmospheric agents, and it may have encountered a variety of molecules that it might combine with. Attempts to isolate allergens from real-life source materials such as house dust have to contend with this. Hard as this may be, it is an important aspect of allergen characterization. For an overview of the recent developments in the characterization of variants of natural allergen, see Chapman and Briza [17].

One aspect is the problem of contaminants. Some contaminants, such as proteins from mites, fleas and yeasts in skin-derived source material, might be considered trivial from a biochemist's perspective in the sense that they just represent some more proteins to monitor and to get rid of. The tougher challenge is how to deal with components forming complexes with the allergen. One issue is the enzymatic activity of some purified natural allergens that is not found in their recombinant counterpart, with the proteolytic activity of Fel d 1 as a well-documented example [18]. Based on the structure of the protein it is unlikely to be a proteolytic enzyme, so a persistent contaminating enzyme is a logical explanation. However, it might be argued that such a persistent contaminant is part of a complex natural allergen.

Another aspect contributing to the complexity of allergen source materials is the existence of large families of closely related proteins that are hard to separate, while their immunological properties may be quite distinct. Well-established examples in the allergen field are the lipocalins (allergens from cow, horse, dog and rodents) and the Fel d 1-related proteins belonging to the secretoglobin family.

4

The Lipocalin Family

Urinary proteins from rodents were studied extensively by Dr. Joan Longbottom, a biochemist working in the lab of Jack Pepys [19]. She had already noticed the presence of allergen variants with distinct but overlapping properties. These proteins were cloned for reasons other than allergy – they are carriers of pheromones and thus important for the social life of rodents. Variants of these pheromone carriers are possibly involved in determining individual scents [20].

When 2 of the major dog allergens were cloned, they were both found to belong to the lipocalin family [21], but they were not closely related (sequence identity was <30%, with little or no obvious cross-reactivity). Whereas Can f 2 was related to the rodent urinary proteins, Can f 1 was not a urinary protein or a product of the major salivary glands, but was instead a lipocalin derived from minor salivary glands on the back of the tongue implicated in taste perception [22].

While many lipocalins are secretory, ligand-binding proteins, this is by no means true for all. Some are sufficiently related to an IgE-inducing lipocalin to be cross-reactive, possibly without being relevant in relation to allergic sensitization or symptoms.

The Secretoglobin Family

In 1973, a major cat allergen was isolated from cat pelt. It was initially named Cat 1 [23], and later became Fel d 1. Biochemical analysis of natural Fel d 1, purified using a monoclonal antibody, had indicated that is was likely to be a homodimer of a heterodimer of a larger and a smaller chain. When it was cloned in 1991 [24], these 2 chains were found to be products of separate genes, rather than produced as a cleaved single-chain protein precursor. Recombinant production was achieved initially by expressing each chain separately [25], with substantial IgE-binding activity to both chains. Currently, it is obtained by recombinant expression of one of various single-chain fusion proteins; for an example, see Kaiser et al. [12].

At the time of cloning only a few distantly related proteins were known, and the 2 Fel d 1 chains were not considered to be homologues. With the recognition of the secretoglobin family of small secreted mammalian proteins, both Fel d 1 chains are now considered to be members. In mice the subfamily of androgen-binding proteins has expanded to 64 members ('evolutionary bloom'), whereas in humans there are only 6 [26].

Perspective: From Dust Back to Dust

The spiral stairs of history have brought us back to a state of confusion, but at a substantially higher level. We need to consider the life cycle of the allergen molecule. The pristine beauty of crystalline allergens will have to be translated back into the dust of real-life allergen exposure. We need to establish which allergens are actually in the airborne dust, and how the environment has changed each of these proteins since the ribosome delivered them into the world. As discussed for the pollen allergens [17], a close collaboration between the fields of molecular biology and quantitative proteomics is needed to obtain qualitative and quantitative information on exposure to real-life allergens. However, for indoor allergens such as mammalian allergens the relevant source material, house dust, is an even bigger challenge than pollen.

References

1 Stanworth DR: The isolation and identification of horse-dandruff allergen. Biochem J 1957;11:170–191.
2 Voorhorst R, Spieksma-Boezeman MI, Spieksma FT: Is a mite (*Dermatophagoides* sp.) the producer of the house-dust allergen? Allerg Asthma (Leipz) 1964;10:329–334.
3 Bleumink E, Berrens L: Synthetic approaches to the biological activity of β-lactoglobulin in human allergy to cows' milk. Nature 1966;212:541–543.
4 Aalberse RC, Hoorweg E, Reerink-Brongers EE: Interactions between IgE and house dust extract as studied by the radioallergosorbent test (RAST). Dev Biol Stand 1975; 29:197–207.
5 Aalberse RC: Allergens in house dust. Acta Otorhinolaryngol Belg 1978;32:25–31.
6 Platts-Mills TA, Thomas WR, Aalberse RC, Vervloet D, Chapman MD: Dust mite allergens and asthma: report of a second international workshop. J Allergy Clin Immunol 1992;89:1046–1060.
7 Ponterius G, Brandt R, Hulten E, Yman L: Comparative studies on the allergens of horse dandruff and horse serum. Int Arch Allergy Appl Immunol 1973;44:679–691.
8 Løwenstein H, Markussen B, Weeke B: Identification of allergens in extract of horse hair and dandruff by means of crossed radioimmunoelectrophoresis. Int Arch Allergy Appl Immunol 1976;51:38–47.
9 Sutton R, Wrigley CW, Baldo BA: Detection of IgE- and IgG-binding proteins after electrophoretic transfer from polyacrylamide gels. J Immunol Methods 1982;52:183–194.
10 Aalberse RC: Monoclonal antibodies in allergen standardization. Arb Paul Ehrlich Inst 1983;78:137–140.
11 Böcskei Z, Groom CR, Flower DR, Wright CE, Phillips SE, Cavaggioni A, Findlay JB, North AC: Pheromone binding to two rodent urinary proteins revealed by X-ray crystallography. Nature 1992;360:186–188.
12 Kaiser L, Velickovic TC, Badia-Martinez D, Adedoyin J, Thunberg S, Hallen D, Berndt K, Gronlund H, Gafvelin G, van Hage M, Achour A: Structural characterization of the tetrameric form of the major cat allergen Fel d 1. J Mol Biol 2007;370:714–727.
13 Ichikawa K, Vailes LD, Pomés A, Chapman MD: Molecular cloning, expression and modelling of cat allergen, cystatin (Fel d 3), a cysteine protease inhibitor. Clin Exp Allergy 2001;31:1279–1286.

14 Goubran-Botros H, Poncet P, Rabillon J, Fontaine T, Laval JM, David B: Biochemical characterization and surfactant properties of horse allergens. Eur J Biochem 2001;268:3126–3136.

15 Smith W, O'Neil SE, Hales BJ, Chai TL, Hazell LA, Tanyaratsrisakul S, Piboonpocanum S, Thomas WR: Two newly identified cat allergens: the von Ebner gland protein Fel d 7 and the latherin-like protein Fel d 8. Int Arch Allergy Immunol 2011;156:159–170.

16 Van Milligen FJ, van Swieten P, Aalberse RC: Structure of the major cat allergen Fel d 1 in different allergen sources: an immunoblotting analysis with monoclonal antibodies against denatured Fel d 1 and human IgE. Int Arch Allergy Immunol 1992;99:63–73.

17 Chapman MD, Briza P: Molecular approaches to allergen standardization. Curr Allergy Asthma Rep 2012;12:478–484.

18 Ring PC, Wan H, Schou C, Kroll Kristensen A, Roepstorff P, Robinson C: The 18-kDa form of cat allergen *Felis domesticus* 1 (Fel d 1) is associated with gelatin- and fibronectin-degrading activity. Clin Exp Allergy 2000;30:1085–1096.

19 Walls AF, Longbottom JL: Quantitative immunoelectrophoretic analysis of rat allergen extracts. 1. Antigenic characterisation of fur, urine, saliva and other rat-derived materials. Allergy 1983;38:419–431.

20 Hurst JL, Payne CE, Nevison CM, Marie AD, Humphries RE, Robertson DH, Cavaggioni A, Beynon RJ: Individual recognition in mice mediated by major urinary proteins. Nature 2001;414:631–634.

21 Flower DR, North AC, Sansom CE: The lipocalin protein family: structural and sequence overview. Biochim Biophys Acta 2000;1482:9–24.

22 Konieczny A, Morgenstern JP, Bizinkauskas CB, Lilley CH, Brauer AW, Bond JF, Aalberse RC, Wallner BP, Kasaian MT: The major dog allergens, Can f 1 and Can f 2, are salivary lipocalin proteins: cloning and immunological characterization of the recombinant forms. Immunology 1997;92:577–586.

23 Ohman JL, Lowell FC, Bloch KJ: Allergens of mammalian origin: characterization of allergen extracted from cat pelts. J Allergy Clin Immunol 1973;52:231–241.

24 Morgenstern JP, Griffith IJ, Brauer AW, Rogers BL, Bond JF, Chapman MD, Kuo MC: Amino acid sequence of Fel d 1, the major allergen of the domestic cat: protein sequence analysis and cDNA cloning. Proc Natl Acad Sci USA 1991;88:9690–9694.

25 Rogers BL, Morgenstern JP, Garman RD, Bond JF, Kuo MC: Expression, purification, IgE binding and reaction with cat-allergic human T cells. Mol Immunol 1993;30:559–568.

26 Jackson BC, Thompson DC, Wright MW, McAndrews M, Bernard A, Nebert DW, Vasiliou V: Update of the human secretoglobin *(SCGB)* gene superfamily and an example of 'evolutionary bloom' of androgen-binding protein genes within the mouse *Scgb* gene superfamily. Hum Genomics 2011;5:691–702.

Dr. R.C. Aalberse
Sanquin Blood Supply Foundation and Academic Medical Centre
Plesmanlaan 125
NL–1066 CX Amsterdam (The Netherlands)
E-Mail r.aalberse@sanquin.nl

Bergmann K-C, Ring J (eds): History of Allergy. Chem Immunol Allergy. Basel, Karger, 2014, vol 100, pp 248–255
DOI: 10.1159/000358863

The Latex Story

Monika Raulf

Institute for Prevention and Occupational Medicine of the German Social Accident Insurance, Institute of the Ruhr University Bochum, Bochum, Germany

Abstract

The milky sap of the rubber tree *Hevea brasiliensis* is the source of the commercial production of natural rubber latex (NRL) devices, and also represents a source of potent allergenic proteins. NRL materials were introduced in the health care field in about 1840 with the advent of technical abilities to produce suitable and flexible NRL materials for medical products, especially gloves. In the late 1980s, with the increase of transmittable diseases, particularly HIV infection, the use of NRL gloves increased dramatically. During the 1990s, NRL emerged as a major cause of clinically relevant allergy in health care workers using NRL gloves and spina bifida patients with operation on the first day. The increased recognition of NRL allergies, the enhanced research on allergen characterization and sensitization mechanisms, and education about this allergy in health care facilities combined with the introduction of powder-free gloves with reduced protein levels are all factors associated with a decline in the number of suspected cases of NRL allergies in the late 1990s. NRL allergy is a very good example of a 'new allergy' that suddenly arises with tremendous health and economic implications, and also of an allergy which becomes history in a relatively short period of time based on successful primary prevention strategies by strict allergen avoidance.

Latex as a Rubber and Protein Source

The word 'latex' is deducted from the Spanish word for milk and relates to the white milky sap synthesized by the specialized laticifer cells of a tree and secreted from the wounded trunk. As Ownby [1] described, the use of latex items (rubber balls, wooden tool handles wrapped with rubber, etc.) in ancient Mesoamerica can be documented as early as 1600 BC. The source of these rubber artifacts was latex from the *Castilla elastica* tree (Panama or Mexican rubber tree) mixed with the juice from a morning glory vine *(Ipomoea alba)* to improve the quality of the material. Over 2,000 plants produce such liquid latex, but nowadays the sap of the rubber tree, *Hevea brasiliensis,* a native of the Amazon

Basin, is the source of commercially produced natural rubber latex (NRL). Most *H. brasiliensis* trees grow commercially in a number of tropical countries, including former British colonies such as Malaysia, Thailand and India. Smaller quantities are produced in the native regions of Central and South America.

In England in about 1770, the dried latex was called 'rubber' because it was well suited to rub out pencil marks. Latex collected from the *H. brasiliensis* tree by scarifying its trunk contains the polymeric hydrocarbon 1,4-*cis*-polyisoprene as the main constituent. Only 1–2% of the fresh weight of *Hevea* latex is made up of proteins, which are heterogeneously distributed in the latex sap [2] and involved in the biosynthesis of the polyisoprene associated with the coagulation of latex and in the defense of the plant against various diseases. After ultracentrifugation of the fresh latex sap [3], three main fractions (the rubber phase, the C-serum and the bottom fraction, B-serum) are easily discerned. The rubber phase comprises the rubber particles and two main, insoluble proteins which are extractable from the surface of the rubber particles. Most of the C-serum and B-serum proteins are water soluble. Latex C-serum contains various proteins (more than 200 polypeptides) and some of them are enzymes associated with the rubber biosynthesis. An alternative source of latex is offered by the North American and Mexican desert shrub, the guayule bush *(Parthenium argentatum)*, which is botanically not related to *H. brasiliensis* and does not appear to contain proteins cross-reactive with the allergens of the *Hevea* latex [4].

In about 1840, Charles Goodyear and Nathaniel Hayward in the USA discovered the process of vulcanization, which solved the problem of instability of rubber items. This method enabled the manufacture of suitable and flexible NRL materials, which were soon used in medical products, especially gloves. Various chemicals, such as accelerators, activators, antioxidants and vulcanizing agents, are used in the production of medical gloves, which were first introduced into surgery in the 1880s. During the development of better and more suitable medical gloves over the next hundred years, various dusting powders were used to prevent the gloves from sticking to each other and to facilitate donning and removal [5].

In addition to medical and household gloves, a huge number of other products are manufactured from NRL. Catheters, condoms, tourniquets, baby pacifiers and toy balloons are only some examples of items which may contain allergenic proteins capable of eliciting immunoglobulin (Ig) E-mediated allergy and probably also causing sensitization of exposed subjects.

History of Latex Allergy – When Did the Problems Start?

Historically, NRL allergy is a disease 'born in Europe' [6]. In 1927, 2 cases were published concerning immediate-type latex allergy in Germany. The first, reported by Stern [7], involved urticaria and laryngeal edema caused by a 'caoutchouc' (rubber) dental prosthesis. The second, reported by Grimm [8], occurred after inhalation of NRL particles from a warmed electric wire isolated by rubber. In contrast to these immediate-type I reactions, physicians had been aware of contact dermatitis (a T cell-mediated type IV reaction) to ingredients of latex products for a long time. The trigger of these reactions can be attributed to low-molecular-weight chemical additives and accelerators used in glove manufacturing, such as thiurams, carbamates and derivatives of thiourea, benzothiazole and amines. Clinical symptoms start 12–48 h after contact with the latex product and worsen within 72 h (the so-called 'crescendo reaction').

The 'renaissance' of the immediate-type latex allergy started in 1979, when Nutter [9] from the UK described immediate wheal-and-flare reactions after wearing latex household gloves. In the following years numerous reports about severe allergic reactions after various NRL contacts and other NRL-related publications appeared in the literature (fig. 1). The first 2 cases of intraoperative anaphylactic reactions in nurses, presumably to latex gloves, were described by Turjanmaa et al. [10]. In addition, Finnish groups demonstrated by using the Prausnitz-Küstner passive transfer test that NRL allergy is an IgE-mediated reaction and also showed the presence of

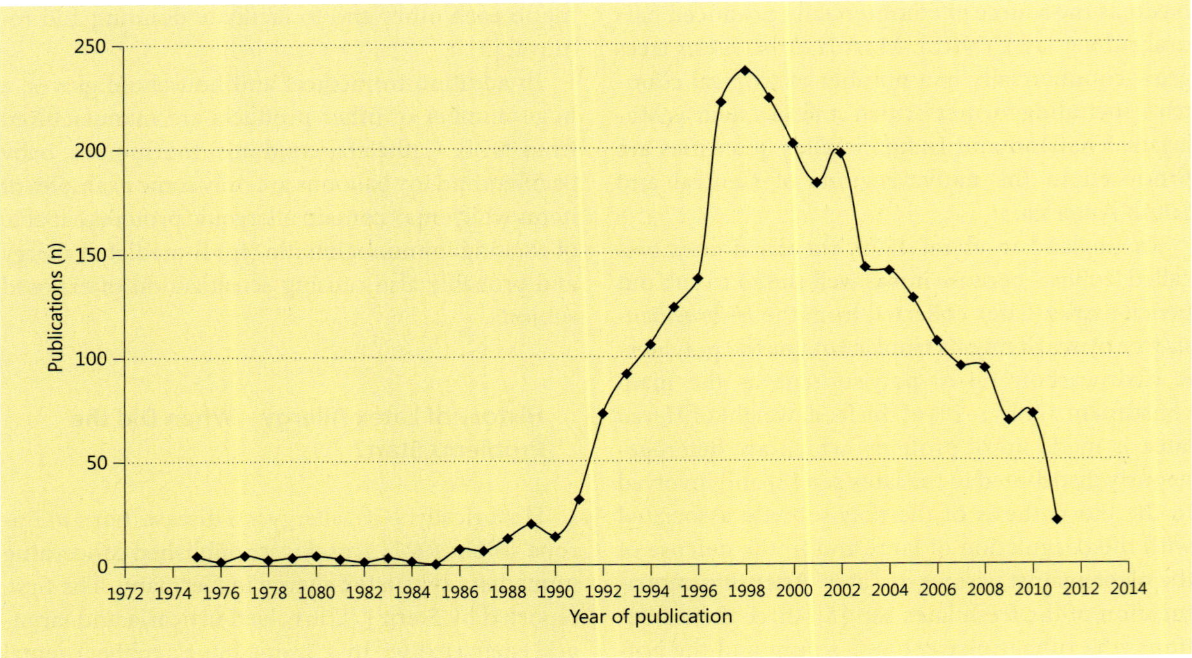

Fig. 1. Number of latex publications between 1975 and 2011.

IgE antibodies specific to NRL [11, 10]. The first reports of latex allergy in the North American literature appeared in 1989 [reviewed in 12]. Slater [13] described two children with spina bifida and a history of urticarial after exposure to rubber products who subsequently experienced intraoperative anaphylaxis.

Many theories have been proposed to explain the sudden increase in the number of individuals affected by latex allergy, starting in the 1980s and extending into the 1990s [1]. Even though not all essential information is available and the key question has been difficult to answer, several factors can be considered. One factor was elevated hygiene standards in medicine in response to transmissible infectious diseases (especially AIDS) and which involved using an increasing number of NRL products, especially NRL gloves. The demand for gloves increased dramatically, resulting in an acute shortage. As manufacturers struggled to meet demands, products of variable quality began to appear on the market, and the magnitude of the allergy problem grew [14]. Gloves of this early era had a wide range of extractable protein content, depending on the manufacturing procedures. It is speculated that changes made in the manufacturing process, such as fewer leaching steps of the NRL to eliminate proteins, were a main factor in the development of NRL allergy (the quality of the latex gloves declined). It was soon apparent that the extractable proteins can produce sensitization on contact with various areas of the body, and the dusting powder on the gloves could facilitate the process. In addition, the NRL allergen-bound powder phenomenon was established in the early 1990s [15–17] describing that proteins attached to cornstarch can become widely disseminated antigens when the particles of the powder become airborne as the gloves are donned and removed. The latex protein-starch particles represented a potential mechanism for exposure and sensitization of health care workers (as directly exposed glove users) and patients (indirectly exposed, for example in operation theaters) to latex allergens. The second important factor related to the increasing recognition of latex allergy was the realization that it actually existed and the dissemination of information about latex allergy amongst health care workers, spina bifida patients and the general public. Independent of clear elucidation of the reasons since the mid 1980s, IgE-mediated hypersensitivity to NRL has been recognized as an important health problem with extensive health and economic implications. This resulted in intense scientific efforts not only to establish preventive strategies, but also to identify the allergen source and improve the diagnosis.

Who Were at Risk? Risk Factors and Epidemiology Aspects

NRL exposure can take place either through direct skin/mucus membrane contact or via inhalation. Before the initiation of a primary NRL prophylaxis around and during surgery, anesthesia of all spina bifida patients and the introduction of powder-free gloves with reduced protein levels in hospitals, the group with a higher risk of developing an NRL allergy included children with spina bifida, health care workers and individuals with a history of multiple surgeries. In addition, high risks were also described for non-health-care workers with exposure to latex, including hairdressers, cleaners and food service workers, as well as workers in rubber industrial companies or subjects with food allergy and atopy.

Depending on the definition of the groups studied and the methods for assessment of latex sensitization and/or allergy, the observed prevalence among children with spina bifida ranged between 25 and 72% [18–20], whereas the prevalence among health care workers ranged between 0 and 30% [21, 22]. Among adult blood donors showing latex-specific IgE antibodies, two separate studies reported a sensitization frequency of about 6% [23, 24]. In contrast, the prevalence in the general population is between 0 and 2.3% [25, 26]. Individuals who are allergic to latex products may experience allergic reactions due to cross-reactivity from a variety of fresh fruits, vegetables and nuts.

Characterization of Relevant Allergens

To date, about 250 different NRL polypeptides have been identified. About 60 are able to bind human IgE [27] and currently 16 allergens have been included in the latest nomenclature list of the International Nomenclature Committee of Allergens (IUIS) and assigned official numbers (http://www.allergen.org; table 1). Most of the allergens are available in recombinant form. There is good evidence that various risk groups are sensitized by different NRL allergens. It is quite obvious that the means of contact with the allergenic proteins is of enormous importance for the development of a sensitization. Some of the major NRL allergens are presented below.

The first major allergen in NRL, the 'rubber elongation factor', was characterized in 1993 by Czuppon et al. [28] and was named according to the IUIS allergen nomenclature as Hev b 1. Hev b 1 is a latex-specific allergen without relevant homology to other plant proteins. Hev b 1 and Hev b 3 are rubber particle proteins strongly associated with latex allergy in spina bifida patients. Using rHev b 1 coupled with ImmunoCAP as a diagnostic tool, 80.6% of all spina bifida sera (n = 31) and 30% of the sera obtained from patients with multiple surgeries were rHev b 1 positive. In contrast, only 11.5% of 104 sera samples from latex-allergic health care workers were Hev b 1-IgE positive [29].

The most important allergen detectable in the C-serum is Hev b 5, an acidic (pI 3.5) and heat-stable 16- to 24-kDa protein, rich in glutamic acid as well as proline residues. Its physiological function is unknown. The native Hev b 5 was characterized by Akasawa et al. [30], whereas the first recombinant Hev b 5 (rHev b 5) was described by Slater et al. [31]. Data demonstrated that in all patient groups (health care workers, spina bifida patients and patients with multiple surgeries) rHev b 5-specific IgE concentrations were the most pronounced [29].

One of the most important NRL allergens for health care workers appears to be prohevein, a 20-kDa precursor protein assigned by the WHO/IUIS as Hev b 6.01 isolated from the B-serum. The maturing process of the mRNA is responsible for the development of a mature prohevein. A post-transla-

Table 1. Immunological and clinical properties of characterized latex allergens of the rubber tree *H. brasiliensis* – IUIS nomenclature list

Latex allergen	Molecular weight, kDa	Protein name, biological function or physiological role	Significance as an allergen
Hev b 1	14	Rubber elongation factor	Major allergen for spina bifida
Hev b 2	34	β-1,3-Glucanase	(Major) allergen
Hev b 3	24	Small rubber particle proteins	Major allergen for spina bifida
Hev b 4	53–55	Lecithinase homolog	Minor allergen
Hev b 5	16	Acidic structural protein	Major allergen for spina bifida as well as for health care workers
Hev b 6.01	20	Prohevein (hevein precursor)	Major allergen (the dominant IgE-binding epitope is Hev b 6.02)
Hev b 6.02	4.7	Hevein	Major allergen
Hev b 6.03	14	C-domain of prohevein	Minor allergen
Hev b 7	44	Patatin-like protein (esterase) from latex B- and C-serum	Minor allergen
Hev b 8	14	Profilin (actin-binding protein)	Minor allergen
Hev b 9	51	Enolase	Minor allergen
Hev b 10	26	Manganese superoxide dismutase	Minor allergen
Hev b 11	30	Class I chitinase	Minor allergen
Hev b 12	9	Non-specific lipid transfer protein	Minor allergen
Hev b 13	42	Esterase	(Major) allergen
Hev b 14	30	Hevamin	Minor allergen

Allergens indicated as being 'major' within parentheses are important in this discussion.

tional cleavage produces two further proteins, the 4.7-kDa hevein (Hev b 6.02) and the 14-kDa C-terminal domain Hev b 6.03. All three allergens exist in the plant although the ratio between Hev b 6.01 and Hev b 6.03 is about 30:1 [2]. Hevein comprises the most important part of IgE-binding epitopes in the prohevein molecule. In addition, hevein shows homology to several chitin-binding lectin domains [32, 33] and may be responsible for certain cross-reactivities to several other plants and food [2].

Latex-Fruit/Plant Syndrome – Problems with Cross-Reactivity

About 30–50% of latex-allergic patients show allergic symptoms to plant-derived foods, especially fresh fruits [34]. The association was called latex-fruit syndrome [35, 36] and a huge and constantly increasing number of fruits are described, and the most commonly involved are avocado, banana, chestnut and kiwi. Several latex allergens have been discussed as being responsible for the latex-fruit cross-reactivity, such as Hev b 2 [37], Hev b 6.02 [38–40], Hev b 7 [41], Hev b 8 [42] and Hev b 12 (fig. 2) [43]. The time course of sensitization is an ongoing subject of discussion. In the literature there are some reports describing a symptomatic fruit allergy (banana) before symptoms of NRL allergy were noted [44], as well as NRL allergic symptoms preceding a banana allergy [45]. In a long-term follow-up study of latex and fruit antibodies in spina bifida patients, Mennicken et al. [46] observed good evidence that latex sensitization usually precedes fruit sensitization. In some cases, use of recombinant single latex allergens for latex-specific IgE mapping is helpful to discriminate between cross-reactivity and co-sensitization of latex and fruits.

Latex as a Model for Molecular Allergology – How to Improve the Diagnosis?

In the past the diagnosis of a latex sensitization was rather difficult because several studies demonstrated that IgE test systems gave false-negative re-

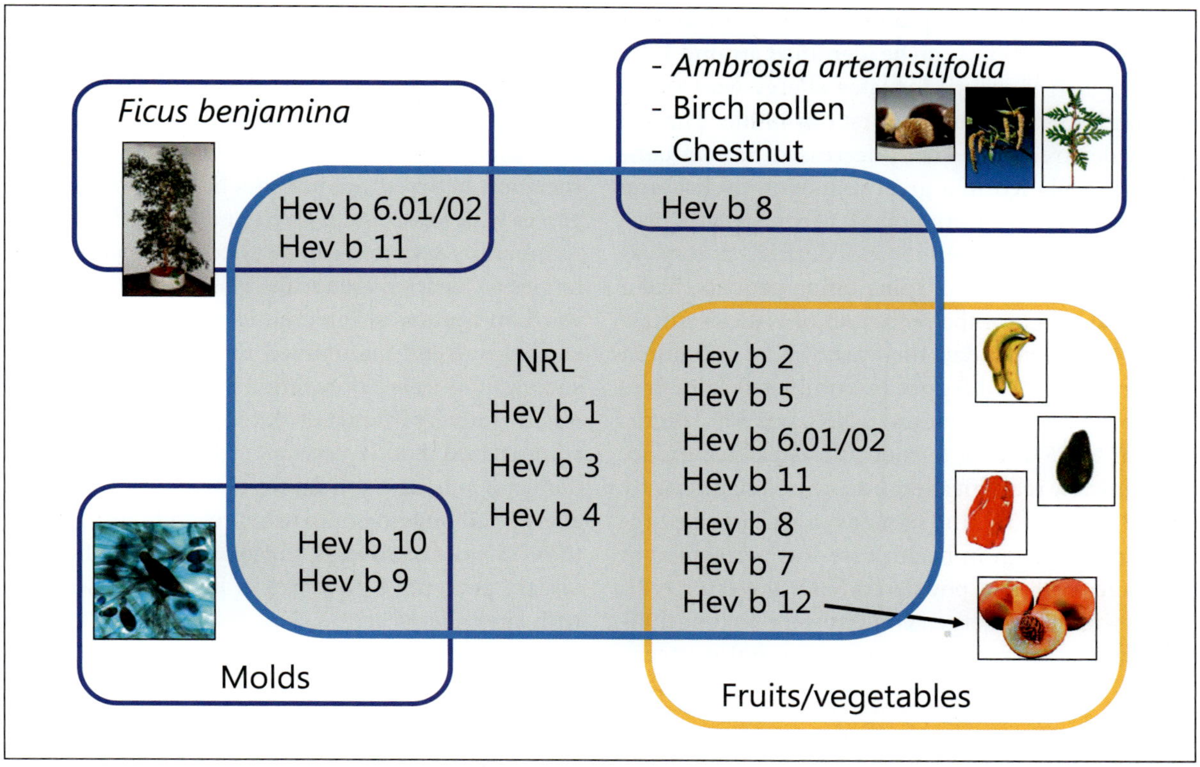

Fig. 2. Molecular association of the latex-fruit/food syndrome – allergens probably responsible for cross-reactivity.

sults in more than 25% of patients with allergic reactions based on NRL and skin test-positive subjects [47]. One reason for these discrepancies was a missing allergen. Indeed, by addition of rHev b 5 to the diagnostic repertoire of latex allergens, 8 out of 16 subjects with clear latex allergy and negative latex-specific IgE values using the Pharmacia CAP system showed significantly elevated IgE levels to Hev b 5 [48]. These findings demonstrated that the latex allergen Hev b 5 may play a special role in diagnostic tests showing false-negative IgE results. The addition of rHev b 5 in sufficient amounts significantly improved the ImmunoCAP used for serological testing [49]. These results indicate a new approach: if relevant allergens are labile to survive all the steps required for the production of a standardized allergen preparation, they can be added as a stable recombinant protein to the allergen preparation during production. In contrast, in cases of false-positive latex-specific IgE results in subjects without clinical symptoms to latex, negative skin prick test based on IgE-binding to N-glycans and/or O-glycans, which are often part of plant-derived allergens such as latex, inhibition studies with 'cross-reactive carbohydrate determinants' can be performed to clarify if protein epitopes (with clinical relevance) or the glyco-epitopes (with low clinical relevance) are responsible for the IgE-binding to latex [29]. In addition component-resolved diagnosis using microarray [50] or single placed ImmunoCAP coupled with recombinant or native allergens [29] are reliable tools for diagnosing latex allergy.

Preventive Measures – Successful Avoidance Strategy

The introduction of powder-free, latex-poor gloves decreased the high frequency of latex allergy in high-risk populations like health care workers

[51] and patients with spina bifida [52, 53]. In general the turning point can be identified around 1994 when high-risk groups for latex allergy were operated on NRL-free from the first day of life. The use of powder-free gloves with decreased protein content especially led to a great reduction in airborne latex allergen [53]. Initiation of a primary NRL prophylaxis program around and during surgery, as well as anesthesia of all spina bifida patients, had a beneficial effect on the reduction of NRL sensitization [54]. The latest data finally show that in children with spina bifida who grew up completely latex-free from birth on, sensitization to NRL was 5% in comparison to 55% for a former non-latex-free group, and clinically relevant allergy decreased significantly from 37 to 1% [55]. In Germany, a nationwide prevention campaign in health care was performed in 1997 and 1998 and powdered NRL gloves or NRL gloves with high allergen content were no longer allowed after a revised version of the compulsory technical regulations for dangerous substances was edited in December 1997 (Ministry of Labour and Social Affairs, 2008). The effectiveness of these measures for primary prevention in Germany has been shown by Allmers et al. [51] through a clear association between the introduction of powder-free gloves with low protein levels and the decline in the number of suspected cases of occupational NRL allergies on a nationwide scale. Therefore, straightforward and practical interventions that are properly carried out and maintained are good examples of successful primary prevention strategies. Nevertheless, a study by Merget et al. [56] published in 2010 summarized that, 10 years after the latex allergy epidemic, a substantial number of subjects with latex allergy had ongoing mild work-related symptoms of the eyes, nose or airways, suggesting that further secondary preventive measures in health care workers with latex allergy are needed.

References

1 Ownby DR: A history of latex allergy. J Allergy Clin Immunol 2002;110:S27–S32.
2 Yeang HY, Arif SA, Yusof F, Sunderasan E: Allergenic proteins of natural rubber latex. Methods 2002;27:32–45.
3 Moir GFJ: Ultracentrifugation and staining of *Hevea* latex. Nature 1959;184:1626–1628.
4 Siler DJ, Cornish K, Hamilton RG: Absence of cross-reactivity of IgE antibodies from subjects allergic to *Hevea brasiliensis* latex with a new source of natural rubber latex from guayule *(Parthenium argentatum)*. J Allergy Clin Immunol 1996;98:895–902.
5 Truscott W: Glove powder reduction and alternative approaches. Methods 2002;27:69–76.
6 Turjanmaa K, Mäkinen-Koljunen S, Reunala T, Alenius H, Palosuo T: Natural rubber latex allergy: the European experience. Immunol Allergy Clin North Am 1995;15:71–88.
7 Stern G: Überempfindlichkeit gegen Kautschuk als Ursache von Urticaria und Quinckeschem Ödem. Klin Wochensch 1927;6:1096–1097.
8 Grimm A: Überempfindlichkeit gegen Kautschuk als Ursache von Urticaria und Quinckeschem Ödem. Klinische Wochensch 1927;6:1479.
9 Nutter AF: Contact urticaria to rubber. Br J Dermatol 1979;101:597–598.
10 Turjanmaa K, Reunala T, Tuimala R, Karkkainen T: Severe IgE-mediated allergy to surgical gloves. Allergy 1984:39:35.
11 Köpman A, Hannuksela M: Contact uritcaria to rubber. Duodecim 1983;3:39.
12 Granady LC, Slater JE: The history and diagnosis of latex allergy. Immunol Allergy Clin North Am 1995;15:21–29.
13 Slater JE: Rubber anaphylaxis. N Engl J Med 1989;320:1126–1130.
14 McFadden ER Jr: Natural rubber latex sensitivity seminar: conference summary. J Allergy Clin Immunol 2002;110:S137–S140.
15 Lagier F, Badier M, Martigny J, Charpin D, Vervloet D: Latex as aeroallergen. Lancet 1990;336:516–517.
16 Beezhold D, Beck WC: Surgical glove powders bind latex antigens. Arch Surg 1992;127:1354–1357.
17 Baur X, Ammon J, Chen Z, Beckmann U, Czuppon AB: Health risk in hospitals through airborne allergens for patients presensitised to latex. Lancet 1993;342:1148–1149.
18 Konz KR, Chia JK, Kurup VP, Resnick A, Kelly KJ, Fink JN: Comparison of latex hypersensitivity among patients with neurologic defects. J Allergy Clin Immunol 1995;95:950–954.
19 Bernardini R, Novembre E, Lombardi E, Mezzetti P, Cianferoni A, Danti DA, Mercurella A, Vierucci A: Risk factors for latex allergy in patients with spina bifida and latex sensitization. Clin Exp Allergy 1999;29:681–686.
20 Yassin MS, Sanyurah S, Lierl MB, Fischer TJ, Oppenheimer S, Cross J, O'Brien K, Steinmetz C, Khoury J: Evaluation of latex allergy in patients with meningomyelocele. Ann Allergy 1992;69:207–211.
21 Yassin MS, Lierl MB, Fischer TJ, O'Brien K, Cross J, Steinmetz C: Latex allergy in hospital employees. Ann Allergy 1994;72:245–249.
22 Garabrant DH, Schweitzer S: Epidemiology of latex sensitization and allergies in health care workers. J Allergy Clin Immunol 2002;110:S82–S95.
23 Kanny G, Moneret-Vautrin DA, Flabbee J, Beaudouin E, Morisset M, Thevenin F: Population study of food allergy in France. J Allergy Clin Immunol 2001;108:133–140.
24 Ownby DR, Ownby HE, McCullough J, Shafer AW: The prevalence of anti-latex IgE antibodies in 1,000 volunteer blood donors. J Allergy Clin Immunol 1996;97:1188–1192.
25 Porri F, Lemiere C, Birnbaum J, Guilloux L, Didelot R, Vervloet D, Charpin D: Prevalence of latex allergy in atopic and nonatopic subjects from the general population. J Allergy Clin Immunol 1995;95:154.

26 Turjanmaa K, Alenius H, Mäkinen-Kiljunen S, Reunala T, Palosuo T: Natural rubber latex allergy. Allergy 1996;51:593–602.

27 Posch A, Chen Z, Raulf-Heimsoth M, Baur X: Latex allergens. Clin Exp Allergy 1998;28: 134–140.

28 Czuppon AB, Chen Z, Rennert S, Engelke T, Meyer HE, Heber M, Baur X: The rubber elongation factor of rubber trees *(Hevea brasiliensis)* is the major allergen in latex. J Allergy Clin Immunol 1993;92:690–697.

29 Raulf-Heimsoth M, Rihs HP, Rozynek P, Cremer R, Gaspar A, Pires G, Yeang HY, Arif SA, Hamilton RG, Sander I, Lundberg M, Brüning T: Quantitative analysis of immunoglobulin E reactivity profiles in patients allergic or sensitized to natural rubber latex *(Hevea brasiliensis)*. Clin Exp Allergy 2007;37:1657–1667.

30 Akasawa A, Hsieh LS, Martin BM, Liu T, Lin Y: A novel acidic allergen, Hev b 5, in latex: purification, cloning and characterization. J Biol Chem 1996;271:25389–25393.

31 Slater JE, Vedvick T, Arthur-Smith A, Trybul DE, Kekwick RG: Identification, cloning, and sequence of a major allergen (Hev b 5) from natural rubber latex *(Hevea brasiliensis)*. J Biol Chem 1996;271:25394–25399.

32 Posch A, Chen Z, Wheeler C, Dunn MJ, Raulf-Heimsoth M, Baur X: Characterization and identification of latex allergens by two-dimensional electrophoresis and protein microsequencing. J Allergy Clin Immunol 1997;99:385–395.

33 Rozynek P, Posch A, Baur X: Cloning, expression and characterization of the major latex allergen prohevein. Clin Exp Allergy 1998;28:1418–1426.

34 Radauer C, Adhami F, Fürtler I, Wagner S, Allwardt D, Scala E, Ebner C, Hafner C, Hemmer W, Mari A, Breiteneder H: Latex-allergic patients sensitized to the major allergen hevein and hevein-like domains of class I chitinases show no increased frequency of latex-associated plant food allergy. Mol Immunol 2011;48:600–609.

35 Blanco C: Latex-fruit syndrome. Curr Allergy Asthma Rep 2003;3:47–53.

36 Wagner S, Breiteneder H: The latex-fruit syndrome. Biochem Soc Trans 2002;30: 935–940.

37 Barre A, Culerrier R, Granier C, Selman L, Peumans WJ, Van Damme EJ, Bienvenu F, Bienvenu J, Rougé P: Mapping of IgE-binding epitopes on the major latex allergen Hev b 2 and the cross-reacting 1,3β-glucanase fruit allergens as a molecular basis for the latex-fruit syndrome. Mol Immunol 2009; 46:1595–1604.

38 Chen Z, Posch A, Cremer R, Raulf-Heimsoth M, Baur X: Identification of hevein (Hev b 6.02) in *Hevea* latex as a major cross-reacting allergen with avocado fruit in patients with latex allergy. J Allergy Clin Immunol 1998;102:476–481.

39 Posch A, Wheeler CH, Chen Z, Flagge A, Dunn MJ, Papenfuss F, Raulf-Heimsoth M, Baur X: Class I endochitinase containing a hevein domain is the causative allergen in latex-associated avocado allergy. Clin Exp Allergy 1999;29:667–672.

40 Raulf-Heimsoth M, Stark R, Sander I, Maryska S, Rihs HP, Brüning T, Voshaar T: Anaphylactic reaction to apple juice containing acerola: cross-reactivity to latex due to prohevein. J Allergy Clin Immunol 2002; 109:715–716.

41 Schmidt MH, Raulf-Heimsoth M, Posch A: Evaluation of patatin as a major cross-reactive allergen in latex-induced potato allergy. Ann Allergy Asthma Immunol 2002;89: 613–618.

42 Raulf-Heimsoth M, Kespohl S, Crespo JF, Rodriguez J, Feliu A, Brüning T, Rihs HP: Natural rubber latex and chestnut allergy: cross-reactivity or co-sensitization? Allergy 2007;62:1277–1281.

43 Beezhold DH, Hickey VL, Kostyal DA, Puhl H, Zuidmeer L, van Ree R, Sussman GL: Lipid transfer protein from *Hevea brasiliensis* (Hev b 12), a cross-reactive latex protein. Ann Allergy Asthma Immunol 2003; 90:439–445.

44 M'Raihi L, Charpin D, Pons A, Bongrand P, Vervloet D: Cross-reactivity between latex and banana. J Allergy Clin Immunol 1991; 88:129–130.

45 Cinquetti M, Peroni D, Zoppi G: Latex allergy in a child with banana anaphylaxis. Acta Paediatr 1995;84:709–710.

46 Mennicken O, Cremer R, Weiss M: Follow-up study on the latex-fruit-syndrome in patients with spina bifida (abstract). Annual Meeting SRSbH, Dublin, 2004.

47 Hamilton RG, Adkinson NF, Mulitcenter Latex Skin Testing Study Task Force: Diagnosis of natural rubber latex allergy: multicenter latex skin testing efficacy study. J Allergy Clin Immunol 1998;102:482–490.

48 Chen Z, Rihs HP, Slater JE, Paupore EJ, Schneider EM, Baur X: The absence of Hev b 5 in capture antigen may cause false-negative results in serologic assays for latex-specific IgE antibodies. J Allergy Clin Immunol 2000;105:S8.

49 Lundberg M, Chen Z, Rihs HP, Wrangsjö K: Recombinant spiked allergen extract. Allergy 2001:56:794–795.

50 Ebo DG, Hagendorens MM, De Knop KJ, Verweij MM, Bridts CH, De Clerck LS, Stevens WJ: Component-resolved diagnosis from latex allergy by microarray. Clin Exp Allergy 2010;40:348–358.

51 Allmers H, Schmengler J, Skudlik C: Primary prevention of natural rubber latex allergy in the German health care system through education and intervention. J Allergy Clin Immunol 2002;110:318–323.

52 Levy DA, Allouche S, Chabane MH, Leynadier F: Powder-free protein-poor rubber latex gloves and latex sensitization. JAMA 1999:281:988.

53 Niggemann B: IgE-mediated latex allergy – an exciting and instructive piece of allergy history. Pediatr Allergy Immunol 2010;21: 997–1001.

54 Cremer R, Kleine-Diepenbruck U, Hoppe A, Bläker F: Latex allergy in spina bifida patients – prevention by primary prophylaxis. Allergy 1998;3:709–711.

55 Blumchen K, Bayer P, Buck, Michael T, Cremer R, Fricke C, Henne T, Peters H, Hofmann U, Keil T, Schlaud M, Wahn U, Niggemann B: Effects of latex avoidance on latex sensitization, atopic status and allergic diseases in patients with spina bifida. Allergy 2010;65:1585–1593.

56 Merget R, van Kampen V, Sucker K, Heinze E, Taeger D, Goldscheid N, Haufs MG, Raulf-Heimsoth M, Komak K, Nienhaus A, Bruening T: The German experience 10 years after the latex allergy epidemic: need for further preventive measures in healthcare employees with latex allergy. Int Arch Occup Environ Health 2010;83:895–903.

4

Prof. Dr. Monika Raulf
Kompetenz-Zentrum Allergologie/Immunologie
Institut für Prävention und Arbeitsmedizin der
Deutschen Gesetzlichen Unfallversicherung
Institut der Ruhr-Universität Bochum (IPA)
Bürkle-de-la-Camp Platz 1
DE–44789 Bochum (Germany)
E-Mail raulf@ipa-dguv.de

Bergmann K-C, Ring J (eds): History of Allergy. Chem Immunol Allergy. Basel, Karger, 2014, vol 100, pp 256–267
DOI: 10.1159/000359916

Peanut Allergens

Wolf-Meinhard Becker[a] · Uta Jappe[a, b]

[a]Division of Clinical and Molecular Allergology, Research Center Borstel, Airway Research Center North (ARCN), German Center for Lung Research, Borstel, and [b]Department of Dermatology, Allergology and Venereology, University of Lübeck, Lübeck, Germany

Abstract

The earliest known evidence of peanut farming dates back 7,600 years. With a prevalence of roughly 1%, peanut allergy is a diagnostic and treatment challenge, but is also a very good model for studying all aspects of food allergy, including its molecular basis and pathomechanisms. Therefore, the very starting point for elucidating all these aspects is the identification of peanut allergens with subsequent clearing of their structure and their preparation as pure recombinant and/or natural allergens. This is the basis for in vitro diagnostic tests as well as the development of immunotherapeutic drugs. With regard to class I food allergy, peanut allergy affects by far the largest group of patients. In peanuts, 12 allergens have been identified and their molecular characteristics are described herein. Ara h 1, Ara h 3.01 and Ara h 3.02 (the former Ara h 4) belong to the cupin superfamily. The conglutins Ara h 2, Ara h 6 and Ara h 7, and the non-specific lipid transfer protein Ara h 9 belong to the prolamin superfamily. Ara h 5 (profilin) and Ara h 8 (Bet v 1-homologous protein) cause class II food allergies and are associated with inhalation allergy to pollen via the sequential and/or conformational similarity of molecules. Two peanut oleosins are listed as Ara h 10 and Ara h 11 and two defensins as Ara h 12 and Ara h 13 by the WHO/IUIS Allergen Nomenclature Subcommittee. The effect of the above-specified allergens has to be considered in the context of their matrix, which is influenced by processing factors and the individual's immune system.

In sensitized individuals peanuts may induce a broad spectrum of allergic reactions, with the degree of severity ranging from mild to fatal anaphylactic symptoms (table 1). After the ingestion of peanuts symptoms that evolve in the gastrointestinal as well as in the respiratory tract may include skin and mucosa and may affect the whole system by expressing all the features of an anaphylactic shock. In highly sensitized patients symptoms occur even after skin contact to peanut allergens [1], aggravating atopic eczema but also inducing symptoms of a type I reaction [2].

Table 1. Manifestation of peanut allergy on different organ compartments and its symptoms with increasing severity

	Symptoms		
Severity:	mild	moderate	severe
Skin	hives, pruritus	atopic dermatitis, urticaria	angioedema
Respiratory tract	rhino-conjunctivitis, wheezing	shortness of breath, asthma	acute severe asthma
Gastrointestinal tract	diarrhea, nausea and vomiting, OAS	abdominal pain	laryngeal edema
Systemic reaction			anaphylactic shock

It has to be considered that all symptoms may occur singularly as well as in combination.

One important aspect of the diagnostic challenge is the variety and severity of clinical symptoms of peanut allergy, which in part can be associated with single peanut allergens, i.e. Ara h 2 or Ara h 6 as marker allergens for severe symptoms [3, 4]. Another point of consideration is the incalculable amount of processed peanut proteins as a source of allergens in complex foodstuff, which relates to the problem of so-called 'hidden' allergens. A third aspect is the fact that an efficacious and – above all – a safe causative treatment of peanut allergy still does not exist. Thus, peanut allergy is a challenge of diagnosis and treatment but also a very good model to study all aspects of food allergy, including its molecular basis and pathomechanisms.

Prevalence of Peanut Allergy

As shown by Sicherer et al. [5], the prevalence of peanut allergy remains steady among adults in the USA, with a rate of 1.3%. In children, however, it increased from 0.4% in 1997 to 1.4% in 2008. Similar results were obtained by Venter et al. [6] in the UK for children aged 3–4 years, whereby the prevalence of peanut allergy first increased but seems to have stabilized since the late 1990s. These studies show why it is so difficult to obtain reliable prevalence data for peanut allergy in general, and in Europe in particular. However, these data are sufficient to give an idea of the impact of peanut allergy.

Geographical Origin of Peanuts

Peanut, *Arachis hypogaea* (in Greek, hypogaea means 'under the earth'), is a seed and belongs to the legume family (Fabacaea) along with beans, peas, lentils and lupines. Thus, peanuts or groundnuts phylogenetically are in fact not nuts like walnuts and hazel nuts are, and are not stone fruits like almonds. It is important to keep that in mind when hypothesizing about allergenic cross-reactivities between foodstuffs.

Peanuts originate from South America, in particular Paraguay and Bolivia, where two different diploid *Arachis* species, *A. duranensis* and *A. ipaensis*, grow even today as wild relatives of *A. hypogaea.* Most probably, the allotetraploid species *A. monticola* originates from both *A. duranensis* and *A. ipaensis*, and has further developed into the domesticated peanut, *A. hypogaea* [7]. The contribution of *A. duranensis* and *A. ipaensis* to the allotetraploid *A. hypogaea* becomes evident when focusing on the two isoforms of the single peanut allergen *A. hypogaea* (Ara h) 2.0101 (16.5 kDa) and Ara h 2.0201 (18 kDa), where Ara h 2.0101 is contributed by *A. duranensis* and Ara h 2.0201 by *A. ipaensis* [8]. The anthropologist Dillehay et al. [9] found the earliest known evidence of peanut farming dating back 7,600 years in northern Peru. The strongest hypotheses regarding the worldwide spread of peanuts are that the Portuguese carried peanuts to Africa and the Spanish via the Philippines to Malaysia, Japan, China and India [10, 11]. In 2011, the top producers of peanuts in the shell were China, followed by India, Nigeria and then the USA (http://faostat.fao.org/site/339/default.aspx; consulted in April 2013).

Table 2. Classification of peanut allergens applying physical and biochemical criteria

Allergen	Protein families	Sedimentation coefficient	Biological function	Alias names/ synonyms in proteomics
Ara h 1	cupin superfamily	7 S vicilin	storage protein	conarachin
Ara h 3	cupin superfamily	11 S legumin, glycinin	storage protein	arachin
Ara h 2	prolamin superfamily	2 S albumin	storage protein, trypsin inhibitor	conglutin
Ara h 6	prolamin superfamily	2 S albumin	storage protein	conglutin
Ara h 7	prolamin superfamily	2 S albumin	storage protein	conglutin
Ara h 9	prolamin superfamily		nsLTP	
Ara h 5	profilin			
Ara h 8	Bet v 1-related protein		PR-10	
Ara h 10	oleosin		oil body forming	
Ara h 11	oleosin		oil body forming	
Ara h 12	defensin		PR-12	
Ara h 13	defensin		PR-12	

Varieties of peanuts from different parts of the world contain similar proteins, including Ara h 1 and Ara h 2, and their immunoglobulin E (IgE)-binding properties have also been reported to be similar to a great extent [12]. Historically, the separation and identification of peanut proteins follows the method of Osborne, originally developed for wheat proteins [13]. The proteins in cereal seeds are usually divided into four groups according to physical criteria (solubility): albumins (water-soluble), globulins (saline-soluble), prolamins (alcohol-soluble proline and glutamine-rich storage proteins) and glutelins [14]. Components of the albumin fraction of peanuts are agglutinins (peanut agglutinin; PNA), protease/α-amylase inhibitors and phospholipases [15]. There is an overlap of these components with the cereal prolamin superfamily, including three major groups of plant food allergens, the 2 S (Swedberg unit) albumins, lipid transfer proteins and cereal α-amylase/trypsin inhibitors, which have related structures in peanut [16]. The globulins were subdivided into arachin and conarachin fractions (the major storage proteins). Conarachin can be separated by ultracentrifugation into 7 S and 11 S components which in turn belong to the vicilins and legumins. Peanut allergens are classified by different terms, as shown in table 2. The classification of peanut allergens is performed according to different criteria representing certain protein families or superfamilies. A further criterion is the Swedberg unit, S, a constant which is still valid, although it is obtained by nowadays obsolete protein separation techniques via centrifugation. Further criteria are protein function and historically delineated substance designations used in proteomics.

Another classification of food allergens relies on their potency to elicit allergic symptoms based on the main route of sensitization [17]. Some foods are able to induce allergies in early childhood via the gastrointestinal tract as the sensitization route, including cow's milk, hen egg, fish, shellfish, tree nuts like walnuts, Brazil nuts or hazel nuts, wheat, legumes like soybean, lupine seeds or peanuts (class I food allergy). In contrast, class II food allergies are induced by foods of plant origin via cross-reactivity between pollen allergens and food allergens (i.e. birch pollen/apple or hazelnut allergy), with the sensitization occurring primarily in the respiratory tract.

Class I Food Allergy

The class I food allergies are induced by allergens which are stable against denaturation via digestion and thermal processing, and, therefore, predominantly induce sensitization via the gastrointestinal tract and elicit systemic clinical symptoms. As a consequence, it is a standard test procedure to investigate the stability of the allergen in question with simulated gastric and pancreatic fluid to determine its allergenic potency. The respective allergens are called class I food allergens. They are characterized by linear or stable conformational IgE-reactive epitopes. Twenty-three [18] linear epitopes were identified for the peanut allergen Ara h 1, whereas there are ten for Ara h 2 [19] and four for Ara h 3 [20]. Moreover, Sen et al. [21] could show that Ara h 2 generates stable fragments under digestion conditions. With the growing number of identified and characterized peanut allergens it has become evident that these allergens must not exclusively be defined as class I, and that some can be class II allergens instead. The latter are Ara h 5 (profilin) and Ara h 8, a pathogenesis-related (PR)-10 protein cross-reactive with Bet v 1. Class II allergens normally cause mild-to-moderate symptoms like the oral allergy syndrome (OAS). However, for the Ara h 8-analogous allergen in soybean *(Glycine maxima)*, Gly m 4 (Sam 22), anaphylactic reactions were observed after ingestion of probably insufficiently heated soy preparations with high Gly m 4 content [22, 23]. In the context of severe reactions, Ara h 9, a non-specific (ns) lipid transfer protein (LTP), is an interesting allergen because of its digestion-resistant nature. Sensitization to Ara h 9 was found in patients living in southern Europe, mostly suffering from peach allergy mediated by IgE antibodies to the peach LTP (*Prunus persica*, Pru p 3) [24–26]. Since these patients primarily suffered from peach allergy and only from mild symptoms after ingestion of peanuts, Ara h 9 seems to fulfil the characteristics of a class II allergen. The reason could be its low concentration in peanuts, which is hypothesized from the fact that Ara h 9 could not be detected in routine peanut extracts but could be detected by more sophisticated methodology [24].

The food allergic 'march' starts with cow's milk and egg allergy which, in contrast to peanut allergy, mostly resolve in accordance with a maturing of the gastrointestinal immune system, whereas only 20% of peanut-allergic children develop a tolerance [27]. In contrast to class I, class II food allergies with an onset in adulthood start with tree or grass pollen allergies.

Class II Food Allergies

Class II food allergies are caused by cross-reactivity in adolescents and adult patients suffering from inhalant allergies such as tree or grass pollen allergies and latex allergy. Typical class II food allergies are the birch pollen-associated apple/hazelnut, the celery/spice allergy or the latex-fruit syndrome. One particular and clinically relevant characteristic feature of class II allergy is that the responsible allergens are not stable to heat processing and digestion whereby the relevant conformational epitopes are destroyed so that patients are able to consume cooked fruit without developing symptoms. On a molecular level the cross-reactive allergen Bet v 1 from birch *(Betula verrucosa)* acts as a primary sensitizer. The class II allergens Mal d 1 (apple) or Cor a 1 (hazel nut) are Bet v 1-homologous allergens, as are Dau c 1 (carrot), Pru av 1 (cherry), Pru p 1 (peach), Pru ar 1 (apricot), Pyr c 1 (pear), Gly m 4 (soybean) and Api g 1 (celery). This explains why some patients with long-lasting birch pollen/apple allergy additionally develop a carrot and/or a cherry allergy. In peanut the Bet v 1-homologous allergen is Ara h 8. As mentioned above, class II food allergens generally cause mild-to-moderate symptoms, such as OAS. Sometimes severe allergic reactions are observed in patients suffering from class II food allergies, for instance to hazelnut. One reason might be that the patient developed a sensitization against hazelnut nsLTP, Cor a 8 [28], or a storage protein (Cor a 11).

Taken together, food allergen sources eliciting a class I food allergy containing class I and also class II allergens in the case of peanut Ara h 5, Ara h 8 and possibly Ara h 9 cause mild-to-moderate symptoms like OAS. Food allergen sources eliciting a class II food allergy additionally containing class I allergens in the case of hazelnut, Cor a 8, have the potency to provoke severe allergic reactions [28].

In contrast to IgE antibody detection on the basis of crude allergen extracts, a component-resolved diagnosis including marker allergens for severe reactions (i.e. Ara h 2 [3], or Ara h 6 [4]) provides the allergologist with more reliable results with which to advise the patients as to whether they should carry an emergency kit or not. The respective clinical studies with regard to more marker allergens are still ongoing.

Allergens of Peanut

As summarized in table 3, 12 peanut allergens have been identified and characterized so far [29, 30]. It is the explicit concern to depict the characteristics of the mature proteins (allergens), which is in contrast to data bank entries, where the proteins are listed with their signal peptides as the basis from which to delineate their molecular weight (MW) and isoelectric point (pI). This does not mirror the features of the mature protein as it is present in the extract. According to size exclusion chromatography (Superdex 200), nearly 90% of the peanut extract protein is located in the void volume containing trimers or oligomers of Ara h 1 and hexamers of Ara h 3 with MWs above 200 kDa [31–33], whereby the extract was obtained with ammonium hydrogen carbonate buffer (pH 8) simulating chewing conditions [34].

Ara h 1 and Ara h 3

Ara h 1 and Ara h 3 are seed storage proteins and belong to the globulins. Ara h 1 is a 7 S vicilin and Ara 3 an 11 S legumin (glycinin). Both allergens possess two conserved cupins, barrel structures, belonging as two-domain bicupins to the cupin superfamily. This is valuable information with regard to the prognosis of possible cross-reactive components in other legumes or nuts. According to our current state of knowledge, Ara h 1 was first described by Barnett and Howden [35].

Ara h 1 is a glycoprotein with a C-terminal N-asparagine (496N) glycosylation site conjugated with different oligosaccharides $Man_{5-6}GlcNAc_2$ or $Man_{3-4}XylGlcNAc_2$ [36]. These saccharides are reactive with the lectin Con A, which proved to be useful for the purification of Ara h 1. As shown by Buschmann et al. [37] for the peanut extract obtained under SDS-PAGE conditions, Ara 1 consists of two isoforms differing in length. The full-length isoform in our hands is resistant to N-terminal sequencing but detectable by Ara h 1-specific monoclonal antibodies as a broad band changing over to the band of the shorter isoform. The latter starts with G-85 (see table 3) as shown by N-terminal sequencing and contains at least one hydroxyproline (p) as a post-translational modification. This kind of modification resulting in a mass shift of 16 Da should be considered when analyzing proteins by proteomics using the trypsin fingerprinting approach because the match of fragments could be improved. The existence of the larger isoform as such is a matter of discussion. Three IgE-reactive epitopes of the described 23 are located in positions 25–34, 48–57 and 65–74 [18] of the N-terminus of the putative larger isoform. However, these epitopes could be generated by fragments, as has been postulated by Wichers et al. [38]. Indeed, we found such fragments identified by N-terminal sequencing and position (MW, pI) in 2D electrophoresis [39]. On the other hand, we found N-terminal fragments of the whole molecule in the proteomics data set of the diploma thesis of Ties Latendorf [39, 40].

Ara h 3 and Ara h 4 are isoallergens with a sequence identity of 91%; consequently, Ara h 4 was renamed Ara h 3.02 in 2012 by the WHO/IUIS Allergen Nomenclature Subcommittee. The confusion in nomenclature started with the unauthorized designation of a 14-kDa fragment as Ara h 3 [41, 42]. The Ara h 3/4 allergens are the products of a multi-gene family. At least twelve isoforms exist as a result of running the basic local alignment search tool (BLAST; http://blast.ncbi.nlm.nih.gov/Blast.cgi). Three isoforms are depicted in table 3 as important prototypes: Ara h 3 and Ara h 4 (now Ara h 3.02) as the originally described allergens, as well as iso-Ara h 3. The MWs of the Ara h 3/4 (now Ara h 3) isoforms are within the range of 58 kDa with a pI of 5.8. The proteins were post-translationally cleaved according to the 11 S signature (fig. 1) in an acidic and basic subunit only joined via a dicysteine (cystine) providing a compact storage of these molecules in the seed [29]. Thus, these molecules are heterodimers which under reducing conditions in 2D electrophoresis leads to a typical pattern of spots within the range of 43 kDa for the acidic subunit and spots at 28 kDa for the basic subunit (fig. 2) [43, 44]. The acidic subunit divides into further fragments. Interestingly, for the recombinant acidic subunit, Dodo et al. [45] could show trypsin inhibitor properties. The resistance against digestion might be one cause for the allergenicity of Ara h 3/4. Rabjohn et al. [20] identified four linear IgE-reactive epitopes in the acidic subunit, whereby three of them are possibly conserved in all isoforms. In peanut-allergic children a further IgE-reactive epitope was found in the basic subunit [46, 47].

Table 3. Characteristics of peanut allergens

Allergen	$MW_{calculated}$, kDa	pI	Special characteristics	N-terminus	Protein family	Function	Accession No.
Ara h 1	68,757	6.36	glycoprotein	K_{26}SSPYQK	7S globulin	storage protein	P43238
	61,882	6.03	glycoprotein truncated isoform	G_{85}SpPGE	vicilin	storage protein	
Ara h 2	17,993	5.51		R_{22}QQEL	2 S albumin	trypsin inhibitor	AY158467
	16,637	5.5		R_{22}QQEL	conglutin	trypsin inhibitor	L77197
Ara h 3	58,697	5.58	isoallergens forming hexamers	I_{21}SF RQQ[a]	11 S globulin	storage protein	AAC63045
iso-Ara h 3	56,241	5.35	isoallergens forming hexamers	V_{19}TFRQGG	legumin	storage protein	AAT39430
Ara h 4	58,849	5.47	isoallergens forming hexamers	I_{21}SFRQQ			AF086821
Ara h 3/4[a]	23,115	6.58	trypsin inhibitor	I_{23}SFRQQ			AF487543
Ara h 5	14,051	4.58	profilin	MSWQTYV	profilin		AF059615
Ara h 6	14,491	5.02		M_{21}RRERGR	conglutin		AF092846
Ara h 7.0101	16,322	5.56		T_{21}RWDPD	conglutin		AF091737
Ara h 7.0201	17,374	7.49		T_{21}RWDPD			EU046325
Ara h 8.0101	16,952	5.03	Bet v 1-homologous protein, PR-10	MGVFTF		PR-10 protein	AY328088
Ara h 8.0201	16,281	5.07	Bet v 1-homologous protein, PR-10	GVHTFEE		PR-10 protein	EF436550
Ara h 9.0101	9,135	9.45	PR-14	I_{25}SCGQVN		nsLTP	EU159429
Ara h 9.0201	9,054	9.25		L_{25}SCGQVN		nsLTP	EU161278
Ara h 10.0101	15,595	9.36		MTDRTQP		oleosin	AY722694
Ara h 10.0102	17,752	9.61		MTDRTQP		oleosin	AY722695
Ara h 11.0101	14,307	9.08		(M)AEALYY		oleosin	DQ097716
Ara h 12	5,184		PR-12			defensin	
Ara h 13	5,472		PR-12			defensin	
Oleosin	18,435	9.8		MATATDRA		oleosin	AF325917
Oleosin 3	16,875	8.99	IgE-reactive epitope, SDQTRTGY	MSDQTRTGY		oleosin	AAU21501
PNA	26,749	5.03	occurs as tetramer	A_{24}ETVSFN		lectin	S42352

Copyright Dustri-Verlag, data modified from Becker et al. [29], reproduced with permission. MW and pI are calculated from the primary structure of the mature protein, i.e. the structure of the accession No. without the signal peptide (signal 4: http://www.cbs.dtu.dk/services/SignalP/) [30]. Iso = Isoform.

[a] N-terminus incomplete.

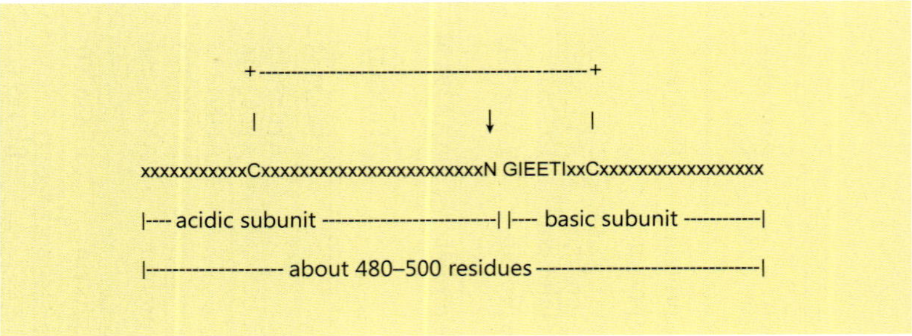

Fig. 1. 11 S seed storage protein signature (Ara h 3) taken from IPR006044 and Becker et al. [29]. Copyright Dustri-Verlag. Reproduced with permission. ↓ indicates cleavage site; x represents any amino acid and C conserved cysteine involved in a disulfide bond.

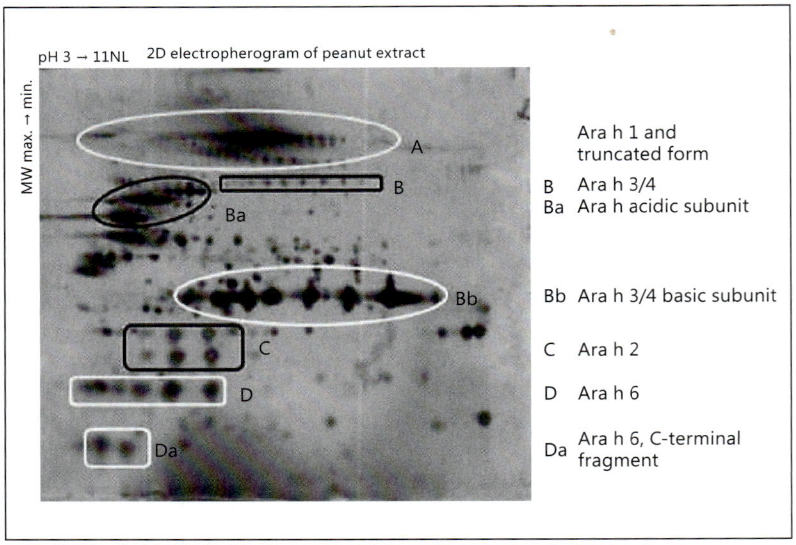

Fig. 2. 2D electropherogram of peanut extract. Taken from figure 4a, modified, in Krause et al. [43]. Copyright Wiley-VCH Verlag GmbH & Co. KGaA. Reproduced with permission. Allocation of the allergens according to figure 3 taken from Schmidt et al. [44]. The first dimension is isoelectric focusing (pH range 3–11, non-linear, 18 cm); the second dimension is 14% SDS-PAGE under reducing conditions. The proteins were visualized by silver staining. Ara h 3/4 was renamed as Ara h 3.01/3.02.

Ara h 2, Ara h 6 and Ara h 7

Ara h 2, Ara h 6 and Ara h 7 are 2 S storage proteins of the conglutin type and belong to the prolamin superfamily. Members of this family are characterized by the presence of a conserved pattern of six or eight cysteine residues that are located within a sequence of about 100 amino acid residues forming three or four intramolecular disulfide bonds and are stable to thermal processing and proteolysis (fig. 3) [48]. Furthermore, they present an α-amylase/trypsin inhibitor motif [48].

Ara h 2 is a major allergen of peanuts and occurs in two isoforms with different MWs, which is due to a 12-amino-acid insert with an MW of 1,414 Da [49]. In peanut extract both isoforms are depicted in the 2D electrophoresis/immunoblot, with at least three spots from each presenting isoallergens (fig. 2). These isoallergens may be generated by amino acid deletion at the C-terminus or amino acid exchanges or site-selective hydroxylation of prolines in positions 46, 53 and 65, as shown by tandem mass spectrometry [50]. Furthermore, Li et al. [50] did not find the N-glycosylation site occupied by oligosaccharides, which is in contrast with previous reports [51]. As experimentally shown, Ara h 2 possesses trypsin inhibitor properties [52]. This explains its resistance to digestion. Moreover, Ara h 2 proved to have the strongest resistance to baking processes when compared to all other peanut allergens [53]. This is in line with the fact that the Maillard reaction (a chemical reaction with sugars) increases the IgE reactivity [52]. One reason might be that some of the ten linear IgE-reactive epitopes improve their immunological fit by the Maillard reaction.

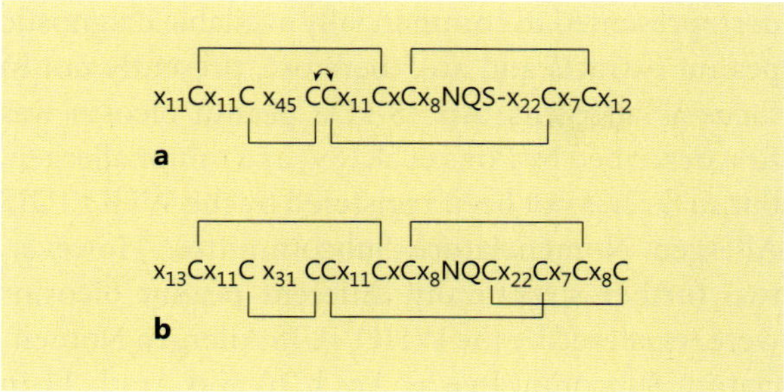

Fig. 3. Structure characteristics of the conglutin: Ara h 2 (**a**) and Ara h 6 (**b**) with conserved cysteines involved in disulfide bonds based on experimental data. Anchor points for disulfide bridges ↷ may be inverted [50, 54]. x represents any amino acid residue. NQS = N-glycosylation site.

In its primary protein sequence, Ara h 6 exhibits an identity with Ara h 2 of 53% and, in comparison with Ara h 2, possesses ten instead of eight cysteines but no N-glycosylation site. Like Ara h 2, Ara h 6 is resistant to digestion and stable against heating, especially in baking processes [55]. The tertiary structure of Ara h 6 (1W2Q) was elucidated, identifying at least four α-helical structures and the location parameters of disulfide bonds (cystine; fig. 3) [54]. In the 2D electrophoresis, at least four spots representing isoallergens of Ara h 6 are detectable (fig. 2). Furthermore, under reducing conditions in the SDS-PAGE/immunoblot an IgE-reactive C-terminal fragment starting with S-48 and an N-terminal fragment of 6 kDa is exclusively detectable by N-terminal sequencing. This is in agreement with the findings of two research groups that identified the described fragments as heterodimers remaining linked via disulfide bonds generated by endogenous cleavage [56, 57]. In digestion experiments under physiological conditions, Ara h 2 and Ara h 6 form stable fragments even under reducing conditions [58]. This supports the idea that cross-reactivities between Ara h 2 and Ara h 6 are mediated by IgE-reactive conformational epitopes. This leads to the question of which of the allergens is the primary sensitizer. Since in Western blotting there are patients who show exclusive IgE reactivities against Ara h 2 or Ara h 6, an independent sensitization pathway by either is to be assumed. The finding that Ara h 2 and Ara h 6 exhibit the biggest part of effector activity in peanut extract is particularly interesting [59].

Ara h 7 was at first identified by the phage display system and cloned, but initially the natural counterpart was not found in peanut extract [60]. Ara h 7.0101 possesses an identity of 42% to Ara h 2, only comes with six cysteines in contrast to the expected eight and contains an N-glycosylation site. These features are in line with findings in the expressed sequence tag (EST) database. However, Schmidt et al. [61] were successful in cloning an Ara h 7.0201 with eight cysteines. In a proteomics project with enriched peanut proteins of an MW below 20 kDa, natural Ara h 7 was identified distributed on six spots in the 2D electrophoresis. By trypsin fingerprinting Ara h 7.0201 was identified as an authentic protein and registered as an allergen by the WHO/IUIS Allergen Nomenclature Subcommittee, and the existence of a second isoallergen, Ara h 7.0202, could be shown [61]. Because of its low content in peanuts its impact on allergy is presently considered to be small.

Ara h 9

The fourth peanut allergen which belongs to the prolamin superfamily is the nsLTP, Ara h 9. Its existence was first described indirectly by Asero et al. [62]. It is difficult to identify Ara h 9 in peanut extract, which is normally obtained by weak basic (pH 8) buffers. Using acidic buffers for extraction we were successful in identifying Ara h 9 by cross-reactive anti-hazelnut LTP rabbit serum [24]. Identifying the N-terminus of peanut nsLTP via Edman degradation and using a peanut EST database we were able to clone two isoforms of Ara h 9.0101 and Ara h 9.0201, which were registered by the WHO/IUIS Allergen Nomenclature Subcommittee. Anti-Ara h 9 IgE-positive patients were mostly found in Mediterranean countries like Italy or Spain and were often suffering from an anti-Pru p 3 IgE-positive peach allergy. Thus, Ara h 9 has features of a class II allergen with Pru p 3 as the primary sensitizer. This is supported by the fact that in those patients the IgE reactivity against classical peanut allergens like Ara h 1, Ara h 2 or Ara h 3 is lacking [24–26]. Probably, the concentration in food is an additional critical factor which determines whether an allergen has the functional properties of a class I or class II allergen.

Ara h 5 and Ara h 8

With regard to their cross-reactivity to inhalant allergens, Ara h 5 and Ara h 8 are typical class II allergens in peanut extract. Their concentration in peanut extract is probably low because in Western blot the respective proteins are not detectable, for instance by India Ink, but are detectable by immunostaining [23, 39]. Ara h 5 has a sequence identity of 72% with the birch pollen profilin Bet v 2 [63]. In Western blot experiments rBet v 2 is not able to inhibit patients' IgE reactivity to Ara h 5 but the vice versa experiment is successful. These findings were supported by homology screening and epitope analysis where Ara h 5 possesses a specific, non-cross-reactive epitope [64]. Mittag et al. [65] investigated the function of Ara h 5 and, especially, Ara h 8. According to their work, the impact of Ara h 5 as a class II food allergen should be low because only 30% of birch pollen-allergic patients are Bet v 2 sensitized. In birch pollen-allergic patients Ara h 8 is a major allergen, which causes a predominantly mild-to-moderate peanut allergy [65]. As shown by Asarnoj et al. [66] the symptoms are mild when ingesting peanuts if the titer of IgE reactivity against birch pollen extract is higher than to peanut extract itself. Riecken et al. [67] were successful in cloning an isoform of Ara h 8.0201 which in its primary structure has a 94% identity with the natural Ara h 8. The authentic structure of Ara h 8.0201 was confirmed by trypsin fingerprinting of isolated nAra h 8. In accordance with the Bet v 1 it was possible to show experimentally that Ara h 8 contains a hydrophobic region [68] in which lipids bind, which, according to preliminary experiments, may prevent the molecule from gastric digestion [68]. All in all these findings spotlight the significance of lipid-protein-(allergen) interaction.

Peanut oleosin, Ara h 10 and Ara h 11

Oleosins are structural proteins that form oil bodies. In SDS-PAGE and subsequently in immunoblot they may occur as dimers and oligomers. Because of their affinity to lipids, oleosins may be underrepresented in commercially available diagnostic peanut extracts and are, therefore, presently not in focus as allergens. An 18-kDa peanut oleosin was first described by Pons et al. [69] as a minor allergen, but so far has not been registered by the WHO/IUIS Allergen Nomenclature Subcommittee. However, two further structurally different peanut oleosins were registered by the WHO/IUIS Allergen Nomenclature Subcommittee as Ara h 10 and Ara h 11 in 2008, but at present (March 2014) a publication is still lacking. Thus, their significance as allergens is unclear. A further candidate as an allergen might be peanut oleosin 3 (accession No. AAU21501) for which an IgE-reactive epitope was found [70].

Ara h 12 and Ara h 13

Peanut defensins were first identified as allergens in 2012 by our group by applying a one-step oleosin extraction method [71] from peanut flour. Using an alkaline (pH 11) aqueous methanol chloroform mixture, when analyzed at 8 kDa by Western blot, the supernatant contained not only oleosins, but also LTP and even defensins as the double band. The defensins presumably occur as dimers [72]. In 2012, the new peanut allergens were assigned by the WHO/IUIS Allergen Nomenclature Subcommittee as Ara h 12 and Ara h 13. Plant defensins are small, highly stable, cysteine-rich peptides primarily directed against fungal pathogens [73].

Peanut Agglutinin and Cross-Reactive Carbohydrate Determinants

PNA, a tetramer, was described as a minor allergen by Burks et al. [74], but so far it has not been accepted as a peanut allergen by the WHO/IUIS Allergen Nomenclature Subcommittee. In our experience patients with IgE reactivity against PNA are rare and, therefore, it seems to be of minor relevance.

In vitro carbohydrate determinant (CCD) reactivity is based on the presence of α1,3-fucose and/or β1,2-xylose residues on N-glycans of plant (xylose/fucose) and insect (fucose) glycoproteins. These IgE-reactive determinants are not present on the canonical peanut allergens known so far. However, there exist glycoproteins with CCDs in peanut extract, which are clinically irrelevant but targets of IgE in CCD-sensitized patients [75]. These CCDs undermine the specificity of serological tests quantifying IgE reactivities. This should be considered when interpreting serological test results for IgE reactivity based on peanut extracts because the IgE concentration against the crude peanut extract may be so high that clinicians regard it as dangerous, not knowing that it is due to basically clinically irrelevant CCD sensitization.

Conclusion

With the identification and preparation of single peanut allergens the foundation for a component-resolved diagnosis is laid and in parts realized. In this context, IgE against Ara h 2 has already been shown to be indicative of a manifest and severe peanut allergy [3]. This also seems to be the case for other storage proteins (Ara h 1, Ara h 6). Furthermore, with the molecular clearance of peanut allergens the possibility of the development of a personalized therapy is provided. In any case it is now possible to study the interaction of single peanut allergens with the gastrointestinal tract and the immune system to elucidate the pathomechanism of peanut allergy. This will provide further insights to answer the question of what makes peanuts so allergenic [76].

Acknowledgements

This review leans on and significantly updates previous reviews published in German [23, 29, 39], with approval given by the Dustri publishing house.

4

References

1 Tan BM, Sher MR, Good RA, Bahna SL: Severe food allergies by skin contact. Ann Allergy Asthma Immunol 2001;86:583–586.

2 Asero R, Antonicelli L: Does sensitization to foods in adults occur always in the gut? Int Arch Allergy Immunol 2010;154:6–14.

3 Nicolaou N, Poorafshar M, Murray C, Simpson A, Winell H, Kerry G, Härlin A, Woodcock A, Ahlstedt S, Custovic A: Allergy or tolerance in children sensitized to peanut: prevalence and differentiation using component-resolved diagnostics. J Allergy Clin Immunol 2010;125:191–197.

4 Asarnoj A, Glaumann S, Elfström L, Lilja G, Lidholm J, Nilsson C, Wickman M: Anaphylaxis to peanut in a patient predominantly sensitized to Ara h 6. Int Arch Allergy Immunol 2012;159:209–212.

5 Sicherer SH, Muñoz-Furlong A, Godbold JH, Sampson HA: US prevalence of self-reported peanut, tree nut, and sesame allergy: 11-year follow-up. J Allergy Clin Immunol 2010;125:1322–1326.

6 Venter C, Hasan Arshad S, Grundy J, Pereira B, Bernie Clayton C, Voigt K, Higgins B, Dean T: Time trends in the prevalence of peanut allergy: three cohorts of children from the same geographical location in the UK. Allergy 2010;65:103–108.

7 Seijo G, Lavia GI, Fernández A, Krapovickas A, Ducasse DA, Bertioli DJ, Moscone EA: Genomic relationships between the cultivated peanut (*Arachis hypogaea*, Leguminosae) and its close relatives revealed by double GISH. Am J Bot 2007;94:1963–1971.

8 Ramos ML, Fleming G, Chu Y, Akiyama Y, Gallo M, Ozias-Akins P: Chromosomal and phylogenetic context for conglutin genes in *Arachis* based on genomic sequence. Mol Genet Genomics 2006;275:578–592.

9 Dillehay TD, Rossen J, Andres TC, Williams DE: Preceramic adoption of peanut, squash, and cotton in northern Peru. Science 2007;316:1890–1893.

10 Phillips SL: The incredible peanut. Ethnobotanical leaflets, 1998. http://opensiuc.lib.siu.edu/ebl/vol1998/iss1/.

11 Purseglove JW: Groundnut; in Purseglove JW (ed): Tropical Crops: Dicotyledons. London, Longmans, Green & Co, 1968, pp 228–237.

12 Koppelman SJ, Vlooswijk RA, Knippels LM, Hessing M, Knol EF, van Reijsen FC, Bruijnzeel-Koomen CA: Quantification of major peanut allergens Ara h 1 and Ara h 2 in the peanut varieties Runner, Spanish, Virginia, and Valencia, bred in different parts of the world. Allergy 2001;56:132–137.

13 Osborne TB: The Proteins of the Wheat Kernel. Washington, Carnegie Institution, 1907.

14 Branlard G, Bancel E: Protein extraction from cereal seeds. Methods Mol Biol 2007;355:15–25.

15 Loza C, Brostoff J: Peanut allergy. Clin Exp Allergy 1995;25:493–502.

16 Mills EN, Jenkins JA, Alcocer MJ, Shewry PR: Structural, biological, and evolutionary relationships of plant food allergens sensitizing via the gastrointestinal tract. Crit Rev Food Sci Nutr 2004;44:379–407.

17 Breiteneder H, Ebner C: Molecular and biochemical classification of plant-derived food allergens. J Allergy Clin Immunol 2000;106:27–36.

18 Shin DS, Compadre CM, Maleki SJ, Kopper RA, Sampson H, Huang SK, Burks AW, Bannon GA: Biochemical and structural analysis of the IgE binding sites on Ara h 1, an abundant and highly allergenic peanut protein. J Biol Chem 1998;273:13753–13759.

19 Stanley JS, King N, Burks AW, Huang SK, Sampson H, Cockrell G, Helm RM, West CM, Bannon GA: Identification and mutational analysis of the immunodominant IgE binding epitopes of the major peanut allergen Ara h 2. Arch Biochem Biophys 1997;342:244–253.

20 Rabjohn P, Helm EM, Stanley JS, West CM, Sampson HA, Burks AW, Bannon GA: Molecular cloning and epitope analysis of the peanut allergen Ara h 3. J Clin Invest 1999;103:535–542.

21 Sen M, Kopper R, Pons L, Abraham EC, Burks AW, Bannon GA: Protein structure plays a critical role in peanut allergen stability and may determine immunodominant IgE-binding epitopes. J Immunol 2002;169:882–887.

22 Kleine-Tebbe J, Vogel L, Crowell DN, Haustein UF, Vieths S: Oral allergy syndrome and anaphylactic reactions caused by a Bet v 1-related PR-10 protein in soybean, SAM22. J Allergy Clin Immunol 2002;110: 797–804.

23 Becker WM , Schocker F, Boldt A: Peanut allergens: structure and characteristics. Allergologie 2005;28:359–366.

24 Krause S, Reese G, Randow S, Zennaro D, Quaratino D, Palazzo P, Ciardiello MA, Petersen A, Becker WM, Mari A: Lipid transfer protein (Ara h 9) as a new peanut allergen relevant for a Mediterranean allergic population. J Allergy Clin Immunol 2009; 124:771–778.

25 Lauer I, Dueringer N, Pokoj S, Rehm S, Zoccatelli G, Reese G, Moncin M, Bahima C, Enrique E, Lidholm J, Vieths S, Scheurer S: The non-specific lipid transfer protein, Ara h 9, is an important allergen in peanut. Clin Exp Allergy 2009;39:1427–1437.

26 Javaloyes G, Goikoetxea MJ, García Núñez I, Sanz ML, Blanca M, Scheurer S, Vieths S, Ferrer M: Performance of different in vitro techniques in the molecular diagnosis of peanut allergy. J Investig Allergol Clin Immunol 2012;22:508–513.

27 Marshall H: 20% of sufferers could outgrow peanut allergy. Trends Immunol 2001;22: 183.

28 Schocker F, Lüttkopf D, Scheurer S, Petersen A, Cistero-Bahima A, Enrique E, San Miguel-Moncin M, Akkerdaas J, van Ree R, Vieths S, Becker WM: Recombinant lipid transfer protein Cor a 8 from hazelnut: a new tool for in vitro diagnosis of potentially severe hazelnut allergy. J Allergy Clin Immunol 2004;113:141–147.

29 Becker WM, Schocker F, Petersen A: Allergene der Erdnuss: Struktur und Charakteristika; in Werfel T, Wüthrich B (eds): Nahrungsmittel und Allergie 3. Munich, Dustri, 2010, pp 156–166.

30 Petersen TN, Brunak S, von Heijne G, Nielsen H: SignalP 4.0: discriminating signal peptides from transmembrane regions. Nat Methods 2011;8:785–786.

31 Maleki SJ, Kopper RA, Shin DS, Park CW, Compadre CM, Sampson H, Burks AW, Bannon GA: Structure of the major peanut allergen Ara h 1 may protect IgE-binding epitopes from degradation. J Immunol 2000;164:5844–5849.

32 van Boxtel EL, van Beers MMC, Koppelman SJ, van den Broek LAM, Gruppen H: Allergen Ara h 1 occurs in peanuts as a large oligomer rather than as a trimer. J Agric Food Chem 2006;54:7180–7186.

33 Mills EN, Jenkins J, Marigheto N, Belton PS, Gunning AP, Morris VJ: Allergens of the cupin superfamily. Biochem Soc Trans 2002; 30:925–929.

34 Becker WM: Characterization of Ara h 1 by two-dimensional electrophoresis, immunoblot and recombinant techniques: new digestion experiments with peanuts imitating the gastrointestinal tract. Int Arch Allergy Immunol 1997;113:118–121.

35 Barnett D, Howden ME: Partial characterization of an allergenic glycoprotein from peanut (*Arachis hypogaea* L.). Biochem Biophys Acta 1986;882:97–105.

36 Kolarich D, Altmann F: N-Glycan analysis by matrix-assisted laser desorption/ionization mass spectrometry of electrophoretically separated nonmammalian proteins: application to peanut allergen Ara h 1 and olive pollen allergen Ole e 1. Anal Biochem 2000;285:64–75.

37 Buschmann L, Petersen A, Schlaak M, Becker WM: Reinvestigation of the major peanut allergen Ara h 1 on molecular level. Monogr Allergy 1996;32:92–98.

38 Wichers HJ, De Beijer T, Savelkoul HF, Van Amerongen A: The major peanut allergen Ara h 1 and its cleaved-off N-terminal peptide; possible implications for peanut allergen detection. J Agric Food Chem 2004;52: 4903–4907.

39 Becker WM, Petersen A, Jappe U: Peanut allergens: new consolidated findings on structure, characteristics and allergome. Allergologie 2011;34:398–411.

40 Latendorf T: Proteom-Analyse von Allergenen unterschiedlicher Erdnussvarietäten; Diplomarbeit, Institut für Immunologie, Christian-Albrechts-Universität zu Kiel, 2007.

41 Burks AW, Sampson HA, Bannon GA: Peanut allergens. Allergy 1998;53:725–730.

42 Eigenmann PA, Burks AW, Bannon GA, Sampson HA: Identification of unique peanut and soy allergens in sera adsorbed with cross-reacting antibodies. J Allergy Clin Immunol 1996;98:969–978.

43 Krause S, Latendorf T, Schmidt H, Darcan-Nicolaisen Y, Reese G, Petersen A, Janssen O, Becker WM: Peanut varieties with reduced Ara h 1 content indicating no reduced allergenicity. Mol Nutr Food Res 2010;54:381–387.

44 Schmidt H, Gelhaus C, Latendorf T, Nebendahl M, Petersen A, Krause S, Leippe M, Becker WM, Janssen O: 2-D DIGE analysis of the proteome of extracts from peanut variants reveals striking differences in major allergen contents. Proteomics 2009;9: 3507–3521.

45 Dodo HW, Viquez OM, Maleki SJ, Konan KN: cDNA clone of a putative peanut (*Arachis hypogaea* L.) trypsin inhibitor has homology with peanut allergens Ara h 3 and Ara h 4. J Agric Food Chem 2004;52:1404–1409.

46 Boldt A, Fortunato D, Conti A, Petersen A, Ballmer-Weber B, Lepp U, Reese G, Becker WM: Analysis of the composition of an IgE-reactive high molecular weight protein complex of peanut extract containing Ara h 1 and Ara h 3/4. Proteomics 2005;5:675–686.

47 Restani P, Ballabio C, Corsini E, Fiocchi A, Isoardi P, Magni C, Poiesi C, Terracciano L, Duranti M: Identification of the basic subunit of Ara h 3 as the major allergen in a group of children allergic to peanuts. Ann Allergy Asthma Immunol 2005;94:262–266.

48 Mills EN, Jenkins JA, Alcocer MJ, Shewry PR: Structural, biological, and evolutionary relationships of plant food allergens sensitizing via the gastrointestinal tract. Crit Rev Food Sci Nutr 2004;44:379–407.

49 Chatel JM, Bernard H, Orson FM: Isolation and characterization of two complete Ara h 2 isoforms cDNA. Int Arch Allergy Immunol 2003;131:14–18.

50 Li J, Shefcheck K, Callahan J, Fenselau C: Primary sequence and site-selective hydroxylation of prolines in isoforms of a major peanut allergen protein Ara h 2. Protein Sci 2010;19:174–182.

51 Burks AW, Williams LW, Connaughton C, Cockrell G, O'Brien TJ, Helm RM: Identification and characterization of a second major peanut allergen, Ara h II, with use of the sera of patients with atopic dermatitis and positive peanut challenge. J Allergy Clin Immunol 1992;90:962–969.

52 Maleki S, Viquez O, Jacks T, Dodo H, Champagne ET, Chung SY, Landry SJ: The major peanut allergen, Ara h 2, functions as a trypsin inhibitor, and roasting enhances this function. J Allergy Clin Immunol 2003;112: 190–195.

53 Gruber P, Becker WM, Hofmann T: Influence of the Maillard reaction on the allergenicity of rAra h 2, a recombinant major allergen from peanut *(Arachis hypogaea)*, its major epitopes, and peanut agglutinin. J Agric Food Chem 2005;53:2289–2296.

54 Lehmann K, Schweimer K, Reese G, Randow S, Suhr M, Becker WM, Vieths S, Rösch P: Structure and stability of 2S albumin type peanut allergens: implications for the severity of peanut allergic reactions. Biochem J 2006;395:463–472.

55 Suhr M, Wicklein D, Lepp U, Becker WM: Isolation and characterization of natural Ara h 6: evidence for a further peanut allergen with putative clinical relevance based on resistance to pepsin digestion and heat. Mol Nutr Food Res 2004;48:390–399.

56 Bernard H, Mondoulet L, Drumare MF, Paty E, Scheinmann P, Thaï R, Wal JM: Identification of a new natural Ara h 6 isoform and of its proteolytic product as major allergens in peanut. J Agric Food Chem 2007;55:9663–9669.

57 Marsh J, Rigby N, Wellner K, Reese G, Knulst A, Akkerdaas J, van Ree R, Radauer C, Lovegrove A, Sancho A, Mills C, Vieths S, Hoffmann-Sommergruber K, Shewry PR, Marsh J, Rigby N, Wellner K, Reese G, Knulst A, Akkerdaas J, van Ree R, Radauer C, Lovegrove A, Sancho A, Mills C, Vieths S, Hoffmann-Sommergruber K, Shewry PR: Purification and characterisation of a panel of peanut allergens suitable for use in allergy diagnosis. Mol Nutr Food Res 2008;52(suppl 2):272–285.

58 Koppelman SJ, Hefle SL, Taylor SL, de Jong GA: Digestion of peanut allergens Ara h 1, Ara h 2, Ara h 3, and Ara h 6: a comparative in vitro study and partial characterization of digestion-resistant peptides. Mol Nutr Food Res 2010;54:1711–1721.

59 Chen X, Zhuang Y, Wang Q, Moutsoglou D, Ruiz G, Yen SE, Dreskin SC: Analysis of the effector activity of Ara h 2 and Ara h 6 by selective depletion from a crude peanut extract. J Immunol Methods 2011;372:65–70.

60 Kleber-Janke T, Crameri R, Appenzeller U, Schlaak M, Becker WM: Selective cloning of peanut allergens, including profilin and 2S albumins, by phage display technology. Int Arch Allergy Immunol 1999;119:265–274.

61 Schmidt H, Krause S, Gelhaus C, Petersen A, Janssen O, Becker WM: Detection and structural characterization of natural Ara h 7, the third peanut allergen of the 2S albumin family. J Proteome Res 2010;9:3701–709.

62 Asero R, Mistrello G, Roncarolo D, Amato S, Caldironi G, Barocci F, van Ree R: Immunological cross-reactivity between lipid transfer proteins from botanically unrelated plant-derived foods: a clinical study. Allergy 2002;57:900–906.

63 Kleber-Janke T, Crameri R, Scheurer S, Vieths S, Becker WM: Patient tailored cloning of allergens by phage display: peanut *(Arachis hypogaea)* profilin, a food allergen enriched from rare mRNA. J Chromatogr B 2001;756:295–305.

64 Cabanos C, Tandang-Silvas MR, Odijk V, Brostedt P, Tanaka A, Utsumi S, Maruyama N: Expression, purification, cross-reactivity and homology modeling of peanut profilin. Protein Expr Purif 2010;73:36–45.

65 Mittag D, Akkerdaas J, Ballmer-Weber BK, Vogel L, Wensing M, Becker WM, Koppelman SJ, Knulst AC, Helbling A, Hefle SL, van Ree R, Vieths S: Ara h 8, a Bet v 1-homologous allergen from peanut, is a major allergen in patients with combined birch pollen and peanut allergy. J Allergy Clin Immunol 2004;114:1410–1417.

66 Asarnoj A, Movérare R, Ostblom E, Poorafshar M, Lilja G, Hedlin G, van Hage M, Ahlstedt S, Wickman M: IgE to peanut allergen components: relation to peanut symptoms and pollen sensitization in 8-year-olds. Allergy 2010;65:1189–1195.

67 Riecken S, Lindner B, Petersen A, Jappe U, Becker WM: Purification and characterization of natural Ara h 8, the Bet v 1 homologous allergen from peanut, provides a novel isoform. Biol Chem 2008;389:415–423.

68 Petersen A, Rennert S, Kull S, Becker WM, Notbohm H, Goldmann T, Jappe U: Roasting and lipid binding provide allergenic and proteolytic stability to the peanut allergen Ara h 8. Biol Chem 2014;395:239–250.

69 Pons L, Chery C, Romano A, Namour F, Artesani MC, Gueant JL: The 18 kDa peanut oleosin is a candidate allergen for IgE-mediated reactions to peanuts. Allergy 2002;57:88–93.

70 Kobayashi S, Katsuyama S, Wagatsuma T, Okada S, Tanabe S: Identification of a new IgE-binding epitope of peanut oleosin that cross-reacts with buckwheat. Biosci Biotechnol Biochem 2012;76:1182–1188.

71 D'Andréa S, Jolivet P, Boulard C, Larré C, Froissard M, Chardot T: Selective one-step extraction of *Arabidopsis thaliana* seed oleosins using organic solvents. J Agric Food Chem 2007;55:10008–10015.

72 Petersen A, Rennert S, Böttger M, Becker WM, Krause S, Gutsmann T, Lindner B, Jappe U: Defensin: a novel allergen in peanuts? European Academy of Allergy and Clinical Immunology Congress 16–20 June 2012 in Geneva. Allergy 2012;67(Suppl 96):374.

73 Sagaram US, Pandurangi R, Kaur J, Smith TJ, Shah DM: Structure-activity determinants in antifungal plant defensins MsDef1 and MtDef4 with different modes of action against *Fusarium graminearum*. PLoS One 2011;6:e18550.

74 Burks AW, Cockrell G, Connaughton C, Guin J, Allen W, Helm RM: Identification of peanut agglutinin and soybean trypsin inhibitor as minor legume allergens. Int Arch Allergy Immunol 1994;105:143–149.

75 Vidal C, Vizcaino L, Díaz-Peromingo JA, Garrido M, Gomez-Rial J, Linneberg A, Gonzalez-Quintela A: Immunoglobulin-E reactivity to a glycosylated food allergen (peanuts) due to interference with cross-reactive carbohydrate determinants in heavy drinkers. Alcohol Clin Exp Res 2009; 33:1322–1328.

76 Petersen A, Becker WM, Jappe U: What makes peanuts so allergenic? J Serb Chem Soc 2013;78:321–331.

4

Dr. rer. nat. Wolf-Meinhard Becker and Prof. Dr. med. Uta Jappe
Research Center Borstel
Parkallee 35
DE–23845 Borstel (Germany)
E-Mail wbecker@fz-borstel.de and ujappe@fz-borstel.de

Bergmann K-C, Ring J (eds): History of Allergy. Chem Immunol Allergy. Basel, Karger, 2014, vol 100, pp 268–277
DOI: 10.1159/000359918

Environmental Pollution and Allergy: Historical Aspects

Heidrun Behrendt[a, c] · Francesca Alessandrini[a, c] · Jeroen Buters[a, c] · Ursula Krämer[d] · Hillel Koren[e] · Johannes Ring[b, c]

[a]Center for Allergy and Environment (ZAUM), [b]Department of Dermatology and Allergology Biederstein, Technical University of Munich (TUM), and [c]Christine Kühne Center for Allergy Research and Education (CK-CARE), Munich, and [d]IUF-Leibniz-Research Institute for Environmental Medicine, Düsseldorf, Germany; [e]Environmental Protection Agency (EPA), Durham, N.C., USA

Abstract

It may be a coincidence, but it is a fact that the first clear characterization of hay fever began in England where modern industrialization started in Europe. Only at the end of the 20th century were associations of the increasing prevalence of allergy with outdoor air pollution discussed. The seminal study came from Japan from the group of T. Miyamoto linking the increase in Japanese cedar pollinosis to an increased prevalence of Diesel cars and probably exposure to Diesel exhaust in epidemiological, animal experimental and in vitro studies. In Germany first epidemiological studies were done in North Rhine-Westphalia and Bavaria in 1987 and 1988 showing a striking prevalence of allergic disease of up to 10–20% in preschool children. After German reunification the most surprising observation was a lower prevalence of hay fever in East German children compared to the West, although there was a much higher air pollution with SO_2 and large particulate matter. Modern smog as found over West German cities most likely originating from traffic exhaust and consisting of fine and ultrafine particles was shown to be associated with higher incidence rates of allergy and allergic sensitization. In the 10 years after reunification there was a steep increase of allergy prevalence in East German children reaching almost the same level as in West Germany. Obviously, a multitude of lifestyle factors – beyond air pollution – may be involved in the explanation of this phenomenon. Surprisingly the skin manifestation of atopy, namely atopic eczema, was more frequent in East German children compared to the West, thus differing from airway allergy. Meanwhile in vitro studies and animal experiments have shown that a variety of air pollutants mostly from environmental tobacco smoke (indoors) and from traffic exhaust (outdoors) can stimulate immune cells inducing a Th2-dominated response besides their irritative effects. While 50 years ago in allergy textbooks a clear distinction was made between 'toxic' or 'allergic', the newly developed concept of allergotoxicology has stimulated research tremendously, meaning 'the investigation of effects of toxic substances upon the induction, elicitation and maintenance of allergic reactions'.

The observation that noxious agents from the environment can affect human health goes back to ancient times [see the chapters by Ring, this vol., pp. 2–20]. While it was mostly infectious agents that threatened whole populations through epidemics such as pests or smallpox, it was already apparent in the Middle Ages that man-made 'pollution', i.e. impurities in the air, could also lead to disease. In 1272, King Edward I of England, for example, gave the order to reduce the coal smoke problem [1].

Regarding indoor air the roots of occupational medicine lie in the discovery of noxious agents associated with certain occupations [2]. Together with the beginning of industrialization this part of environmental hygiene became more and more apparent. Maybe it is no coincidence that the first actual descriptions and real research on hay fever began in England, where modern industrialization started in Europe.

Only in the 20th century were public health measures taken, especially after the 'big smog' episodes in the city of London in the 1950s [3], and finally leading to the 'Clean Air Acts' introduced in the USA in 1970 and followed by several amendments [1].

While the role of environmental pollutants in the development of allergy was only slowly taken up by the scientific community, it was lay groups, the press and certain developments of alternative medicine which brought the problem to the attention of the public. Especially in the USA, the theory of clinical ecology had derived from American allergists in the 1920s, leading to a concept that almost any kind of 'impairment of feeling well' might be an 'allergy' against some environmental noxious substances, most commonly pollutant chemicals; the clinical symptoms were often psychological abnormalities or psychiatric diseases after the ingestion of foods or contact with chemicals [4–7].

In the 1970s, large areas of woodland in Germany were suffering from an unknown disease leading to the death of thousands of trees – the phenomenon called 'Waldsterben' ('dying forests') aroused tremendous public interest. It might be mentioned that the forest plays an essential role in German culture, philosophy and art, especially with regard to the German romanticism in the 19th century with the popular movement of hiking through forests. The phenomenon of 'Waldsterben' paved the way for studies investigating environmental pollutant effects upon human health. It was attributed mainly to the so-called 'acid rain' originating from high sulfur dioxide emissions from old power plants.

Table 1. Classification of particle air pollutants

Compartment:
- Indoor
- Outdoor

Sources:
- Industrial sources
- Traffic exhaust
- Emission of pollutants by catastrophes, illegal practices or exceptional circumstances

Development:
- Primary, directly emitted into the atmosphere
- Secondary, only developing in the air by chemical processes

Aggregate state:
- Gaseous
- Particulate

Size:
- Large/coarse particulate matter 2.5–10 μm (PM 10)
- Fine particles 0.1–2.5 μm (PM 2.5)
- Ultrafine particles <0.1 μm

Origin:
- Biogenic (by nature; e.g. pollen, molds)
- Anthropogenic (by human activity)

Scientific investigations accepting the influence of environmental pollutants as relevant for allergic diseases or as worthwhile to be studied only seriously began at the end of the 1970s and beginning of the 1980s. These investigations primarily comprised epidemiological trials, in vitro studies of cell culture systems, clinical studies and finally animal experiments, but also aerobiological studies.

With regard to indoor air, exposure to environmental tobacco smoke was primarily studied. With regard to outdoor air pollution one had to differentiate between different kinds of particles according to size (table 1) and quality, as well as its origin from either industrial sources or traffic exhaust.

In many countries (as for example in Germany) this research was not very much appreciated by the mainstream authorities. Scientists trying to study the effect of environmental pollutants with regard to allergy were often regarded as 'political' or seen to be

Table 2. Prevalence of hay fever associated with allergy to Japanese cedar pollen in various environments in the Nikko area [12]

People living within 200 m from heavy traffic and densely planted cedar trees	13.2%
People living in areas near cedar tree forests with considerable car traffic	8.8%
People living near cedar tree forests with limited traffic	5.1%
People living in mountain areas with almost no cedar trees	1.7%
People living in areas with high traffic, but sparse cedar growth	9.6%

in contact with the newly developing 'green' parties in Europe, so that official funding by research authorities was very difficult to obtain.

In the following the authors will give a short review of some personal experiences, which will also touch on the work of other groups. However, we would like to stress that this is not a scientific-historic analysis describing developments all over the world in detail, but rather a subjective summary.

One of the authors (H.B.) clearly remembers a lecture of the German allergist Karlheinz Schulz from Hamburg at a WHO meeting 1983 where he clearly demonstrated that apparently toxic substances can also induce allergic reactions [8]. He even postulated that in order to induce allergy, a substance should have some 'toxic' properties [Schulz, pers. commun.]. This lecture may have started the development of the concept of 'allergotoxicology', as will be described later in this chapter.

Epidemiological Studies

Early Studies in Japan

There were reports of associations of the increasing prevalence of allergies with outdoor air pollution in 1966 [9, 10], yet the real epidemiology of allergy with regard to environmental pollution started in Japan in the 1980s with studies performed by the group of Miyamoto.

Terumasa Miyamoto noticed in the 1960s that there was a high and increasing prevalence of hay fever in Japan on the basis of allergy to Japanese cedar pollen *(Cryptomeria japonica)*. Miyamoto concluded that the increase in Japanese cedar pollen allergy could not be attributed to an increased prevalence of cedar trees in Japan which had been there for centuries.

In 1974, the prevalence of Japanese cedar pollen allergy was below 3.8%, in the year 1981 it was 9.4% [11, 12]. This phenomenon gave birth to the idea of an epidemiological study in Japan in five different areas around the famous town of Nikko. Miyamoto's group compared the following populations: (1) people living within 200 m of intercity roads with high traffic volumes and densely planted with Japanese cedar trees; (2) areas in or near cedar forests with limited traffic; (3) areas with cedar forests and considerable car traffic; (4) areas in the Japanese mountains with almost no cedars, and (5) areas in small towns where Japanese cedar trees were less common but there was a rather high car traffic volume.

The results of these studies were impressive (table 2). It became apparent that the highest prevalence of Japanese cedar pollinosis was found along roads lined with Japanese cedar trees (13.2%), whereas hay fever and Japanese cedar pollen allergy was almost absent (1.7%) in mountain areas with no cedar growth. The other populations showed prevalence rates between 5.1 and 9.6% [12].

In the discussion of their findings, Miyamoto mentioned that in the same decades between 1951 and 1988 the number of diesel cars registered in Japan had shown a dramatic increase from 20,000 to 7,600,000. In 1988, the total number of automobiles in Japan was 53,000,000. This led the group to study more intensively the effects of diesel exhaust particles in animal experiments and in in vitro studies (see below).

Early Studies in Germany

In Germany, the epidemiology of allergy started in two different places, namely in Düsseldorf in North Rhine-Westphalia in 1986 and in Munich in Bavaria in 1987. The two groups did not know each other and only met at the congress of the European Academy of Allergy and Clinical Immunology (EAACI) in September 1989 in Berlin, where they were surprised that they had found similar results showing a rather high prevalence of allergy (16–

20%) in pre-school children [13, 14]. The history of each of these initiatives is shortly described in the following paragraphs.

In the 1950s and 1960s, the Ruhr area in North Rhine-Westphalia was heavily polluted and extremely high SO_2 and particle concentrations were measured, and even visibility was affected. Therefore, at the end of the 1960s Chancellor Willy Brandt declared that the sky above the Ruhr area should be blue again. Clean air plans, which were enforced by law (Bundesimmissionsschutzgesetz), were introduced. At first they mainly consisted of huge measurement campaigns of air-borne pollutants to control whether concentrations were below the limit values. In the mid-1970s, the state government with Heinz Kühn and Johannes Rau as prime ministers decided that the clean air plans should not only include air pollution concentration registries, but also so-called 'Wirkungskataster' (registration of effects) whereby health parameters of the population were also studied in the same areas as where air pollution measurements were made. In the first years allergies were explicitly excluded from these registries of effects because they were considered as diseases too rare to be relevant. Health effects in children entering primary school were investigated from 1985 and only in 1987 were parameters of allergic diseases included in these 'Wirkungskataster' examinations [15] due to the initiative of Heidrun Behrendt, then a member of the Medizinisches Institut für Umwelthygiene (headed by Hans-Werner Schlipköter), which conducted the 'Wirkungskataster' on behalf of the local government.

In Bavaria, prime minister Franz-Josef Strauss wanted to build a nuclear recycling plant ('Wiederaufbereitungsanlage') in order to solve the problem of nuclear waste near the town of Schwandorf in the Upper Palatinate, close to the Czech border. There was increasing opposition in the population with protests and demonstrations against the government. Franz-Josef Strauss decided on a very simple procedure: to examine the population in the area of Schwandorf prior to the establishment of the nuclear plant and to repeat this examination in regular intervals after the recycling facility had begun operating, thus providing scientific evidence as to whether or not there was a hazard to human health. He then called an expert committee existing of nuclear physicists, radiation biologists, epidemiologists, microbiologists and several clinical disciplines. One of the authors (J.R.) had to replace his boss at this meeting and was surprised that almost all the experts were totally uninterested; they concluded that such a study would be a waste of money since 'with all likelihood nothing really serious could occur'. The meeting took place in the Ministry of Environment of the State of Bavaria (Bavaria was the first state to officially found such a ministry in Germany) and the moderator of the session, the chemist Dr. Vogel, being a highly ranked ministry official, was trying to motivate the experts to do something. Finally, the only two groups making a commitment were the Department of Dermatology (Otto Braun-Falco, Johannes Ring) and the Department of Epidemiology of Ludwig Maximilian University (with Karl Überla). Thus, the first epidemiological study investigating the parameters of allergy, both of immediate type and delayed type (contact allergy), was started in several areas in Upper Palatinate with control regions in Upper Franconia and Upper Bavaria (Bad Reichenhall, Berchtesgaden in the alpine region).

Strikingly, these investigations showed a high prevalence of atopic diseases (asthma, rhinoconjunctivitis, atopic eczema) in 5- to 6-year-old preschool children both in North Rhine-Westphalia and Bavaria, with prevalence rates between 10 and 20%! Many parents were not even aware of the disease, so it became clear that the high prevalence of allergy was not due to increased public awareness, but was indeed a true fact. Comparing the various regions, there were no significant differences within Bavaria, and high rates were also found in the Upper Bavarian region of Berchtesgaden, known as a tourist resort. There was a trend towards higher prevalence rates for atopic eczema in areas near the Czech or East German border with high air pollution.

In North Rhine-Westphalia it was found that there were significant differences between certain areas, with children in rural areas less affected. Furthermore, for the first time it was found in German children that there was a clear-cut association with exposure to traffic exhausts. The prevalence of sensitization against pollen was significantly higher for children spending more than 1 h per day in heavy traffic than for those spending less time in traffic. Such an association was only found in Cologne but not in rural Borken [15].

East/West Comparison Studies in Germany and Europe

Six weeks after the EAACI congress in Berlin in 1989, the Berlin Wall was knocked down and the reunification of East and West Germany started. Nobody would have seriously envisaged this, except, perhaps, the British allergist Thomas Platts-Mills who, sitting in front of a beer in a street café said to one of the authors the prophetic words: 'The last time I was in Berlin was in 1961 when they built this crazy wall, it's really time now they tear it down!'

This political change allowed epidemiological studies in populations of different regions with the same ethnic background, climatic characteristics and cultural heritage, with the only difference being that these parts were divided by communist dictatorship ('experimentum dictaturae'). Six groups in Germany immediately started to plan epidemiological investigations in East and West Germany, namely the group of Dennis Nowak and Joachim Heinrich, who compared Hamburg in West Germany with Erfurt in East Germany in the frame of the European Community Respiratory Health Survey (ECRHS), and the group of Heinz-Erich Wichmann and Joachim Heinrich, who observed health trends in the villages of Bitterfeld, Hettstedt and Zerbst in Saxony-Anhalt, part of the former East Germany. Erika von Mutius from Munich studied children in the city of Leipzig (former East Germany) and compared the results with children from Munich. The group of Ulrich Keil and Stephan Weiland compared results from Münster (West Germany) with those in Greifswald (East Germany) in the frame of the ISAAC project, and the West German federal health survey conducted by the Robert Koch Institute was extended to places in East Germany. The group around Heidrun Behrendt, Ursula Krämer and Johannes Ring compared different regions both in East and West Germany selected according to air pollution parameters in North Rhine-Westphalia (West Germany), Saxony and Saxony-Anhalt (former East Germany). Here both rural and urban areas were included.

Here are some personal recollections of the study which was conducted by the Institute for Environmental Hygiene at the Heinrich Heine University in Düsseldorf (director, Hans-Werner Schlipköter) and the Department of Dermatology and Allergy at the University of Hamburg (director, Johannes Ring) in co-operation with several groups of the former 'Bezirkshygieneinstitute' (district hygiene institutes) in Halle, Magdeburg, and several towns in the 'Altmark' region. For such studies there was no special funding and it would have taken too long to apply for official grants. The study was funded from the budget of the institutes in Düsseldorf and Hamburg. The first visits to Saxony and Saxony-Anhalt were like an 'expedition' into a foreign country. The concrete walls and frontier buildings were still existent along the border, although the fences had no function any longer and the watch towers from where machine guns had been fired had been vacated only recently. When we got out of the car in Halle, one of us suffered a severe attack of coughing due to the obvious high content of sulfur oxide in the air, which could also be clearly smelled. Sometimes we met in rooms formerly used by the 'Stasi' (State Security, the secret police of the German Democratic Republic). However, we were in an enthusiastic mood and we met many excellent and friendly colleagues from East Germany who had a lot of experience in environmental medicine.

At the level of the district hygiene institutes, water, soil, air and health were combined in one institute, whereas in West Germany for the same measurements we usually had to contact four different institutes. The only difference was that these institutes in East Germany had not been allowed to publish the results of their measurements, or had done so only with great difficulties.

In addition to questionnaires we examined every single child and, uniquely, we not only studied the airway, but also the skin by dermatologically trained physicians from Hamburg University. At a certain point in time there were 16 physicians from the department busy with the field work in various locations in West and East Germany. The remaining physicians at home had to work twice as hard. The same held true for the researchers in Düsseldorf. This whole endeavor was only possible on the basis of the tremendous enthusiasm of all the young colleagues involved, so that in the winter of 1990/1991 we could already start with our work. The official reunification of East and West Germany occurred on October 3, 1990. A little later, Bengt Björkstén from Linköping carried out a study comparing children from the Eastern European country of Estonia with children from Sweden.

The results of these studies have filled books and thick volumes of reports and have been published in many articles [16–26]. There were three striking findings: (1) there was a significantly higher amount of air pollution with regard to sulfur dioxide and large particles in East Germany compared to West Germany, but more traffic-related pollution in West Germany; (2) there was less airway allergy and sensitization in East German children compared to their West German counterparts, and (3) the prevalence of eczema did not follow the pattern of airway allergy; it was even higher in East German children [27]. Furthermore, in this study we found that children in East Germany had significantly higher total serum immunoglobulin (Ig) E levels, while at the same time they suffered less from airway allergy [16].

The striking finding of less hay fever in the higher polluted East German area became known worldwide and led to some – maybe premature and unjustified – 'conclusions', culminating in the sentence 'environment has nothing to do with the increase in allergies', which has been uttered by some researchers from that time until today.

It was obvious that the type of air pollution prevalent in Eastern Europe was not associated with increased allergy prevalence rates. However, in the study comparing East and West German areas with varying air pollution it was found that the 'modern' type of air pollution over West German cities with fine particles and ozone most likely originating from traffic exhaust was associated with high allergy prevalence rates; so it was important not only to measure the quantity, but also to characterize the quality of air pollution!

There were of course many other variables of lifestyle parameters which differed between East and West Germany besides air pollution [28]. One factor was that children in East Germany, compared to West German children, more often and from a younger age (already during the first year of life) attended childcare facilities ('Kinderkrippen'). Children attending day care centers very early in life had less asthma and sensitization (but not eczema) later in life than those not attending day care centers at a young age. Thus, immune stimulation by microbial contact might have exerted a protective effect [29]. In 1989, David Strachan coined the term 'hygiene hypothesis' when he found that younger children in large families had less allergies than the eldest siblings, maybe attributed to more infectious stimuli with protective effects regarding allergy development [30].

One could write a whole book on the possible mechanisms for explanation of the differences between East and West Germany with regard to allergy. Until now all these concepts are hypothetical in nature and we do not know for sure what caused the difference (e.g. much lower and decreased mobility, less freedom to move, slower pace of daily life, more old-fashioned living conditions and household equipment, different types of cars and traffic exhaust, differences in vaccination strategies and compliance) [see the chapter by Gassner, this vol., pp. 278–286]. However, after carefully following and comparing the trends in allergy prevalence over 10 years, some possible explanations have emerged. Hay fever and sensitization against pollen were the most sensitive allergic manifestations to changes experienced specifically in East Germany. Increasing numbers of only children, less single-room heating with fossil fuels and the increasing importance of traffic-related pollution in East Germany partly explained the differences in time trends between East and West Germany [31]. Interestingly, in the context of a later study the still higher eczema prevalence in East (Leipzig) than in West Germany (Munich) could be completely explained by differences in early day care attendance (still very often in the East and very rare in the West) because children with early day care attendance had much more eczema at the age of 6 years than children without [32]. This is at least an explanation for the East-West German differences in eczema prevalence of today. Possibly this same explanation also holds for the differences in eczema prevalence between 1991 and 2000.

In 1985, the family practitioner Dr. Gassner found in the small village of Grabs in the Rhine valley that

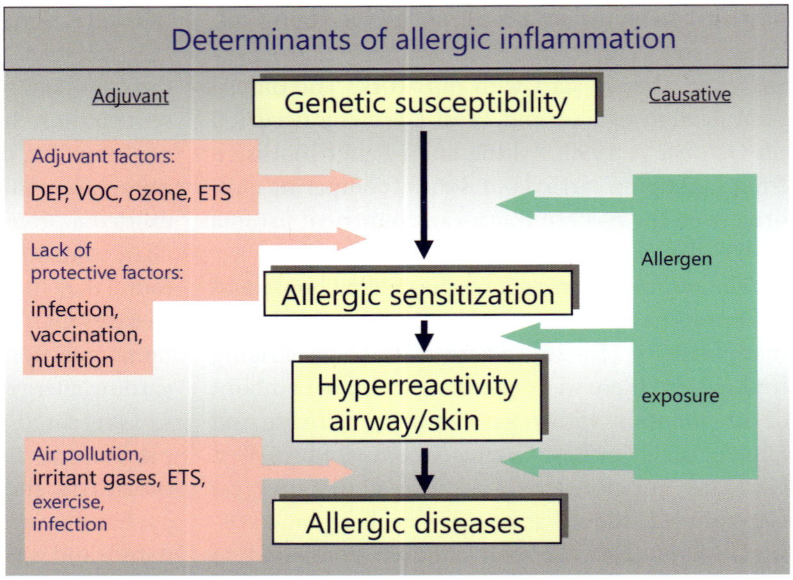

Fig. 1. Determinants of the biogenic and anthropogenic environment influencing the development of an allergic reaction [according to 42]. DEP = Diesel exhaust particles; VOC = volatile organic compounds; ETS = environmental tobacco smoke.

the children of farmers had hay fever significantly less often than the children of teachers or other people living in the same village and breathing the same air [33, 34]. From these observations the famous studies in alpine farmers in Bavaria, Switzerland and Austria originated which proved that farmers' children indeed suffer much less frequently from allergy (respiratory allergy) than other children in the same villages. In trying to explain this phenomenon, early immune stimulation already in the womb – when the mother is working in the stable and when she is drinking unprocessed cow's milk – has been suggested to be an important allergen-protective factor [35].

It has to be kept in mind that the term 'environment' became more and more restricted to the anthropogenic factors, while natural constituents of ambient aerosols, like pollen and molds, were rather forgotten until the early 1990s. It is interesting that in most of these older epidemiological investigations generally no effort was made to quantify the allergen exposure of the children examined. All this only came much later with measurements of house dust mite allergen in the indoor air [36] and again very much later with measurement of free pollen allergen in the outdoor air [37].

Furthermore, in large epidemiological trials including the cities of Hamburg in Northern Germany and Augsburg in Southern Germany it became apparent that within Germany there was not only an East-West gradient, but also a North-South gradient in allergen prevalence. Incidentally, the city of Leipzig is not so much to the east, but rather to the north of Munich. This might help to explain why the most striking differences between East and West German children were found in the study performed by Erika von Mutius comparing Leipzig and Munich [26, 38].

Aerobiological Studies

Only at the end of the 1970s were pollen counts regularly measured over large areas within North America and Europe, and only in the 1990s did scientists start to study the interactions between pollutant particles and pollen. It was found that pollen from highly polluted urban aerosols showed agglomeration of fine dust particles; these interactions led to morphological changes of the pollen surface and also altered the release patterns of pollen constituents [39] (fig. 1).

In 1981, Burrows [40] found relevant associations between allergen exposure, air pollution in the form of environmental tobacco smoke and parameters of allergic sensitization. The process of pollen grain activation and allergen release was found to be influenced by environmental pollutants, both gaseous (e.g. ozone) and particulate in nature [41]. Sulfur dioxide as a gaseous pollutant was shown to have a clear inhibitory effect on allergen release from pollen, an effect which also might help to explain the East-West differences in hay fever prevalence.

Studying allergen release from pollen and mechanisms of pollen activation, it was found that pollen are more than allergen carriers: under humid conditions they also release potent biologically active mediators like pollen-associated lipid mediators with pro-inflammatory and immunomodulatory effects [42–44].

In vitro Studies

Parallel to the epidemiological trials in several groups the effects of environmental pollutants were studied in in vitro cellular systems using macrophages, lymphocytes, mast cells and eosinophils [12, 45–47]. It was found that some air pollutants, especially diesel exhaust particles, were able to induce Th2 immune deviation and secretion of interleukin-4 and interleukin-13 in the cell culture [48].

Animal Experiments

The group of Miyamoto had already collected diesel exhaust particles and injected them together with ovalbumin as allergen into Balb/c mice and found enhanced IgE production when diesel exhaust particles were applied together with the allergen [49]. They could also show similar effects with particles collected from the ambient air [50]. Similar results were observed by the group of Saxon and Diaz-Sanchez [51] as well as Salvi et al. [52].

When Balb/c mice were sensitized with ovalbumin, Alessandrini et al. [53] could show that exposure to elemental carbon ultrafine particles prior to allergen challenge exhibited a strong enhancing effect upon the severity of airway inflammation. This effect was dose and time dependent and could be demonstrated when the particles had been inhaled up to 4 days before allergen exposure. Further investigations on the mechanisms underlying these effects showed that oxidative stress plays a critical role in carbon ultrafine particle-induced augmentation of allergen-induced airway inflammation [54].

Clinical Studies

Following the animal experiments of Shields [55] on the effect of ozone on the lung, the group of Hillel Koren, working at the laboratories of the environmental protection agency (EPA) of the USA in the Research Triangle Park, performed studies on the effect of ozone upon airway allergy induction using clinical exposure chambers and showing that exposure to ozone can enhance the reactivity to allergen challenge [56–59]. Other groups performed challenge studies with environmental tobacco smoke as well as diesel exhaust particles and found similar effects besides the clear-cut irritative-toxic effect at higher doses [52].

The group of Jack Pepys studied the allergy-enhancing effects of platinum salts used for car catalytic converters and found IgE-mediated reactions against platinum salts in workers engaged in the production of these catalyzers [60]. This belongs more to occupational medicine, but should be mentioned here with regard to effect of metal salts upon allergic reactions.

While it has been known for decades that metal salts like nickel sulfate and potassium chromate belong to the most potent contact sensitizers, the role of metal salts upon IgE-mediated reactions was studied by groups in Düsseldorf [61] and in France [62], where they found an increased rate of autoimmune diseases like glomerulonephritis or lupus erythematosus after mercury exposure.

The Concept of 'Allergotoxicology'

While in classical allergy textbooks there is usually a clear distinction made between 'toxic' or 'allergic' with regard to incompatibility reactions to environmental substances, it soon became clear when studying the effects of pollutants that they can not only produce organ damage, such as to the liver, kidney or lung, but they can also influence the development of allergic reactions. Thus, the concept of 'allergotoxicology' was developed by Heidrun Behrendt and defined as 'the investigation of effects of toxic substances upon the induction, elicitation and maintenance of allergic reactions' [42].

Research in this field comprises studies at all levels, from epidemiology, in vitro culture systems and animal experiments up to clinical studies in humans, volunteers and patients. It is still a fascinating field of research. The debate concerning whether air pollutants play a role in allergy development or not has become less intense. It is obvious that not only one factor plays a role and can explain the rising prevalence of allergies, but that it is a complex interaction of both protective (e.g. infectious stimuli, hygiene hypothesis) and enhancing factors (e.g. environmental tobacco smoke, traffic exhausts) from the environment which determines the development of allergy (fig. 1).

References

1 Lioy PJ, Zhang J: Air pollution; in Swift DL, Foster WM (eds): Air Pollutants and the Respiratory Tract. New York, Dekker, 1999, pp 1–38.
2 Ramazzini B: De morbis artificum diatriba. Padova, 1713.
3 Swift DL, Foster WM (eds): Air Pollutants and the Respiratory Tract. New York, Dekker, 1999.
4 Feingold BF: Recognition of food additives as a cause of symptoms of allergy. Ann Allergy 1968;26:309–313.
5 Rinkel HJ: Migraine. Some considerations of allergy as a factor in familial recurrent headaches. J Allergy 1933;4:1933.
6 Rowe AH: Gastrointestinal food allergy. A study based on 100 cases. J Allergy 1930;1:172.
7 Randolph TG: Blood studies in allergy; variations in eosinophiles following test feeding of foods. J Allergy 1947;18:199–211.
8 World Health Organisation: Allergy and hypersensitivity to chemicals: interim document 12. Copenhagen, WHO, 1983/1986.
9 Yoshida K, Oshima H, Imai M: Air pollution and asthma in Yokkaichi. Arch Environ Health 1966;13:763–768.
10 Osebold JW, Gershwin LJ, Zee YC: Studies on the enhancement of allergic lung sensitization by inhalation of ozone and sulfuric acid aerosol. J Environ Pathol Toxicol 1980;3:221–234.
11 Kaneko Y, Motohashi Y, Nakamura H, et al: Increasing prevalence of Japanese cedar pollinosis: a meta-regression analysis. Int Arch Allergy Immunol 1995;107:236–238.
12 Miyamoto T, Takafuji S: Environment and allergy; in Ring J, Przybilla B (eds): New Trends in Allergy III. Berlin, Springer, 1991, pp 459–468.
13 Oberbarnscheidt J, Stiller-Winckler R, Krämer U, Dolgner R, Behrendt H: Untersuchungen zum Einfluss von Luftschadstoffen auf die Sensibilisierung und den Immunstatus 6 jähriger Kinder. Allergologie 1990;13:316–317.
14 Kunz B, Ring J, Dirschedl P, Przybilla B, Vieluf D, Greif A, Gries A, Huber HC, Kapsner T, Letzel H, Römmelt H, Michel R, Schotten K, Stickl H, Vogl-Vosswinckel E, Überla K: Innenraumluftbelastung und atopische Erkrankungen bei Kindern; in Ring J (ed): Epidemiologie allergischer Erkrankungen. Munich, MMW Medizin, 1991, pp 202–220.
15 Ministerium für Umwelt, Raumordnung und Landwirtschaft des Landes Nordrhein-Westfalen: Wirkungskataster zu den Luftreinhalteplänen Rheinschiene Süd und Rheinschiene Mitte. Düsseldorf, 1990.
16 Behrendt H, Krämer U, Dolgner R, Hinrichs J, Willer HJ, Hagenbeck H, Schlipköter HW: Elevated levels of total serum IgE in East German children: atopy, parasites, or pollutants? A comparative study among 2,054 preschool children in East and West Germany. Allergo J 1993;3:31–40.
17 Björkstén B: Genetic and environmental interaction in children. Prog Allergy Clin Immunol 1993;3:97–103.
18 Duhme H, Weiland SK, Rudolph P, Wienke A, Kramer A, Keil U: Asthma and allergies among children in West and East Germany: a comparison between Münster and Greifswald using the ISAAC phase I protocol. Eur Respir J 1998;11:840–847.
19 Heinrich J, Hoelscher B, Frye C, et al: Trends in prevalence of atopic diseases and allergic sensitization in children in Eastern Germany. Eur Respir J 2002;19:1040–1046.
20 Hirsch T, Weiland SK, von Mutius E, et al: Inner city air pollution and respiratory health and atopy in children. Eur Respir J 1999;14:669–677.
21 Krämer U, Altus C, Behrendt H, Dolgner R, Gutsmuths FJ, Hille J, Hinrichs I, Mangold M, Paetz B, Ranft U, Röpke H, Teichmann S, Willer HJ, Schlipköter HW: Epidemiologische Untersuchungen zur Auswirkung der Luftverschmutzung auf die Gesundheit von Schulanfängern. Forum Städte Hyg 1992;43:82–87.
22 Krämer U, Behrendt H, Dolgner R, et al: Airway diseases and allergies in East and West German children during the first 5 years after reunification: time trends and the impact of sulphur dioxide and total suspended particles. Int J Epidemiol 1999;28: 865–873.
23 Nicolai T, Bellach B, von Mutius E, Thefeld W, Hoffmeister H: Increased prevalence of sensitization against aeroallergens in adults in West compared with East Germany. Clin Exp Allergy 1997;27:886–892.
24 Nowak D, Heinrich J, Jörres R, Wassmer G, Berger J, Beck E, Boczor S, Claussen M, Wichmann HE, Magnussen H: Prevalence of respiratory symptoms, bronchial hyperresponsiveness and atopy among adults: West and East Germany. Eur Respir J 1996; 9:2541–2552.
25 von Mutius E, Martinez F, Fritzsch C, Nicolai T, Roell G, et al: Prevalence of asthma and atopy in two areas of West and East Germany. Am J Respir Crit Care Med 1994; 149:358–364.
26 von Mutius E, Weiland SK, Fritzsch C, et al: Increasing prevalence of hay fever and atopy among children in Leipzig, East Germany. Lancet 1998;351:862–866.
27 Schäfer T, Krämer U, Vieluf D, Abeck D, Behrendt H, Ring J: The excess of atopic eczema in East Germany is related to the intrinsic type. Br J Dermatol 2000;143:992–998.
28 Wichmann H: Environment, life-style and allergy: the German answer. Allergo J 1995; 6:315–316.
29 Krämer U, Heinrich J, Wjst M, Wichmann HE: Age of entry to day nursery and allergy in later childhood. Lancet 1999;353:450–454.
30 Strachan DP: Hay fever, hygiene, and household size. BMJ 1989;299:1259–1260.
31 Krämer U, Oppermann H, Ranft U, Schäfer T, Ring J, Behrendt H: Differences in allergy trends between East and West Germany and possible explanations. Clin Exp Allergy 2010;40:289–298.

32 Cramer C, Link E, Bauer CP, Hoffmann U, von Berg A, Lehmann I, Herbarth O, Borte M, Schaaf B, Sausenthaler S, Wichmann H-E, Heinrich J, Krämer U: Association between attendance of day care centres and increased prevalence of eczema in the German birth cohort study LISAplus. Allergy 2011;66:68–75.
33 Gassner M: Immunologisch-allergologische Reaktionen unter veränderten Umweltbedingungen. Schweiz Rundsch Med Prax 1992;81:426–430.
34 Braun-Fahrländer C, Gassner M, Grize L, et al: Prevalence of hay fever and allergic sensitization in farmer's children and their peers living in the same rural community: Swiss Study on Childhood Allergy and Respiratory Symptoms with Respect to Air Pollution (SCARPOL). Exp Allergy 1999;29:28–34.
35 Waser M, Michels KB, Bieli C, Floistrup H, Pershagen G, von Mutius E, Ege M, Riedler J, Schram-Bijkerk D, Brunekreef B, van Hage M, Lauener R, Braun-Fahrlander C: Inverse association of farm milk consumption with asthma and allergy in rural and suburban populations across Europe. Clin Exp Allergy 2007;37:661–670.
36 Krämer U, Lemmen C, Bartusel E, Link E, Ring J, Behrendt H: Current eczema in children is related to Der f 1 exposure but not to Der p 1 exposure. Br J Dermatol 2006;154: 99–105.
37 Buters JT, Weichenmeier I, Ochs S, Pusch G, Kreyling W, Boere AJ, Schober W, Behrendt H: The allergen Bet v 1 in fractions of ambient air deviates from birch pollen counts. Allergy 2010;65:850–858.
38 Cramer C, Ranft U, Ring J, Möhrenschlager M, Behrendt H, Oppermann H, Wilhelm M, Krämer U: Allergic sensitisation and disease in mother-child pairs from Germany: role of early childhood environment. Int Arch Allergy Immunol 2007;143:282–289.
39 Behrendt H, Ewers HJ, Hüttl RF, Jänicke M, Plassmann E, Rehbinder E, Sukopp H: Sondergutachten des Rates der Sachverständigen für Umweltfragen: Umwelt und Gesundheit – Risiken richtig einschätzen. Stuttgart, Metzler Poeschel, 1999.
40 Burrows B, Halonen M, Barbee A, Lebowitz MD: The relationship of serum immunoglobulin E to cigarette smoking. Am Rev Respir Dis 1981;124:523–525.
41 Risse U, Tomczok J, Huss-Marp J, Darsow U, Behrendt H: Health-relevant interaction between airborne particulate matter and aeroallergens (pollen). J Aerosol Sci 2000; 31:27–28.
42 Behrendt H: Grundlagen der Allergie und mögliche Angriffspunkte für Umweltchemikalien. Allergologie 1989;12:95–99.
43 Traidl-Hoffmann C, Jakob T, Behrendt H: Determinants of allergenicity. J Allergy Clin Immunol 2009;123:558–566.
44 Traidl-Hoffmann C, Mariani V, Hochrein H, et al: Pollen-associated phytoprostanes inhibit dendritic cell interleukin-12 production and augment T helper type 2 cell polarization. J Exp Med 2005;201:627–636.
45 Seemayer NH, Hadnagy W, Behrendt H, Tomingas R: Indicators of petential health risks by airborne particulates: cytotoxic, mutagenic and carcinogenic effects on mammalian cells in vitro; in Seemayer NH, Hadnagy W (eds): Environmental Hygiene. Berlin, Springer, 1988, pp 54–59.
46 Behrendt H, Friedrich KH, Kainka-Stänicke E, Darsow U, Becker WM, Tomingas R: Allergens and pollutants in the air – A complex interaction; in Ring J, Przybilla B (eds): New Trends in Allergy III. Berlin, Springer, 1991, pp 467–478.
47 Diaz-Sanchez D, Rumold R, Gong H Jr: Challenge with environmental tobacco smoke exacerbates allergic airway disease in human beings. J Allergy Clin Immunol 2006;118:441–446.
48 Diaz-Sanchez D, Tsien A, Fleming J, Saxon A: Combined diesel exhaust particulate and ragweed allergen challenge markedly enhances human in vivo nasal ragweed-specific IgE and skews cytokine production to a T helper cell 2-type pattern. J Immunol 1997;158:2406–2413.
49 Muranaka M, Suzuki S, Koizumi K: Adjuvant activity of diesel-exhaust particulates for the production of IgE antibody in mice. J Allergy Clin Immunol 1986;77:616–623.
50 Maejima K, Tamura K, Taniguchi Y, Nagase S, Tanaka H: Comparison of the effects of various fine particles on IgE antibody production in mice inhaling Japanese cedar pollen allergens. J Toxicol Environ Health 1997;52:231–248.
51 Saxon A, Diaz-Sanchez D: Air pollution and allergy: you are what you breathe. Nat Immunol 2005;6:223–226.
52 Salvi S, Blomberg A, Rudell B, Kelly F, Sandstrom T, Holgate ST, Frew AJ: Acute inflammatory responses in the airways and peripheral blood after short-term exposure to diesel exhaust in healthy human volunteers. Am J Respir Crit Care Med 1999;159:702–709.
53 Alessandrini F, Schulz H, Takenaka S, Lentner B, Karg E, Behrendt H, Jakob T: Effects of ultrafine carbon particle inhalation on allergic inflammation of the lung. J Allergy Clin Immunol 2006;117:824–830.
54 Alessandrini F, Beck-Speier I, Krappmann D, Weichenmeier I, Takenaka S, Karg E, Kloo B, Schulz H, Jakob T, Mempel M, Behrendt H: Role of oxidative stress in ultrafine particle-induced exacerbation of allergic lung inflammation. Am J Respir Crit Care Med 2009;179:984–991.
55 Shields TG, Smith G, Ledingham IM: Proceedings: mechanisms of oxygen toxicity. Br J Anaesth 1975;47:904.
56 Hazucha MJ, Ginsberg JF, McDonnell WF, Haak ED Jr, Pimmel RL, Salaam SA, House DE, Bromberg PA: Effects of 0.1 ppm nitrogen dioxide on airways of normal and asthmatic subjects. J Appl Physiol Respir Environ Exerc Physiol 1983;54:730–739.
57 McDonnell WF, Horstman DH, Salaam SA, Raggio LJ, Green JA: The respiratory responses of subjects with allergic rhinitis to ozone exposure and their relationship to nonspecific airway reactivity. Toxicol Ind Health 1987;3:507–517.
58 Koren HS, Bromberg PA: Respiratory responses of asthmatics to ozone. Int Arch Allergy Immunol 1995;107:236–238.
59 Koren HS: Environmental risk factors in atopic asthma. Int Arch Allergy Immunol 1997;113:65–68.
60 Pepys J, Pickering CAC, Hughes EG: Asthma due to inhaled chemical agents-complex salts of platinum. Clin Allergy 1972;2:391–396.
61 Gleichmann E, Kimber I, Purchase IF: Immunotoxicology: suppressive and stimulatory effects of drugs and environmental chemicals on the immune system. A discussion. Arch Toxicol 1989;63:257–273.
62 Prouvost-Danon A, Abadie A, Sapin C, Bazin H, Druet P: Induction of IgE synthesis and potentiation of anti-ovalbumin IgE antibody response by HgC12 in the rat. J Immunol 1981;126:699–702.

Prof. Dr. med. Heidrun Behrendt
ZAUM – Zentrum Allergie und Umwelt
Technische Universität München
Biedersteinerstrasse 29
DE–80802 München (Germany)
E-Mail heidrun.behrendt@lrz.tum.de

Bergmann K-C, Ring J (eds): History of Allergy. Chem Immunol Allergy. Basel, Karger, 2014, vol 100, pp 278–286
DOI: 10.1159/000359961

Farmers and Their Environment: Protective Influences of the Farming Environment against the Development of Allergies

Markus Gassner

Institute of Allergology and Dermatology and Institute for Family Medicine, University of Zurich, Zurich, Switzerland

Abstract

Compared with other population groups, the way of life of farmers can be viewed as being similar to that of our ancestors. The settled continuation of generations within certain critical geographical and environmental conditions requires a special local network of knowledge and experience. The immune system provides protection against microbes and their toxins. Each strong reaction impedes an active adaptation. Allergy is therefore a harmful intolerance and represents one of many different paradoxes. The aim of this chapter is to demonstrate some of the interactions of tolerance and adaptation from a historical background.

Farmers and Their Environment

Nature gives a certain time period to each living organism. The length of life depends on the genes and the environmental factors on the era and geographic site of where and when organisms are living. These very trivial aspects of dependence on time and place are crucial if we want to understand the influence of social and hygiene conditions in the history of medicine. This has been true for the past and will be for the future. As the future is unknown, it might be worthwhile comparing present differing living conditions in societies and countries, and comparing them with the situations of our predecessors (fig. 1).

Agriculture, the Art of Adaptation

In early history, when agriculture developed, it was an art aimed at achieving an optimal local adaptation, to reduce the need for migration by producing more food or wood for buildings and energy, as well as fibers for clothes. Agriculture led to the development of adaptation technologies in different areas. Tolerance of local conditions instead of migration is the first partial aspect of an active adaptation for long-term survival. It is only possible to harvest what grows under the climatic and geographic conditions. Human beings used seeds from grasses which were selected and bred into diverse cereal species in order to render better harvests of less perishable grains. By good care of plants and animals – ac-

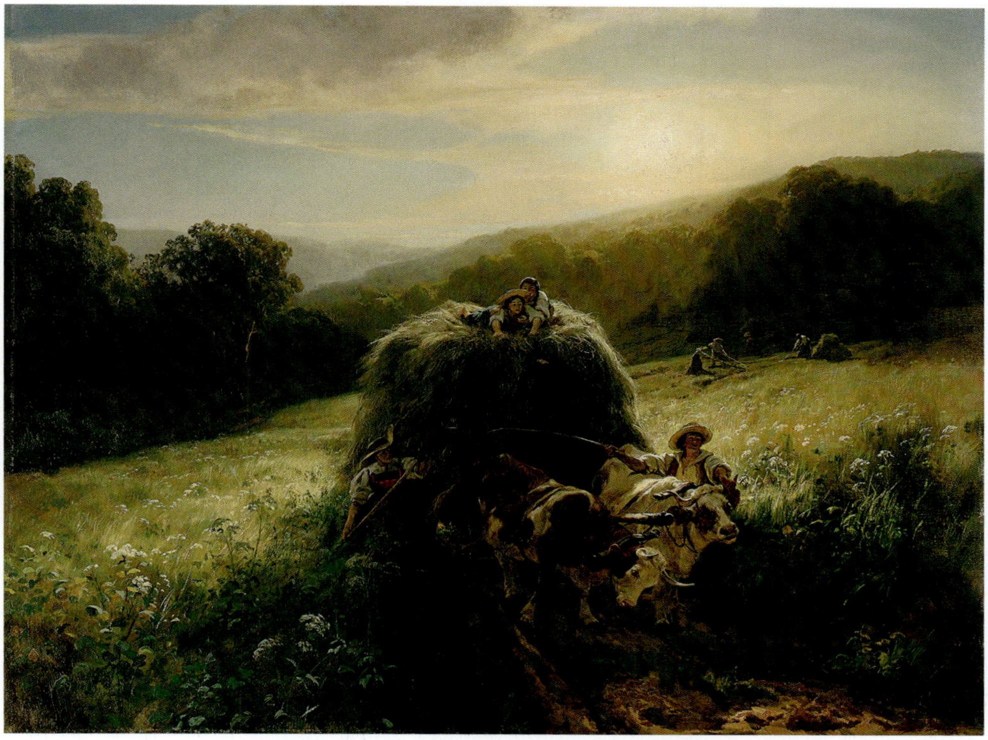

Fig. 1. The 'Heuwagen' by Rudolf Koller (1826–1906) shows many aspects of historical cross-linked situations in the agriculture of Switzerland: co-working of many family members, rapid harvesting before a thunder storm by knowledge of local meteorological conditions, use of cows (horses) for food (milk, meat, leather, etc.) and transportation with 'the archaic biodiesel' as food energy. Grass and cereals were the only primary energy for all local overland transportation and represented a significant competition to the production of every food for humans as well all farm animals.

tive adaptation – survival is possible for more human beings and animals under otherwise intolerable life conditions.

In central Europe, especially in mountainous areas, the change of seasons was the primary specific difficulty for survival. Harvest time was limited to summer and early autumn. Survival in winter was impossible without the preservation of food. The best harvest is useless when the fruits cannot be eaten at the right time. Conservation of food was one of the first conditions determining that more people could live in the same area. The property of more and better food gave and gives rise to envy and greed among human beings and can be the reason for robbery, social conflicts and wars.

In this medical-historic article, we cannot comment on the effects of agricultural products on consumers, or on the economic conditions regarding the distribution of goods, i.e. politics. However, with regard to public health the prophylaxis in the production of food is crucial: one aspect here is occupational diseases in farmers. The following pages will focus upon the effects of 'battles' between farmers and microorganisms with immunologic 'weapons'. The technologies of preservation (drying and packing) were of immense importance for our ancestors as well as their domestic animals prior to the efficient use of altered temperature (boiling and freezing). This was especially crucial for human beings who not only had to adapt their own life, but also the life of the domestic animals to the seasonal climatic conditions.

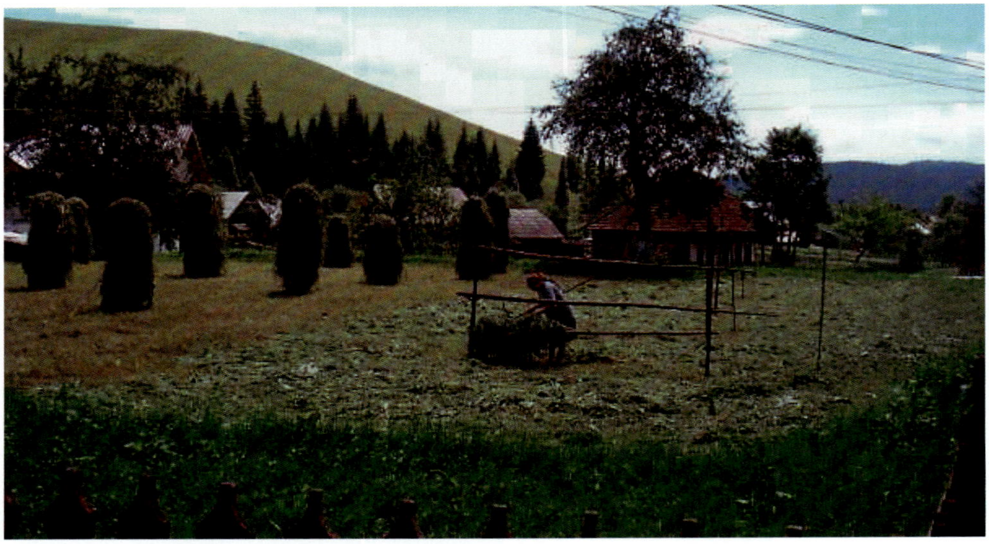

Fig. 2. Drying hay needs long blades of grass. That is why grass could only be cut once to thrice a year in mountain areas. The photo shows two archaic techniques still used in 2009 on a farm in Romania. The same techniques were commonly used in Switzerland in the last century, now replaced by different kinds of silage techniques [2], which allows the grass to be cut up to six times every year in some places, and for some grasses to be cut before they are flowering and release there allergenic pollen!

Drying

The life of microorganisms is impaired by a reduction of water content, which can be used for preservation. This mechanism was used for the preservation of cereals and grasses as basic food, and also as feed for domestic animals in winter (hay). Ramazzini, the father of occupational medicine, reported on an illustrative example of this technology, the disease of the sifters of cereals:

> Almost all persons who earned their bread by sieving and measuring cereals, are short-winded, cachectic and rarely reach a great age. [1]

We do not know whether this 'fever' of the grain sifters was asthma according to modern medicine, organic dust toxic syndrome via endotoxins and glucans, or chronic obstructive pulmonary disease (COPD). In those times farmers did not have cigarettes!

The harvesting of hay requires exact knowledge of meteorology. Grass and cereals had to be cut at an optimal point of time and dried rapidly in order to be preserved. When the soil was too wet, the cut grass would rot. Grass could be dried either by hanging it on poles or long stalks (fig. 2), which was time consuming and energy sapping. Moist hay in the stable was a catastrophe. The fermentation process caused heat, sometimes self-inflammation and fires, and in former times many stables burnt down. Fermentation via thermophilic spores spoilt the hay even for animals and caused severe diseases in cattle and farmers, such as pneumoconioses (farmer's lung). Meadows in shadowy areas presented more problems in the production of less dangerous hay.

Wrapping

Most microorganisms need oxygen for survival. Liquids could be preserved via fermentation in closed vessels, as for instance wine or must. Partly, this was also possible for solid foods (e.g. sauerkraut). The preservation of milk in the form of cheese in different variations is one of the ancient and highly developed arts of agriculture. The bark of the cheese was the wrapping material.

A milestone in agriculture was the discovery of the technique of silage by Virtanen [2]. This technique not only prevented rotting and improved the nutritional qualities compared to dried hay, but also allowed an earlier and more frequent cutting of the grass. Consequently, most grasses could then be cut prior to blooming. Therefore, it might be possible that pollen emission and also immission was then reduced. It remains uncertain which grasses might be less or more affected by the lack of seeding. Therefore, it is unclear what influence this technique has on the immission of allergenic molecules from grass pollen in different regional conditions.

Mechanical Technology

The tractor with a gasoline motor can be regarded as a symbol of the development of modern technology, replacing domestic animals like horses and oxen in the production (ploughing) and transport of foods. Tractors, trucks and railway engines replaced classical transportation by horses. Horse breeding for this purpose became obsolete. The whole transport business in the countryside became 'dismicrobiologized'. Zoonotic epidemic infectious diseases were no longer a problem for the transport of goods. Coal and oil allowed the production of engines and railways, leading to a gigantic outsourcing of agriculture. The same technology also opened up new vast and very fertile areas used for agriculture by corrective measures applied to the water supplies from mountains and river plains down to the sea. Concerning the supply of energy, coal made the cities independent from woods and forests. For this reason, forests disappeared as a result of cultivation, while others recovered or were endangered by air pollutants of fossil fuels. Cities, however, could grow 'infinitely', thereby causing the exponential growth of the population on Earth.

There is a certain irony in this story: the energy consumption of mankind is setting new limits, both geographically and biologically. Agriculture today is abused worldwide in order to produce 'biological fuels' instead of foods. In former times, it was politically essential who the owner of land or a territory was. Wars were started during the last millennia in order to keep or gain the productivity of farmers. Today, values in the globalized, economized and commercialized world have changed. As a consequence, health has also been affected. The epidemiologic rise of allergy seems to be an indicator of this development.

Allergology

Our immune system evolved in order to defend the organism against microbial dangers. In this endeavor, compromises and adaptation processes are necessary. By definition, to react with an allergy means to react in an immunologically paradoxical way against natural environmental factors.

In 1981, we started a seroepidemiological investigation in the village of Grabs in the upper Swiss Rhine valley, after a boy presented with hay fever. He wanted to become a baker and his mother asked me what his risk for developing baker's asthma would be. In those days, there were no epidemiologic data regarding the prevalence of allergic sensitization in school kids. Therefore, we started to investigate routinely all pupils who had to come obligatorily for medical school examinations. We did this with the informed consent of their parents (fig. 3) [3]. From these studies, we learned a great deal, especially concerning certain obviously paradoxical phenomena, as are outlined in the following sections of this review.

The Paradox of Dose Effect

The first analysis of these school kids showed that amongst the children of 80 farmers none were suffering from hay fever. However, it was obvious that these children were exposed to pollen quite extensively. The physicochemical dose-effect principle did not seem to be relevant for the development of a specific sensitization.

This was not a new phenomenon. In 1873, Charles Blackley [4] published his observation that farmers' children suffered less frequently from hay fever. Richard Rehsteiner [5] observed the same when he examined school children in Switzerland in 1926. This phenomenon was largely interpreted as indolence of farmers with regard to this sometimes mild

4

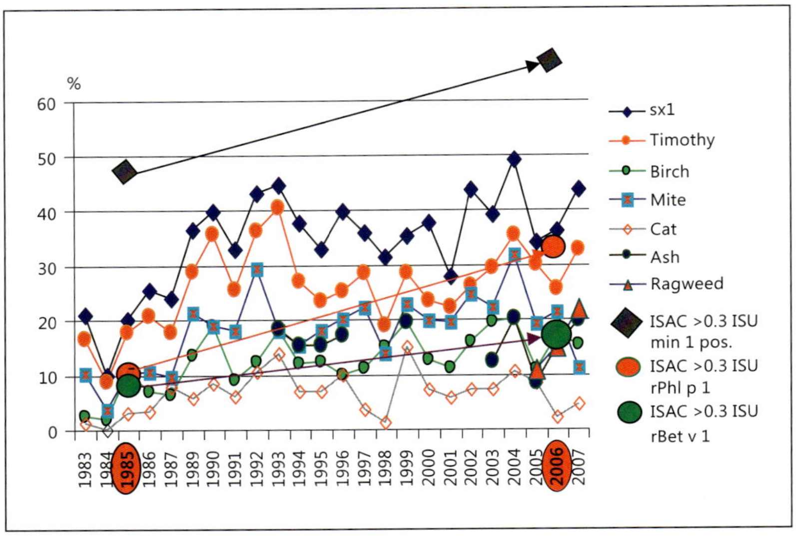

Fig. 3. Time trend in the sensitization rate, 1983–2007, of the school children from Grabs at the age of 15 years: RAST/CAP test >70 kU/ml. The sera of 1986 and 2006 were retested in 2008 with molecular allergens (ISAC test).

symptomatology, or based on genetic reasons, or it was explained by a healthy worker effect, i.e. those individuals in villages who became allergic would leave the countryside and move to the cities and only the tolerant children would stay and become farmers.

The Paradox of Toxic Interactions

High sensitization rates against pollen in cities in spite of less exposure led to the idea of an adjuvant effect of pollutants. In Germany, the death of forests ('Waldsterben') was associated with smog in the eastern German states prior to reunification and everybody expected a higher prevalence of hay fever there. However, there was the paradox that East German children had a lower prevalence of hay fever and asthma compared to West German children, as was found in two independent studies by the group led by Erika von Mutius [6] who compared Munich and Leipzig, and the group led by Heidrun Behrendt and Ursula Krämer [7] who compared several regions in West Germany and former East Germany. Also, similar to the studies on farmers' children, the effect was present only in respiratory allergy, while atopic eczema was either equally or more often prevalent among East German children. The East-West difference within Germany or Europe in allergy prevalence cannot be explained only by the farming environment, since classical farmers did not exist in the communist German Democratic Republic. Different patterns of air pollution seem to be of relevance with regard to traffic exhaust emissions, showing an allergy-enhancing effect [8].

Farmers used wood more often, representing their own traditional energy source, for preparing foods and for heating. Their neighbors in Grabs more frequently used a central oil-fired heating and electrical cooking stove.

Considering 'summer smog', farmers' children inhaled more ozone, since they often helped during hay harvesting around noon, the time of high sun and ozone exposure, as well as on a longer walk to school. It can also be considered that at this time children were also hard working, meaning they were forced to ventilate more of all the toxic substances in the air.

The Paradox of Tolerance or Adaption

Farmers' children show distinct quantitative differences in the sensitization pattern compared to the children of parents not associated with agriculture. Children who only occasionally help on a farm or children of parents who do farming as a part-time job react intermediately. The differences are most significant between farmers' children with regard to specific immunoglobulin (Ig) E levels against timo-

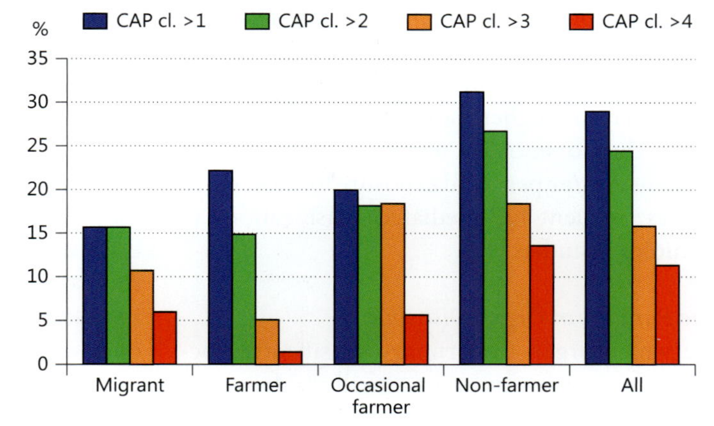

Fig. 4. Patterns of the quantitative sensitization to timothy grass pollen (CAP g6) according to the paternal profession (farmers) or nationality (migrants) in 1,297 serum samples, 1983–2002. CAP class 1: 0.35–69, class 2: 0.7–3.49, class 3: 3.45–17.49, class 4 >5.3 kU/l IgE g6.

thy grass *(Phleum pratense)* pollen (fig. 4) [9]. Continuous quantitative and allergen-specific differences argue for adaptation and against tolerance. Adaptation means getting used to a foreign substance by habituation under continuous exposure and can be compared with callus of the skin under chronic irritation or increases in muscle strength by physical training. The term 'tolerance' was coined in 1945 by R.D. Owen [10] when he found that dizygotic twin calves tolerate the blood group of the respective twin. Adaptation should be used for a quantitative and not a permanent reaction to an environmental condition, and tolerance should relate to a clear genetic variation or an acquired cause with a permanent reaction pattern.

The Paradox of Chronic Obstructive Lung Disease

With fewer allergies and less asthma amongst farmers' children, one might expect lower mortality and morbidity from chronic obstructive lung diseases in their fathers. However, in Switzerland the mortality statistics for the years 1988–1992 in dairy farmers showed the highest and highly significant age-standardized proportional mortality rate (127 for ICD-8 460–519) for all lung diseases, bronchitis and asthma, but not for lung cancer. This phenomenon was not found in farmers who exclusively produce cereals, vegetables or wine [11].

The Paradox of Endotoxins

In his book written in 1906, Alfred Wolff-Eisner [12], a pioneer of hay fever research, described a lot of aspects related to endotoxins which had been discovered by Richard Pfeiffer in 1904. Analogies to the diphtheria toxin were made; Philipps Dunbar in Hamburg created a serum therapy with 'Pollantin', a horse antipollen serum. The word 'fever', which was also used by Charles Blackley, is older than the discovery of the thermometer. Endotoxins are heat-resistant lipopolysaccharides of bacterial cell walls and can cause elevations in body temperature in human beings and mammals. As pyrogenic impurities, they are present in a variety of biological products. While they were difficult to detect some decades ago, when the pyrogen test was only applied in rabbits, it is easier to detect them using the limulus test where endotoxins coagulate the hematolymph of the horseshoe crab *(Limulus polyphemus)*.

A typical feverish disease in dairy farmers is the organic dust toxic syndrome which occurs when mold-contaminated hayricks are emptied and cleaned or when hay is restacked in spring ('Heuschroten'). These well-known reactions in farmers are mostly caused by endotoxins and glucans. Endotoxins can also modify the immune reaction. They possibly stimulate TNF-α production, which might explain antitumor effects with regard to lung cancer, which in turn might explain the lower mortality due

4

to lung cancer in farmers [13]. Cigarettes obviously do not play a role here. It is a pity that young smokers lose the irritative intolerance reaction of their bronchi, occurring with their first cigarette! There is no proof that the higher mortality of farmers from COPD is due to smoking. Farmers' children with continuous and/or perinatal exposure to endotoxins show less frequent IgE-mediated sensitizations in epidemiologic studies [14].

The Paradox of Organ Distribution

Via which organ the primary sensitization occurs remains an open question. Small children usually develop the first sensitization against foods with symptoms of the skin and airways; the most prominent sensitizations are against hen's egg, cow's milk or fish, many of which are lost over time until puberty. Why the sensitization against aeroallergens only occurs later is unclear. Only 30 years ago cross-reactions between pollen and food allergens were discovered; molecular allergology can explain the basis of this first purely clinical phenomenon. Still there is a paradox in explaining the correlations of these infectious diseases. One could expect that common airborne infectious diseases of the airways, such as influenza, respiratory syncytial virus, measles, mumps and rubella, should influence the development of allergic reactions of the lungs like asthma. Matricardi [15], however, showed that the risk is influenced by gastrointestinal infections like hepatitis A, toxoplasmosis and cytomegalovirus.

Helicobacter pylori can obviously cause macroscopically and microscopically visible 'pores' or even ulcera in the gut wall. However, this infection is also more protective with regard to allergies against aeroallergens. In our village of Grabs the seroreactivity of *H. pylori* showed a distinct correlation with the origin of the mother, especially when she came from south-east Europe. This can explain the low prevalence of hay fever in children from migrant populations in spite of a lack of exposure to domestic animals [16].

From these findings one might speculate that the immunity of the airways can be influenced pharmacologically via the gut. Contact with a cow during pregnancy can prevent hay fever at least partially, but keeping a cow is not a good practical recommendation for people living in a city. Therefore, one tries to identify certain germs, especially lactobacilli or other bacteria, with less harmful 'endotoxins'. The first results of clinical trials were scientifically disappointing, although this was not the case commercially speaking, considering the boom of 'healthy' food additives, especially in yoghurt, such as prebiotics and probiotics [17]. The question of which route of application of the allergen might be optimal in allergen-specific immunotherapy remains an open debate today.

The Paradox of Gnotobiotics

Forty years ago a new strain of mice was discovered which in homozygous animals had no hair (nude mice) and no thymus, and, therefore, no T cell reactivity. These mice had quite a reduced life expectancy even under sterile conditions. When they were living in a gnotobiotic situation, i.e. intestinal flora with harmless germs, they survived much longer. In such a condition they could be better used as hosts for transplanted human cancer cells which could not be rejected, since they had no thymus.

In the human intestinal tract we find a quite diverse biotope of multiple germs which is essential for a variety of functions, such as destruction of animal and plant cell walls, degradation of biochemicals and 'delegated' production of essential substances like vitamins. Many people are quite sensitive to alterations of this intestinal flora, e.g. after the use of antibiotics.

The individual constancy of bacterial colonization is striking. It is generally thought that newborns profit from the enteral environmental experience of their mothers and colonize their sterile neonatal gut during birth with well-known harmless maternal germs. Certain strains of lactobacilli may have a preventive effect in atopic eczema which is short-lasting and does not influence the prevalence of sensitizations in school children. However, there is little epidemiologic information [17], and the pathophysiology is also not well understood. Another relevant question is wherefrom the children born by cesarean section develop their individual gut flora.

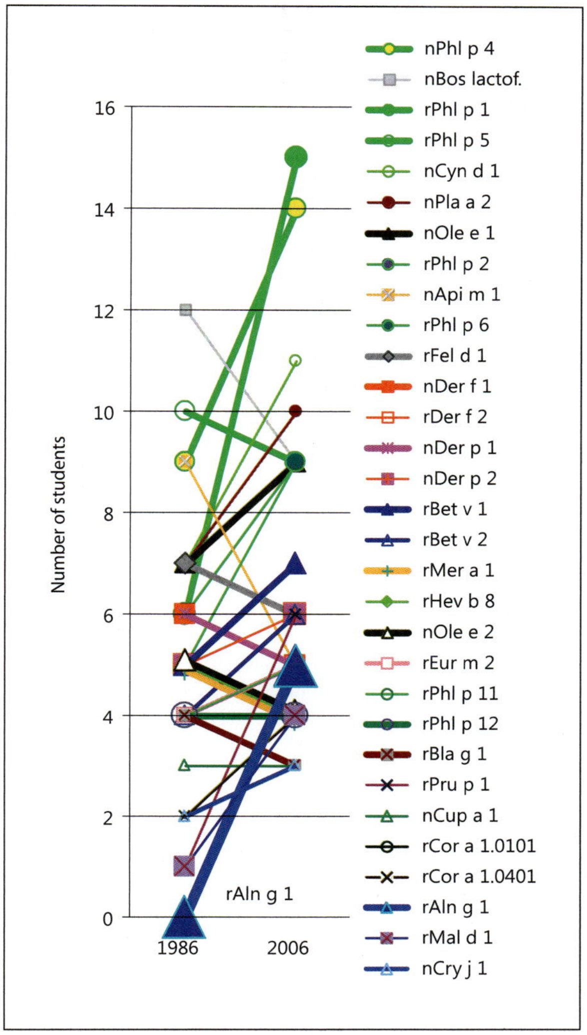

Fig. 5. Changes of IgE seroprevalence (>0.3 ISU) to some molecular antigens in unselected school children of Grabs between 1986 (n = 54) and 2006 (n = 46). Particularly striking is the rise of sensitizations to rAln g 1 from 0 to 5 (10.9%) of the pupils in 2006.

The Paradox of Genetics

In human society power is always also dependent upon political genetics. Noble people had to marry within adequate political circles. Equally, the agricultural community preferred the stability of their inhabitants. Heritage laws with regulated consanguinity optimized the long-term richness of generations over generations.

The farmer also depended upon the genetics of his products: which kind of cereal and cattle would yield the most harvest on what area of land? The classical gene technology of ancient times was breeding by selection both in plants and animals. Today, with modern technology, we can introduce heterozygous DNA into animals and plants with all risks and chances. Gene technology is of immense diagnostic help in the epidemiology of microorganisms. The genetic code of a virus gives information about its origin. Monoclonal antibodies allow molecular allergy diagnostics. Farmers' children not only show quantitative differences in sensitizations, but also qualitative specific sensitization patterns against various recombinant allergens.

By molecular analytics new information can be obtained regarding allergen cross-linking. The school children investigated in 2006 in Grabs showed much higher sensitization rates against rAln g 1 than those from the year 1986 (fig. 5). Looking at regional sources we found that 15 years ago a main street was newly planted with alders. These alders *(Alnus spaethii)* probably originated from Kew (London) in 1894 and were cultivated in Berlin. They were first described by Callier in 1908 as a hybrid of *A. japonica* and *A. subcordata* [18]. Without a natural habitat they seem to be man-made, created through cross-pollination. It was clearly a voluntary outdoor experiment conducted by man by planting a genetically altered large organism. The tree looks beautiful, but is already pollinating in December! Its PR-10 protein shows a different homology to rBet v 1, otherwise it would not have been detected in this epidemiological study. Will this imported tree propagate Japanese or Caucasian genes among the domestic alders?

The Paradox of Migration

Migrants do not change their genes, but rather their environment. Consequently, they represent a film negative of the farmers' 'stabilitas loci'. They do not breed animals, and even tend not to keep pets, because kept animals impede mobility. Their spectrum of sensitization reflects partly their origin and partly the actual interaction with their new environment.

As for allergies, it is interesting that children from migrants react quantitatively in a similar way to farmers' children in the northern Alps (fig. 4). They are also quantitatively less frequently sensitized towards aeroallergens.

The Paradox of Slums

All the paradoxes mentioned show that the so-called hygiene hypothesis can only explain partial aspects of the 'allergy' phenomenon. Dirt is not healthy, even if traditional lifestyle in Europe can have protective advantages regarding the development of allergies. Children in marginal countries of the world, especially in slums, show quite different reaction patterns in their IgE systems; they react less frequently to various pollen, but more often to aeroallergens of animal origin, especially mites.

The internet has changed our attitude towards books and libraries, yet the knowledge of a single individual is still rather limited. Our immune system can be compared to the nervous system not only in weight, but also in its interaction with the environment, its talent for specificity and its remarkably good memory. Our brain is only able to recognize a certain relation, either as images, like the eye of an insect, or like a mirror and in fragments. Let us hope that these short reflections on historical developments regarding the influences of the farming environment may have beneficial effects for our children with regard to preventive strategies and risk avoidance.

References

1 Ackermann JC-G: Bernhard Ramazzinis (1633–1714) Abhandlungen von den Künstlern und Handwerkern. Stendal, Franzen und Grosse, 1780.

2 Steiner W: Untersuchungen über die Konservierung von Grünfutter nach dem Verfahren von A.I. Virtanen; Dissertation. Zürich, Leemann & Co., 1936.

3 Gassner M: Häufigkeit allergologischer Erkrankungen bei Schulkindern einer Landbevölkerung im Hinblick auf die Berufsberatung. Zbl Haut Geschlechtskrankheiten 1985;150:649.

4 Blackley C: Experimental Researches on the Causes and Nature of Catarrhus Aestivus (Hay Fever or Hay Asthma). London, Ballière, Tindal and Cox, 1873 (facsimile: Abington, Oxford Historical Books, 1988, pp 155–156).

5 Rehsteiner R: Beiträge zur Kenntnis der Verbreitung des Heufiebers; Dissertation. Zürich, Hans Gutzwiller, 1926.

6 von Mutius E, Weiland SK, Fritsch C, Duhme H, Keil U: Increasing prevalence of hay fever and atopy among children in Leipzig, East Germany. Lancet 1998;351:862–866.

7 Krämer U, Behrendt H, Dolgner R, Ranft U, Ring J, Willer H, Schlipköter HN: Airway diseases and allergies in East and West German children during the first 5 years after reunification: time trends and the impact of sulphur dioxide and total suspended particles. Int J Epidermiol 1999;28:865–873.

8 Behrendt H, Becker WM: Localization, release and bioavailability of pollen allergens: the influence of environmental factors. Curr Opin Immunol 2001;13:709–715.

9 Braun-Fahrländer C, Gassner M, Grize L, Neu U, Sennhauser FH, Varonier HS, Vuille JC, Wüthrich B, SCARPOL Team: Prevalence of hay fever and allergic sensitization in farmer's children and their peers living in the same rural community. Clin Exp Allergy 1999;29:28–34.

10 Owen RD: Immunogenic consequence of vascular anastomosis between bovine twins. Science 1945;102:400.

11 Gassner M, Spuhler T: Warum sterben Bauern häufiger an Lungenkrankheiten? Schweiz Med Wochenschr 1995;125:667–675.

12 Wolff-Eisner A: Das Heufieber, sein Wesen und seine Behandlung. München, Lehmanns, 1906, pp 130–131.

13 Rylander R, Peterson Y: Organic dusts and lung disease. Am J Int Med 1990;17:1–148.

14 von Mutius E, Braun-Fahrländer C, Schierl R, Riedler J, Erlenmann S, Maisch S, Waser M, Nowak D: Exposure to endotoxin or other bacterial components might protect against the development of allergy. Clin Exp Allergy 2000;30:1230–1234.

15 Matricardi PM, Rosmini F, Ferrigno L, Nisini R, Rapicetta M, Chionne P, Stroffolini T, Pasquini P, D'Amelio R: Cross sectional retrospective study of prevalence of atopy among Italian military students with antibodies against hepatitis A virus. BMJ 1977;314:999–1003.

16 Heuberger F, Pantoflickova D, Gassner M, Oneta C, Grehn M, Blum A, Dorta G: *Helicobacter pylori* infection in Swiss adolescents: prevalence and risk factors. Eur J Gastroenterol Hepatol 2003;15:179–183.

17 Bischoff S (ed): Probiotica, Präbiotica und Symbiotica. Stuttgart, Georg Thieme, 2009.

18 Callier AS: Neue Gehölze: *Alnus spaethii*. Mitteil Deutsch Dendrol Ges 1908:215–216.

Dr. med. Markus Gassner
General Practitioner and School Physician
CH–9472 Grabs (Switzerland)
E-Mail m.gassner@hin.ch

5 Progress in Allergy Management

Progress in Allergy Management

Bergmann K-C, Ring J (eds): History of Allergy. Chem Immunol Allergy. Basel, Karger, 2014, vol 100, pp 288–301
DOI: 10.1159/000359962

History of Catecholamine Research

Klaus Starke

Department of Experimental and Clinical Pharmacology and Toxicology, Albert-Ludwigs-Universität, Freiburg im Breisgau, Germany

Abstract

The prominence of catecholamines and their congeners in allergic diseases rests chiefly on their use in asthma and acute hypersensitivity reactions, such as anaphylaxis. They act in these indications by activating both α- and β-adrenoceptors. Adrenaline, the prototype, was discovered in the adrenals in 1893/1894. In 1939, dopa decarboxylase was the first enzyme in the biosynthesis of catecholamines to be described. Later other catecholamines like noradrenaline and dopamine were characterized. The identification of the active chemicals went along with studies regarding catecholamine receptors. It took until 1948 before the existence of at least two different receptors for the different effects was accepted. Meanwhile, genes from all mammalian catecholamine receptors have been cloned.

The prominence of catecholamines and their congeners in allergic diseases rests chiefly on their use in asthma and acute hypersensitivity reactions, such as systemic anaphylaxis where they may save life. They act in these indications by activation of both α- and β-adrenoceptors. The research conducted up until 1924 has been carefully compiled by Paul Trendelenburg [1], and research histories were written by Hermann Blaschko in 1972 [2] and 1987 [3], by Zénon Bacq in 1983 [4], Maxwell Richard Bennett in 1999 [5] and Josef Donnerer and Fred Lembeck in 2006 [6]. Adrenaline, the prototype, was discovered in the adrenals in 1893/1894. This – the first extraction of a hormone from its gland, before the term 'hormone' was coined [7] – caused a sensation, but there had been forerunners.

Adrenaline in the Adrenal Medulla: Preludes

In the best book on asthma of the 19th century [8], first published in 1860, the British physician and physiologist Henry Hyde Salter (1823–1871) included a chapter on treatment 'by stimulants'. Strong coffee was very helpful, presumably because it dispelled sleep, which favored asthma. Even more impressive, however, was the response to a 'strong mental emotion':

> The cure of asthma by violent emotion is more sudden and complete than by any other remedy whatever; indeed, I know few things more striking and curious in the whole history of therapeutics. ... The cure ... takes *no* time; it is instantaneous, the intensest paroxysm ceases on the instant ...

As upon injection of adrenaline or terbutaline, we might add and thus interpret Salter's observations on, for example, the effect of fire in the house next door.

At the same time as Salter unwittingly made use of the adrenal medulla, the French physician Alfred Vulpian (1826–1887) found that there was something unique about it [9]: material scraped from it colored green when ferric chloride was added. This did not occur with the cortex or with any other tissue. The adrenal medulla hence contained 'une matière spéciale, inconnue jusqu'ici et qui constitue le signe particulier de ces organes'. Vulpian even came to the insight that the substance entered 'le torrent circulatoire', since blood from the adrenal veins did show the ferric chloride reaction.

In the early 1890s, the German pharmacologist Carl Jacobj [10] (1857–1944), in the laboratory of Oswald Schmiedeberg (1838–1921) in Strasbourg, studied the relationship between the adrenals and the intestine. Electrical stimulation of the vagus nerve or injection of muscarine elicited peristalsis, which was promptly abolished by electrical stimulation of the adrenals. The experiment has been called 'the first indirect demonstration of the role of the adrenal medulla as an endocrine organ', and 'actually a more sophisticated demonstration of the adrenal medullary function than the classic study of Oliver and Schäfer' [11]. While this may be true, Jacobj did not envisage a chemical signal secreted into the blood to influence distant organs, in other words a hormone, but instead envisaged nerves running from the adrenals to the gut, which he termed 'Hemmungsbahnen für die Darmbewegung'.

Adrenaline in the Adrenal Medulla: Oliver and Schäfer, 1893/1894

George Oliver (1841–1915) was a physician practicing in the spa town of Harrogate in North Yorkshire. Edward Albert Schäfer (1850–1935) was professor of physiology at University College London. In 1918, he prefixed the surname of his physiology teacher William Sharpey (1802–1880) to his own to become Edward Albert Sharpey Schäfer. The canonical story, told by Henry Hallett Dale [12] (1875–1968), who worked at University College London from 1902 to 1904, runs as follows:

> Dr. Oliver, I was told, ... had a liking and a 'flair' for the invention of simple appliances, with which observations and experiments could be made on the human subject. Dr. Oliver had invented a small instrument with which he claimed to be able to measure, through the unbroken skin, the diameter of a living artery, such as the radial artery at the wrist. He appears to have used his family in his experiments, and a young son was the subject of a series, in which Dr. Oliver measured the diameter of the radial artery, and observed the effect upon it of injecting extracts of various animal glands under the skin. ... We may picture, then, Professor Schafer, in the old physiological laboratory at University College, ... finishing an experiment of some kind, in which he was recording the arterial blood pressure of an anaesthetised dog. ... To him enters Dr. Oliver, with the story of the experiments on his boy, and, in particular, with the statement that injection under the skin of a glycerin extract from calf's suprarenal gland was followed by a definite narrowing of the radial artery. Professor Schafer is said to have been entirely sceptical, and to have attributed the observation to self-delusion. ... He can hardly be blamed, I think; knowing even what we now know about the action of this extract, which of us would be prepared to believe that injecting it under a boy's skin would cause his radial artery to become measurably more slender? Dr. Oliver, however, is persistent; he ... suggests that, at least, it will do no harm to inject into the circulation, through a vein, a little of the suprarenal extract, which he produces from his pocket. So Professor Schafer makes the injection, expecting a triumphant demonstration of nothing, and finds himself standing 'like some watcher of the skies, when a new planet swims into his ken', watching the mercury rise in the manometer with amazing rapidity and to an astounding height.

However often this tale has been reiterated, it is not beyond doubt. Dale himself said that it was handed down in University College, and showed

5

some surprise that the constriction of the radial artery was measurable. Of Oliver's descendants, none recalled experiments on his son [13]. Dale's report of subcutaneous injections contradicts the parties concerned. The following is an account from Oliver [14]:

> During the winter of 1893–1894, while prosecuting an inquiry as to ... agents that vary the calibre of ... arteries ... I found that the administration by the mouth of a glycerine extract of the adrenals of the sheep and calf produced a marked constrictive action on the arteries.

The following is a version of events according to Schäfer [15]:

> In the autumn of 1893 there called upon me in my laboratory in University College a gentleman who was personally unknown to me. ... I found that my visitor was Dr. George Oliver, [who] was desirous of discussing with me the results which he had been obtaining from the exhibition by the mouth of extracts from certain animal tissues, and the effects which these had in his hands produced upon the blood vessels of man.

Systemic effects of orally given adrenaline are highly unlikely. So some details of the canonical text may be legend.

Regardless, on March 10, 1884, Oliver and Schäfer presented their findings to the Physiological Society in London [16]. A 47-page account followed a year later, in the style of the time without statistics, but with precise descriptions of many individual experiments and 25 recordings on kymograph smoked drums, showing, besides the blood pressure increase, reflex bradycardia and contraction of the spleen [17] (fig. 1):

> It appears to be established as the result of these investigations that ... the suprarenal capsules are to be regarded although ductless, as strictly secreting glands. The material which they form and which is found, at least in its fully active condition, only in the medulla of the gland, produces striking physiological effects upon the muscular tissue generally, and especially upon that of the heart and arteries. Its action ... is produced mainly if not entirely by direct action.

Oliver was not slow to try adrenal extracts in patients, once again orally and rather indiscriminately, from Addison's disease and 'loss of vasomotor tone' to diabetes mellitus, diabetes insipidus and 'exophthalmic goitre' [14].

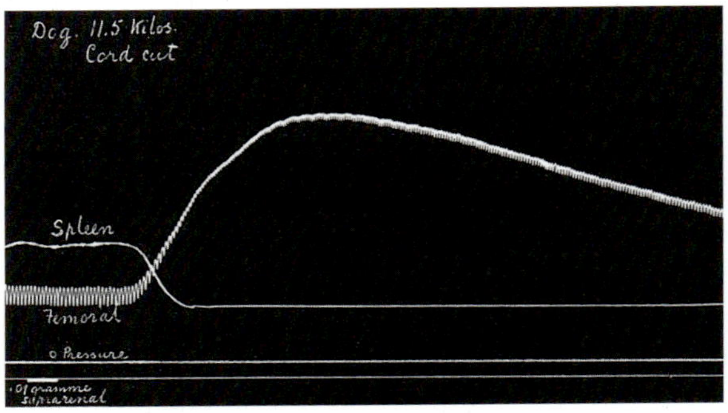

Fig. 1. Effect of an adrenal extract on arterial pressure and spleen volume of an anesthetized dog.

Why, we may ask, this tampering with tissue extracts and subsequently with patients? Oliver probably had become interested in 'organotherapy', believing that powerful substances existed in tissues and ought to be discovered for medicinal use [18].

The first use in asthma, in 1903 in New York, was not based on the bronchospasmolytic effect of adrenaline, which was discovered later [19, 20], but instead on the vasoconstrictor effect, which was hoped to alleviate the 'turgidity of the bronchial mucosa' – presumably vascular congestion and edema [21]. 'Given hypodermatically, adrenalin chloride is capable of cutting short attacks of asthma in from two to twenty minutes.' Adrenalin chloride was obtained from Parke, Davis & Co., see below.

Adrenaline in the Adrenal Medulla: Independent Discoverers

A year after Oliver and Schäfer, Władysław Szymonowicz [22] (1869–1939) and Napoleon Cybulski (1854–1919) of the Jagiellonian University in Kraków reported essentially similar findings and conclusions. In one aspect, they went beyond the work that had been conducted in England: blood from the adrenal veins caused hypertension when injected intravenously in a recipient dog, whereas blood from other veins did not. This showed that the adrenal pressor substance was in fact secreted into the blood and, thus, confirmed Vulpian.

The Polish authors freely acknowledged the priority of Oliver and Schäfer, and the British authors acknowledged the independence of Szymonowicz and Cybulski. The main difference was in the location of the action: to the periphery by Oliver and Schäfer and to the central nervous system by Szymonowicz and Cybulski. In 1896, Rudolf Gottlieb [23] (1864–1924) in Heidelberg confirmed that the action was directly on the heart and blood vessels.

Another year later, the American physician William Bates [24] (1860–1931), perhaps motivated like Oliver, instilled adrenal extracts into the eye and found that 'the conjunctiva of the globe and lids whitened in a few minutes'. He correctly explained the effect to be due to vasoconstriction, and administered the extracts in various eye diseases. Later catecholamine research has not done him justice: none of the histories mentioned above cite him, although an attentive asthma historian does [25].

Chemistry

The 'extraordinary active principle' [12] of the adrenal medulla challenged contemporary chemistry. In Baltimore, John Jacob Abel [26] (1857–1938) partially purified it to what he called 'epinephrine', and Otto von Fürth [27] (1867–1938) in Strasbourg purified it to what he called 'suprarenin'. Starting with Abel's procedure, the Japanese chemist Jokichi Takamine [28] (1854–1922), who had set up his own laboratory in New York, obtained it in pure form in 1901 and arranged for Parke, Davis & Co. to market it as 'Adrenalin', spelt without the terminal 'e'. In 1903, natural adrenaline was found to be optically active and levorotary; in 1905 synthesis of the racemate was achieved by Friedrich Stolz (1860–1936) at Hoechst AG in Höchst near Frankfurt am Main and by Henry Drysdale Dakin (1880–1952) at the University of Leeds; in 1906 the chemical structure was elucidated by Ernst Joseph Friedmann [29] (1877–1956) in Strasbourg, and in 1908 the dextrorotary enantiomer was shown to be almost inactive by Arthur Robertson Cushney [30] (1866–1926) at the University of Michigan, leading him to brilliantly conclude that 'the "receptive substance" affected by adrenalin' is able to discriminate between the optical isomers and, hence, is itself optically active. Overall, 32 designations have been coined, of which 'adrenaline', preferred in the UK, and 'epinephrine', preferred in the USA, persist as generic names in the scientific literature [31].

Catecholamine Neurotransmitters: Adrenaline

A new chapter was opened in 1899 when Max Lewandowsky [32] (1876–1918), working in Berlin, observed that adrenal extracts acted on the smooth muscle of the eye and orbit of cats – as the iris dilator muscle and the nictitating membrane – in the same way as sympathetic nerve stimulation. The correspondence was extended by John Newport Langley (1852–1925) and, under his supervision, Thomas Renton Elliott (1877–1961) in Cambridge. In four papers published in 1904 in volume 31 of *Journal of Physiology*, Elliott described the similarities organ by organ. For example, electrical sympathetic nerve stimulation contracted the ileocolic sphincter of the cat but relaxed the circular muscle in the adjoining ileum and colon, and 'Adrenalin' (again the Parke, Davis & Co. product) did precisely the same [33]. His visionary hypothesis stands in the abstract [34] of a presentation to the Physiological Society of May 21, 1904, a little over 10 years after Oliver and Schäfer's presentation:

> Adrenalin does not excite sympathetic ganglia when applied to them directly, as does nicotine. Its effective action is localised at the periphery. ... I find that even after ... complete denervation, whether of three days' or ten months' duration, the plain muscle of the dilatator pupillae will respond to adrenalin and that with greater rapidity and longer persistence than does the iris whose nervous relations are uninjured. Therefore it cannot be than adrenalin excites any structure derived from, and dependent for its persistence on, the peripheral neurone. ... The point at which the stimulus of the chemical excitant is received, and transformed into what may cause the change of tension of the muscle fibre, is perhaps a mechanism developed out of the muscle cell in response to its union with the synapsing sympathetic fibre, the function of which is to receive and transform the nervous impulse. Adrenalin might then be the chemical stimulant liberated on each occasion when the impulse arrives at the periphery.

This abstract is the 'birth certificate' of chemical neurotransmission [35]. Elliott was never so explicit again. It seems he was discouraged by the lack of a favorable response from his seniors, Langley in particular, and a few years later he left physiological research.

The breakthrough for chemical neurotransmission came when, in 1921, Otto Loewi (1873–1961), working in Graz, demonstrated the 'humorale Übertragbarkeit der Herznervenwirkung' in amphibians [36]. 'Vagusstoff' transmitted inhibition from the vagal nerves, and 'Acceleransstoff' transmitted stimulation from the sympathetic nerves to the heart [37]. Loewi took some years to commit himself with respect to the nature of the 'Stoffe', but in 1926 he was sure that Vagusstoff was acetylcholine, and in 1936 he wrote [38]: 'I no longer hesitate to identify the Sympathicusstoff with adrenaline.'

He had luck in the latter statement. In most amphibian organs, including the heart, the concentration of adrenaline far exceeds that of noradrenaline and adrenaline is indeed the main transmitter. In mammals, however, difficulties arose. In 1910, in a comprehensive structure-activity study of adrenaline-like compounds, Dale and the chemist George Barger [39] (1878–1939) pointed out that Elliott's hypothesis assumed a stricter parallelism between the effects of sympathetic nerve impulses and adrenaline than actually existed. For example, sympathetic impulses shared with adrenaline contractile effects in the cat's bladder trigon, but not relaxant effects in the cat's bladder fundus. In this respect, 'amino-ethanol-catechol' – noradrenaline – mimicked sympathetic nerves more closely than adrenaline did. The Harvard Medical School physiologist Walter Bradford Cannon (1871–1945), who had popularized the idea of a sympatho-adrenal system preparing the body for fight and flight, and his colleague Arturo Rosenblueth (1900–1970) developed an elaborate but 'queer' [4] theory of two 'sympathins', sympathin E (excitatory) and sympathin I (inhibitory). The Belgian pharmacologist Zénon Bacq (1903–1983), as well as Canadian and American pharmacologists between 1934 and 1938, suggested that noradrenaline might be the – or at least one – postganglionic sympathetic transmitter [2, 4]. However, nothing definite was brought to light until after the Second World War.

In 1936, the year of Loewi's final acceptance of adrenaline as the (amphibian) sympathetic transmitter, Dale and Loewi received the Nobel Prize in Physiology or Medicine 'for their discoveries relating to chemical transmission of nerve impulses'.

Formation and Destruction

The German-British biochemist Hermann Blaschko (1900–1993), the chief witness here, who, in 1933, had left Germany because he was Jewish, wrote the following in 1987 in Oxford, looking back on 'a half-century of research on catecholamine biosynthesis':

> Our modern knowledge of the biosynthetic pathway for the catecholamines begins in 1939, with the publication of a paper by Peter Holtz and his colleagues: they described the presence in the guinea-pig kidneys of an enzyme that they called dopa decarboxylase, because it catalysed the formation of dopamine and carbon dioxide from the amino acid L-dopa. [3]

The paper by Peter Holtz (1902–1970) et al. [40] originated from the Institute of Pharmacology in Rostock. In that same year, 1939, both Blaschko [41], then in Cambridge, and Holtz [42] in Rostock predicted the entire sequence of tyrosine → l-DOPA → oxytyramine = dopamine → noradrenaline → adrenaline. Edith Bülbring [43] (1903–1990), who had also fled National Socialist racism in 1933, demonstrated methylation of noradrenaline to adrenaline in adrenal tissue in Oxford in 1949, and Julius Axelrod [44] (1912–2004) detected phenylethanolamine N-methyltransferase in Bethesda in 1962. The two remaining enzymes, tyrosine hydroxylase and dopamine β-hydroxylase, were also characterized around 1960.

Even before contributing to the formation pathway, Blaschko had discovered a destruction mechanism. In 1937, he showed with his co-workers that a 'tyramine oxidase' described in 1928 [45] also oxidized dopamine, noradrenaline and adrenaline [46]. It was later named monoamine oxidase. This seemed to clarify the fate of the catecholamines in the body, but in 1956 Blaschko [cited in 2] suggested that, because the oxidation was slow, 'other mechanisms of inactivation … will be found to play an important part. Here is a gap in our knowledge which remains to be filled'. Within a year, Axelrod had narrowed the gap by showing that dopamine, noradrenaline and adrenaline were O-methylated by catechol O-methyltransferase [47]. To fill the gap completely, however, the role of membranes had to be appreciated (see below).

Catecholamine Neurotransmitters: Noradrenaline

Thanks to Holtz and Blaschko it was clear that animals synthesized noradrenaline. What was lacking in order to attribute a transmitter role to it was proof of its presence in tissues at effective concentrations and not only as a short-lived intermediate. On April 16, 1945, Ulf von Euler (1905–1983) of Karolinska Institutet in Stockholm, who had already discovered or co-discovered substance P and prostaglandins, submitted to *Nature* the first of a series of papers that gave this proof [48]. After many bioassays and chemical assays conducted on organ extracts, he concluded [49] that mammalian sympathetically innervated tissues as well as, in small amounts, the brain, but not the nerve-free placenta, contained noradrenaline and that noradrenaline was the 'sympathin' of Cannon and Rosenblueth, the 'physiological transmitter of adrenergic nerve action in mammals'. Overflow of noradrenaline into the venous blood of the cat's spleen upon sympathetic nerve stimulation 2 years later bore out this conclusion [50]. In amphibian hearts, on the other hand, the transmitter role of adrenaline was confirmed [49].

The war prevented Peter Holtz and his group in Rostock from being recognized alongside von Euler as the discoverers of the second catecholamine transmitter noradrenaline. Their approach was different. They sought for catecholamines in human urine and found a blood pressure-increasing material 'Urosympathin' that they identified as a mixture of dopamine, noradrenaline and adrenaline [51]:

> As to the origin of Urosympathin we would like to suggest the following. Dopamine in urine is the fraction that was not consumed for the synthesis of sympathin E and I. ... Sympathin E and I, i.e. noradrenaline and adrenaline, are liberated in the region of the sympathetic nerve endings when these are excited; by way of the blood stream they can also act on remote parts of the body. An additional source of adrenaline is the adrenal medulla, its major formation and storage site. The question arises whether the adrenals are also a formation and storage site for noradrenaline.

The manuscript was received by Springer-Verlag in Leipzig on October 8, 1944. On October 15, the printing office in Braunschweig was destroyed by an airstrike. Publication was delayed to volume 204 of *Naunyn-Schmiedebergs Archiv für experimentelle Pathologie und Pharmakologie* [51], which was published in 1947. Peter Holtz later used to cite the paper as 'Holtz et al. 1944/47' or 'Holtz, Credner and Kroneberg 1944/47', for example when he and Hans Joachim Schümann (1919–1998) reported that the adrenal medulla indeed contained noradrenaline as a second hormone [52].

Remembering his and Barger's structure-activity analysis of 1910 [39], Dale [53] wrote in 1953:

> Doubtless I ought to have seen that nor-adrenaline might be the main transmitter – that Elliott's theory might be right in principle and faulty only in this detail. ... It is easy, of course, to be wise in the light of facts recently discovered; lacking them I failed to jump to the truth, and I can hardly claim credit for having crawled so near and then stopped short of it.

The next step led to the central nervous system. It was taken by Marthe Vogt (1903–2003), who, after Blaschko and Bülbring, is the third refugee from Germany in this history and at that time was working with John Henry Gaddum (1900–1965) in the Institute of Pharmacology of the University of Edinburgh:

> The presence of noradrenaline and adrenaline in the brain has been demonstrated by von Euler (1946) and Holtz (1950). These substances were supposed, undoubtedly correctly, to occur in the cerebral vasomotor nerves. The present work is concerned with the question whether these sympathomimetic amines, besides their role as transmitters at vasomotor endings, play a part in the function of the central nervous tissue itself. In this paper, these amines will be referred to as 'sympathin', since they were found invariably to occur together, with noradrenaline representing the major component, as is characteristic for the transmitter of the peripheral sympathetic system. [54]

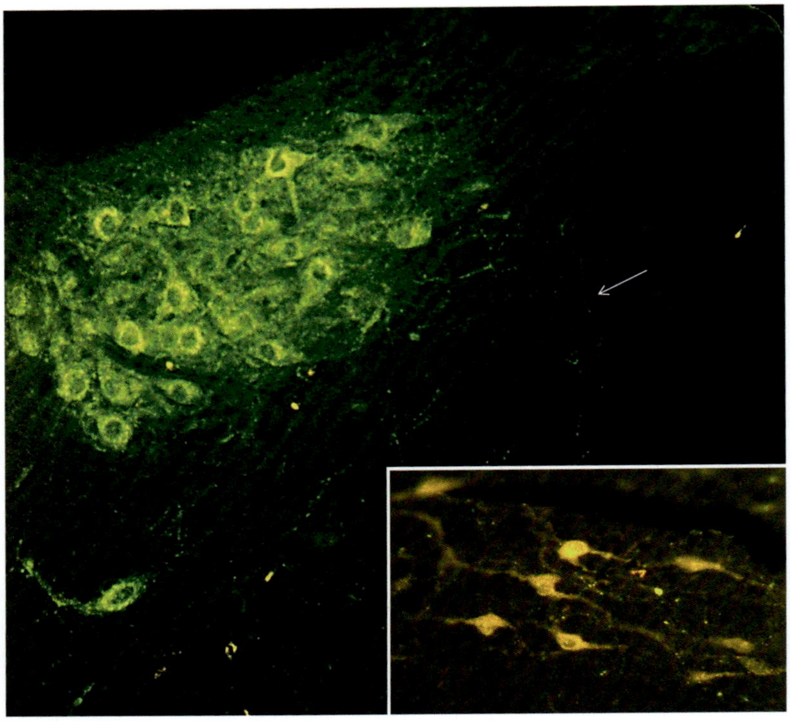

Fig. 2. Noradrenaline neurons in locus coeruleus and (inset) serotonin neurons in nucleus raphe obscurus of the rat. The arrow indicates a varicose axon. From Dahlström and Fuxe [55].

Vogt created a detailed map of noradrenaline in the dog brain. Its uneven distribution, not reflecting the distribution of vasomotor nerves, and its persistence after removal of the superior cervical ganglia made it 'tempting to assign to the cerebral sympathin a transmitter role like that which we assign to the sympathin found in the sympathetic ganglia and their postganglionic fibres'. Her assignment was confirmed, the finishing touch being the visualization of the noradrenaline as well as adrenaline and (see below) dopamine pathways in the central nervous system with the histofluorescence technique developed by Nils-Åke Hillarp (1916–1965) and Bengt Falck (born 1927) in Sweden in 1962 (fig. 2).

Catecholamine Neurotransmitters: Dopamine

The noradrenaline story recurred. As noradrenaline lies on the path to adrenaline, dopamine lies on the path to noradrenaline (and hence adrenaline). In 1958/1959, Arvid Carlsson (born 1923) and his group in the Pharmacology Department of the University of Lund, including the medical students Åke Bertler and Evald Rosengren, not only found dopamine in the brain, but also – like noradrenaline in Marthe Vogt's exemplary study – in uneven distribution, quite different from the distribution of noradrenaline, with the highest concentration, 80% of total brain dopamine, in the corpus striatum, which contained only traces of noradrenaline. Carlsson's group had previously found that reserpine, which was known to cause a parkinsonism syndrome, depleted dopamine (as well as noradrenaline and serotonin) from the brain. They concluded that 'dopamine is concerned with the function of the corpus striatum and thus with the control of motor function' [56, 57]. Thus, for the first time the reserpine-induced parkinsonism in laboratory animals and, by implication, Parkinson's disease in humans, was related to depletion of striatal dopamine. A year later, Oleh Hornykiewicz (born 1926), who had been introduced to dopamine by Blaschko and was carrying out a color reaction on extracts of human corpus striatum in the Pharmacological Institute of the University of Vienna, saw the brain dopamine deficiency in Parkinson's disease 'with [his] own naked eye: instead of the pink colour given by the comparatively high concentrations of dopamine in the control samples, the reaction vials containing the extracts of the Parkinson's disease striatum showed hardly a tinge of pink discoloration' [58, 59].

In 1970, von Euler and Axelrod were two of three winners of the Nobel Prize in Physiology or Medicine, 'for their discoveries concerning the humoral transmitters in the nerve terminals and the mechanism for their storage, release and inactivation', and in 2000 Carlsson was one of three winners of the prize 'for their discoveries concerning signal transduction in the nervous system'.

Membrane Passage

Membranes are essential in the life of catecholamines: catecholamines must pass through membranes, and must deliver their chemical message at membrane receptors.

Catecholamines are synthesized inside cells and sequestered in intracellular vesicles. This was first shown – by Blaschko and Arnold Welch (1908–2003) [60] in Oxford, and by Hillarp et al. [61] in Lund – for the adrenal medulla and later for sympathetic nerves [62] and the brain [63]. In addition to catecholamines the vesicles contained ATP, with a molar noradrenaline:ATP ratio in bovine splenic sympathetic nerve vesicles of 5.2:1, as was determined by Schümann and Grobecker [64] in 1958 in Frankfurt am Main. Looking ahead, Blaschko and Welch [60] asked: 'What happens inside the cell when nervous impulses reach it?' Exocytosis was not among the possibilities they considered. To establish exocytosis, it required the analogy of the quantal release of acetylcholine at the neuromuscular junction shown by Bernard Katz (1911–2003), the third winner of the 1970 Nobel Prize in Physiology or Medicine, the demonstration of the co-release with catecholamines of other vesicle constituents such as ATP and dopamine β-hydroxylase, and the unquestionable electron microscopic images of vesicles fusing with the plasma membrane [65].

Acetylcholine, once released, is degraded in the extracellular space by acetyl cholinesterase, which faces that space. In the case of the catecholamines, however, the enzymes of degradation, monoamine oxidase and catechol O-methyltransferase, like the enzymes of synthesis, are intracellular. Therefore, uptake through cell membranes, rather than metabolism, is the primary means of their clearance from the extracellular space. Beginning in 1959, the mechanisms started to be deciphered. Axelrod's group in Bethesda wished to clarify the in vivo fate of catecholamines using radioactively labelled catecholamines of high specific activity, which had just become available. ^{3}H-adrenaline and ^{3}H-noradrenaline given intravenously to cats were partly O-methylated, but another part was taken up in the tissues and stored unchanged [66, 67]. Erich Muscholl [68] (born in 1926) in Mainz, who had worked with Marthe Vogt in Edinburgh, wished to know how cocaine sensitized tissues to catecholamines. Intravenous noradrenaline was taken up into the heart and spleen of rats, and cocaine prevented the uptake, 'thus increasing the amount of noradrenaline available for combination with the adrenergic receptors'. The uptake of ^{3}H-noradrenaline was severely impaired after sympathectomy, indicating that it occurred mainly into sympathetic nerve terminals. In support of this, Georg Hertting (born in 1925) and Axelrod [69] elegantly showed that freshly incorporated ^{3}H-noradrenaline was re-released from the cat spleen when the sympathetic nerves were stimulated. A few years later, Leslie Iversen (born in 1937) in Cambridge found that other cells also took up catecholamines. He called uptake into noradrenergic neurons, which was cocaine-sensitive, uptake$_1$, and uptake into other cells, which was cocaine-resistant, uptake$_2$. With the reserpine-sensitive uptake from the cytoplasm into the storage vesicles there were thus three catecholamine membrane passage mechanisms. Iversen's book of 1967, entitled *The Uptake and Storage of Noradrenaline in Sympathetic Nerves* [70], was very successful, demonstrating the fascination of the field and its rich pharmacology.

With the advent of molecular genetic techniques, the three transport mechanisms have been traced to the proteins since 1990. They now comprise the plasma membrane noradrenaline transporter, NAT or

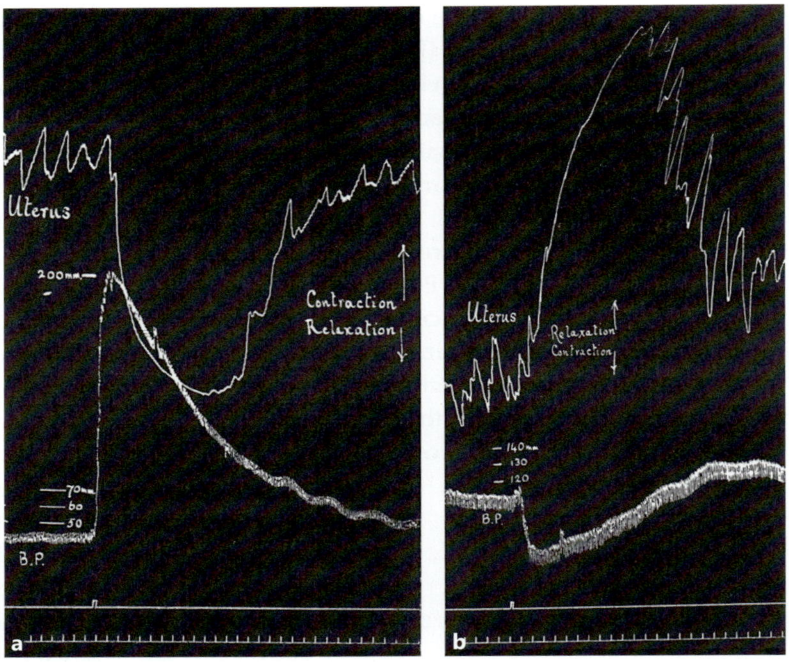

Fig. 3. Adrenaline reversal in a cat. Before ergot (**a**) adrenaline causes an increase in arterial pressure and contraction of the (early pregnant) uterus; after injection of an ergot extract (**b**) adrenaline lowers blood pressure and relaxes the uterus.

NET, the classical uptake$_1$, and the analogous dopamine transporter DAT; the plasma membrane 'extraneuronal monoamine transporter', EMT, also known as 'organic cation transporter 3', Iversen's uptake$_2$, and the 'vesicular monoamine transporter', VMAT, with two isoforms VMAT1 and VMAT2.

Receptors

Research on the catecholamines was interwoven with research on their receptors. In 1904, Dale became head of the Wellcome Physiological Research Laboratory in London and started research on ergot extracts. The relevance of his communication in 1906 [71] 'On some physiological actions of ergot' lies less in the effects of the extracts given alone than in their interaction with adrenaline: they reversed the normal pressor effect of adrenaline to a depressor effect and the normal contraction effect on the early-pregnant cat's uterus to relaxation: the famous 'adrenaline reversal' (fig. 3). The pressor and uterine contraction effects of pituitary extracts, in contrast, remained unchanged, as did the effects of adrenaline on the heart and effects of parasympathetic nerve stimulation. Dale clearly saw the specificity of the 'paralytic' effect of ergot for 'the so-called myoneural junctions connected with the true sympathetic or thoracic-lumbar division of the autonomic nervous system' – the adrenoceptors. He also saw its specificity for the 'myoneural junctions' mediating smooth muscle contraction as opposed to those mediating smooth muscle relaxation. But there he stopped. He did not conceive any close relationship between the smooth muscle-inhibitory and the cardiac sites of action of catecholamines.

Catecholamine receptors persisted in this wavering state for more than 40 years. Additional blocking agents became available, but only for the smooth muscle excitatory receptors. Additional agonists were also synthesized. Outstanding among them became isoprenaline, N-isopropyl-noradrenaline, of Boehringer Ingelheim, studied pharmacologically alongside adrenaline and other N-substituted noradrenaline derivatives by Richard Rössler (1897–1945) and Heribert Konzett (1912–2004) in Vienna. The Viennese pharmacologists used their 'Konzett-Rössler test' [72] to examine bronchodilation. Intravenous injection of pilocarpine to induce bronchospasm was followed by intravenous injection of the agonists [73]. 'Arrangement of all amines according to their bronchospasmolytic effect yields a series from the most potent, isopropyl-adrenaline, via the approximately equipotent bodies adrenaline, propyl-adrenaline and butyl-adrenaline, to the weakly active isobutyl-adrenaline.' Isoprenaline also exerted marked positive chronotropic and inotropic effects. Boehringer introduced it for use in asthma in 1940. After the war it became available to Germany's former enemies and over the years was traded under about 50 names. In addition to this therapeutic success it was one of the agonists with which Ahlquist solved the 'myoneural junction' riddle. 'By virtue of this property the reputation of the substance spread all over the world and it became a tool for many investigations on different aspects of pharmacology and therapeutics' [74]. However, the story had a dark side: overdosage caused numerous deaths due to cardiac side effects, an estimated three thousands in the UK alone [75].

Raymond P. Ahlquist (1914–1983) was head of the Department of Pharmacology at the University of Georgia School of Medicine, now Georgia Health Sciences University. In 1948, he saw what had escaped Dale in 1906:

> The adrenotropic receptors have been considered to be of two classes, those whose action results in excitation and those whose action results in inhibition of the effector cells. Experiments described in this paper indicate that although there are two kinds of adrenotropic receptors they cannot be classified simply as excitatory or inhibitory since each kind of receptor may have either action depending on where it is found. [76]

Ahlquist chose six agonists, including adrenaline, noradrenaline, α-methylnoradrenaline and isoprenaline, and examined their effects on several organs. He found that the six substances possessed two – and only two – rank orders of potency in these organs. For example, the rank order of potency was 'adrenaline > noradrenaline > α-methylnoradrenaline > isoprenaline' in promoting the contraction of blood vessels, but 'isoprenaline > adrenaline > α-methylnoradrenaline > noradrenaline' in stimulating the heart. The receptors with the first rank order (for example for blood vessel contraction) he called α-adrenoceptors ('alpha adrenotropic receptor'), while the receptors with the second rank order (for instance for stimulation of the heart, but also for bronchodilation) he called β-adrenoceptors ('beta receptor'):

> This concept of two fundamental types of receptors is directly opposed to the concept of two mediator substances (sympathin E and sympathin I) as propounded by Cannon and Rosenblueth and now widely quoted as 'law' of physiology. ... There is only one adrenergic neuro-hormone, or sympathin, and that sympathin is identical with epinephrine. [76]

The haze surrounding the receptors was thus blown away. Yet, perhaps because Ahlquist dismissed Cannon and Rosenblueth rather harshly, his manuscript was rejected by the *Journal of Pharmacology and Experimental Therapeutics*, and only in a second submission accepted by the *American Journal of Physiology*. Moreover, although he was right in his 'one transmitter – two receptors' postulate, he was wrong in the identification of the transmitter with adrenaline. Lastly, Ahlquist failed to adduce the selectivity of the then-known antagonists for the α-adrenoceptors to support his concept.

These may have been reasons why the α,β-terminology was slow to spread. The change came with two publications in 1958. In the first, from Lilly Research Laboratories, dichloroisoprenaline selectively blocked some smooth muscle inhibitory effects of adrenaline and isoprenaline [77]; in the second, it blocked cardiac excitatory effects of adrenaline and isoprenaline as well [78]. In the first, which does not mention Ahlquist, dichloroisoprenaline blocked 'certain adrenergic inhibitory receptor sites' [77]; but in the second the results:

> support the postulate of Ahlquist (1948) that the adrenotropic inhibitory receptors and the cardiac chronotropic and inotropic adrenergic receptors are functionally identical, i.e. that both are *beta* type receptors. ... It is suggested that this terminology be extended to the realm of adrenergic blocking drugs, e.g. that blocking drugs be designated according to the receptor for which they have the greatest affinity, as either *alpha* or *beta* adrenergic blocking drugs. [78]

Dichloroisoprenaline was the first 'β-blocker' (with some intrinsic activity). Pronethalol followed in 1962 and propranolol in 1964 [79], both invented by James Black (1924–2010) and his colleagues at Im-

5

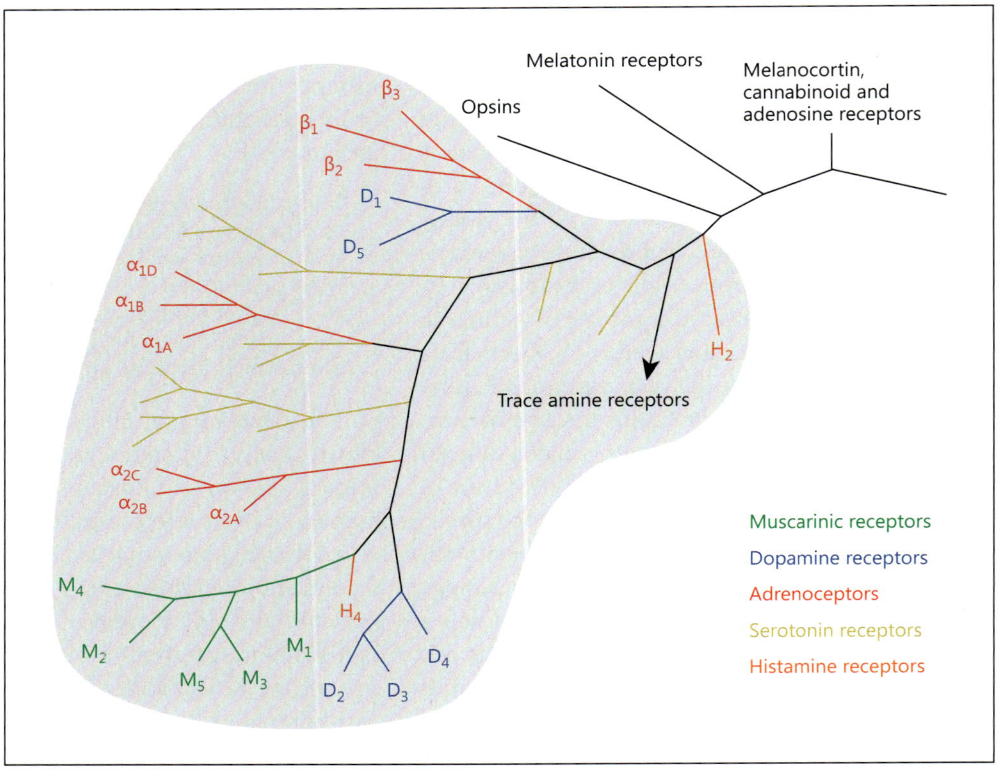

Fig. 4. The amine receptor cluster, with nine adrenoceptors and five dopamine receptors, in the phylogenetic tree of human G-protein-coupled receptors. Based on Frederiksson et al. [89].

perial Chemical Industries Pharmaceuticals in the UK. In 1967, β-adrenoceptors were subdivided into β_1 and β_2 [80], and a third β-type began to be suspected in the late 1970s, above all in adipocytes [81].

α-Adrenoceptor subclassification began in 1971 with the discovery of the self-regulation of noradrenaline release through α-adrenoceptors on noradrenergic synaptic terminals, presynaptic α-autoreceptors [5]. Their existence was initially combated but is now established, for example by the demonstration of their messenger RNA in noradrenergic neurons [82, 83]. They differed from α-receptors on effector cells and in 1974 became the prototype α_2-receptors, the long-known smooth muscle contraction-mediating receptors becoming α_1 [84].

Even before dopamine was identified as the third catecholamine transmitter, Blaschko [3] suspected it might possess receptors of its own. The first hint, he wrote, was the finding by Peter Holtz et al. [85] in 1942 that small doses of dopamine lowered the blood pressure of rabbits and guinea pigs, whereas adrenaline always increased the blood pressure. Holtz erred in his interpretation, but Blaschko had 'no doubt that his observations are of the greatest historical importance, as the first indication of an action of dopamine that characteristically and specifically differs from those of the two other catecholamines' [3]. A re-investigation of the blood pressure-lowering effect in dogs in 1964 proposed 'specific dopamine receptors for dilation' [86], and at the same time evidence for dopamine receptors distinct from α- and β-adrenoceptors accrued from other experimental approaches.

In 1986, the first gene coding for a catecholamine receptor, the β_2-adrenoceptor from hamster lung, was cloned by a group of sixteen scientists, among them Robert Lefkowitz (born in 1943) and Brian Kobilka (born in 1955) of Duke University in Durham,

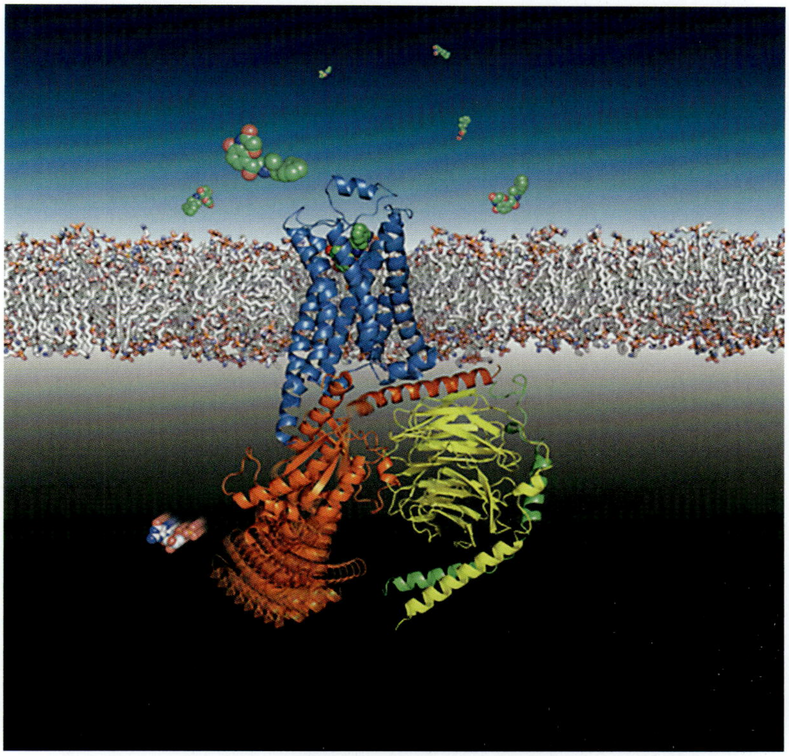

Fig. 5. The β_2-adrenoceptor and its coupling to the G-protein G_s.

N.C., USA [87]. Genes for all mammalian catecholamine receptors have now been cloned: for the nine adrenoceptors α_{1A}, α_{1B}, α_{1D}, α_{2A}, α_{2B}, α_{2C}, β_1, β_2 and β_3 and the five dopamine receptors D_1, D_2, D_3, D_4 and D_5 (fig. 4). Their fine structure, either without agonist or agonist-activated, begins to be understood at high resolution [88].

Earl Wilbur Sutherland (1915–1974) won the 1971 Nobel Prize in Physiology or Medicine 'for his discoveries concerning the mechanisms of the action of hormones', in particular the discovery of cyclic adenosine monophosphate as the second messenger in the action of catecholamines at β-adrenoceptors and of glucagon at glucagon receptors, which led to the discovery of G-protein-coupled receptors. In 1988, James Black was one of three winners of the Nobel Prize in Physiology or Medicine 'for their discoveries of important principles for drug treatment', Black's 'important principles' being the blockade of β-adrenoceptors and of histamine H_2-receptors. In 2012, Robert Lefkowitz and Brian Kobilka shared the Nobel Prize in Chemistry 'for studies of G-protein-coupled receptors' (fig. 5).

References

1 Trendelenburg P: Adrenalin und adrenalinverwandte Substanzen; in Hefter A (ed): Handbuch der experimentellen Pharmakologie. Berlin, Springer, 1924, vol 2, part 2, pp 1130–1293.

2 Blaschko H: Catecholamines 1922–1971; in Blaschko H, Muscholl E (eds): Catecholamines: Handbuch der experimentellen Pharmakologie XXXIII. Berlin, Springer, 1972, pp 1–15.

3 Blaschko H: A half-century of research on catecholamine biosynthesis. J Appl Cardiol 1987;2:171–183.

4 Bacq ZM: Chemical transmission of nerve impulses; in Parnham MJ, Bruinvels J (eds): Discoveries in Pharmacology. Amsterdam, Elsevier, 1983, vol 1, pp 49–103.

5 Bennett MR: One hundred years of adrenaline: the discovery of autoreceptors. Clin Auton Res 1999;9:145–159.

6 Donnerer J, Lembeck F: Adrenaline, noradrenaline and dopamine: the catecholamines; in Donnerer and Lembeck (eds): The Chemical Languages of the Nervous System. Basel, Karger, 2006, pp 150–160.
7 Henderson J: Ernest Starling and 'Hormones': an historical commentary. J Endocrinol 2005;184:5–10.
8 Salter HH: On Asthma: Its Pathology and Treatment. Philadelphia, Blanchard, 1864.
9 Vulpian A: Note sur quelques réactions propres à la substance des capsules surrénales. CR Acad Sci 1856;43:663–665.
10 Jacobj C: Beiträge zur physiologischen und pharmakologischen Kenntnis der Darmbewegungen mit besonderer Berücksichtigung der Beziehung der Nebenniere zu denselben. Arch Exp Pathol Pharmakol 1892;29:173–211.
11 Carmichael SW: The history of the adrenal medulla. Rev Neurosci 1989;2:83–99.
12 Dale H: Natural chemical stimulators. Edinburgh Med J 1938;45:461–480.
13 Barcroft H, Talbot JF: Oliver and Schäfer's discovery of the cardiovascular action of suprarenal extract. Postgrad Med J 1968;44: 6–8.
14 Oliver G: On the therapeutic employment of the suprarenal glands. Br Med J 1895;2: 653–655.
15 Schäfer EA: On the present condition of our knowledge of the functions of the suprarenal capsules. Br Med J 1908;1:1277–1281.
16 Oliver G, Schäfer EA: On the physiological action of extract of the suprarenal capsules. J Physiol 1894;16:I–IV.
17 Oliver G, Schäfer EA: The physiological effects of extracts of the suprarenal capsules. J Physiol 1895;18:230–276.
18 Borell M: Organotherapy, British physiology, and discovery of the internal secretions. J Hist Biol 1976;9:235–286.
19 Kahn RH: Zur Physiologie der Trachea. Arch Anat Physiol Arch Physiol 1907:398–426.
20 Januschke H, Pollak L: Zur Pharmakologie der Bronchialmuskulatur. Arch Exp Pathol Pharmakol 1911;66:205–220.
21 Bullowa JGM, Kaplan DM: On the hypodermatic use of adrenalin chloride in the treatment of asthmatic attacks. NY Med J 1903; 83:787–790.
22 Szymonowicz L: Die Function der Nebenniere. Pflügers Arch Ges Physiol 1895;64: 97–164.
23 Gottlieb R: Ueber die Wirkung der Nebennierenextrakte auf Herz und Blutdruck. Arch Exp Pathol Pharmakol 1896;38:99–112.
24 Bates WH: The use of extract of suprarenal capsule in the eye. NY Med J 1896:647–650.
25 Persson CGA: Astute observers discover anti-asthma drugs. Pharmacol Toxicol 1995; 77(suppl 3):7–15.
26 Abel JJ: Ueber den blutdruckerregenden Bestandtheil der Nebenniere, das Epinephrin. Z Physiol Chem 1899;28:318–361.
27 von Fürth O: Zur Kenntniss der brenzcatechinähnlichen Substanz der Nebennieren. 3. Mittheilung. Z Physiol Chem 1900;29: 105–123.
28 Takamine J: Adrenalin, the active principle of the suprarenal glands and mode of preparation. Am J Pharmacy 1901;73:523–535.
29 Friedmann E: Die Konstitution des Adrenalins. Beitr Z Chem Physiol Pathol 1906;8: 95–120.
30 Cushny AR: The action of optical isomers. 3. Adrenalin. J Physiol 1908;37:130–138.
31 Tansey EM: What's in a name? Henry Dale and adrenaline, 1906. Med Hist 1995;39: 459–476.
32 Lewandowsky M: Ueber die Wirkung des Nebennierenextractes auf die glatten Muskeln, im Besonderen des Auges. Arch Physiol 1899;360–366.
33 Elliott TR: On the innervation of the ileocolic sphincter. J Physiol 1904;31:157–168.
34 Elliott TR: On the action of adrenalin. J Physiol 1904;31:XX–XXI.
35 Stjärne L, Hedqvist P, Lagercrantz H, Wennmalm Å (eds): Chemical Neurotransmission: 75 years. London, Academic Press, 1981, p XIII.
36 Loewi O: Über humorale Übertragbarkeit der Herznervenwirkung. 1. Mitteilung. Pflügers Arch Ges Physiol 1921;189:239–242.
37 Loewi O: Über humorale Übertragbarkeit der Herznervenwirkung. 2. Mitteilung. Pflügers Arch Ges Physiol 1922;193:201–231.
38 Loewi O: Quantitative und qualitative Untersuchungen über den Sympathicusstoff. Pflügers Arch Ges Physiol 1936;237:504–514.
39 Barger B, Dale HH: Chemical structure and sympathomimetic action of amines. J Physiol 1910;41:19–59.
40 Holtz P, Heise R, Lüdtke K: Fermentativer Abbau von l-Dioxyphenylalanin (Dopa) durch Niere. Naunyn Schmiedebergs Arch Exp Pathol Pharmakol 1939;191:87–118.
41 Blaschko H: The specific action of L-dopa decarboxylase. J Physiol 1939;96:50–51.
42 Holtz P: Dopadecarboxylase. Naturwissenschaften 1939;27:724–725.
43 Bülbring E: The methylation of noradrenaline by minced suprarenal tissue. Br J Pharmacol 1949;4:234–244.
44 Axelrod J: Purification and properties of phenylethanolamine-N-methyltransferase. J Biol Chem 1962;237:1657–1660.
45 Hare MLC: Tyramine oxidase. 1. A new enzyme system in liver. Biochem J 1928;22: 968–979.
46 Blaschko H, Richter D, Schlossmann H: The oxidation of adrenaline and other amines. Biochem J 1937;31:2187–2196.
47 Axelrod J: O-Methylation of epinephrine and other catechols in vitro and in vivo. Science 1957;126:400–401.
48 von Euler US: A sympathomimetic pressor substance in animal organ extracts. Nature 1945;156:18–19.
49 von Euler US: A specific sympathomimetic ergone in adrenergic nerve fibres (sympathin) and its relations to adrenaline and nor-adrenaline. Acta Physiol Scand 1946;12:73–97.
50 Peart WS: The nature of splenic sympathin. J Physiol 1948;108:491–501.
51 Holtz P, Credner K, Kroneberg G: Über das sympathicomimetische pressorische Prinzip des Harns ('Urosympathin'). Naunyn Schmiedebergs Arch Exp Pathol Pharmakol 1947;204:228–243.
52 Holtz P, Schümann HJ: Arterenol – ein neues Hormon des Nebennierenmarks. Naturwissenschaften 1948;35:159.
53 Dale H: Adventures in Physiology. London, Pergamon Press, 1953, p 98.
54 Vogt M: The concentration of sympathin in different parts of the central nervous system under normal conditions and after the administration of drugs. J Physiol 1954;123: 451–481.
55 Dahlström A, Fuxe K: Evidence for the existence of monoamine neurons in the central nervous system. 1. Demonstration of monoamines in the cell bodies of brain stem neurons. Acta Physiol Scand 1964;62(suppl 247):1–55.
56 Bertler Å, Rosengren E: Occurrence and distribution of dopamine in brain and other tissues. Experientia 1959;15:10–11.
57 Carlsson A: The occurrence, distribution and physiological role of catcholamines in the nervous system. Pharmacol Rev 1959; 11:490–493.
58 Ehringer H, Hornykiewicz O: Verteilung von Noradrenalin und Dopamin (3-Hydroxytyramin) im Gehirn des Menschen und ihr Verhalten bei Erkrankungen des extrapyramidalen Systems. Klin Wochenschr 1960;38:1236–1239.
59 Hornykiewicz O: From dopamine to Parkinson's disease: a personal research record; in Samson F, Adelman G (eds): The Neurosciences: Paths of Discovery II. Basel, Birkhäuser, 1992, pp 125–147.
60 Blaschko H, Welch AD: Localization of adrenaline in cytoplasmic particles of the bovine adrenal medulla. Naunyn Schmiedebergs Arch Exp Pathol Pharmakol 1953; 219:17–22.
61 Hillarp NÅ, Lagerstedt S, Nilson B: The isolation of a granular fraction from the suprarenal medulla, containing the sympathomimetic catechol amines. Acta Physiol Scand 1953;29:251–263.

62 von Euler US, Hillarp NÅ: Evidence for the presence of noradrenaline in submicroscopic structures of adrenergic axons. Nature 1956;177:44–45.
63 de Robertis E, Pellegrino de Iraldi A, Rodríguez de Lores Arnaiz G, Zieher LM: Synaptic vesicles from the rat hypothalamus. Isolation and norepinephrine content. Life Sci 1965;4:193–201.
64 Schümann HJ, Grobecker H: Über den Noradrenalin- und ATP-Gehalt sympathischer Nerven. Naunyn Schmiedebergs Arch Exp Pathol Pharmakol 1958;233:296–300.
65 Thureson-Klein Å: Exocytosis from large and small dense cored vesicles in noradrenergic nerve terminals. Neuroscience 1983; 10:245–252.
66 Axelrod J, Weil-Malherbe H, Tomchick R: The physiological disposition of H^3-epinephrine and its metabolite metanephrine. J Pharmacol Exp Ther 1959;127:251–256.
67 Whitby LG, Axelrod J, Weil-Malherbe H: The fate of H^3-norepinephrine in animals. J Pharmacol Exp Ther 1961;132:193–201.
68 Muscholl E: Effect of cocaine and related drugs on the uptake of noradrenaline by heart and spleen. Br J Pharmacol 1961;16: 352–359.
69 Hertting G, Axelrod J: Fate of tritiated noradrenaline at the sympathetic nerve-endings. Nature 1961;192:172–173.
70 Iversen LL: The Uptake and Storage of Noradrenaline in Sympathetic Nerves. Cambridge, University Press, 1967.
71 Dale HH: On some physiological actions of ergot. J Physiol 1906;34:163–206.
72 Konzett H, Rössler R: Versuchsanordnung zu Untersuchungen an der Bronchialmuskulatur. Naunyn Schmiedebergs Arch Exp Pathol Pharmakol 1940;195:71–74.
73 Konzett H: Neue broncholytisch hochwirksame Körper der Adrenalinreihe. Naunyn Schmiedebergs Arch Exp Pathol Pharmakol 1941;197:27–40.
74 Konzett H: On the discovery of isoprenaline. Trends Pharmacol Sci 1981;2:47–49.
75 Sneader W: Drug Discovery: The Evolution of Modern Medicines. Chichester, Wiley & Sons, 1985, p 103.
76 Ahlquist RP: A study of the adrenotropic receptors. Am J Physiol 1948;153:586–600.
77 Powell CE, Slater IH: Blocking of inhibitory adrenergic receptors by a dichloro analog of isoproterenol. J Pharmacol Exp Ther 1958; 122:480–488.
78 Moran NC, Perkins ME: Adrenergic blockade of the mammalian heart by a dichloro analog of isoproterenol. J Pharmacol Exp Ther 1958;124:222–237.
79 Black JW, Crowther AF, Shanks RG, Dornhorst AC: A new adrenergic beta-receptor antagonist. Lancet 1964;i:1080–1081.
80 Lands AM, Arnold A, McAuliff JP, Luduena FP, Brown TG: Differentiation of receptor systems activated by sympathomimetic amines. Nature 1967;214:597–598.
81 Zaagsma J, Nahorski SR: Is the adipocyte β-adrenoceptor a prototype for the recently cloned 'β_3-adrenoceptor'? Trends Pharmacol Sci 1990;11:3–7.
82 Nicholas AP, Pieribone V, Hökfelt T: Distribution of mRNAs for alpha-2 adrenergic receptor subtypes in rat brain: an in situ hybridization study. J Compar Neurol 1993; 328:575–594.
83 Starke K: Presynaptic autoreceptors in the third decade: focus on α_2-adrenoceptors. J Neurochem 2001;78:685–693.
84 Langer SZ: Presynaptic regulation of catecholamine release. Biochem Pharmacol 1974;23:1793–1800.
85 Holtz P, Credner K, Koepp W: Die enzymatische Entstehung von Oxytyramin im Organismus und die physiologische Bedeutung der Dopadecarboxylase. Naunyn Schmiedebergs Arch Exp Pathol Pharmakol 1942;200:356–388.
86 Eble JN: A proposed mechanism for the depressor effect of dopamine in the anesthetized dog. J Pharmacol Exp Ther 1964;145: 64–70.
87 Dixon RAF, Kobilka BK, et al: Cloning of the gene and cDNA for mammalian β-adrenergic receptor and homology with rhodopsin. Nature 1986;321:75–79.
88 Rosenbaum DM, Zhang C, et al: Structure and function of an irreversible agonist-β_2 adrenoceptor complex. Nature 2011;469: 236–240.
89 Frederiksson R, Lagerström MC, Lundin LG, Schiöth HB: The G-protein-coupled receptors in the human genome form five main families: phylogenetic analysis, paralogon groups, and fingerprints. Mol Pharmacol 2003;63:1256–1272.

5

Prof. Klaus Starke
Institut für Experimentelle und Klinische Pharmakologie und Toxikologie
Albert-Ludwigs-Universität Freiburg
Albertstrasse 25
DE–79104 Freiburg (Germany)
E-Mail klaus.starke@pharmakol.uni-freiburg.de

Progress in Allergy Management

Bergmann K-C, Ring J (eds): History of Allergy. Chem Immunol Allergy. Basel, Karger, 2014, vol 100, pp 302–310
DOI: 10.1159/000359963

Antihistamines

Martin K. Church · Marcus Maurer

Department of Dermatology and Allergy, Allergy Center Charité, Universitätsmedizin, Berlin, Germany

Abstract

The discovery of histamine, its physiological role and reversal of its pharmacological effects by antihistamines takes us on a journey through the origins of modern physiology and the rising understanding of pharmacology at the end of the 19th and the early part of the 20th centuries. This journey, which has been traced in the excellent historical review by Michael Emanuel [Clin Exp Allergy 1999;29:1–11], is populated by some of the greatest scientists of the era, including six Nobel laureates – Bovet, Dale, Ehrlich, Richet, Windaus and Black. In addition, it laid the basis of medicinal chemistry not only for antihistamines, but also for the discovery of a plethora of drugs still in use today.

At the beginning of the 20th century, scientists had a reasonably clear idea of the anatomy of the nervous system and that individual nerve cells formed the basis of the system. They also knew that nerve messages travelled in the form of minute electrical currents along the length of a neuron and then passed from the axon of one cell to the dendrites of a nearby cell. It was suggested that this transmission involved biologically active amines. Indeed, epinephrine (adrenaline) had already been discovered [1, 2]. Then, in 1910, Dale [3] published his studies on β-iminazolylethylamine, a putrefaction product of histidine. Believing this amine, which was later to be named histamine, to be a transmitter in the autonomic nervous system, Dale performed detailed comparisons with adrenaline. In his discussion, Dale concluded:

> The action of β-iminazolylethylamine appears a somewhat complicated one. It cannot be summarised with reference to any division of the autonomic system, like that of some other amines.

Although Dale was also studying anaphylaxis [4], it was not until his paper in 1919 on histamine shock [5] that he finally tied histamine and anaphylaxis together, and it was another 8 years [6] before histamine was extracted from tissues. In that paper, Dale concluded that histamine 'must have some important function in the control and adjustment of the circulation through the small blood vessels'.

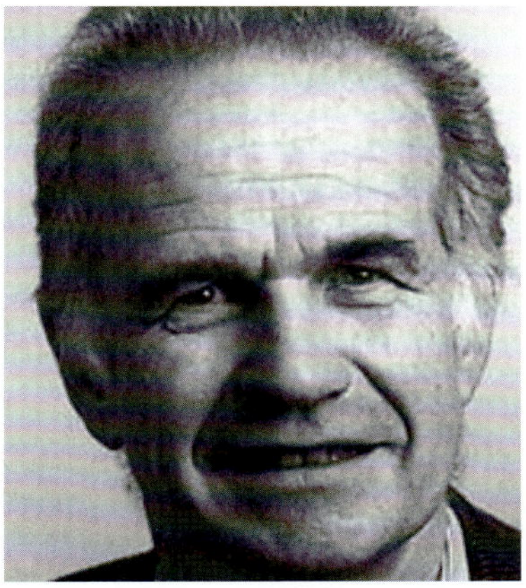

Fig. 1. Daniel Bovet.

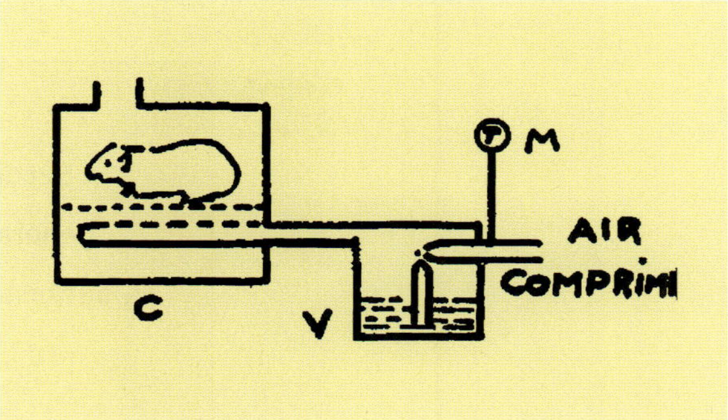

Fig. 2. Diagram of an apparatus in which bronchospasm in guinea pigs is produced by inhalation of histamine aerosol. C = Closed box in which the animal is observed; V = aerosolizer containing a solution of histamine hydrochloride; M = manometer.

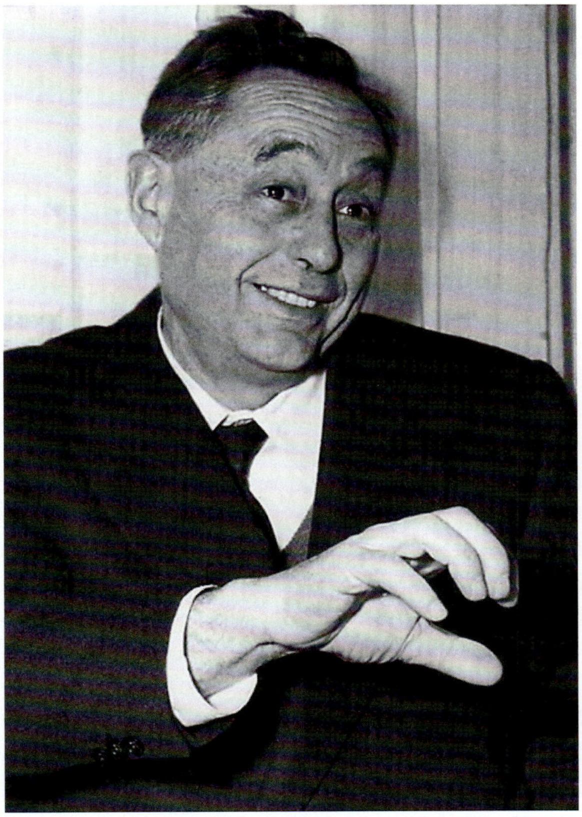

Fig. 3. Bernard Halpern.

The Discovery of Antihistamines

It was against this background that Daniel Bovet (fig. 1) started his quest to find an antihistamine. In his 1950 review of his quest to discover an antihistamine [7], Bovet wrote:

> Three naturally occurring amines, acetylcholine, epinephrine, and histamine, may be grouped together because they have a similar chemical structure, are all present in the body fluids, and exert characteristically strong pharmacologic activities. There are alkaloids which interfere with the effects of acetylcholine. Similarly, there are sympathicolytic poisons which neutralize or reverse the effects of epinephrine. It seemed possible to me, therefore, that some substance might exist which exerts a specific antagonism toward histamine. With this hypothesis in mind, I began an investigation in 1937 to determine the effect upon the susceptibility toward histamine of various substances of known activity on the autonomic nervous system.

Bovet, together with Anne-Marie Staub, who was preparing her doctorate thesis in his laboratory, used three types of laboratory methods for the evaluation of the degree of activity of the various compounds [7]. In the first test, they determined the action against the lethal effects of histamine in guinea pigs. This test they believed to be 'perfectly specific'. In the second test (fig. 2, reproduced together with its original legend), they determined the protection against histamine administered in the form of an aerosol.

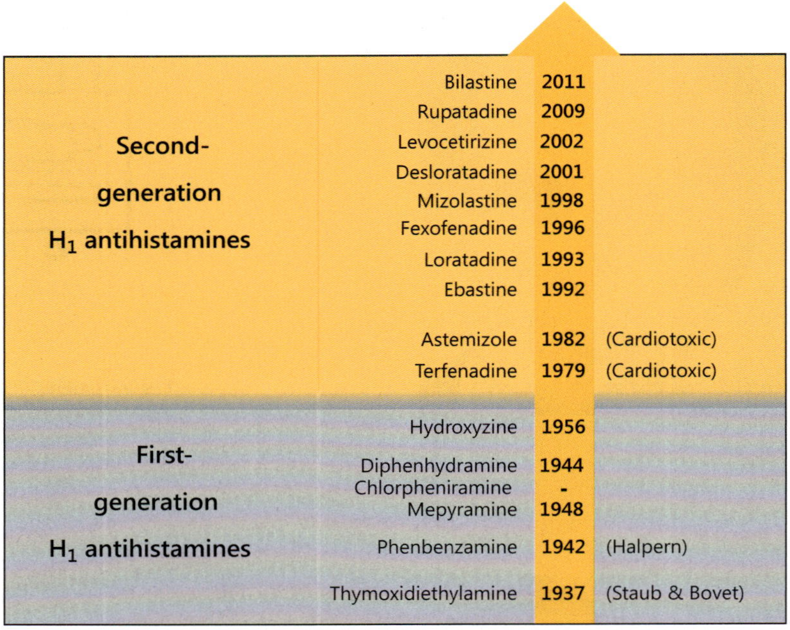

Fig. 4. The dates of introduction of the most common H_1 antihistamines.

Here, they believed that symptoms similar to asthma were produced. In the third test for determining antihistaminic activity, which they believed to be the least specific one, they ascertained the effect of compounds on histamine-induced spasm of the isolated guinea pig ileum.

Thymoxyethyldiethylamine (929 F) was the first of the substances in which antihistamine properties were recognized [8, 9]. From the chemical standpoint, compound 929 F belonged to a series of amines with a phenolic ether function which included substances that possessed either anti-epinephrine or antihistaminic activity. Another group of compounds in which sympathomimetic, sympatholytic and antihistaminic amines were found side by side were aniline compounds. It was the study of one of this group that led to the discovery of diethylaminoethyl-N-ethylaniline (1571 F) [10]. A derivative of 1571 F, N-diethylaminoethyl-N-benzylaniline (Antergan), was the first antihistamine to be introduced clinically in 1942 by Bernard Halpern from the Institute Pasteur in Paris [11] (fig. 3). This was followed by diphenhydramine in 1945 [12] and chlorpheniramine, brompheniramine and promethazine [13] later in the same decade (fig. 4).

The Discovery of H_2, H_3 and H_4 Antihistamines

While the classical antihistamines discovered in the 1940s and 1950s, such as mepyramine, suppressed the effects of histamine in contracting the smooth muscle of various organs, such as the gut and bronchi, actions such as increased gastric acid secretion, increased heart rate and contraction of the rat uterus were 'mepyramine resistant'. This observation led Ash and Schild [14] to hypothesize that histamine exerted its effects through more than one receptor and led them to define the classical 'mepyramine-sensitive' receptor as the histamine H_1 receptor.

In order to find drugs which antagonized the 'mepyramine-resistant' effects of histamine, particularly its stimulation of gastric acid secretion, in 1964 Sir James Black and his colleagues at The Research Institute of Smith Kline and French Laboratories began to synthesize and test over 700 compounds which were closely related to the structure of histamine [15]. This work led to the definition of the histamine H_2 receptor and the discovery of burimamide and cimetidine [16], the forerunners of the H_2 antihistamines for the treatment of gastric ulcers.

Work by Jean-Charles Schwartz et al. [17] in Paris in the early 1980s demonstrated that histamine was not only a transmitter in the periphery, but also in the brain. Furthermore, they showed that the postsynaptic effects were mediated primarily by histamine. However, they also realized that histamine, like other neurotransmitters, may modulate its own release through a presynaptic receptor, an action they suggested to be mediated by a class of receptor, designated as H_3, which was pharmacologically distinct from the previously characterized histamine H_1 and H_2 receptors [18]. This discovery and the realization that histamine H_3 receptors are located almost exclusively in the brain led to the investigation of H_3 antihistamines for the treatment of cognitive disorders and Alzheimer's disease [19].

Using the DNA sequence of the histamine H_3 receptor, several research groups independently identified a previously unexplored G-protein-coupled receptor sequence in the human genome as a new histamine receptor, the histamine H_4 receptor [20]. The identification of histamine H_4 receptors on hematopoietic cells, eosinophils, mast cells and dendritic cells, and its potential role in chemotaxis and activation of these cells has stimulated widespread research into the possible use of H_4 antihistamines in allergic disease [21].

First- and Second-Generation H_1 Antihistamines

While the earliest antihistamines resembled histamine in their basic chemical structure consisting of an ethylamine group linking aromatic and aliphatic substituents, similar or greater activities have been found in compounds of many different chemical series, including ethanolamines, ethylene diamines, alkylamines, piperazines, piperidines and phenothiazines.

While all these groups of compounds contain drugs with H_1 antihistaminic activity, they also contain compounds with other 'anti-amine' actions, either as antagonists or interfering with their re-uptake mechanisms. Not only does this explain the diverse adverse effects of first-generation H_1 antihistamines, but it also provided the pharmaceutical industry with a platform to search for other drugs. Two examples are given. First, a systematic chemical synthesis of phenothiazine derivatives in an attempt to find a substance resembling promethazine, but with a more marked antipsychotic action, led to the discovery of chlorpromazine, a drug with many actions in the central nervous system, including antidopaminergic, anticholinergic and anti-α-adrenergic activity [22]. Second, following the discovery of chlorpromazine another antihistaminic agent, imipramine, was investigated for its potential antipsychotic activity. However, while it was noted that imipramine had little antipsychotic action, elevation of the mood of depressed patients was evident. This observation led to the introduction of tricyclic antidepressants [23]. It is hardly surprising, therefore, that these first-generation antihistamines had poor receptor selectivity and significant unwanted side effects.

A major advance in antihistamine development occurred in the 1980s with the introduction of second-generation H_1 antihistamines [24], which are minimally or non-sedating because of their limited penetration of the blood-brain barrier. In addition, these drugs are highly selective for the histamine H_1 receptor and have no anticholinergic effects (fig. 4).

H_1 Antihistamines and the Central Nervous System

Perhaps the greatest drawback of first-generation H_1 antihistamines is their ability to cross the blood-brain barrier and interfere with histaminergic transmission. Histamine is an important neuromediator in the human brain which contains approximately 64,000 histamine-producing neurons, located in the tuberomamillary nucleus. When activated these neurons stimulate H_1 receptors in all of the major parts of the cerebrum, cerebellum, posterior pituitary and spinal cord [25] where they increase arousal in the circadian sleep/wake cycle, reinforce learning and memory, and have roles in fluid balance, suppression of feeding, control of body temperature, control of the cardiovascular system and mediation of stress-triggered release of ACTH and δ-endorphin from the pituitary gland [26]. It is not surprising then that antihistamines crossing the blood-brain barrier interfere with all of these processes.

Physiologically, the release of histamine during the day causes arousal whereas its decreased production at night results in a passive reduction of the arousal response. When taken during the day, first-generation H_1 antihistamines, even in the manufacturers' recommended doses, frequently cause daytime somnolence, sedation, drowsiness, fatigue, and impaired concentration and memory [27, 28]. When taken at night, first-generation H_1 antihistamines increase the latency to the onset of rapid eye movement (REM) sleep and reduce the duration of REM sleep [29–31]. The residual effects of poor sleep, including impairment of attention, vigilance, working memory and sensorimotor performance, are still present the next morning [30, 32]. The detrimental central nervous system effects of first-generation H_1 antihistamines on learning and examination performance in children, and on the impairment of the ability of adults to work, drive and fly aircraft, have been reviewed in detail in a recent review [33].

In contrast to first-generation H_1 antihistamines, second-generation H_1 antihistamines have a reduced penetration of the brain. The major reason for this is because their translocation across the blood-brain barrier is under the control of active transporter proteins, of which the ATP-dependent efflux pump, P-glycoprotein, is the best known [34, 35]. It has also become apparent that antihistamines differ in their substrate specificity for P-glycoprotein, with fexofenadine being a particularly good substrate [36]. In the brain, the H_1 receptor occupancy of fexofenadine assessed using positron emission tomography (PET) scanning is negligible at <0.1%, and, in psychomotor tests, fexofenadine is not significantly different from placebo [37]. Furthermore, fexofenadine has been shown to be devoid of central nervous effects even at supraclinical doses of up to 360 mg [38].

While fexofenadine is devoid of central nervous system effects, many other second-generation H_1 antihistamines still penetrate the brain to a small extent where they have the potential to cause some degree of drowsiness or somnolence, particularly when used in higher doses. For example, PET scanning of the human brain has shown that single oral doses of 10 and 20 mg of cetirizine caused 12.5 and 25.2% occupancy of the H_1 receptors in prefrontal and cingulate cortices, respectively [39]. These results would explain the repeated clinical findings that the incidence of drowsiness or fatigue is greater with cetirizine than with placebo [40–43]. Recent publications have suggested that, at the manufacturer's recommended doses, levocetirizine is less sedative than cetirizine [44] and desloratadine causes negligible somnolence [45, 46]. However, it should be pointed out that 'mean results' do not reveal everything as some patients may show considerable somnolence whereas others are unaffected.

H_1 Antihistamines and Cardiotoxicity

The introduction of the first non-sedating H_1 antihistamines in the late 1970s and 1980s brought new and unexpected problems, with an increasing number of reports showing an association between the consumption of astemizole and terfenadine and cardiotoxicity. Both of these are essentially prodrugs which are metabolized by the cytochrome P450 enzyme, CYP3A4, to their active form. However, it was soon realized that if this metabolism was blocked by the concomitant use of inhibitors of CYP3A4, such as ketoconazole, itraconazole and macrolide antibiotics, or by grapefruit juice, which causes post-translational downregulation of CYP3A4, then this could cause the prolongation of the QT interval, leading to the appearance of polymorphic ventricular arrhythmias, syncope and even cardiac arrest in susceptible individuals [47]. The main mechanism underlying this acquired QT syndrome and a potentially fatal torsade de pointes arrhythmia is the inhibition of the potassium channel encoded by hERG (the human ether-a-go-go-related gene).

Astemizole and terfenadine are no longer approved by regulatory agencies in most countries. However, some first-generation H_1 antihistamines, such as promethazine [48], brompheniramine [49] and chlorpheniramine [50], may also be associated with a prolonged QTc and cardiac arrhythmias when taken in large doses or overdoses. Today, the concentration of a drug to produce a half-maximal block of the hERG potassium current (IC_{50}) is used as a surrogate marker for proarrhythmic properties of compounds and is the primary test for cardiac safety of drugs [51]. No clinically significant cardiac effects have been reported for the second-generation H_1 antihistamines fexofenadine, the metabolite of terfenadine, desloratadine, loratadine, cetirizine, levocetirizine, azelastine, ebastine, mizolastine, rupatadine or bilastine [52–56].

The Anti-Inflammatory Properties of H_1 Antihistamines

The potential of H_1 antihistamines to exert anti-inflammatory properties has been debated for over half a century ever since Arunlakshana and Schild [57] in 1953 demonstrated their ability to inhibit histamine release from mast cells. With the advancing knowledge about the molecular mechanisms underlying the effects of H_1 antihistamines, it is pertinent to reassess this possibility and comment on its possible clinical relevance. In order to put these comments on a scientific basis, we have postulated that some anti-inflammatory effects of H_1 antihistamines are subsequent to their interaction with H_1 receptors while others are receptor independent.

Receptor-Independent Mechanisms

The early studies of Mota and Dias de Silva [58] in 1960 using guinea pig and rat mast cells showed clearly that not only do antihistamines have the capacity to inhibit histamine release, but at higher concentrations they may also stimulate a drug-induced release of histamine. From the many studies done with first-generation and some early second-generation H_1 antihistamines to explore the mechanisms of this biphasic effect, the following conclusions may be drawn [47]. First, there is no correlation between the concentrations of drugs which inhibit histamine release and their H_1 antihistaminic potency. The most likely mechanism lies in their lipophilic cationic structure which allows them to exert a direct inhibitory effect on calcium ion channels, reducing the inward Ca^{2+} current activated by intracellular Ca^{2+} store depletion. Second, the concentrations of drugs required to prevent mast cell and basophil histamine release in vitro are in the order of 1–10 μM, much higher than those likely to occur systemically in vivo following oral dosage.

To test the clinical significance of this effect, two H_1 antihistamines, cetirizine and loratadine, were administered at a dose of 10 mg orally, 4 h before the provocation of histamine release by intradermal injections of 3 and 10 mg/ml of codeine [59]. The results showed a clear inhibition of the ensuing weal and flare responses, demonstrating that the drugs had been absorbed and were bioactive. However, the use of dermal microdialysis to recover histamine release from the extracellular fluid showed that neither drug reduced histamine release. Thus, it is unlikely that inhibition of mast cell histamine release by H_1 antihistamines contributes to their beneficial therapeutic effects following systemic administration in the treatment of allergic and inflammatory reactions. Similar results have been obtained with fexofenadine following nasal allergen challenge [60]. However, these effects may be clinically relevant following the topical administration of drugs which enables higher concentrations to be achieved locally. An example of this is the administration of olopatadine eyedrops which significantly reduce histamine release into tears [61].

Receptor-Dependent Mechanisms

The first clue that H_1 antihistamines may have receptor-dependent anti-inflammatory effects came in 1987 from the observation that cetirizine reduced the influx of eosinophils into the sites of allergic reactions [62]. Initially this was claimed to be an 'additional' effect of cetirizine which was not related to the histamine H_1 receptor, but it soon became apparent that these anti-inflammatory effects were not solely confined to cetirizine but were shared by other H_1 antihistamines [63]. Subsequent studies have shown the anti-inflammatory effect to result from the ability of H_1 antihistamines to downregulate the activation of NF-κB [64], an ubiquitous transcription factor which binds to promoter/enhancer regions of many genes regulating the production of a number of pro-inflammatory cytokines and adhesion proteins, including IL-1β, IL-6, IL-8, TNF-α and GM-CSF. Because this effect is mediated by H_1 receptors it will occur with all clinically used H_1 antihistamines, the degree of effect being dependent on their H_1 antihistaminic potency and the dose at which the drugs are used [47].

H_1 Antihistamines Are Not Receptor Antagonists but Are Inverse Agonists

The human histamine H_1 receptor is a member of the superfamily of G-protein-coupled receptors. This superfamily represents at least 500 individual membrane proteins that share a common structural motif of seven transmembrane α-helical segments. The histamine H_1 receptor gene encodes a 487-amino-acid protein with a molecular mass of 55.8 kDa [65]. The histamine H_1 receptor, like other G-protein-coupled receptors, may be viewed as 'cellular switch' which exists as an equilibrium between the inactive or 'off' state and the active or 'on' state. In the case of the histamine H_1 receptor, histamine cross-links sites on transmembrane domains III and V to stabilize the receptor in its active conformation, thus causing the equilibrium to swing to the 'on' position. H_1 antihistamines, which are not structurally related to histamine, do not antagonize the binding of histamine but bind to different sites on the receptor to produce the opposite effect [47]. For example, cetirizine cross-links sites on transmembrane domains IV and VI to stabilize the receptor in the inactive state and swing the equilibrium to the 'off' position. Thus, H_1 antihistamines are not receptor antagonists but are inverse agonists in that they produce the opposite effect on the receptor to histamine. Consequently, the preferred term to define these drugs is 'H_1 antihistamines' rather than 'histamine antagonists'.

Conclusions

Clearly, the last 70 years have seen great advances in the development of antihistamines; but what of the future? The further development of H_1 antihistamines for the treatment of allergic diseases appears to be limited to completely preventing penetration into the brain so that higher doses can be used in absolute safety in conditions such as severe urticaria. Research into H_4 antihistamines is still in its infancy and the efficacy of these is yet to be established. Finally, it is now becoming apparent that many histamine-induced events may be caused by the activation of multiple histamine receptor subtypes and, thus, the development of drugs with activity at more than one receptor subtype may offer a new approach to antihistamine therapy.

References

1 Abel JJ: Ueber den blutdruckerregenden Bestandtheil der Nebenniere, das Epinephrin. Z Physiol Chem 1899;28:318–324.

2 Takamine J: The isolation of the active principle of the suprarenal gland. J Physiol 1902; 27:xxix–xxx.

3 Dale HH, Laidlaw PP: The physiological action of β-iminazolylethylamine. J Physiol 1910;41:318–344.

4 Dale HH: The anaphylactic reaction of plain muscle in the guinea-pig. J Pharmacol 1913; 4:167–223.

5 Dale HH, Laidlaw PP: Histamine shock. J Physiol 1919;52:355–390.

6 Best CH, Dale HH, Dudley HW, Thorpe WV: The nature of vasodilator constituents of certain tissue extracts. J Physiol (Lond) 1927;62:397–417.

7 Bovet D: Introduction to antihistamine agents and antergan derivative. Ann NY Acad Sci 1950;50:1089–1126.

8 Bovet D, Staub A: Action protectrice des éthers phénoliques au cours de l'intoxication histaminique. CR Seances Acad Sci 1937; 124:527–549.

9 Staub AM, Bovet D: Action de la thymoxyethyldiethylamine (929F) et des éthers phénoliques sur le choc anaphylactique. Compt Rend Soc Biol 1937;125:818–821.

10 Staub AM: Recherches sur quelques bases synthétiques antagonistes de l'histamine. Ann Inst Pasteur 1939;63:400–436.

11 Halpern BN: Les antihistaminiques de synthèse. Essais de chimiothérapie des états allergiques. Arch Int Pharmacodyn Ther 1942;681:339–408.

12 Loew ER, Macmillan R, Kaiser M: The antihistamine properties of benadryl, B dimethylaminoethyl benzhydryl ether hydrochloride. J Pharmacol Exp Ther 1946;86:229–238.

13 Halpern BN, Hamburger J: A new synthetic anti-histamine substance derived from phenothiazine (Phenergan, 3,277 R.P.). Can Med Assoc J 1948;59:322–326.

14 Ash AS, Schild HO: Receptors mediating some actions of histamine. Br J Pharmacol Chemother 1966;27:427–439.

15 Black JW, Duncan WA, Durant CJ, Ganellin CR, Parsons EM: Definition and antagonism of histamine H_2-receptors. Nature 1972;236:385–390.

16 Brimblecombe RW, Duncan WA, Durant GJ, Ganellin CR, Parsons ME, Black JW: The pharmacology of cimetidine, a new histamine H_2-receptor antagonist. Br J Pharmacol 1975;53:435P-436P.

17 Schwartz JC, Pollard H, Quach TT: Histamine as a neurotransmitter in mammalian brain: neurochemical evidence. J Neurochem 1980;35:26–33.

18 Arrang JM, Garbarg M, Schwartz JC: Autoinhibition of brain histamine release mediated by a novel class (H_3) of histamine receptor. Nature 1983;302:832–837.
19 Brioni JD, Esbenshade TA, Garrison TR, Bitner SR, Cowart MD: Discovery of histamine H_3 antagonists for the treatment of cognitive disorders and Alzheimer's disease. J Pharmacol Exp Ther 2011;336:38–46.
20 Leurs R, Chazot PL, Shenton FC, Lim HD, de Esch IJ: Molecular and biochemical pharmacology of the histamine H_4 receptor. Br J Pharmacol 2009;157:14–23.
21 Smits RA, Leurs R, de Esch IJ: Major advances in the development of histamine H_4 receptor ligands. Drug Discov Today 2009;14:745–753.
22 Dundee JW. A review of chlorpromazine hydrochloride. Br J Anaesth 1954;26:357–379.
23 Klerman GL, Cole JO: Clinical pharmacology of imipramine and related antidepressant compounds. Pharmacol Rev 1965;17:101–141.
24 Holgate ST, Canonica GW, Simons FE, Taglialatela M, Tharp M, Timmerman H, Yanai K: Consensus Group on New-Generation Antihistamines (CONGA): present status and recommendations. Clin Exp Allergy 2003;33:1305–1324.
25 Haas H, Panula P: The role of histamine and the tuberomamillary nucleus in the nervous system. Nat Rev Neurosci 2003;4:121–130.
26 Brown RE, Stevens DR, Haas HL: The physiology of brain histamine. Prog Neurobiol 2001;63:637–672.
27 Simons FE: Advances in H_1-antihistamines. N Engl J Med 2004;351:2203–2217.
28 Juniper EF, Stahl E, Doty RL, Simons FE, Allen DB, Howarth PH: Clinical outcomes and adverse effect monitoring in allergic rhinitis. J Allergy Clin Immunol 2005;115:S390–S413.
29 Adam K, Oswald I: The hypnotic effects of an antihistamine: promethazine. Br J Clin Pharmacol 1986;22:715–717.
30 Boyle J, Eriksson M, Stanley N, Fujita T, Kumagi Y: Allergy medication in Japanese volunteers: treatment effect of single doses on nocturnal sleep architecture and next day residual effects. Curr Med Res Opin 2006;22:1343–1351.
31 Rojas-Zamorano JA, Esqueda-Leon E, Jimenez-Anguiano A, Cintra-McGlone L, Mendoza Melendez MA, Velazquez MJ: The H_1 histamine receptor blocker, chlorpheniramine, completely prevents the increase in REM sleep induced by immobilization stress in rats. Pharmacol Biochem Behav 2009;91:291–294.
32 Kay GG, Berman B, Mockoviak SH, Morris CE, Reeves D, Starbuck V, Sukenik E, Harris AG: Initial and steady-state effects of diphenhydramine and loratadine on sedation, cognition, mood, and psychomotor performance. Arch Intern Med 1997;157:2350–2356.
33 Church MK, Maurer M, Simons FE, Bindslev-Jensen C, van Cauwenberge P, Bousquet J, Holgate ST, Zuberbier T: Risk of first-generation H_1-antihistamines: a GA(2)LEN position paper. Allergy 2010;65:459–466.
34 Schinkel AH: P-Glycoprotein, a gatekeeper in the blood-brain barrier. Adv Drug Deliv Rev 1999;36:179–194.
35 Chen C, Hanson E, Watson JW, Lee JS: P-glycoprotein limits the brain penetration of nonsedating but not sedating H_1-antagonists. Drug Metab Dispos 2003;31:312–318.
36 Cvetkovic M, Leake B, Fromm MF, Wilkinson GR, Kim RB: OATP and P-glycoprotein transporters mediate the cellular uptake and excretion of fexofenadine. Drug Metab Dispos 1999;27:866–871.
37 Tashiro M, Sakurada Y, Iwabuchi K, Mochizuki H, Kato M, Aoki M, Funaki Y, Itoh M, Iwata R, Wong DF, Yanai K: Central effects of fexofenadine and cetirizine: measurement of psychomotor performance, subjective sleepiness, and brain histamine H_1-receptor occupancy using ^{11}C-doxepin positron emission tomography. J Clin Pharmacol 2004;44:890–900.
38 Hindmarch I, Shamsi Z, Kimber S: An evaluation of the effects of high-dose fexofenadine on the central nervous system: a double-blind, placebo-controlled study in healthy volunteers. Clin Exp Allergy 2002;32:133–139.
39 Tashiro M, Kato M, Miyake M, Watanuki S, Funaki Y, Ishikawa Y, Iwata R, Yanai K: Dose dependency of brain histamine H_1 receptor occupancy following oral administration of cetirizine hydrochloride measured using PET with $[^{11}C]$doxepin. Hum Psychopharmacol 2009;24:540–548.
40 Meltzer EO, Weiler JM, Widlitz MD: Comparative outdoor study of the efficacy, onset and duration of action, and safety of cetirizine, loratadine, and placebo for seasonal allergic rhinitis. J Allergy Clin Immunol 1996;97:617–626.
41 Howarth PH, Stern MA, Roi L, Reynolds R, Bousquet J: Double-blind, placebo-controlled study comparing the efficacy and safety of fexofenadine hydrochloride (120 and 180 mg once daily) and cetirizine in seasonal allergic rhinitis. J Allergy Clin Immunol 1999;104:927–933.
42 Salmun LM, Gates D, Scharf M, Greiding L, Ramon F, Heithoff K: Loratadine versus cetirizine: assessment of somnolence and motivation during the workday. Clin Ther 2000;22:573–582.
43 Mann RD, Pearce GL, Dunn N, Shakir S: Sedation with 'non-sedating' antihistamines: four prescription-event monitoring studies in general practice. BMJ 2000;320:1184–1186.
44 De Vos C, Mitchev K, Pinelli ME, Derde MP, Boev R: Non-interventional study comparing treatment satisfaction in patients treated with antihistamines. Clin Drug Investig 2008;28:221–230.
45 Day JH, Briscoe MP, Rafeiro E, Ratz JD: Comparative clinical efficacy, onset and duration of action of levocetirizine and desloratadine for symptoms of seasonal allergic rhinitis in subjects evaluated in the Environmental Exposure Unit (EEU). Int J Clin Pract 2004;58:109–118.
46 Devillier P, Roche N, Faisy C: Clinical pharmacokinetics and pharmacodynamics of desloratadine, fexofenadine and levocetirizine: a comparative review. Clin Pharmacokinet 2008;47:217–230.
47 Leurs R, Church MK, Taglialatela M: H_1-antihistamines: inverse agonism, anti-inflammatory actions and cardiac effects. Clin Exp Allergy 2002;32:489–498.
48 Jo SH, Hong HK, Chong SH, Lee HS, Choe H: H_1 antihistamine drug promethazine directly blocks hERG K^+ channel. Pharmacol Res 2009;60:429–437.
49 Park SJ, Kim KS, Kim EJ: Blockade of HERG K^+ channel by an antihistamine drug brompheniramine requires the channel binding within the S6 residue Y652 and F656. J Appl Toxicol 2008;28:104–111.
50 Hong HK, Jo SH: Block of HERG K^+ channel by classic histamine H_1 receptor antagonist chlorpheniramine. Korean J Physiol Pharmacol 2009;13:215–220.
51 Polak S, Wisniowska B, Brandys J: Collation, assessment and analysis of literature in vitro data on hERG receptor blocking potency for subsequent modeling of drugs' cardiotoxic properties. J Appl Toxicol 2009;29:183–206.
52 Ten Eick AP, Blumer JL, Reed MD: Safety of antihistamines in children. Drug Saf 2001;24:119–147.
53 Du Buske LM: Second-generation antihistamines: the risk of ventricular arrhythmias. Clin Ther 1999;21:281–295.
54 Simons FE, Prenner BM, Finn A Jr: Efficacy and safety of desloratadine in the treatment of perennial allergic rhinitis. J Allergy Clin Immunol 2003;111:617–622.
55 Hulhoven R, Rosillon D, Letiexhe M, Meeus MA, Daoust A, Stockis A: Levocetirizine does not prolong the QT/QTc interval in healthy subjects: results from a thorough QT study. Eur J Clin Pharmacol 2007;63:1011–1017.

56 Izquierdo I, Merlos M, Garcia-Rafanell J: Rupatadine: a new selective histamine H_1 receptor and platelet-activating factor (PAF) antagonist: a review of pharmacological profile and clinical management of allergic rhinitis. Drugs Today (Barc) 2003;39: 451–468.
57 Arunlakshana O, Schild HO: Histamine release by antihistamines. J Physiol (Lond) 1953;119:47P–48P.
58 Mota I, Dias da Silva W: The antianaphylactic and histamine releasing properties of the anti-histamines: their effect on mast cells. Br J Pharmacol 1960;15:396–404.
59 Perzanowska M, Malhotra D, Skinner SP, Rihoux JP, Bewley AP, Petersen LJ, Church MK: The effect of cetirizine and loratadine on codeine-induced histamine release in human skin in vivo assessed by cutaneous microdialysis. Inflamm Res 1996;45:486–490.
60 Allocco FT, Votypka V, deTineo M, Naclerio RM, Baroody FM: Effects of fexofenadine on the early response to nasal allergen challenge. Ann Allergy Asthma Immunol 2002;89:578–584.
61 Leonardi A, Abelson MB: Double-masked, randomized, placebo-controlled clinical study of the mast cell-stabilizing effects of treatment with olopatadine in the conjunctival allergen challenge model in humans. Clin Ther 2003;25:2539–2552.
62 Fadel R, Herpin-Richard N, Rihoux JP, Henocq E: Inhibitory effect of cetirizine 2HCl on eosinophil migration in vivo. Clin Allergy 1987;17:373–379.
63 Townley RG: Antiallergic properties of the second-generation H_1 antihistamines during the early and late reactions to antigen. J Allergy Clin Immunol 1992;90:720–725.
64 Bakker RA, Schoonus SB, Smit MJ, Timmerman H, Leurs R: Histamine H_1-receptor activation of nuclear factor-kappa B: roles for $G\beta\gamma$- and $G\alpha_{q/11}$-subunits in constitutive and agonist-mediated signaling. Mol Pharmacol 2001;60:1133–1142.
65 Fukui H, Fujimoto K, Mizuguchi H, Sakamoto K, Horio Y, Takai S, Yamada K, Ito S: Molecular cloning of the human histamine H_1 receptor gene. Biochem Biophys Res Commun 1994;201:894–901.

Prof. Martin K. Church
Allergie-Centrum-Charité, Department of Dermatology and Allergy
Charité – Universitätsmedizin
Charitéplatz 1
DE–10117 Berlin (Germany)
E-Mail mkc@southampton.ac.uk

Progress in Allergy Management

Bergmann K-C, Ring J (eds): History of Allergy. Chem Immunol Allergy. Basel, Karger, 2014, vol 100, pp 311–316
DOI: 10.1159/000359984

Glucocorticoids

Peter J. Barnes

Airway Disease Section, National Heart and Lung Institute, Imperial College, London, UK

Abstract

Glucocorticoids are the most effective anti-inflammatory treatment for allergic diseases, and inhaled glucocorticoids have now become the first-line treatment for asthma. Glucocorticoids were discovered in the 1940s as extracts of the adrenal cortex and this was followed by the isolation of adrenocorticotropic hormone (ACTH) from pituitary gland extracts. Cortisone and ACTH were found to be very beneficial in the treatment of rheumatoid arthritis and Kendall, Reichstein and Hench received the Nobel Prize in Physiology and Medicine for this work in 1950. Bordley and colleagues first showed that ACTH was very beneficial in the treatment of allergic diseases in 1949, but the use of systemic glucocorticoids was limited by side effects. Inhaled glucocorticoids were discovered from topical steroids developed for skin inflammation and beclomethasone dipropionate was introduced in 1972, initially in low doses but later in higher doses, and became the standard treatment for persistent asthma. Subsequently, inhaled glucocorticoids were combined with long-acting β_2-agonists in combination inhalers for even greater therapeutic benefit. There is now a good understanding of the molecular basis for the anti-inflammatory effects of glucocorticoids in allergic diseases. The search for even safer glucocorticoids based on the dissociation of anti-inflammatory and side effect mechanisms is currently ongoing.

Glucocorticosteroids (also known as glucocorticoids or corticosteroids) are the most effective treatment for asthma and other allergic diseases and it has proven extraordinarily difficult to find any new treatment that comes close to their therapeutic benefit. Glucocorticoids are naturally occurring hormones and their remarkable anti-inflammatory effects were first discovered in the early 1950s, shortly after the synthesis of cortisol, the main glucocorticoid secreted by the adrenal cortex.

Early Studies with Glucocorticoids

Solomon Solis-Cohen, a physician from Philadelphia, first reported in 1900 that orally administered adrenal gland extract (adrenal substance pills) was beneficial in asthma [1]. It was assumed that the clinical benefit of adrenal extract was explained by the adrenaline from the adrenal medulla and the direct

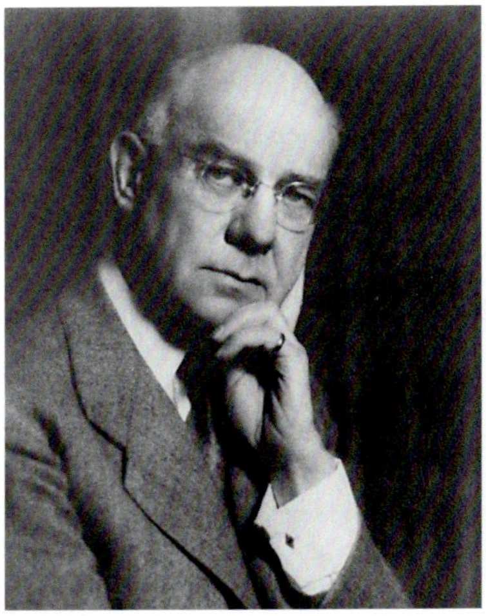

1

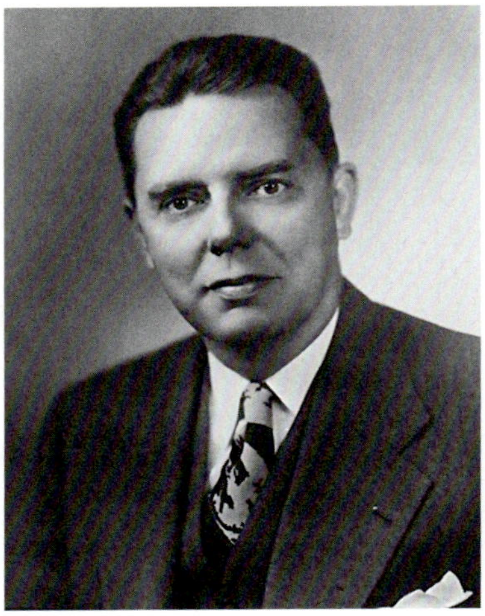

2

Fig. 1. Dr. Edward C. Kendall (1886–1972), chemist who received the Nobel Prize in Physiology and Medicine in 1950 for the discovery of glucocorticoids.

Fig. 2. Philip Showalter Hench (1896–1965), rheumatologist from the Mayo Clinic who shared the Nobel Prize for the discovery of glucocorticoids.

bronchodilator effect of adrenaline (epinephrine) was first demonstrated by Kahn in 1907 using precontracted tracheal strips in vitro [2]. However, since adrenaline is not significantly absorbed after oral administration it is very likely that the benefits of orally administered adrenal extract described by Solis-Cohen were due to its glucocorticoid content [3]. This was not recognised at the time and it was not until cortisol was isolated from the adrenal cortex that the idea of glucocorticoids as a therapy for asthma became clear. The Nobel Prize in Physiology and Medicine was awarded in 1950 to Edward Kendall, a chemist working at the Mayo Foundation, Tadeus Reichstein, a Swiss biochemist, and Philip Hench, a clinician working at the Mayo Clinic, for 'discoveries relating to the hormones of the adrenal cortex, their structure and biological effects'. Edward Kendall (fig. 1) isolated several steroids from the adrenal cortex during the 1940s, including cortisone (initially known as compound E) and subsequently adrenocorticotropic hormone (ACTH), which was isolated from pituitary gland extracts. Philip Hench (fig. 2), a rheumatologist at the Mayo Clinic, was keen to test these drugs in patients with rheumatoid arthritis, but this was delayed by the difficulty in preparing enough compound E for administration and also by his military service. Compound E (cortisone) was first given by intravenous injection to patients with rheumatoid arthritis in 1948 and shown to be very beneficial. This was followed by the demonstration that ACTH was equally effective. Merck and Company first produced cortisone commercially in 1949. Shortly after Hench's demonstration of the clinical efficacy of cortisone and ACTH in rheumatoid patients, John Bordley (fig. 3), an ENT specialist, and colleagues at Johns Hopkins University showed that ACTH had equally dramatic effects in patients with asthma and allergic rhinitis [4]. They described 5 patients with asthma, interestingly all of whom had eosinophilic sputum, who improved rapidly with intramuscular injections of ACTH over a 3-week period, with disappearance of the sputum. They went on to confirm these observations in a larger group of patients. As a replacement for the injections it was subsequently shown that oral cortisone, widely used at the time to treat several inflammatory diseases, was an effective therapy in patients with difficult-to-control asthma.

First Controlled Trial of Glucocorticoid in Asthma

However, there was scepticism in the UK about the efficacy of cortisol, leading to a Medical Research Council multicentre trial of cortisone in asthma patients, which was in fact the first placebo-controlled trial ever performed in asthma [5]. Surprisingly, the results were disappointing with little clinical improvement, which was not sustained during the 2

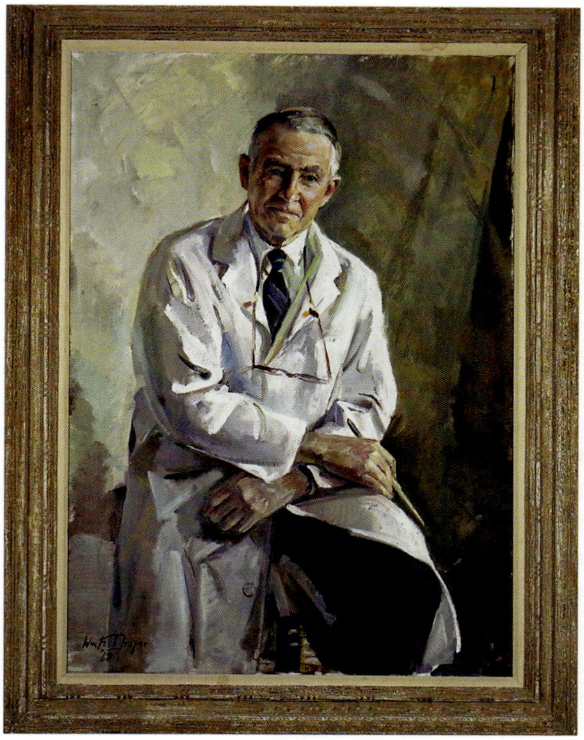

Fig. 3. Dr. John E. Bordley (1903–1993) – chaired the Department of Otolaryngology at Johns Hopkins University in Baltimore and first demonstrated the beneficial effects of ACTH in treating allergic disease.

months of therapy. This may have reflected the low dose of cortisone used, the lack of objective measurements of lung function and most likely the inclusion of many patients who had chronic obstructive pulmonary disease (COPD), who show little clinical improvement with even high doses of glucocorticoids. The Brompton Hospital in London was one of the participating centres in this trial and Jack Pepys, who was professor of allergy and one of the investigators, carefully selected asthma patients with no evidence of COPD, showing marked clinical improvement in these patients.

Despite this poor result oral glucocorticoids became increasingly used in patients with severe asthma, but it was clear that side effects were a major problem resulting in the stunting of growth in children, osteoporosis and metabolic disturbances. This immediately suggested the need to give glucocorticoids by inhalation as a way of reducing the systemic side effects.

Inhaled Glucocorticoids

When the severe metabolic and endocrine side effects of oral glucocorticoid became apparent, it was thought that a way to reduce this problem was to deliver the glucocorticoid by inhalation. However, cortisone and dexamethasone given by inhalation proved to be of little benefit. This later turned out to be because of their lack of topical efficacy and led to a search for topically active steroids. McKenzie and Stoughton [6] had discovered that this topical efficacy was correlated with skin blanching, although the cellular basis for this test is still uncertain. Hydrocortisone turned out to be weak in the McKenzie test, but two synthetic glucocorticoids, beclomethasone dipropionate (BDP) and betamethasone 17-valerate, gave good skin blanching responses. Both of these steroids were effective as topical treatments for eczema and psoriasis, predicting that they may also be effective by inhalation.

Both of these new steroids were developed for inhalation. BDP was developed in an inhaled formulation by the team of Sir David Jack (fig. 4) at Allen & Hanburys/Glaxo, and clinical trials in asthma were begun in about 1970 [7]. An important paper by Harry Morrow Brown et al. [8] in 1972 established that inhaled BDP was very effective in reducing the need for oral glucocorticoids and in many patients achieved better control. Interestingly, Brown reported that the patients who did best had high numbers of eosinophils in their sputum, an observation that has been confirmed in many subsequent (and much more recent) studies [9]. BDP inhalers became available for the treatment of asthma in 1972. Low doses of inhaled BDP (100 μg four times daily) were initially used as a way to reduce the requirement for oral glucocorticoids. High doses of BDP (250 μg/puff) were subsequently introduced in order to more effectively treat patients with more severe asthma [10]. About this time it became clear that inhaled BDP twice daily was as effective as administration four times daily and was more convenient for patients [11]. In addition to BDP other topical glucocorticoids were developed for treating asthma. Budesonide was developed by Ralph Brattsand and colleagues working for Astra in Sweden, and was the first glucocorticoid optimised for inhaled use, with a favourable

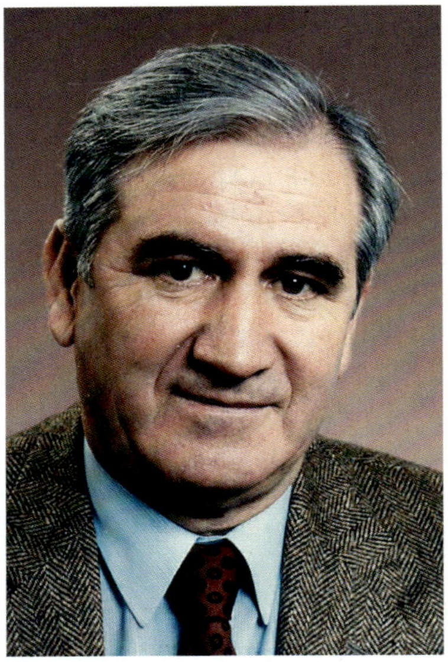

Fig. 4. Sir David Jack FRS (1923–2011), chemist who developed the first inhaled glucocorticoid for the treatment of asthma.

ratio of topical to systemic effect as a result of the efficient hepatic metabolism of any swallowed glucocorticoid, and was introduced in the early 1980s [12]. Budesonide therefore had a therapeutic advantage over BDP since systemic side effects were less likely. This was followed by the development of fluticasone propionate by Jack's group at Glaxo, which had an even more efficient first pass metabolism. Other glucocorticoids were subsequently introduced and, although all work focussed on activating glucocorticoid receptors, there were differences in the pharmacodynamic effects. Mometasone and ciclesonide also have reduced systemic effects and may be suitable for once daily dosing in mild asthma patients. Ciclesonide is a prodrug that is activated by esterases in the lower airways so may also have less risk of upper airway side effects [13].

In parallel with the development of inhaled glucocorticoids for asthma, the same drugs were developed either as nasal sprays or drops for the treatment of rhinitis. While inhaled glucocorticoids were initially used in patients with relatively severe asthma, with the growing recognition that even patients with mild asthma have chronic inflammation of the airways, inhaled glucocorticoid came to be used in the majority of patients with persistent asthma, from mild to severe patients [14]. With the recognition that the doses of inhaled glucocorticoids needed to control asthma in the majority of patients were not associated with significant systemic side effects, their use was also extended to children. Indeed, inhaled glucocorticoid gradually came to replace the widely used cromoglycate that was subsequently found in controlled trials to be relatively ineffective. The widespread use of inhaled glucocorticoids in asthma has almost certainly been the major reason why asthma morbidity, hospital admissions and mortality have progressively fallen over the last decade. Inhaled glucocorticoids have now become amongst the most widely used therapies in the world given the high prevalence of asthma and, to a lesser extent, COPD. There is now a search for inhaled glucocorticoids with even better therapeutic ratios and less systemic side effects, including the development of selective glucocorticoid receptor activator drugs and dissociated steroids that may not even have a classical steroid structure [15].

Combination Inhalers

A major breakthrough was the discovery that adding an inhaled long-acting β_2-agonist (LABA – salmeterol or formoterol) to an inhaled glucocorticoid produced greater clinical benefit than increasing the dose of inhaled glucocorticoids. This was fist demonstrated in a study in general practice patients in the UK by GlaxoSmithKline in 1994, when it was shown that patients who were not controlled with 400 µg daily of BDP were better controlled and showed better lung function when salmeterol was added to this dose rather than increasing the dose of BDP to 1,000 µg daily [16]. At first the results seemed counterintuitive since it was believed that if asthma was not controlled at a low dose of glucocorticoid it was because the dose was insufficient and a higher dose would be effective. It was also known that LABA, unlike glucocorticoids, did not have any anti-inflammatory effects. This study became one of the most highly cited papers in respiratory medicine and allergy. The unexpected findings were subsequently confirmed in scores of other studies, all of which showed that adding a LABA was more effective than increasing the dose of inhaled glucocorticoid. For example, the FACET study, which was the largest controlled trial in asthma patients at its time of publication, showed that adding formoterol was more effective than a 4-fold increase in dose of inhaled glucocorticoids and that this combination was very effective in severe exacerbations [17]. These studies led to the development of combination inhalers containing a glucocorticoid with a LABA and these have now become the most effective and convenient means of controlling asthma. Indeed, fluticasone propionate/salmeterol (Seretide, Advair) has now become the third biggest selling drug worldwide, with a market that is increasing throughout the world. The reasons for the greater efficacy of combination inhalers compared to inhaled glucocorticoids alone relate to their complementary effects in asthma and there is also a synergy between the glucocorticoid and β_2-agonist effects [18]. Another reason is the shallow dose-response to inhaled glucocorticoids. Although inhaled glucocorticoids (BDP) have been used to treat asthma since the early 1970s, it is only relatively recently that dose-response studies have been conducted in asthma patients. This occurred because it was mandated by the Food and Drug Administration (FDA) when inhaled glucocorticoids were introduced in the USA in the early 1990s. These dose-response studies require approximately 100 patients for each dose of inhaled glucocorticoid, which is why the studies were only conducted when the FDA requested this information. The flat dose-response study was with inhaled budesonide [19], but similar dose-responses were subsequently shown with all other inhaled glucocorticoids [20].

Mechanisms of Action

When cortisol was first discovered it was believed to function mainly as a stress hormone involved in maintaining body homeostasis and regulating glycogen metabolism. However, its anti-inflammatory effects became rapidly apparent when Hench studied its effects in rheumatoid arthritis patients. It was then shown to reduce the infiltration of inflammatory cells into tissues, but its molecular mechanism of action has proved difficult to elucidate. It was shown that radiolabelled cortisol and other glucocorticoids bound to specific macromolecular complexes that were subsequently identified as glucocorticoid receptors [21], and that these glucocorticoid receptors interacted with DNA molecules in the nucleus to affect gene expression. During the 1970s it was established that the glucocorticoid binding and DNA sites were distinct as they could be separated by proteolysis. Around this time it was also shown that glucocorticoid receptors could activate several genes and it was therefore assumed that the anti-inflammatory effects of glucocorticoids were due to the activation of genes that had anti-inflammatory effects. Although several anti-inflammatory genes were identified this was unlikely to account for the marked anti-inflammatory effects of glucocorticoids in suppressing multiple activated inflammatory genes. Another possibility was that glucocorticoid receptors could directly inactivate inflammatory genes, although this was never convincingly demonstrated and direct inhibition of cytokine genes, for example, was not found. A more likely explanation was that glucocorticoids directly inhibited transcription factors, such as activator protein-1 or nuclear factor-κB, which were responsible for the activation of multiple inflammatory genes [22, 23]. However, these direct interactions turned out to be more an artefact of the overexpression systems that were used to demonstrate these molecular interactions [24]. More recently it has been found that low concentrations of glucocorticoids switch off inflammatory genes through the recruitment of histone deacetylase-2, HDAC2, a nuclear enzyme that deacetylates the hyperacetylated histones associated with activated inflammatory genes, such as cytokines. In addition, HDAC2 deacetylates glucocorticoid receptors which is necessary for them to suppress activated inflammatory genes [25].

Future Directions

Glucocorticoids remain the most effective anti-inflammatory drugs available for the treatment of allergic diseases and it has been difficult to find any other drugs anywhere near as effective. The main limitation of glucocorticoids is their side effects at high doses. To a large extent this has been overcome by topical administration, although systemic effects may be seen at high doses. There have been attempts to improve glucocorticoid safety by dissociating anti-inflammatory effects from side effect mechanisms and this has resulted in the identification of several 'dissociated steroids' [15]. These drugs are now in development and it is hoped that the side effects of oral glucocorticoids may be considerably reduced. Another approach is to develop non-steroidal anti-inflammatory treatments. So far this has proven to be very difficult as most of the drug classes developed, such as phosphodiesterase-4 and p38 MAP kinase inhibitors, have dose-limiting side effects.

References

1 Solis-Cohen S: The use of adrenal substances in the treatment of asthma. JAMA 1900; 34:1164–1169.

2 Brewis RAL: Classical Papers in Asthma. London, Science Press, 1990.

3 Barnes PJ: Drugs for asthma. Br J Pharmacol 2006;147(suppl 1):S297–S303.

4 Bordley JE, Carey RA, Harvey AM: Preliminary observations on the effect of adrenocorticotropic hormone in allergic diseases. Bull Johns Hopkins Hosp 1949;85:396–410.

5 Medical Research Council: Controlled trial of effects of cortisone acetate in status asthmaticus; report to the Medical Research Council by the subcommittee on clinical trials in asthma. Lancet 1956;271:803–806.

6 McKenzie AW, Stoughton RB: Method for comparing percutaneous absorption of steroids. Arch Dermatol 1962;86:608–610.

7 Barnes PJ, Breckenridge A: David Jack (1924–2011) who revolutionised the treatment of asthma. Thorax 2012;67:266–267.

8 Brown HM, Storey G, George WH: Beclomethasone dipropionate: a new steroid aerosol for the treatment of allergic asthma. Br Med J 1972;1:585–590.

9 Green RH, Brightling CE, McKenna S, Hargadon B, Parker D, Bradding P, Wardlaw AJ, Pavord ID: Asthma exacerbations and sputum eosinophil counts: a randomised controlled trial. Lancet 2002;360:1715–1721.

10 Smith MJ, Hodson ME: High-dose beclomethasone inhaler in the treatment of asthma. Lancet 1983;i:265–269.

11 Toogood JH, Baskerville JC, Jennings B, Lefcoe NM, Johansson SA: Influence of dosing frequency and schedule on the response of chronic asthmatics to the aerosol steroid budesonide. J Allergy Clin Immunol 1982; 70:288–298.

12 Thalen A, Brattsand R: Synthesis and anti-inflammatory properties of budesonide, a new non-halogenated glucocorticoid with high local activity. Arzneimittelforschung 1979;29:1687–1690.

13 Derendorf H: Pharmacokinetic and pharmacodynamic properties of inhaled ciclesonide. J Clin Pharmacol 2007;47:782–789.

14 Barnes PJ: Inhaled glucocorticoids for asthma. N Engl J Med 1995;332:868–875.

15 Clark AR, Belvisi MG: Maps and legends: the quest for dissociated ligands of the glucocorticoid receptor. Pharmacol Ther 2012; 134:54–67.

16 Greening AP, Ind PW, Northfield M, Shaw G: Added salmeterol versus higher-dose corticosteroid in asthma patients with symptoms on existing inhaled corticosteroid. Lancet 1994;344:219–224.

17 Pauwels RA, Lofdahl C-G, Postma DS, Tattersfield AE, O'Byrne PM, Barnes PJ, Ullman A: Effect of inhaled formoterol and budesonide on exacerbations of asthma. N Engl J Med 1997;337:1412–1418.

18 Barnes PJ: Scientific rationale for inhaled combination therapy with long-acting β2-agonists and corticosteroids. Eur Respir J 2002;19:182–191.

19 Busse WW, Chervinsky P, Condemi J, Lumry WR, Petty TL, Rennard S, Townley RG: Budesonide delivered by Turbuhaler is effective in a dose-dependent fashion when used in the treatment of adult patients with chronic asthma. J Allergy Clin Immunol 1998;101:457–463.

20 Adams NP, Jones PW: The dose-response characteristics of inhaled corticosteroids when used to treat asthma: an overview of Cochrane systematic reviews. Respir Med 2006;100:1297–1306.

21 Hackney JF, Gross SR, Aronow L, Pratt WB: Specific glucocorticoid-binding macromolecules from mouse fibroblasts growing in vitro: a possible steroid receptor for growth inhibition. Mol Pharmacol 1970;6:500–512.

22 Yang-Yen H-F, Chambard J-C, Sun Y-L, Smeal T, Schmidt TJ, Drovin J, Karin M: Transcriptional interference between c-Jun and the glucocorticoid receptor: mutual inhibition of DNA binding due to direct protein-protein interaction. Cell 1990;62: 1205–1215.

23 Barnes PJ, Karin M: Nuclear factor-κB: a pivotal transcription factor in chronic inflammatory diseases. N Engl J Med 1997; 336:1066–1071.

24 Barnes PJ: Glucocorticosteroids: current and future directions. Br J Pharmacol 2011; 163:29–43.

25 Ito K, Yamamura S, Essilfie-Quaye S, Cosio B, Ito M, Barnes PJ, Adcock IM: Histone deacetylase 2-mediated deacetylation of the glucocorticoid receptor enables NF-kB suppression. J Exp Med 2006;203:7–13.

Prof. P.J. Barnes
Airway Disease Section, National Heart and Lung Institute, Imperial College
Dovehouse Street
London SW3 6LY (UK)
E-Mail p.j.barnes@imperial.ac.uk

Progress in Allergy Management

Bergmann K-C, Ring J (eds): History of Allergy. Chem Immunol Allergy. Basel, Karger, 2014, vol 100, pp 317–322
DOI: 10.1159/000359986

Chromones

Alan M. Edwards

The David Hide Asthma and Allergy Research Centre, St. Mary's Hospital, Newport, UK

Abstract

The chromones are a class of chemical compounds characterised by the presence of the structure *5:6 benz-1:4-pyrone* in their chemical make-up. The first chromone in clinical use, khellin, was extracted from the seeds of the plant *Ammi visnaga*, and had been used for centuries as a diuretic and as a smooth muscle relaxant. Its use in bronchial asthma was reported in 1947. In the 1950s, Benger's Laboratories embarked on a research programme to synthesise and develop modifications of khellin for the treatment of asthma. New compounds were screened using animal models to test the ability of the compound to prevent the anaphylactic release of histamine and SRS-A (leukotrienes) from sensitised guinea pig lung, and a human model to check the ability to reduce the bronchoconstriction induced by inhaled antigen bronchial challenge. For initial screening the human work was undertaken by Dr. R.E.C. Altounyan, who suffered from allergic bronchial asthma and was employed by Benger's Laboratories. After 8 years and more than 600 challenges using over 200 compounds, in 1965 Altounyan arrived at disodium cromoglycate (DSCG), the chromone that met the criteria of providing more than 6 h of protection. DSCG is still used today as a mast cell stabiliser.

5

Background

The chromones are a class of chemical compounds characterised by the presence of the structure *5:6 benz-1:4-pyrone* (fig. 1) in their chemical make-up. As drugs used in clinical medicine they are classified as mast cell stabilisers: their primary pharmacological activity is to prevent the release of inflammatory mediators from mast cells. Although cells containing granules had been described by Friedrich von Recklinghausen in 1863, these cells were first called mast cells (Mastzellen) by Paul Ehrlich in his thesis from the University of Leipzig in 1878.

In 1921, Prausnitz and Küstner [1] described details of the antigen/antibody reaction in a sensitised individual in their paper translated from German by

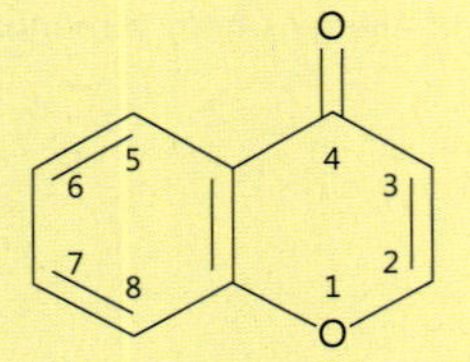

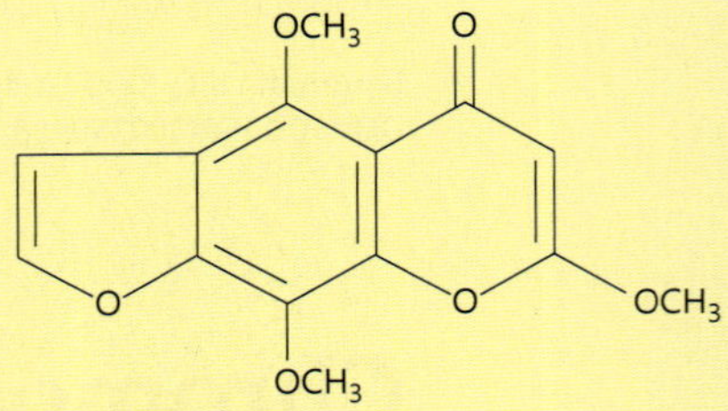

Fig. 1. Chromone chemical structure.
Fig. 2. The structure of khellin.

Prausnitz as 'Studies on supersensitivity'. In 1932, Bartosch et al. [2] reported that a substance, probably identical to histamine, appeared in the perfusion fluid from the lungs of sensitised guinea pigs after the addition of antigen. In 1952, Riley and West [3] showed that the amount of histamine in tissues correlated with the number of mast cells. In 1940, Kellaway and Trethewie [4] described another substance found in the perfusate of the lungs of sensitised animals after the anaphylactic response. This substance differed from histamine, with the contraction it caused having a short latency and being less rapid. They called this substance the 'slow reacting substance' or SRS, and it was called the slow reacting substance of anaphylaxis, SRS-A, by later authors. The time course of the release of histamine and SRS-A from sensitised guinea pig lung after the introduction of antigen was described in detail by Brocklehurst [5] in 1960. Together with his co-worker Austen, Brocklehurst showed that the release of histamine could be inhibited by a number of substances [6].

The Chromones

It was against this background that work to develop the chromones as new drugs began in the 1950s at Benger's Pharmaceutical Laboratories in Holmes Chapel, Cheshire, UK. A chromone, khellin (fig. 2), extracted from the seeds of the plant *Ammi visnaga*, had been used for centuries as a diuretic and as a smooth muscle relaxant, particularly for the relief of ureteric colic. Benger's had large supplies of this extract which they marketed as a smooth muscle relaxant and a coronary artery dilator in the form of a tablet (Benecardin®).

In 1947, Anrep et al. [7] reported that intramuscular khellin could provide complete and prolonged relief in bronchial asthma. Benger's then embarked on a research programme to synthesise and develop modifications of khellin that could be administered either orally or by inhalation for the treatment of asthma.

One of the first chromone analogues they synthesised was designated as soluble khellin, or K18. To screen compounds as potential bronchodilators they used guinea pigs treated with an aerosol of the new compound and then challenged with an aerosol of histamine. Figure 3 shows a trace of the respiratory movements of a guinea pig in such an experiment carried out in 1954 by Philip Sheard, a senior pharmacologist. This shows that the increase in bronchoconstriction caused by histamine was prevented by pre-treatment with K18.

Following the appointment of W.E. Brocklehurst as a consultant, the company began to use his guinea pig model as part of the screening programme for new chromones, synthesised in the laboratory. A report from the Research Department dated October 22, 1957, states:

> The perfusate from a shocked guinea pig lung has been shown to contain (i) histamine – a known bronchoconstrictor, (ii) SRS-A – a potent bronchoconstrictor, even in the presence of effective anti-histamine coverage. K18 has been shown to be a specific antagonist of SRS-A, having this property in common with other members of the K series including khellin itself. K18 is not an anti-histamine.

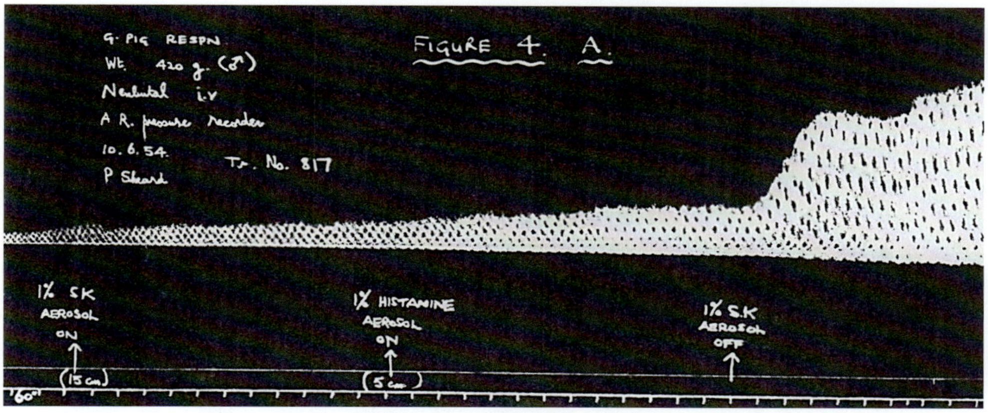

Fig. 3. The effect of inhaled 1% soluble khellin on the bronchoconstrictive effects of inhaled 1% histamine in guinea pigs. Experiment carried out by Philip Sheard at Benger's Laboratories on June 10, 1954.

In 1956, Dr. Roger E.C. Altounyan (fig. 6, 7) joined the Research Department. Roger Altounyan qualified in medicine in 1952 from Emmanuel College, Cambridge, and the Middlesex Hospital Medical School in London. He was atopic and as a child had suffered from severe eczema and mild attacks of wheezing. His first severe attack was of nocturnal asthma when a medical student and progressed to become severe chronic asthma. He knew he was allergic to grass pollen and guinea pig hair, and soon realized the potential of the ability of the compounds being synthesised and screened to inhibit allergic reactions. He also recognised the limitations and problems of animal models in asthma, once commenting that 'the only thing guinea pigs and humans have in common is that neither of us have a tail'.

He began to investigate the potential of new khellin-derived chromones on a human model – himself. He carried out bronchial antigen challenges on himself and tested the ability of prior administration of new compounds to prevent the induced asthmatic reactions.

All new compounds synthesised were now screened using animal models, i.e. the ability of the compound to prevent the anaphylactic release of histamine and SRS-A from sensitised guinea pig lung, and a human model (Altounyan), i.e. antigen bronchial challenge. On the basis of these experiments, Altounyan wrote a report (fig. 4) dated June 1961 which stated:

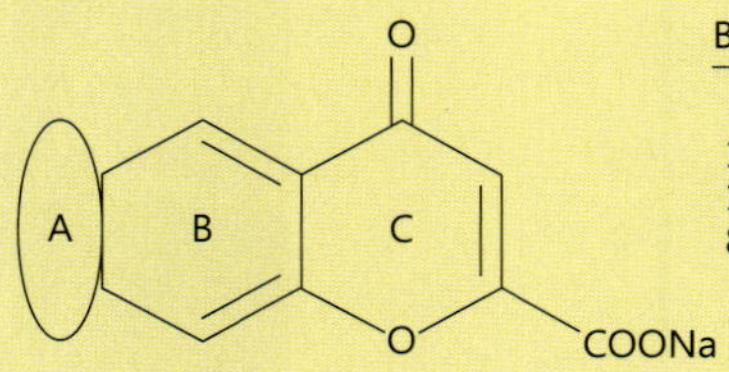

BLA	Ring A
8	Cyclohexane
13	Pyran
14	Dioxan
80	Benzene

Fig. 4. From a report by Dr. Roger Altounyan to the R&D Director at Benger's Laboratories on the effects of different chromones, dated June 1961.

5

To date over 130 BLA compounds have been synthesised. On the basis of human studies a clear structure-activity relationship is apparent. Chromone-2-carboxylic acid derivatives have by far the greatest activity of the compounds tested, the most active of these compounds being BLA8, 13, 14, 80 of which BLA8 is probably the best.

The designation of new compounds had now been given the BLA prefix, standing for Benger's Laboratories anti-anaphylaxis project. The report showed that, in the animal model, BLA8 gave 83% inhibition of histamine release and 78% inhibition of SRS-A release when used at a concentration of 2,660 μg/ml.

In human prophylactic experiments it gave >70% protection administered 1 h before challenge, 57% at

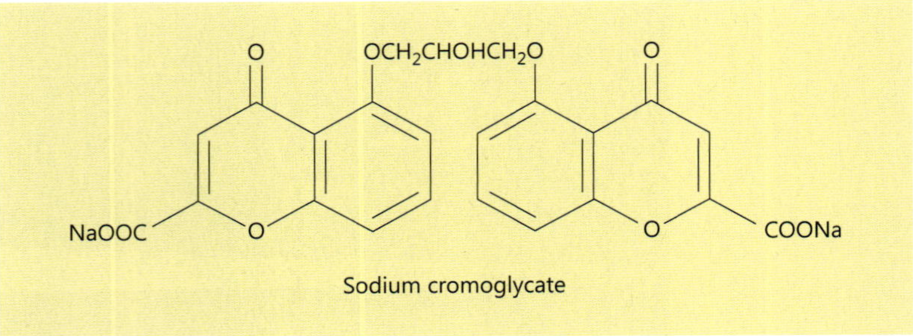

Fig. 5. The structure of disodium cromoglycate.

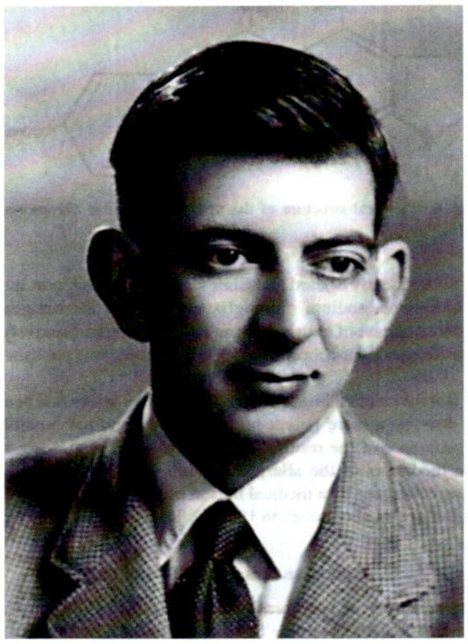

6

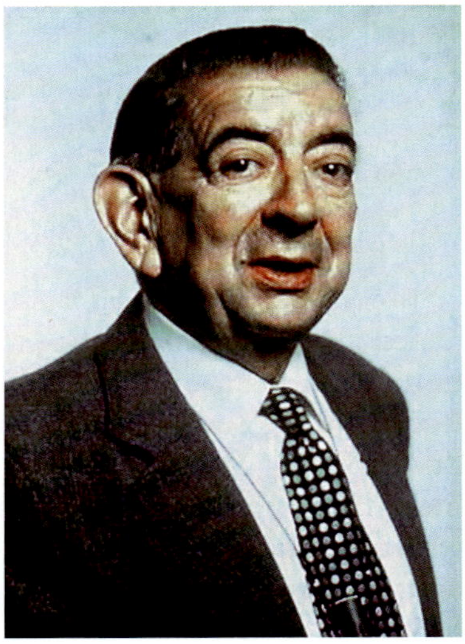

7

Fig. 6. Roger E.C. Altounyan in younger years.
Fig. 7. Roger E.C. Altounyan.

3 h and 30% at 6 h. It was also probably the first chromone to be investigated in the Clinical Immunology Department at the Brompton Hospital by Dr. (later Prof.) Jack Pepys. He reported in 1961 that, when injected into the skin, BLA8 significantly inhibited the skin weal response to pollen extract in sensitised subjects at a dose of 10 mg/ml, but not at 1 mg/ml. BLA13, also designated GR4, had also been investigated at the Brompton Hospital. Ten asthmatic patients were given 200 mg of GR4 at 2, 4 and 6 h before a bronchial antigen challenge. The results were analysed by Dr. Peter Armitage, the honorary statistician to the Institute of Diseases of the Chest at that time, who reported that the compound gave significant protection against antigen challenge at all the time points with no evidence of reduced protection over time. They reported 44% protection at 2 h, 45% at 4 h and 63% at 6 h, but with very wide 95% confidence limits. Altounyan himself had demonstrated >60% protection at 1 h, 56% at 3 h and 43% at 6 h. Incidentally, the prefix GR stands for George Ramage, who had been one of the chemists who synthesised khellin in 1949, became professor of organic chemistry at the University of Salford, and synthesised more chromones and gave them to Benger's Laboratories.

Neither BLA8 nor BLA13 were progressed and work to identify a chromone that would provide >50% protection for 6 h continued. After many pitfalls, a bis-chromone, disodium cromoglycate, DSCG (BL670; fig. 5), was synthesised late in 1964. Altounyan first tested it in February 1965 when it gave 72% protection at 2 h and >50% at 6 h. It therefore met the profile identified by the research group and a programme started culminating in the launch of Intal Compound (20 mg of disodium cromoglycate with 0.1 mg of isoprenaline and 20 mg lactose) for the treatment of asthma in January 1968.

The pharmacologists had continued to test all compounds on animal models but had also moved to tests based on the effects of drugs on the antigen-induced release of histamine and SRS-A from passively sensitised human chopped lung. In 1970, Sheard and Blair [8] reported that DSCG significantly reduced the antigen-induced release of histamine and SRS-A from passively sensitised human chopped lung. Previously, in 1967, Parish [9] had shown that the release of the same mediators was associated with a significant change in altered mast cells from human lung. The final piece of work that confirmed the mast cell stabilising properties of DSCG came from Goose and Blair [10], who showed that the percentage of disrupted mast cells in rats sensitised and challenged with *Nippostrongylus brasiliensis* was significantly reduced with DSCG.

Since those days a large number of manuscripts have been published confirming that the primary mode of action of the chromones, and of DSCG in particular, is the stabilisation of mast cells in both animal and man. Since the launch of DSCG, a large number of additional chromones have been synthesised and investigated in animals and man, all of them by Altounyan. Only one has been made available for clinical use – nedocromil sodium. Although claimed to be more effective than DSCG, the evidence is not convincing and DSCG remains the principal chromone used today.

The use of inhaled DSCG in asthma has declined in recent years, but it remains widely used in allergic conjunctivitis, allergic rhinitis, food allergy and systemic mastocytosis. If a pathological condition is thought to be mast cell related, DSCG is used to show that this is probably the case. Recent examples have been gastrointestinal dysfunction induced by early weaning in guinea pigs [11], and formation of atherosclerotic plaques [12]. Other important recent findings have been the identification of the chromone receptor on mast cells, GPR 35 [13], and that both DSCG and nedocromil sodium inhibit histamine and eicosanoid release from activated human mast cells by releasing annexin A1 [14].

The chromones also affect sensory nerves [15], but their main use is mast cell stabilisation, in which the efficacy is both dose dependent and dependent on the efficiency with which they are applied to the tissue being treated. This is best illustrated by the first published trial of Intal Compound in asthma [16]. A restricted sequential analysis trial conducted in adult patients with severe steroid-dependent asthma showed a highly significant effect after only 9 patients – not a patient profile recognised today. The small amount of isoprenaline had been added by Altounyan to counteract the irritant effect caused in some patients as DSCG is a sodium salt. It is now known that the addition of a short-acting bronchodilator will result in better distribution of the drug throughout the bronchial tree, thus affecting mast cells in both the central and peripheral airways. It is unfortunate that the manufacturers removed the isoprenaline after criticism from clinicians and licensing authorities. Over the years this has probably led to the perception that DSCG is not a very effective treatment for asthma, due to a less efficient distribution of the drug in the bronchial tree. Perhaps in the future someone will revive this effective and useful asthma treatment.

References

1 Prausnitz C, Küstner H: Studien über die Überempfindlichkeit. Zentralbl Bakteriol 1921;86:160–169.

2 Bartosch R, Feldberg W, Nagel E: Das Freiwerden eines histaminähnlichen Stoffes bei der Anaphylaxie des Meerschweinchens. Pflügers Arch Eur J Physiol 1932; 230:129–153.

3 Riley JF, West GB: Histamine in tissue mast cells. J Physiol 1952;117:72–73.

4 Kellaway CE, Trethewie ER: The liberation of a slow-reacting smooth muscle-stimulating substance in anaphylaxis. Quart J Exp Physiol 1940;30:121–145.

5 Brocklehurst WE: The release of histamine and formation of a Slow-Reacting Substance (SRS-A) during anaphylactic shock. J Physiol 1960;151:416–435.

6 Austen KF, Brocklehurst WE: Inhibition of the anaphylactic release of histamine from chopped guinea pig lung by chymotrypsin substrates and inhibitors. Nature 1960;186: 866–868.

7 Anrep GV, Barsoum GS, Kenawy MR, et al: Therapeutic uses of khellin. Lancet 1947; 249:557–558.

8 Sheard P, Blair AM: Disodium cromoglycate: activity in three in vitro models of the immediate hypersensitivity reaction in lung. Int Arch Allergy Appl Immunol 1970; 38:217–224.
9 Parish WE: Release of histamine and slow reacting substance with mast cell changes after challenge of human lung sensitized passively with reagin in vitro. Nature 1967; 215:738–739.
10 Goose J, Blair AMJN: Passive cutaneous anaphylaxis in the rat, induced with two homologous reagin-like antibodies and its specific inhibition with disodium cromoglycate. Immunology 1969;16:749–760.
11 Moeser AJ, Ryan KA, Prashant KN, Blikslager AT: Gastrointestinal dysfunction induced by early weaning is attenuated by delayed weaning and mast cell blockade in pigs. Am J Physiol Gastrointest Liver Physiol 2007;293:G413–G421.
12 Bot I, de Jager SCA, Zernecke A, Lindstedt KA, van Berkel TJC, Weber C, Biessen EAL: Perivascular mast cells promote atherogenesis and induce plaque destabilization in apolipoprotein E-deficient mice. Circulation 2007;115:2516–2525.
13 Yang Y, Lu JY, Wu X, Summer S, Whoriskey J, Sarls C, Reagan JD: G-protein-coupled receptor 35 is a target of the asthma drugs cromolyn disodium and nedocromil sodium. Pharmacology 2010;86:1–5.
14 Yazid S, Sinniah A, Solito E, Calder V, Flower RJ: Anti-allergic cromones inhibit histamine and eicosanoid release from activated human and murine mast cells by releasing annexin A1. PLoS One 2013;8:1–10.
15 Edwards AM, Stevens MT, Church MK: The effects of topical sodium cromoglicate on itch and flare in human skin induced by intradermal histamine: a randomised double-blind vehicle controlled intra-subject design trial. BMC Res Notes 2011;4:47.
16 Howell JBL, Altounyan REC: A double-blind trial of disodium cromoglycate in the treatment of allergic bronchial asthma. Lancet 1967;539–542.

Dr. Alan M. Edwards
Cranbrooke
Moor Lane, Brighstone
Newport, PO30 4DL (UK)
E-Mail alan.edwards@cantab.net

Progress in Allergy Management

Bergmann K-C, Ring J (eds): History of Allergy. Chem Immunol Allergy. Basel, Karger, 2014, vol 100, pp 323–332
DOI: 10.1159/000359989

Characterization and Standardization of Allergen Extracts

Henning Løwenstein

Nødebo, Denmark

Abstract

This paper summarizes the development of the extraction and characterization of allergens responsible for the induction of immunoglobulin (Ig) E-induced allergies from the beginning of the 20th century, including the nomenclature of allergens. The majority of papers characterizing allergens and allergen extracts state that the lack of standardization of allergen extracts is the reason for the paper, and so it has been for more than 100 years. A natural part of that process might be the isolation of an allergen molecule and this starts the speculation of 'what makes that allergen an allergen?' To achieve the perfect standardization is a desirable end that is still awaited. So far none of these problems have been finally solved. I started in allergy shortly after the discovery of IgE in 1967. Since that time the history as I remember it is based on the literature, my interpretation of it, and of course may be a little biased due to personal prejudice! The history of the last 10–15 years has still not matured and it might be a little early to draw conclusions. However, at the end of this chapter I do dare to make a few conclusions after having followed the development in this field for 40 years. As this is history it is not meant to be either comprehensive or technically and scientifically precise in all aspects, but rather draws on some thoughts as to what in my mind have been important developments until now. Specific techniques are only mentioned by name and not intended to be discussed in depth. This activity has, however, pushed me to reflect on my hopes and speculations at the time of my introduction to the field of allergen chemistry. To my surprise I realize that far more than I ever expected at that time has been fulfilled. It has been extremely exciting to be a part of that development.

5

The Beginning

Ever since the 'first' specific immunotherapy injection was performed 100 years ago, in 1911 by Noon [1], the question has been raised of how to characterize allergen extracts in order to be able to faithfully reproduce the treatment. This inevitably required attempts to define allergen extract parameters that would consequently have to be fulfilled – standardization. These parameters were in one or another way a measure of dose and expected to relate the patients' response to the treatment.

From the very beginning it became clear that standardization would only be possible provided intensive knowledge of the composition of the allergen extract was available, as well as the need for isolation and characterization of the main components. The biochemical techniques available for the characterization of a biological extract were quite limited and often reduced to a careful measurement of dry weight of biological material and the volume of the solvent used for extraction, i.e. weight/volume. The Dunbar [2] method of extraction with distilled water was followed by several cycles of repeated freezing and thawing of a 20 mg/ml suspension of pollen *(Phleum pratense)*. Noon [1] used this method after further filtration and boiling for 10 min. A 1 µg/ml dilution of this solution was later named 1 Noon unit per milliliter. Extracts of other pollens were standardized against the *Phleum pratense* extract by comparative tests on the eyes of hay fever patients. This was probably the first attempt to standardize allergen extracts [1].

Shortly after the Noon publication, Kammann [3, 4] reported the protein nature of the allergen (active material) from pollen. Later Cooke [5] exchanged Noon's distilled water with physiological salt solution and added phenol for preservation, thus balancing on the fine line between bacterial growth and protein denaturation. Finally, the preparations were standardized according to their nitrogen content – the protein nitrogen unit (PNU; see below). There were of course already at that time chemical methods available which could determine the content in extracts of protein, carbohydrate, lipid, etc., but these methods were regarded as only of limited use for the characterization of complex biological mixtures.

When, in 1922, Coca [6] established a cookbook for 'the preparation of fluid extracts and solutions for the use in the diagnosis and treatment of the allergies with notes on the collections of pollens', the importance of buffering solutions was revealed and, among others, the 'Coca solution' was proposed and later used quiet broadly. Another buffer often used for the extraction of allergens was the Evans buffer [7]. In a series of studies [5–12] reported by Stull et al. [8] it was realized (again) that allergens from ragweed and grasses were of a protein nature and, consequently, they used ammonium sulfate precipitation, extraction with water, ether and ethanol, as well as temperature shift and proteolytic degradation in their attempts to characterize and isolate the allergens.

Acknowledgement of the significance of proteins in allergen extracts resulted in protein content being expressed in PNUs (1 PNU = 10 ng of protein nitrogen) as a measurement of potency by Cooke [9]. Cooke also compared PNUs with Noon units for purposes of standardization. He used PNUs in his immunotherapy studies where they used ethyl ether-extracted pollen in alkaline saline fluid and estimated the ratio between PNUs and Noon units. The combination of carefully measured PNU, weight/volume and skin tests performed on well-selected patients using high-quality raw material might be used as a batch-to-batch standardization, but the activity might have only little relation to allergen extracts from other allergen sources or the same source produced by another manufacturer. The general results of characterization of allergen extracts up to World War II was that these were complex biological mixtures with properties that included the active material of protein, 'albuminous' nature, degradable to various degrees by enzymes and susceptible to thermal changes. Within the group of grass pollen extracts it had already at that time been clearly shown that a high degree of cross-reactivity existed between the active materials from the various grass species.

The First Purified Allergen Molecules

A new era in the study of characterization and standardization of allergen extracts and specific immunotherapy started with the collaboration between Augustin and Frankland after the World War II. Through the work of Augustin [10], who showed that the absolute majority of allergenic molecules had molecular weights above 10,000 Da, it was (once more) realized that the active material in allergen extracts were proteins. Frankland [11] took advantage of this knowledge and performed his clinical experiment with both full extract and extract with a molecular weight above 10,000 Da – obtained by ultrafiltration – and showed no significant difference. In contrary to the original experiment performed by Noon [1] and as a consequence of the established knowledge that allergens are proteins, these extracts, which had both been extracted from acetone defatted pollens, were not boiled.

Of importance for later attempts to characterize and standardize allergen extracts, in the 1960s an increasing number of protein chemists appeared in allergy. These included, in particular, T.P. King at Rockefeller, New York, in collaboration with Johns Hopkins, Baltimore [reviewed in 12], and David Marsh (in collaboration with Johnson) who was initially based in Cambridge in the UK, and later in the USA (in collaboration with Campbell) [reviewed in 13]. These scientists applied their skills to isolate active allergen molecules from crude extracts. Also, in Norway, intensive studies were performed by Elsayed in collaboration with Aas [14]. Through their research it became clear that allergen sources contained one or more well-defined allergen molecules which accounted for a great part of the allergen activity as shown by skin tests. In their search for active allergy components they both used protein chemical separation methods followed by immunoassays, like Mancini [15] and Ouchterlony techniques [16] using animal antibodies that had been raised against these active allergenic materials. The most significant result of their research was the isolation and characterization of allergen molecules which could be used in clinical studies in a quantitative manner. A few years later, in his review entitled 'Allergens and the genetics of allergy', David Marsh [13] concluded that 'allergens were mainly proteins within a low molecular weight range, large enough to act immunogenic and small enough to easily penetrate the human mucosa'. Holland Berrens [17] came up with a more speculative hypothesis for molecules acting as allergens by postulating that allergenicity was due to molecular rearrangements, the 'amadori' rearrangement. However, nobody was ever able to prove it.

At the same time 'reagins' were very much discussed. The existence of reagins as the factors reacting with allergens in allergy had already been elegantly shown by Prausnitz and Küstner [18] in 1921. Finally, in 1966, immunoglobulin (lg) E was discovered independently by the Ishizakas [19] and Johansson and Bennich [20], thus making it possible to measure patient's 'allergy-reactive' molecules, or 'reagins'. Shortly after the discovery of IgE an in vitro allergy test, the radioallergosorbent test (RAST) [21], which measured the patient's level of allergen-specific serum IgE, was developed. For standardization purposes it became important that 'RAST inhibition' (inhibition of RAST with allergen molecules) [22] was introduced and subsequently proposed as a potency measurement for the purpose of allergen standardization.

At that time in vitro immunoelectrophoretic methods were also being increasingly used for analyses of complex protein mixtures which, when combined with protein chemical separation methods, exhibited unique analytical opportunities. These quantitative immunoelectrophoretic methods, QIE, were developed by Laurell, Clarke and Freeman and further elaborated by the group around Niels Harboe at The Protein Laboratorium, University of Copenhagen [23], where the methods were intensively used for the analyses of primarily human serum proteins.

In 1972, Weeke and Løwenstein introduced these analytical tools into allergy research in general, and in particular into the characterization of allergen extracts. A novel method, crossed radioimmunoelectrophoresis, CRIE, was invented. CRIE enabled the identification of the individual's serum IgE responses against separate allergen components within crude extracts [reviewed in 24]. Using these methods it was revealed that allergen extracts generally contained multiple allergens and most often several major allergens[1].

Characterization of allergen extracts critically depended on the extraction method used and there seemed to be an unofficial consensus among scientists that only 'natural' (i.e. comparable to extraction on the human mucosa) extraction procedures were acceptable. Because the aim was to identify and iso-

[1] The term 'major allergen' was first introduced by Marsh [13] who defined it as an allergen towards which >90% of allergic individuals reacted; this was later modified to >50% by Løwenstein [24].

Table 1. The first allergens

Biological source	Old names	Names according to nomenclature
Short ragweed *(Ambrosia artemisiifolia)*	Ragweed AgE Ragweed AgK	Amb a 1[a] Amb a 2
Rye grass *(Lolium perenne)*	Rye group I Rye group II Rye group III	Lol p 1[a] Lol p 2 Lol p 3
Codfish *(Gadus callarius)*	Cod allergen M	Gad c 1
Timothy grass *(Phleum pratense)*	Timothy Ag25	Phl p 5[a]
House dust mite *(Dermatophagoides pteronyssinus)*	Mite antigen P1, Pp Ag42, Ag12 Dp AgX	Der p 1[a] Der p 2[a]
Domestic cat	Cat I, Cat Ag4	Fel d 1[a]
Birch	Birch Ag23	Bet v 1[a]

[a] Fulfils the eight criteria for defining 'allergens that make a difference' according to Chapman and Aalberse [38].

late individual allergenic components, assays measuring allergenic potency were also needed. Prior to the discovery of IgE various forms of skin tests were used either directly or indirectly, such as the Prausnitz-Küstner test [18]. Thus, the use of RAST [21] and even more the use of RAST inhibition tests [22] represented a clear advantage as allergen extract fractionation assays. It became easy to define the fractions with high allergenic activity. However, the most rational approach was the use of immunoelectrophoretic methods as they could reveal not only major activities, but also the individual allergenic component molecules [24].

The introduction of new activity assays and immunoassays increased the number of isolated and well-characterized allergen molecules. After King's isolation of AgE (Amb a 1) and AgK (Amb a 2) came Marsh's isolation of Rye group I, II and III (Lol p 1, 2 and 3), and Elsayed's isolation of Allergen M (Gad c 1) in the late 1960s. This was followed by Timothy Ag25 (Phl p 5), P1, Dp Ag42, Ag12 (Der p 1), Dp AgX (Der p 2), Cat-I, cat Ag4 (Fel d 1) and Birch Ag23 (Bet v 1) in the 1970s. All of these were later shown to be very important major allergens or 'allergens that make a difference' (table 1).

It was at that time amazing to realize how various research groups using quiet different methods independently isolated identical major allergens: at the IAACI congress in Jerusalem in 1979, the groups of Chapman and Platt-Mills from the USA, Lind and Løwenstein from Denmark, and Stewart and Turner from Australia all presented a major allergen from mite and agreed that it was the same, later named Der p 1. Another early example was the long-standing discussion between Marsh with his Rye group I and Løwenstein with his Timothy Ag25, who both insisted to have the major grass pollen allergen from their respective species. However, these molecules did not cross-react although the scientists knew that there was an overwhelming cross-reactivity between the two species. They never solved the problem, but fortunately continued their life-long collaboration and friendship; the problem was later solved by Aalberse who showed that they represented the later-named grass group 1 and 5 (Lol p 1 and Phl p 5), so they were both right and had identified major grass pollen allergens. It was situations like these that called for an international allergen nomenclature.

The appearance of purified allergen molecules as a result of the characterization of allergen extracts made it possible to use these molecules in quantitative tests not only for clinical immunological studies and standardization purposes, but also for the quantification of allergens within the natural environment. The latter was started in Denmark in the late 1970s [25] and subsequently introduced to Baltimore, where, at that time, investigators considered that there were very few if any house dust mites in their homes. However, an investigation revealed that mite levels were at least as high as in many places in Europe [26].[2]

Standardization Becomes International

Standardization was at that time (approx. 1970–1980) discussed whenever the characterization and isolation of allergens was published, and many national allergy societies had their own discussion group. In the Nordic countries, allergy researchers headed by Kjell Aas proposed allergen standardization to be performed using a combination of skin prick tests (SPT) and RAST inhibition. These methods, combined with a measure of concentrations of the individual allergen molecules by means of quantitative immunoelectrophoretic methods, gave rise to the idea of developing a model for the standardization of allergen extracts [27].[3] The model was a combination of the measurement of the concentration of major allergen molecules, total potency of the extract, qualitative composition of the extract and skin tests performed on a selected number of patients.

Internationally, the IAACI (International Association of Allergy and Clinical Immunology) and IUIS (International Union of Immunological Society) had their standardization committees, the latter with an affiliation to the WHO. In 1977, Alain de Weck, Europe's leading 'immunopolitician' took the initiative to form a joint allergen standardizing committee from these two organizations with the aim of practically solving the problem of standardization to the benefit of the end users: the patients. At that time any allergen manufacturer selected their own unit and methods for control of the quality and potency of allergen extracts and the national regulators were in most cases not well equipped to perform a control, if any at all. In 1980, this was reorganized under the name 'IUIS/WHO Allergen Standardisation Committee' by Alain de Weck, with Henning Løwenstein appointed as the chairman. The new committee was composed of representatives from legal authorities (regulators), experienced allergists (clinicians), independent allergy researchers (scientists) and researchers from many allergen-producing companies. The funding came partly from allergy-related international societies and mainly from the allergen manufacturers. The committee met 1–2 times a year from 1980 to 1988 at the WHO in Geneva, and had a number of fruitful discussions about various assays or combinations of these, requirements to candidate standard extracts and, of course, how to perform skin tests. It appeared at that time that the majority of the committee members would prefer to use a combination of potency measurement (RAST inhibition or similar), qualitative composition (isoelectric focusing or similar) and then of course in vivo skin tests (SPT or intradermal tests), but a minority insisted that quantitative data for major allergen molecules

5

[2] After having collected the samples in the Baltimore area these were shipped by air to the laboratory in Denmark. Unfortunately, they were somehow sent to India and Denmark instead received a package containing nails. To figure this out took about 4 weeks. The paper explained this diplomatically, as follows: 'Since the package went astray in shipment, it is estimated that the samples stayed at ambient temperature for about 4 weeks. Because the mites were killed by placing in a freezer and because the antigens for which the tests were being made are quite stable, no artefacts should have been introduced.' Later results confirmed that statement.

[3] DAS 76 (Danish Allergen Standardization 1976) [27] was a collaboration between Danish clinical allergists, the local allergen manufacturer, Allergologisk Laboratorium København (later ALK), and a research institute, The Protein Laboratory, University of Copenhagen. Allergen extracts were produced for the 14 most used allergen sources from well-selected raw material and stored under optimal conditions. The allergenic activity in wasted as well as maintained material was measured and storage stability was controlled. Patients responding to the various allergen sources were selected based upon case history, SPT, RAST and, in a few cases, challenge test, and sera from these patients were consequently used with the relevant extract for crossed radioimmunoelectrophoresis and for all allergen extracts 'allergograms' defining major and minor allergen molecules being revealed. Subsequently, the allergen extracts could be used as standards for quantitative measurement of major allergen molecule content, for measurement of potency (by RAST inhibition using serum pools from the selected patients), SPT on selected panels of patients and for qualitative control of the extract composition. This model was first presented at the IAACI congress in Buenos Aires in 1976 and later at the first Paul Ehrlich meeting in Frankfurt in 1979.

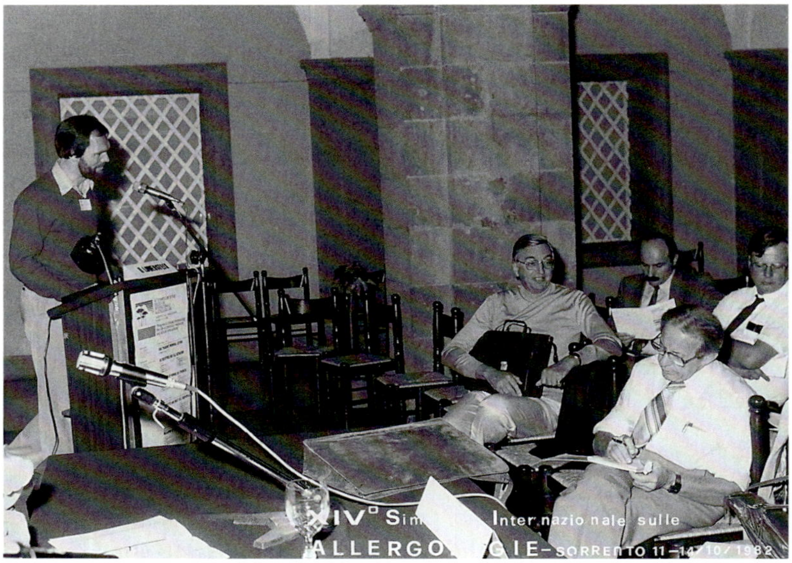

Fig. 1. The situation at a scientific meeting (Collegium Allergologicum Internationale, Sorento, Italy, 1982) where the author gives a presentation on the topic of standardization. This might not keep everybody awake. In the auditorium from the left: de Weck, Ring, Sehon and Schmutzler.

were essential and should be included. However, it was also realized that there existed general rules for testing and applying candidate standards of biological origin to the WHO [28], and that these as a principle would include as many independent tests as possible. Thus, the committee set the task of producing optimal allergen extract standards for the most important allergen sources worldwide and having these approved by the WHO. Companies volunteered for preparing candidate allergen extracts and laboratories for performing relevant in vitro assays for comparison. The candidate extract preparations were glass sealed and the 5–10 assays were all performed in a blind manner at 10–20 laboratories distributed worldwide. As a result of these activities, over a period of 5–6 years, the committee managed to test, select, publish and have approved by the WHO 8 allergen extract standards [29–36] which were stored either by the NIBSC (National Institute for Biological Science and Control) in the UK or by the ATCC (American Type Culture Collection) in the USA. The majority of scientists who had been involved in the isolation and characterization of major allergens from the selected allergen sources also became members of the committee and testing group. Thus, the content of major allergen molecules in the glass-sealed standards could also be stated. The international standards, IS, made it possible to compare with any native allergen extract. When measured by a stated method the potency and content of major allergens relative to the standard (used as a yardstick) could then be expressed and the amount could be given in international units, IU. It also became clear that a common unit should not be used due to the risk that non-identical extracts (extracts with the same IU and from two different companies) could then be used in the same treatment schedule.

The total project was in many ways unique. For the first time it prompted allergen manufacturers, clinical allergists, allergen chemists and regulators from both Europe and North America to collaborate and obtain consensus about a common aim. The results were presented at scientific meetings and raised considerable enthusiasm (fig. 1).

Unfortunately, these WHO-approved international standards never came into use due to the American non-acceptance of WHO standards and their insistence at that time of using skin tests as a 'primary' method in standardization. The limited acceptance among many manufactures of the significance of major allergen molecules in standardization also played a role. From that time on, first with Phillip S. Norman and later Jean Bousquet as the chairmen for the IUIS/WHO Allergen Standardiza-

Table 2. Recommended maintenance doses

Allergen source	Reference	Major allergen	Doses, μg
Cat	42–45		
Felis catus		Fel d 1	14.6
House dust mite	46, 47		
Dermatophagoides pteronyssinus		Der p 1	9.8
Dermatophagoides farinae		Der f 1	13.8
Short ragweed	48		
Ambrosia artimisiifolia		Amb a 1	10.0
Grasses	49, 50		
Dactylis glomerata		Dac g 5	12.0
Festuca pratense		Fes p 5	18.6
Lolium perenne		Lol p 5	12.5
Phleum pratense		Phl p 5	20.5
Tree	51		
Betula verrucosa		Bet v 1	13.0

tion Committee, there continued a long-lasting discussion about skin testing the standards. The next generation of allergen standards began with the introduction of the CREATE Project, detailed below.

The Nomenclature of Allergens

The number of (major) allergens isolated and characterized had increased considerably and, owing to the problem of the use of different names for the same compound, an initiative was taken by David G. Marsh to propose a novel system of nomenclature for allergens. The actual proposal came during a Collegium Internationale Allergologicum (CIA) meeting in 1980 in Constance, where David Marsh, Tom Platts-Mills and Henning Løwenstein came up with the system while having a few beers in a rowing boat on Lake Constance. A committee, the WHO/IUIS Nomenclature Sub-Committee, was subsequently formed by Marsh, Løwenstein, Platts-Mills, T.P. King and Larry Goodfriend and the system (table 1) has from that time on been used with minimal changes and was published in the WHO Bulletin [37]. Since then, and especially after the first introduction of molecular biology in allergen research by the Austrian group headed by Dietrich Kraft and subsequently Rudi Valenta, the number of isolated allergens has increased exponentially and is now well over 1,000 (see www.allergen.org). However, it is interesting to note that those allergen molecules identified and purified prior to the start of the molecular biology era within allergy cover the majority of clinically relevant allergies. A comprehensive review of allergen nomenclature is given by Chapman [38].

New Attempts for Allergen Standardization

The CREATE Project (development of certified reference materials for allergenic products and validation of methods for their quantification) was supported with generous funding from the European Union and headed by the new generation of allergen researchers, in particular Ronald van Ree, Martin Chapman, Stefan Vieths and Fatima Ferreira [39]. The background for this was that from 1985 onwards it became increasingly easy to prepare natural and recombinant allergen molecules, and to analyze these down to the submolecular level. This was due to the revolutionary development of DNA technology including genetic engineering, the facilitated ability to sequence isolated proteins and the ultimate goal for any allergen chemist to also reveal 3-dimensional structures of the proteins by X-ray crystallography and NMR technology (fig. 2). The understanding and acceptance of the significance of the standardization of major allergen molecules constantly grew and was finally acknowledged in the 'WHO position paper – allergen immunotherapy: therapeutic vaccines for allergic diseases', published in 1998 [40]. Historically, allergen standardization was mostly discussed in relation to skin reactivity and not to clinical efficacy. Ideally, the potency of allergen extracts should be expressed in units describing clinical efficacy, rather than as surrogates such as skin test potency. In the years 1980–1996, a number of clinical trials (table 2) using allergen extracts with known content of major allergen molecules were performed and it became evident that effective treatment results were related to the content of major allergen molecules. For all clinically effi-

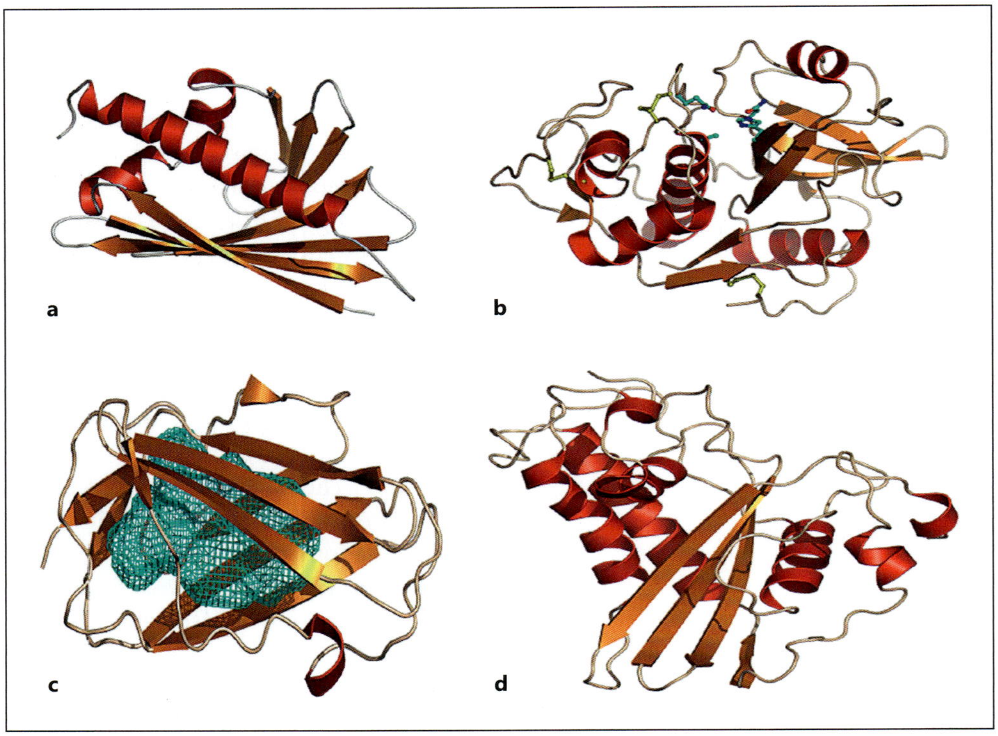

Fig. 2. The three-dimensional structure of 4 major allergens. The red coils illustrate α-helices; the orange arrows β-sheets, and the other parts random coils; the blue part inside Der f 2 illustrates the unusual 'open space'. **a** Bet v 1 [52]. **b** Der p 1 [53]. **c** Der f 2 [54]. **d** Ves v 5 [55].

cient treatments the annual maintenance doses were found to be between 50 and 200 μg of major allergen. This breakthrough was finally acknowledged in the recommendations of the WHO position paper [40].

In the CREATE Project 8 major allergen molecules representing 4 major allergen sources (birch, grass and olive pollen and house dust mites) were selected and the certified reference material developed was intended to serve as primary standards for immunoassays. In addition, monoclonal antibody-based ELISAs for measurement of the allergens were developed, evaluated and validated. The final aim was to provide materials and methods which would make it possible to express a common unit system in absolute mass units of major allergen molecules. This project has been very successful in the characterization of natural and corresponding recombinant allergen molecules, but has suffered from problems in defining material that can fulfil the final aim of the project. This is mainly due to problems in some allergens with finding recombinant allergen molecules representative of all corresponding natural allergen molecules together with the necessary certified ELISAs [41].

The ability to express a common unit system within an allergen extract still remains to be solved due to the contributions to extract potency from non-controlled allergens, such that there will always be a requirement for additional biologic potency assessments. The allergy world is still left with many different and non-convertible unit systems.

Concluding Remarks

In the meantime, leading allergen manufacturers have started to develop allergen vaccines as pharmaceutical products which fulfil registration requirements through the regulatory bodies, including the EMA, FDA and SFDA, etc. – i.e. procedures in line with any other registered pharmaceutical medical product. Within the next decades this development may well reduce the interest for standardization among end users, i.e. allergists and patients, with their interest being directed towards the route of vaccine administration, design and pharma-economy, all of which are related to compliance.

However, all the efforts made in the characterization of allergen extracts and molecules will continue to benefit the whole field of allergy research, a process that has been greatly facilitated by the availability of modern molecular biology and the availability of pure recombinant molecules. Throughout the whole development it has been an indispensable part of allergy research as a quantitative foundation for a huge number of both in vivo and in vitro experiments, without which much knowledge about allergy would never have developed.

In the history of allergen extract characterization and standardization, of which I am also a part, many colleagues have strongly influenced me. In particular I would like to mention Paul Kallos, Alain de Weck and David G. Marsh, as well as all my scientific colleagues and friends in Denmark and abroad.

References

1 Noon L: Prophylactic inoculation against hay fever. Lancet 1911;i:1572–1573.
2 Dunbar WP: Zur Ursache und spezifischen Heilung des Heufiebers. Dtsch Med Wochenschr 1903;9:24–28.
3 Kammann O: Zur Kenntnis des Roggen-Pollens und des darin enthaltenen Heufiebergiftes. Beitr Chem Physiol Path 1904;5: 346–354.
4 Kammann O: Weitere Studien über das Pollentoxin. Biochem Zeitschr 1912;46:151.
5 Cooke RA: The treatment of hay fever by active immunization. Laryngoscope 1915;25: 108–112.
6 Coca AF: Studies in specific hypersensitiveness. 5. The preparation of fluid extracts and solutions for use in the diagnosis and treatment of the allergies with notes on the collection of pollens. J Immunol 1922;7: 163–178.
7 Evans AC: A buffered physiologic salt solution. J Infect Dis 1922;30:95–98.
8 Stull A, Cooke RA, Chobot R: The allergically active substance in pollen: a chemical and biologic study of *Phleum pratense* (Timothy) pollen. J Allergy 1932;3:341–351.
9 Cooke RA, Stull A: The preparation and standardization of pollen extracts for the treatment of hay fever. J Allergy 1933;4:87–91.
10 Augustin FR: Chemical and immunological properties of timothy grass pollen extracts and problems of standardization. Quart Rev Allergy 1952;6:290–314.
11 Frankland AW, Augustin FR: Prophylaxis of summer hay-fever and asthma: a controlled trial comparing crude grass-pollen extracts with the isolated main protein component. Lancet 1954;i:1055–1057.
12 King TP: Chemical and biological properties of some atopic allergens. Adv Immunol 1976;23:77–105.
13 Marsh DG: Allergens and the genetics of allergy; in Sela M (ed): The Antigens. New York, Academic Press, 1975, pp 271–359.
14 Elsayed SK, Aas K: Characterization of a major allergen (cod.) chemical composition and immunological properties. Int Arch Allergy Appl Immunol 1970;38:536–548.
15 Mancini G, Carbonara AO, Heremans JF: Immunochemical quantitation of antigens by single radial immunodiffusion. Immunochemistry 1964;2:235–254.
16 Ouchterlony Ö: Antigen-antibody reactions in gels. Acta Pathol Microbiol Scand 1949; 26:507–515.
17 Berrens L: The Chemistry of Atopic Allergens. Basel, Karger, 1971.
18 Prausnitz C, Küstner H: Studien über die Überempfindlichkeit. Zentralbl Bakt (Orig) 1921;86:160–169.
19 Ishizaka K, Ishizaka T, Hornbrook MM: Physicochemical properties of reagenic antibody. 5. Correlation of reagenic activity with γE-globulin antibody. J Immunol 1966;97:840–853.
20 Johansson SGO, Bennich H: Immunological studies of an atypical (myeloma) immunoglobulin. Immunology 1967;13:381–394.
21 Wide L, Bennich H, Johansson SGO: Diagnosis of allergy by an in vitro test for allergen antibodies. Lancet 1967;ii:1105–1107.
22 Ceska M, Eriksson R, Varga JM: Radioimmunosorbent assay of allergens. J Allergy Clin Immunol 1972;49:1–9.
23 Clarke HGM, Freeman T: A quantitative immunoelectrophoresis method (Laurell electrophoresis); in Peeters H (ed): Protides of the Biological Fluids. Amsterdam, Elsevier Biochemical Press, 1967, p 503.
24 Løwenstein H: Quantitative immunoelectrophoretic methods as a tool for the analysis and isolation of allergens. Prog Allergy 1978;25:1–62.
25 Lind P, Korsgaard J, Løwenstein H: Detection and quantitation of Dermatophagoides antigens in house dust by immunochemical techniques. Allergy 1979;34:319–326.
26 Lind P, Norman PS, Newton M, Løwenstein H, Schwartz B: The prevalence of indoor allergens in the Baltimore area: house dust-mite and animal-dander antigens measured by immunochemical techniques. J Allergy Clin Immunol 1987;80:541–547.
27 Løwenstein H: Physico-chemical and immunochemical methods for the control of potency and quality of allergenic extracts; in Brede HO, Göing H (eds): Regulatory Control and Standardization of Allergenic Extracts. Stuttgart, Gustav Fischer, 1980, pp 122–132.
28 WHO Expert Committee on Biological Standardization: Guidelines for the preparation and establishment of reference materials and reference reagents for biological substances. WHO Tech Rep Ser 1978;626: 101.
29 Helm RM, Gauerke MB, Baer H, Løwenstein H, Ford A, Levy DA, Norman PS, Yunginger JW: Production and testing of an international reference standard of short ragweed pollen extract. J Allergy Clin Immunol 1984;73:790–800.
30 Gjesing B, Jäger L, Marsh DG, Løwenstein H: The international collaborative study establishing the first international standard for timothy *(Phleum pratense)* grass pollen allergenic extract. J Allergy Clin Immunol 1985;75:258–267.

31 Ford A, Seagroatt V, Platts-Mills TAE, Løwenstein H: A collaborative study on the first international standard of *Dermatophagoides pteronyssinus* (house dust mite) extract. J Allergy Clin Immunol 1985;75:676–686.
32 Arntzen FC, Wilhelmsen TW, Løwenstein H, Gjesing B, Maasch HJ, Stromberg R, Einarsson R, Backman A, Makinen-Kiljunen S, Ford A: The international collaborative study on the first international standard of birch *(Betula verrucosa)* pollen extract. J Allergy Clin Immunol 1989;83:66–82.
33 Larsen JN, Ford A, Gjesing B, Levy D, Petrunov B, Silvestri L, Løwenstein H: The collaborative study of the international standard of dog, *Canis domesticus*, hair/dander extract. J Allergy Clin Immunol 1988; 82:318–330.
34 Helm RM, Squillace DL, Yunginger JW, et al: Production of a proposed international reference standard *Alternaria* extract II: results of a collaborative trial. J Allergy Clin Immunol 1988;81:651–663.
35 Baer H, Anderson MC, Helm RM, Yunginger JW, Løwenstein H, Gjesing B, White W, Douglass G, Phillips PR, Schumacher M, Hewitt B, Guerin BG, Charpin J, Carreira J, Lombardero M, Ekramoddoullah AKM, Kisil F, Einarsson R: The preparation and testing of the proposed international reference (IRP) Bermuda grass *(Cynodon dactylon)*-pollen extract. J Allergy Clin Immunol 1986; 78:624–631.
36 Stewart GA, Turner KJ, Baldo BA, Cripps AW, Ford A, Seagroatt V, Løwenstein H, Ekramoddoullah AKM: Standardization of rye-grass pollen *(Lolium perenne)* extract: an immunochemical and physicochemical assessment of six candidate international reference preparations. Int Arch Allergy Appl Immunol 1988;86:9–18.
37 Marsh DG, Goodfriend L, King TP, Løwenstein H, Platts-Mills TAE: Allergen nomenclature. Bull WHO 1986;64:767–774.
38 Chapman MD: Allergen nomenclature; in Kaliner MA, Lockey RF (eds): Allergens and Allergen Immunotherapy. New York, Informa Healthcare, 2008, pp 47–58.
39 van Ree R: A new start for allergen references and standardization based on purified (natural or recombinant) allergens and monoclonal and monospecific polyclonal antibodies. Arb Paul Ehrlich Inst Bundesamt Sera Impfstoffe Frankfurt AM 1999;93: 87–90.
40 Bousquet J, Lockey R, Malling HJ: WHO position paper: allergen immunotherapy: therapeutic vaccines for allergic diseases. Allergy 1998;53(suppl 4):1–42.
41 van Ree R, Chapman MD, et al: The CREATE project: development of certified reference materials for allergenic products and validation of methods for their quantification. Allergy 2008;63:310–326.
42 Sundin B, Lilja G, Graff-Lonnevig V, Hedlin G, Heilborn H, Norrlind K, Pegelow K-O, Løwenstein H: Immunotherapy with partly purified and standardized animal dander extracts. 1. Clinical results from a double-blind study on patients with animal dander asthma. J Allergy Clin Immunol 1986;77: 478–487.
43 van Metre TE, Marsh DG, Adkinson NF, Kagey-Sobotka A, Khattignavong A, Norman PS, Rosenberg GL: Immunotherapy for cat asthma. J Allergy Clin Immunol 1988;82:1055–1068.
44 Hedlin G, Graff-Lonnevig V, Heilborn H, Lilja G, Norrlind K, Pegelow K, Sundin B Løwenstein H: Immunotherapy with cat- and dog-dander extracts. 5. Effects of 3 years of treatment. J Allergy Clin Immunol 1991;87:955–964.
45 Hedlin G, Heilborn H, Lilja G, Norrlind K, Pegelow K-O, Schou C, Løwenstein H: Long-term follow-up of patients treated with a three-year course of cat or dog immunotherapy. J Allergy Clin Immunol 1995;96:879–885.
46 Wahn U, Schweter C, Lind P, Løwenstein H: Prospective study on immunologic changes induced by two different *Dermatophagoides pteronyssinus* extracts prepared from whole mite culture and mite bodies. J Allergy Clin Immunol 1988;82:360–370.
47 Haugaard L, Dahl R, Jacobsen L: A controlled dose-response study of immunotherapy with standardized, partially purified extract of house dust mite: clinical efficacy and side effects. J Allergy Clin Immunol 1993;91:709–722.
48 Creticos P, Reed CE, Norman PS, Khoury J, Adkinson NF, Buncher CR, Busse WW, Bush RK, Gadde J, Li JT: Ragweed immunotherapy in adult asthma. N Engl J Med 1996; 334:501–506.
49 Østerballe O: Immunotherapy in hay fever with two major allergens 19, 25 and partially purified extract of timothy grass pollen. Allergy 1980;35:473–489.
50 Varney GA, Gaga M, Frew AJ, Aber VR, Kay AB, Durham SR: Usefulness of immunotherapy in patients with severe summer hay fever uncontrolled by antiallergic drugs. Br Med J 1991;302:265–269.
51 Petersen BN, Janniche H, Munch EP, Wihl JA, Böwadt H, Ipsen H, Løwenstein H: Immunotherapy with partially purified and standardized tree pollen extracts. 1. Clinical results from a three-year double-blind study of patients treated with pollen extracts either of birch or combinations of alder, birch and hazel. Allergy 1988;43:353–362.
52 Gajhede M, Osmark P, Poulsen FM, Ipsen H, Larsen JN, van Neerven RJ, Schou C, Løwenstein H, Spangfort MD: X-ray and NMR structure of Bet v 1, the origin of birch pollen allergy. Nat Struct Biol 1996;12: 1040–1045.
53 Meno K, Thorsted PB, Ipsen H, Kristensen O, Larsen JN, Spangfort MD, Gajhede M, Lund K: The crystal structure of recombinant pro Der p 1, a major house dust mite proteolytic allergen. J Immunol 2005;175: 3835–3845.
54 Johannessen BR, Skov LK, Kastrup JS, Kristensen O, Bolwig C, Larsen JN, Spangfort MD, Lund K, Gajhede M: Structure of the house dust mite allergen Der f 2: implications for function and molecular basis of IgE cross-reactivity. FEBS Lett 2005;579: 1208–1212.
55 Henriksen A, King TP, Mirza O, Monsalve RI, Meno K, Ipsen H, Larsen JN, Gajhede M, Spangfort MD: Major venom allergen of yellow jackets, Ves v 5: structural characterization of a pathogenesis-related protein superfamily. Proteins 2001;45:438–448.

Dr. Henning Løwenstein
Winthersvej 8A
Nødebo
DK–3480 Fredensborg (Denmark)
E-Mail hl@henninglowenstein.com

Bergmann K-C, Ring J (eds): History of Allergy. Chem Immunol Allergy. Basel, Karger, 2014, vol 100, pp 333–338
DOI: 10.1159/000360047

Allergen-Specific Immunotherapy

Harold S. Nelson[a] · Philip S. Norman[b]

[a]National Jewish Health and University of Colorado School of Medicine, Denver, Colo., and [b]Johns Hopkins Asthma and Allergy Center, Johns Hopkins University School of Medicine, Baltimore, Md., USA

Abstract

Specific immunotherapy was introduced for the treatment of grass pollen-induced hay fever in 1911. The treatment was soon extended to other pollens as well as perennial allergens, and to the treatment of bronchial asthma. Definitive studies of its efficacy for both rhinitis and asthma came only many decades later. Understanding gradually emerged of the underlying immunologic mechanisms that include the generation of regulatory T lymphocytes, immune deviation from allergen-specific Th2 to Th1 responses, and a shift in allergen-specific antibody production from immunoglobulin (Ig) E to IgG4. Along with understanding of the immune basis came an appreciation that immunotherapy modifies allergic disease expression, producing protection against disease progression and symptomatic improvement that persists for years after the treatment is discontinued. Recent new directions for immunotherapy include sublingual administration of inhalant allergens and use of the oral route to treat food allergy.

Spread of Immunotherapy

The recognition by John Bostock of the regular occurrence of symptoms of rhinitis, conjunctivitis and asthma each June in himself and a few others, which he termed hay fever, and the establishment of grass pollen as a cause of these symptoms by Charles Blackley provided the necessary basis for the introduction of immunotherapy by Leonard Noon. Noon [1] believed that the symptoms of hay fever, which had by then become rather common, were caused by a toxin in the grass pollen to which only hay fever sufferers were susceptible. With the intention of inducing an antitoxin, he initiated treatment with subcutaneous injections of low doses of timothy pollen extract and increased the dose initially at 3- to 4- and later 10- to 14-day intervals, employing the increasing conjunctival tolerance to the extract to guide the dosing. Noon was unable to continue his work due to tuberculosis, so a colleague, John Freeman [2], continued the studies and observed the patients through the ensuing grass pollen season. Freeman reported the results in 20 treated patients and observed that the majority of patients experienced fewer symptoms than in previous years or, if treatment was initiated when already symptomatic, a prompt reduction in symptoms.

The method of subcutaneous injections of increasing doses of allergen extracts was rapidly applied in North America to the respiratory symptoms in August and September termed 'autumnal catarrh', which had been recognized for several decades to be due to ragweed pollen. By the 1920s the practice of allergen injections had been extended to include injections of extracts of other pollens and animal danders and for the treatment of asthma as well as rhinoconjunctivitis [3]. It was not, however, until 1968 that these regimens became known as 'immunotherapy' [4]. An important extension of the role of immunotherapy was the recognition in the early 1920s of a substance in house dust as a cause of inhalant allergy [5].

Proof of Efficacy

The acceptance of subcutaneous immunotherapy was for decades based on the anecdotal experience of patients and physicians. Some 4 decades following the publications of Noon and Freeman, several controlled studies were undertaken using house dust or grass pollen extracts. Frankland and Augustin [6] treated 200 patients with pre-seasonal injections of one of four extracts: unmodified mixed grass pollen, the ultrafiltrate of the pollen extract, the concentrated pollen proteins remaining after ultrafiltration and phenol saline. At the end of the grass pollen season patients were asked for their overall impression. Of those receiving either unmodified extract or the concentrated proteins 77% reported good or excellent results compared to only 24% of those receiving the ultrafiltrate or phenol saline. There were methodological problems with this and other early controlled trials of immunotherapy [7]. Lowell and Franklin [7] sought to address these by very careful selection of subjects, developing a diary for assessing the subjects' symptoms, and particularly by employing a placebo that produced local reactions similar to those induced by the active treatment. Without the latter, they felt that the study would become unblinded. In their definitive study, Lowell and Franklin [7] followed patients receiving subcutaneous immunotherapy to mixtures of ragweed and other extracts through one ragweed season. They identified 24 patients who had symptoms, despite immunotherapy, and matched them by their symptom and medication scores into 12 pairs. In March of the following year, fresh extract mixtures were prepared and ragweed was omitted from the mixture of one of each pair, being replaced by an equal volume of caramelized glucose. Symptom/medication scores recorded during the following ragweed pollen season revealed significantly lower scores over 6 consecutive weeks in those receiving ragweed in their treatment mixture. Thus, in this small but carefully crafted study, the investigators had established that immunotherapy with ragweed pollen reduced allergic symptoms during the ragweed pollen season, that the treatment was effective when administered in a mixture with multiple other pollens, that the effect was allergen specific, and that under the conditions of the study, the results of immunotherapy were lost within a period of 5 months following discontinuation.

In the mid-1950s, a remarkable study was undertaken by Douglas Johnstone [8] at the Pediatric Allergy Clinic at the University of Rochester in the USA. Consecutive children referred to the clinic with perennial bronchial asthma were entered into a study comparing injections of buffered saline or extract mixtures containing all the inhalant allergens to which the child reacted on skin testing. The children receiving active treatment were divided into those receiving a maximum dose of each individual component of 1:10,000,000 weight by volume (w/v), 1:5,000 w/v, or the highest tolerated dose (usually not exceeding 1:250 w/v of each extract). The criticism of this study is the adequacy of blinding. In that regard, the parents and children did not know that a study was being conducted, while those who evaluated the results were unaware of the group allocation of the children. A total of 210 children were randomized to the four groups; 173 remained under treatment after 4 years and 130 remained on treatment until they were 16 years of age. The principal outcome was freedom from asthma during the preceding year. After 4 years, this was reported by 18% of the saline and 1:10,000,000 w/v groups, 58% of the 1:5,000 w/v group, and 81% of the highest tolerated dose group. Similar results were reported in those continuing to 16 years of age. This study again established several principles of immunotherapy: that it is effective in treating bronchial asthma, that the results are dose dependent, and that immunotherapy with multiple allergen mixes is effective.

The study by Lowell and Franklin [7] had suggested that the response to allergen immunotherapy was allergen specific, since all subjects continued to receive injections of multiple other allergen extracts, yet removal of the ragweed extract caused loss of protection during the ragweed season. The definitive demonstration of the specificity of immunotherapy came from a study by Norman and Lichtenstein [9]. They identified patients sensitive to and symptomatic with exposure to both grass and ragweed pollens. Half received injections of ragweed extract and half received matching placebos, but none were treated for their grass allergy. In the three subsequent ragweed seasons, those who received ragweed fared significantly better during the ragweed pollen season, but there was no difference between the treated patients and controls during the three grass pollen seasons.

Improvement in Allergen Extracts

The studies for the first 50 years had employed crude or somewhat purified extracts. In 1962, King and Norman [10] isolated the predominant allergen of short ragweed, which they termed antigen E, representing 80–99% of the allergenicity of the whole extract. Studies were undertaken at Johns Hopkins University to examine the safety and efficacy of immunotherapy with antigen E [11]. From 1963 to 1966, a group of subjects with ragweed-allergic rhinitis received pre-seasonal courses of injection immunotherapy with annually increasing doses of antigen E and crude ragweed extract. By the third and fourth seasons results with both active treatments were significantly superior to placebo.

Another advance in immunotherapy was the development of standardized extracts. These have the advantage of greater lot-to-lot and manufacturer-to-manufacturer consistency resulting in improved patient safety. Also for the first time, knowledge of effective doses determined in controlled trials could be applied in clinical practice. Methods of standardization vary, with some extract manufacturers having 'in house' standards, while in the USA the methods of standardization are set by the Food and Drug Administration (FDA). There is some agreement that the most practical unit for standardization is the content of one or more major allergens in the extract. Attempts to set up internationally recognized reference standardized extracts and in vitro tests for these major allergens are underway [12]. In addition to the studies at Johns Hopkins with antigen E, a number of double-blind, placebo-controlled studies of immunotherapy have expressed the doses employed by the content of the major allergen of the extract [13]. A pattern has emerged that suggests that somewhere between 7 and 20 μg of the major allergen is sufficient to provide clinically meaningful improvement with the extracts that have been studied, while one 10th to one 20th of these effective doses have provided less or even no improvement.

Disease Modification by Immunotherapy

Although effective symptomatic medications have become available for the treatment of both rhinoconjunctivitis and asthma, they all share the shortcoming that their beneficial effect is lost within days to months after they are discontinued. Immunotherapy, on the other hand, modifies the underlying immunologic response to the allergen administered, resulting in benefits that often persist for years after it is discontinued. Three lines of evidence have evolved that indicate that immunotherapy modifies the course of the allergic disease. The longstanding perception that clinical improvement with immunotherapy persisted long after its discontinuation was confirmed in a double-blind discontinuation study [14]. Subjects who had been receiving immunotherapy with timothy extract for 3 or 4 years were randomized to continue monthly maintenance injections of timothy extract or to receive placebo for the ensuing 3 years. There were no differences between those continuing and those discontinuing treatment in symptoms or rescue medication use during any of the following three grass pollen seasons. Further evidence of a persisting effect was seen in a study of house dust mite immunotherapy in children aged 5–8 years with mild asthma who were monosensitized to house dust mite [15]. Some of the children received immunotherapy for 3 years, while the others were treated only with symptomatic medications. Three years after the immunotherapy was discontinued there was a significant difference in the development of new skin test sensitivities: 67% in the control group versus only 25% in those who had received house dust mite immunotherapy. Also demonstrating persisting disease modification was the PAT study [16]. Children allergic to timothy and/or birch pollen who only had allergic rhinitis during an observational year were randomized to receive immunotherapy for 3 years or to serve as an observational control group. The outcome of interest was the development of asthma. Those in the observational group were 2.52 times as likely to have developed asthma during the 3 years of treatment and this increased risk persisted without change during 7 further years of post-treatment observations [16].

Immunologic Mechanisms

The studies of Prausnitz and Küstner provided the basis for the demonstration of the antibody responsible for immediate hypersensitivity by passive transfer into the skin. Cooke et al. [17] employed this technique to compare pre- and post-immunotherapy sera for their ability to decrease the activity of ragweed pollen extract at sites of passive cutaneous sensitization. Levels of this blocking antibody measured in vitro, later shown to be predominantly immunoglobulin (Ig) G4, have not been found to correlate well with clinical response. Functional assays of IgG4 activity correlate better, but probably not to a degree to make them a useful surrogate for clinical assessments [18].

For many years after the description of the antibody of immediate hypersensitivity its demonstration depended on passive transfer to a donor's skin: the Prausnitz-Küstner test. The discovery of IgE by the Ishizakas in the USA and Johansson and Benich in Sweden allowed more quantitative assessments in vitro of the response of this antibody to immunotherapy. It was determined that in untreated patients allergen-specific IgE rose with seasonal stimulation, then fell until the next season. With the initiation of immunotherapy there was a prompt increase in allergen-specific IgE, but the subsequent seasonal rises were blunted, resulting in a gradual decline in specific IgE over ensuing years [19].

Attention then turned to the role of the T lymphocyte in the response to immunotherapy. T lymphocytes of allergic patients undergo proliferation on exposure to the relevant allergen. When patients were treated with immunotherapy, there was allergen-specific suppression of this proliferative response that could be shown to be mediated by a subset of their peripheral mononuclear cells [20]. In patients who had received 70 days of immunotherapy with house dust mite extract, this suppressor activity was subsequently shown to be mediated by regulatory CD4+ T lymphocytes secreting interleukin (IL)-10 and transforming growth factor (TGF)-β [21]. IL-10 is responsible for the switch from IgE to IgG4 production and TGF-β for a switch from IgE to IgA. The overall effect is to mimic the immune response to the allergen in non-allergic individuals [21]. Other immunologic changes have been described in patients on more prolonged immunotherapy [22]. Timothy pollen extract was injected into the skin of patients allergic to grass, some of whom had received timothy extract immunotherapy for 3 or 4 years and others who had not. Twenty-four hours later the site of timothy extract injection was biopsied and tissue was assessed for the presence of messenger ribonucleic acid (mRNA) for various cytokines. In the tissue of the patients who had received immunotherapy, but not the controls, there were increased numbers of cells positive for mRNA for IL-12 and interferon-γ, but decreased cells positive for mRNA of IL-4. These findings indicated an alteration in the response to the allergen from Th2 to Th1. Other studies have confirmed that the regulatory T lymphocyte response occurs early but wanes somewhat with time, while the immune deviation is dominant later.

Alternative Approaches to Immunotherapy

Due to the occurrence of reactions to subcutaneous immunotherapy, as well as the prolonged course of clinic visits it entails, alternative methods of application have been investigated. Oral and intranasal immunotherapy have been investigated, but the method that has enjoyed the most success is sublingual immunotherapy. Although there are still some issues to be resolved, including dosing, use of multiple allergen mixes and use in allergic diseases other than allergic asthma and rhinitis, sublingual immunotherapy has been demonstrated to be clinically effective and to share the disease-modifying properties of subcutaneous immunotherapy [23].

Additional Allergic Conditions Treated with Immunotherapy

Immunotherapy was introduced for the treatment of allergic rhinitis and asthma caused by inhalant allergens. It was soon used to treat hymenoptera venom sensitivity employing an extract derived from whole bodies of the insects. Definitive studies in the 1970s demonstrated that the whole body extract provided no more protection than placebo, but injections of the specific venom provided protection against subsequent stings [24].

There were periodic reports of patients with atopic dermatitis responding to immunotherapy. Recently, controlled trials with both subcutaneous and sublingual immunotherapy have suggested that immunotherapy with house dust mite extract may be beneficial in selected patients with atopic dermatitis [25, 26].

Subcutaneous immunotherapy has also occasionally been employed for treating patients with food allergy but, at least for peanut allergy, it proved to be associated with too many systemic reactions to be clinically acceptable [27]. Currently, promising controlled studies are being conducted with oral and sublingual immunotherapy in patients allergic to several foods [28].

References

1 Noon L: Prophylactic inoculation against hay fever. Lancet 1911;i:1572–1573.
2 Freeman J: Further observations on the treatment of hay fever by hypodermic inoculations of pollen vaccine. Lancet 1911;ii: 814–817.
3 Walker IC: Studies on the sensitization of patients with bronchial asthma. Study series III–XXXVI. J Med Res 1917;35–37.
4 Lichtenstein LM, Norman PS, Winkenwerder WL: Clinical and in vitro studies on the role of immunotherapy in ragweed hay fever. Am J Med 1968;44:514–524.
5 Cooke RA: Studies in specific hypersensitiveness. 4. New etiologic factors in bronchial asthma. J Immunol 1922;7:147–162.
6 Frankland AW, Augustin R: Prophylaxis of summer hay-fever and asthma: a controlled trial comparing crude grass-pollen extracts with the isolated main protein component. Lancet 1954;i:1055–1057.
7 Lowell FC, Franklin W: A double-blind study of the effectiveness and specificity of injection therapy in ragweed hay fever. N Engl J Med 1965;273:675–679.
8 Johnstone DE, Dutton A: The value of hyposensitization therapy for bronchial asthma in children: a 14-year study. Pediatrics 1968;42:793–802.
9 Norman PS, Lichtenstein LM: The clinical and immunologic specificity of immunotherapy. J Allergy Clin Immunol 1978;61: 370–377.
10 King TP, Norman PS: Isolation studies of allergens from ragweed pollen. Biochemistry 1962;1:709–720.
11 Norman PS, Winkenwerder WL, Lichtenstein LM: Immunotherapy of hay fever with ragweed antigen E: comparisons with whole pollen extract and placebos. J Allergy Clin Immunol 1968;42:93–108.
12 van Ree R, Chapman MD, Ferreira F, et al: The CREATE project: development of certified reference materials for allergenic products and validation of methods for their quantification. Allergy 2008;63:310–326.
13 Nelson HS: Subcutaneous injection immunotherapy for optimal effectiveness. Immunol Allergy Clin North Am 2011;31:211–226.
14 Durham SR, Walker SM, Varga E-M, Jacobson MR, O'Brien F, Noble W, Till SJ, Hamid QA, Nouri-Aria K: Long-term clinical efficacy of grass-pollen immunotherapy. N Engl J Med 1999;341:468–475.
15 Pajno GB, Barberio G, De Luca F, Morabito L, Parmiani S: Prevention of new sensitizations in asthma children monosensitized to house dust mite by specific immunotherapy: a six-year follow-up study. Clin Exp Allergy 2001;31:1392–1397.
16 Jacobsen L, Niggemann B, Dreborg S, Ferdousi HA, Halken S, Høst A, Koivikko A, Norberg LA, Valovirta E, Wahn U, Möller C: Specific immunotherapy has long-term preventive effect of seasonal and perennial asthma: 10-year follow-up on the PAT study. Allergy 2007;62:943–948.
17 Cooke RA, Bernard JH, Hebald S, Stull A: Serological evidence of immunity with coexisting sensitization in a type of human allergy (hay fever). J Exp Med 1935;62:733–750.

18 Shamji MH, Ljørring C, Francis JN, Calderon MA, Larché M, Kimber I, Frew AJ, Ipsen H, Lund K, Würtzen PA, Durham SR: Functional rather than immunoreactive levels of IgG4 correlate closely with clinical response to grass pollen immunotherapy. Allergy 2012;67:217–226.
19 Lichtenstein LM, Ishizaka K, Norman PS, Sobotka AK, Hill BM: IgE antibody measurements in ragweed hay fever: relationship to clinical severity and the results of immunotherapy. J Clin Invest 1973;52:472–482.
20 Rocklin RE, Sheffer AL, Greineder DK, Melmon KL: Generation of antigen-specific suppressor cells during allergy desensitization. N Engl J Med 1980;302:1213–1219.
21 Jutel M, Akdis M, Budak F, Aebischer-Casaulta C, Wrzyszcz M, Blaser K, Adkis CA: IL-10 and TRGF-β cooperate in the regulatory E cell response to mucosal allergens in normal immunity and specific immunotherapy. Eur J Immunol 2003;33:1205–1214.
22 Hamid QA, Schotman E, Jacobson MR, Walker SM, Surham SR: Increases in IL-12 messenger RNA^{+} cells accompany inhibition of allergen-induced late skin responses after successful grass pollen immunotherapy. J Allergy Clin Immunol 1997;99:254–260.
23 Canonica GW, Bousquet J, Casale T, et al: Sublingual immunotherapy: World Allergy Organization Position Paper 2009. Allergy 2009;64(suppl 91):1–59.
24 Hunt KJ, Valentine MD, Sobotka AK, Benton AW, Amodio FJ, Lichtenstein LM: A controlled trial of immunotherapy in insect hypersensitivity. N Engl J Med 1978;299: 157–161.
25 Werfel T, Breuer K, Ruéff F, Przybilla B, Worm M, Grewe M, Ruzicka T, Brehler R, Wolf H, Schnitker J, Kapp A: Usefulness of specific immunotherapy in patients with atopic dermatitis and allergic sensitization to house dust mites: a multi-centre, randomized, dose-response study. Allergy 2006;61:202–205.
26 Pajno GB, Caminiti L, Vita D, Barberio G, Salzano G, Lombardo F, Canonica GW, Passalacqua G: Sublingual immunotherapy in mite-sensitized children with atopic dermatitis: a randomized, double-blind, placebo-controlled study. J Allergy Clin Immunol 2007;120:164–170.
27 Nelson HS, Lahr J, Rule R, Bock A, Leung D: Treatment of anaphylactic sensitivity to peanuts by immunotherapy with injections of aqueous peanut extract. J Allergy Clin Immunol 1997;99:744–751.
28 Land MH, Kim EH, Burks AW: Oral desensitization for food hypersensitivity. Immunol Allergy Clin North Am 2011;31:367–376.

Prof. Harold S. Nelson
National Jewish Health
1400 Jackson Street
Denver, CO 80206 (USA)
E-Mail nelsonh@njhealth.org

6 Pioneers of Allergy: Personal Reflections

Bergmann K-C, Ring J (eds): History of Allergy. Chem Immunol Allergy. Basel, Karger, 2014, vol 100, pp 340–341
DOI: 10.1159/000360050

K. Frank Austen

Boston, Mass., USA

Year of birth
1928

Place(s) of university education
Amherst College, Amherst, Mass., USA
Harvard Medical School, Boston, Mass., USA

Who were your most important teachers in allergology?
Elmer L. Becker, MD, PhD and Albert L. Sheffer, MD

Please list your 5 most important publications

Orange RP, Murphy RC, Karnovsky ML, Austen KF: The physicochemical characteristics and purification of slow-reacting substance of anaphylaxis. J Immunol 1973;110:760–770.

Fearon DT, Austen KF: Activation of the alternative complement pathway with rabbit erythrocytes by circumvention of the regulatory action of endogenous control proteins. J Exp Med 1977;146:22–33.

Lam BK, Penrose JF, Freeman GJ, Austen KF: Expression cloning of a cDNA for human leukotriene C_4 synthase, a novel integral membrane protein conjugating reduced glutathione to leukotriene A_4. Proc Natl Acad Sci USA 1994;91:7663–7667.

Gurish MF, Tao H, Abonia JP, Arya A, Friend DS, Parker CM, Austen KF: Intestinal mast cell progenitors require CD49dβ7 (α4β7 integrin) for tissue-specific homing. J Exp Med 2001;194:1243–1252.

Barrett NA, Rahman OM, Fernandez JM, Parsons MW, Xing W, Austen KF, Kanaoka Y: Dectin-2 mediates Th2 immunity through the generation of cysteinyl leukotrienes. J Exp Med 2011;208:593–604.

Have you ever had a function as a President and/ or Secretary General of an allergological society?
President of the American Academy of Allergy, Asthma & Immunology
President of the American Association of Immunologists

Which position has had the greatest impact on your professional life?
Chairman of the Department of Rheumatology and Immunology, Harvard Medical School and Robert B. Brigham Hospital

Questions about your professional life

What brought you to allergy?

The possibility that the biochemical response to immunologic activation, the generation of slow-reacting substance of anaphylaxis (SRA-A/cysteinyl leukotrienes) and the in vivo biology of allergic inflammation could be studied with mast cells were the basis for my laboratory program 50 years ago. A chance meeting with Albert L. Sheffer prompted me to seek certification in the subspecialty and to establish an enduring collaboration for clinical application of studies of the mast cell in physical allergy, the cysLTs in asthma and the complement system in hereditary angioedema.

From whom (academic, teacher) did you learn the most?

Three postdoctoral experiences interrupted my 4 years of clinical training at the Massachusetts General Hospital. Each laboratory experience was with a mentor with a passion for probing as deep as technology permitted and a willingness to develop the technical advances needed for the next level. These mentors were Elmer Becker at the Walter Reed Army Institute of Research, Walter Brocklehurst at the National Institute of Health in the UK, and Manfred Mayer at Johns Hopkins.

What was your greatest achievement in allergy?

Among a number of milestones, I would include the cloning of human LTC_4 synthase, the enzyme response for the generation of the cysteinyl leukotrienes, the unraveling of the proteins involved in the integrated function of the amplification loop of the alternative (properdin) complement pathway with Doug Fearon, and the purification of tetrameric human mast cell tryptase with Larry Schwartz.

What was your greatest disappointment?

I can think of no major disappointment, but rather of my surprise when I declined the opportunity to take a distinguished chairmanship of medicine.

What was your most funny experience?

An imitation of the conservative, discreet, impatient Albert L. Sheffer by a young faculty member, David Sloane, at our annual reunion.

Who would you list among the top 10 allergists of the world? (Please only mention individuals already deceased.)

Roy Paterson, Frank Lowell, who provided laboratory space while I was an MGH house officer, Ken Mathews, John Sheldon, Francis Rackerman, Bill Franklin, Bill Sherman, Richard Farr, Frank Dixon, Walter Brocklehurst.

Who would you list among the top 10 living allergists?

Joshua Boyce, Albert L. Sheffer, Mariana Castells, Alain de Weck[1], Steve Wasserman, Allan Kaplan, Dean Metcalfe, Phil Norman, Larry Lichtenstein, Barry Kay.

What do you see as the greatest problem for allergy in the next 10 years?

The continuing funding for development of physician investigators who can probe into the molecular basis of the allergic diseases with insight into their integrated biology.

What will be the next great breakthrough in allergy in the next 10 years?

The development of biologics that can interrupt the innate signals by which allergens drive both asthma phenotypes.

[1] Alain de Weck sadly deceased in the course of the preparation of this book in 2013.

Bergmann K-C, Ring J (eds): History of Allergy. Chem Immunol Allergy. Basel, Karger, 2014, vol 100, pp 342–343
DOI: 10.1159/000360057

John Bienenstock

Hamilton, Ont., Canada

Year of birth
1936

Place(s) of university education
King's College, University of London
Westminster Hospital Medical School

Who were your most important teachers in allergology?
Kurt Bloch, Frank Austen and Tom Tomasi

Please list your 5 most important publications

Bravo JA, Forsythe P, Chew MV, et al: Ingestion of *Lactobacillus* strain regulates emotional behavior and central GABA receptor expression in a mouse via the vagus nerve. Proc Natl Acad Sci USA 2011; 108:16050–16055.

Stead RH, Tomioka M, Quinonez G, et al: Intestinal mucosal mast cells in normal and nematode-infected rat intestines are in intimate contact with peptidergic nerves. Proc Natl Acad Sci USA 1987;84: 2975–2979.

MacQueen G, Marshall J, Perdue M, et al: Pavlovian conditioning of rat mucosal mast cells to secrete rat mast cell protease II. Science 1989;243:83–85.

Befus AD, Pearce FL, Gauldie J, et al: Mucosal mast cells. I. Isolation and functional characteristics of rat intestinal mast cells. J Immunol 1982;128: 2475–2480.

McDermott MR, Bienenstock J: Evidence for a common mucosal immunologic system. I. Migration of B immunoblasts into intestinal, respiratory, and genital tissues. J Immunol 1979;122:1892–1898.

Bienenstock J, Johnston N, Perey DY: Bronchial lymphoid tissue. I. Morphologic characteristics. Lab Invest 1973;28:686–692.

Have you ever had a function as a President and/or Secretary General of an allergological society?
Canadian Society for Immunology (1985–1987)
Society for Mucosal Immunology (1990–1992)
Collegium Internationale Allergologicum (1998–2002)

Which position has had the greatest impact on your professional life?
Positions themselves had less of an impact than my continuing involvement in research and publications at McMaster University.

Questions about your professional life

What brought you to allergy?

I began my immunological career in 1964 as a postdoc for Kurt Bloch at the MGH and Harvard. He was working with Frank Austen who was in turn trying to isolate and learn about slow-reacting substance of anaphylaxis (SRS-A), later described as cysteinyl leukotrienes. I spent time with both of them trying to learn some immunology.

From whom (academic, teacher) did you learn the most?

Many people, students, postdocs and faculty members, but maybe the most productive learning was as a postdoc with Tom Tomasi in Buffalo, 1966–1968, where I had the chance to learn about the emerging field of mucosal immunology and begin to contribute to it.

What was your greatest achievement in allergy?

We (Dean Befus, Fred Pierce, Jack Gauldie) were the first to describe, isolate and characterize mucosal mast cells and show that they were different structurally and functionally from connective tissue mast cells. Later we described the intimate physical association of mucosal mast cells with enteric nerves (Ron Stead), and began to examine the cross-talk between mast cells and nerves (Mike Blennerhassett and many others).

What was your greatest disappointment?

When I ran out of ideas for how to delineate the basis of what we had described as the 'common mucosal immune system' in which mucosal lymphocytes were shown to retain a homing capacity to mucosal tissues, thus differing from lymphocytes in other tissues.

What was your most funny experience?

Many wonderful ones, especially at Collegium Internationale Allergologicum (CIA) meetings, e.g. a most famous allergy professor in his bathrobe coming from the beach thinking his wife was ahead of him going up the stairs, reaching the top and flashing (full frontal exposure of his manly body) to a lady he did not know.

Who would you list among the top 10 allergists of the world? (Please only mention individuals already deceased.)

Carl Prausnitz, Zoltan Ovary, Merrill Chase, Elmer Becker, James Riley, Geoffrey West, Charles Richet, Clemens von Pirquet, Bengt Samuelsson, Jerry Dolovich, Freddy Hargreave.

Who would you list among the top 10 living allergists?

Frank Austen, Kimi and Teri Ishizaka, Alain de Weck[1], Stephen Holgate, Gunnar Johansson, Hans Bennich, Larry Lichtenstein, Steve Galli, Hugh Sampson, Pat Holt.

What do you see as the greatest problem for allergy in the next 10 years?

To establish better treatments and also sustainable prevention strategies for allergies.

What will be the next great breakthrough in allergy in the next 10 years?

The evidence that it is possible to vaccinate against allergens in early childhood and to establish the role that microbial imbalance plays in the development of allergies.

[1] Alain de Weck sadly deceased in the course of the preparation of this book in 2013.

6

Bergmann K-C, Ring J (eds): History of Allergy. Chem Immunol Allergy. Basel, Karger, 2014, vol 100, pp 344–345
DOI: 10.1159/000360059

Kurt Blaser

Davos, Switzerland

Year of birth
1940

Place(s) of university education
University of Bern, Switzerland

Who were your most important teachers in allergology?
Alain de Weck, H.N. Eisen, C.H. Heusser

Please list your 5 most important publications

Walker C, Virchow JC Jr, Bruijnzeel PL, Blaser K: T cell subsets and their soluble products regulate eosinophilia in allergic and nonallergic asthma. J Immunol 1991;146:1829–1835.

Müller U, Akdis CA, Fricker M, Akdis M, Blesken T, Bettens F, Blaser K: Successful immunotherapy with T cell epitope peptides of bee venom phospholipase A2 induces specific T cell anergy in patients allergic to bee venom. J Allergy Clin Immunol 1998; 101:747–754.

Akdis CA, Akdis M, Blesken T, Wymann D, Alkan SS, Müller U, Blaser K: Epitope-specific T cell tolerance to phospholipase A2 in bee venom immunotherapy and recovery by IL-2 and IL-15 in vitro. J Clin Invest 1996;98:1676–1683.

Carballido JM, Faith A, Carballido-Perrig N, Blaser K: The intensity of T cell receptor engagement determines the cytokine pattern of human allergen-specific T helper cells. Eur J Immunol 1997;27:515–521.

Mantel PY, Kuipers H, Boyman O, Rhyner C, Ouaked N, Rückert B, Karagiannidis C, Lambrecht BN, Hendriks RW, Crameri R, Akdis CA, Blaser K, Schmidt-Weber CB: GATA3-driven Th2 responses inhibit TGF-β1-induced FOXP3 expression and the formation of regulatory T cells. PLoS Biol 2007; 5:e329.

Have you ever had a function as a President and/or Secretary General of an allergological society?
No

Which position has had the greatest impact on your professional life?
Director, Swiss Institute of Allergy and Asthma Research

Questions about your professional life

What brought you to allergy?

I was accidentally brought to allergy as a chemist, when I had to synthesize defined model allergens to study molecular pre-requisites and of IgE-dependent mediator release mechanisms. Doing this, I became fascinated by the open field of immunobiology, which was more open and free than chemistry at that time and full of interesting novel biological concepts. Thus, with the help of my teachers, I decided to stay in the field of molecular chemistry and biology, in particular of immunology.

From whom (academic, teacher) did you learn the most?

My former Professor in Organic Chemistry at the University of Bern (Dr. H. Schaltegger) opened my mind decisively towards biology. Professor Alain de Weck encouraged me decisively to start a scientific carrier in immunology and allergy, and provided me the space and promoted my academic carrier at the University of Bern. Later as a postdoctoral fellow at MIT, Dr. Herman Eisen taught me how to plan and perform scientific research projects in immunobiology. He showed me how to critically review data, results and controls in biological research and to publish only if the results were absolutely proven, solid and clear.

What was your greatest achievement in allergy?

Among other important findings in T cell-driven allergy, we have demonstrated that immunotherapy results from specific tolerance, which is induced by IL-10 and/or TGF-β. In humans we demonstrated that a mixture of minimal-length peptides, representing the major T cell epitopes of allergen, is sufficient to induce specific tolerance in T cells and successful allergen-specific immunotherapy. These findings provided the first original knowledge of the basic mechanism of successful immunotherapy and tolerance induction to allergen. Furthermore, they demonstrated that successful allergen-specific immunotherapy results from defined immunological mechanisms.

In bronchial asthma we have generated very early results that different types of asthmatic inflammations are driven by activated T helper cells and governed by different cytokines. We showed that IL-5 and GM-CSF, mostly from activated T cells, protect short-living inflammatory effector cells from apoptosis and prolong their life span in the blood and tissues.

What was your greatest disappointment?

It was a great disappointment to realize how strong clinical opinions and wrong views of a clinical problem can obstruct or impede progress of clinical knowledge, despite new scientific findings demonstrating other facts.

Who would you list among the top 10 allergists of the world? (Please only mention individuals already deceased.)

Clemens von Pirquet, C. Prausnitz and C. Küstner, Ilja Iljitsch Metschnikow, Paul Ehrlich, Leonard Noon and John Freeman, Alain de Weck.

Who would you list among the top 10 living allergists?

John Bienenstock, Stephen Galli, Stephen T. Holgate, Barry A. Kay.

What do you see as the greatest problem for allergy in the next 10 years?

A great problem in allergy is the development of the field away from the specialized allergologists and the decreasing acceptance of allergy as an own specialty in medicine, together with the low financial expectations of allergologists.

What will be the next great breakthrough in allergy in the next 10 years?

A decisive breakthrough will be the defined molecular understanding of allergy development and early avoidance. The impact of epigenetic mechanisms in the development of the disease needs to be molecularly pinpointed and maximally defined.

Bergmann K-C, Ring J (eds): History of Allergy. Chem Immunol Allergy. Basel, Karger, 2014, vol 100, pp 346–349
DOI: 10.1159/000360061

Alain de Weck (1928–2013)

Fribourg, Switzerland

Year of birth
1928

Place(s) of university education
Medical studies, 1947–1953, at the universities of Fribourg (Switzerland), Lausanne (Switzerland), Paris (France) and Geneva (Switzerland)
Swiss Federal Physician Diploma, Geneva, 1953

Who were your most important teachers in allergology?
Werner Jadassohn (dermatology/allergy, Geneva), Herman Eisen (immunochemistry/immunology, St. Louis)

Please list your 5 most important publications
de Weck AL, Eisen HN: Some immunochemical properties of penicillenic acid: an antigenic determinant derived from penicillin. J Exp Med 1960;112:1227–1247.

de Weck AL, Girard JP: Specific inhibition of allergic reactions to penicillin in man by a monovalent hapten. II. Clinical studies. Int Arch Allergy Appl Immunol 1972;42:798–815.

Frey JR, de Weck AL, Geleick H, Polak L: The induction of immunological tolerance during the primary response. Int Arch Allergy Appl Immunol 1972;42:278–299.

Geczy CL, Geczy AF, de Weck AL: Antibodies to guinea pig lymphokines. II. Suppression of delayed hypersensitivity reactions by a 'second generation' goat antibody against guinea pig lymphokines. J Immunol 1976;117:66–72.

Geczy AF, de Weck AL, Geczy CL, Toffler O: Suppression of reaginic antibody formation in guinea pigs by anti-idiotypic antibodies. J Allergy Clin Immunol 1978;62:261–270.

Nakagawa T, Stadler BM, de Weck AL: Flow-cytometric analysis of human basophil degranulation. I. Quantification of human basophils and their degranulation by flow-cytometry. Allergy 1981;36:39–47.

Blaser K, de Weck AL: Regulation of the IgE antibody response by idiotype-anti-idiotype network. Prog Allergy 1982;32:203–264.

de Weck AL, Kristensen F, Joncourt F, Bettens F, Walker C, Wang Y: Lymphocyte proliferation, lymphokine production, and lymphocyte receptors in ageing and various clinical conditions. Springer Semin Immunopathol 1984;7:273–289.

Kurimoto Y, de Weck AL, Dahinden CA: Interleukin 3-dependent mediator release in basophils triggered by C5a. J Exp Med 1989;170:467–479.

Alain de Weck sadly deceased in the course of the preparation of this book in 2013.

Bischoff SC, Baggiolini M, de Weck AL, Dahinden CA: Interleukin 8-inhibitor and inducer of histamine and leukotriene release in human basophils. Biochem Biophys Res Commun 1991;179: 628–633.

de Weck AL: The Carl Prausnitz Memorial Lecture: what can we learn from the allergic zoo? Int Arch Allergy Immunol 1995;107:13–18.

Sanz ML, Maselli JP, Gamboa PM, Oehling A, Diéguez I, de Weck AL: Flow cytometric basophil activation test: a review. J Investig Allergol Clin Immunol 2002;12:143–154.

de Weck AL, Sanz ML: Cellular allergen stimulation test (CAST) 2003, a review. J Investig Allergol Clin Immunol 2004;14:253–273.

Sanz ML, Gamboa PM, de Weck AL: Cellular tests in the diagnosis of drug hypersensitivity. Curr Pharm Des 2008;14:2803–2808.

Have you ever had a function as a President and/ or Secretary General of an allergological society?

Swiss Society of Allergy and Immunology: President

International Association of Allergology and Clinical Immunology (IAACI): Treasurer, Vice-President, President (1985–1988)

International Union of Immunological Societies (IUIS): Secretary General (Founder 1970–1982), President (1983–1986)

Collegium Internationale Allergologicum: Secretary General, President

Honorary Fellow of several allergological and immunological societies (American Academy of Allergy, American College of Allergy, American Academy of Physicians, Deutsche Gesellschaft für Allergologie, Gesellschaft of Immunologie, Société Française d'Immunologie, Österreichische Gesellschaft für Allergologie und Immunologie, etc.)

Which position has had the greatest impact on your professional life?

Doubtlessly, thanks to my double appointments in the main international societies for allergology and immunology over almost 2 decades, I had unique opportunities to influence both fields and to create bridges between the two disciplines with the help of many scientists. My main objectives during that time (1970–1995), particularly within the IAACI, were to foster basic research in allergology and its applications to clinical practice, e.g. through standardization of allergens and allergy diagnostic practices.

Under my successors, particularly under the impulse of Gunnar Johansson, the priorities of the IAACI have switched somewhat to education of allergologists and allergic patients, professional endeavors and co-operation with the pharmaceutical industry in allergy, tasks which are all also important for the development of allergy in a changing world.

Questions about your professional life

What brought you to allergy?

What brought me to allergy was in fact a hazard. Around 1952, after obtaining my diploma as a physician at the University of Geneva, I started an internship in dermatology but had to present a thesis in order to obtain an MD degree. Werner Jadassohn, the chairman of dermatology and quite famous at the time, suggested that I should repeat the seminal experiment of Merrill Chase, who had been the first to transfer specific contact dermatitis to haptens in guinea pigs with lymphoid cells and proved thereby that delayed-type hypersensitivity is caused by sensitized lymphocytes. However, he had not confirmed by histology that the skin sensitivity transferred was really contact dermatitis.

For the first 6 months, I used many guinea pigs in my free time, but was unable to reproduce Chase's experiment. This hurt my self-pride and pushed me to persist. After some technical improvements, I finally succeeded and could confirm histologically the experimental transfer of contact dermatitis, which formed the topic of one of my first publications.

After completion of the internship and clinical training in dermatology/allergy, I continued with experimental allergy and immunology at the Department of Pathology in Geneva and then, in 1958, started a postdoc fellowship at the Division of Dermatology, Washington University, St. Louis, USA, under Herman Eisen.

From whom (academic, teacher) did you learn the most?

After my basic teachers Werner Jadassohn (dermatology) and Erwin Rutishauser (pathology), who taught me the basic tools of academic research (sense of observation, intellectual curiosity, requirements for exactitude, clarity of writing), the man who had the most profound influence on my scientific development was doubtlessly Herman Eisen. Gifted with a brilliant imagination, an exacting and patient request for the truth as well as a humility contrasting with the rush to publication all too frequent at the time, Herman really implanted in me the passion for basic and applied research, a bridge function which has sustained the rest of my academic life.

Later on, as I was on my own in the small Allergy Division I created in Bern upon my return from the USA, were probably Jack Pepys, chief of allergy at the Brompton Hospital, and Michael Sela, chief of immunochemistry at the Weizman Institute.

What was your greatest achievement in allergy?

Due to my work within several institutions (Institute of Clinical Immunology, Bern, Switzerland; Department of Allergology, University of Navarra, Spain; Sandoz/Novartis Research Institute, Vienna, Austria; Roche Research, Basel, Switzerland, and research departments of several pharmaceutical companies) over many years, I have addressed several topics and cannot choose one arbitrarily as the greatest achievement. This also reflects a deliberate choice: I have always considered that meaningful or door-opening contributions to several aspects of the discipline and the building-up of a 'school' of future young leaders is a more important achievement for a scientist than the lifelong exploitation of a single discovery or theme.

Accordingly, I, together with my groups, consider that we have made contributions to:

(1) The immunochemical and immunobiochemical mechanisms of penicillin and other drug allergies. After identifying the penicilloyl antigenic determinant mainly responsible for penicillin allergy, it became possible to investigate systematically the molecular mechanism triggering the anaphylactic reaction in man and to confirm the so-called bridging theory, namely the required linkage of specific antibodies at the surface of the effector cells of allergic inflammation. This also paved the way to the first application of univalent hapten inhibition of clinical allergic reactions in man.

(2) The early recognition of lymphokines as basic intercellular messengers in immediate and delayed reactions. Since the early 1970s, we could study the role of cell-produced molecules in the development and regulation of IgE-mediated and delayed-type reactions, in particular through the first reported specific antibodies against some lymphokines and the use of flow cytometry to investigate the role of some lymphokines (IL-2) on the cell cycle and various clinical conditions, and also the identification of several lymphokines such as IL-3, IL-5 and IL-8 on basophil functions. This early phase culminated in the organization of the 2nd International Lymphokine Workshop in 1979 in Switzerland, where the word 'interleukin' was coined for the first time. This really opened a very vast field for the next 30 years of immunology.

(3) Comparative human and veterinary allergy. Through the study of atopy and IgE-mediated reactions in various species, such as rodents, dogs, cats, horses and monkeys, we have been able to make progress in the understanding of atopy development, genetics and immunobiological mechanisms of allergic diseases.

(4) Development of diagnostic cellular tests in allergy. Studies on allergic lymphocyte reactions in vitro have enabled a better understanding and diagnosis of drug allergies. Similarly, development of tests for leukotrienes and flow cytometric evaluation of basophil activation have provided new diagnostic tools in several allergic conditions.

What was your greatest disappointment?

The greatest disappointment in my professional life is the reverse side of the medal described above: to have started too many things and opened many other interesting doors which I have not been able to exploit and finish. Also, particularly in the field of cellular diagnostic tests in allergy, to have failed to convince the allergologist community, particularly in the USA, of their interest in clinical routine practice. I have seen too often a new but demanding technology being simply rejected by the majority of people not even prepared to try it.

What was your most funny experience?

If you are a scientist working in an interesting field, you are bound to have some competitor(s). In the early 1960s, my main competitor in the field of penicillin allergy was Bernard B. Levine from New York, who has made many very valuable contributions to that topic. One day, I saw his latest paper which described a new technique for the detection of anti-penicillin antibodies, apparently much more efficient than mine. My first reaction was of course to try that technique right away. I called my chief technician and gave her the recipe. A few hours later, she came back, all pale and shaky, and told me: 'Professor, it has exploded!!!'

This made me realize that, obviously, here was the perfect scientific crime. If you describe and publish a technique with deadly consequences, you can be sure that your competitors will try it and be smoothly eliminated.

Who would you list among the top 10 allergists of the world? (Please only mention individuals already deceased.)

I will abstain from nominating past historical figures but rather mention more recent pioneers whom I have personally known and appreciated since 1950. Among these, due to my own orientation, figure less clinical allergists than scientists active in allergy research and immunology related to allergy: Merrill Chase, Zoltan Ovary, Jack Pepys, Bernard Halpern, Jacques Charpin, Otto Westphal, Roy Patterson, Mario Ricci.

Who would you list among the top 10 living allergists?

My priority goes to those who have contributed to the field by continuous and varied contributions and who have built a 'school' of young leaders rather than to those who have become known by a single discovery: Frank Austen, Allen Kaplan, Barry Kay, Jean Bousquet, Johannes Ring, Terumasa Miyamoto, Dietrich Kraft, Gianni Marone, Alberto Oehling, Mike Kaliner.

What do you see as the greatest problem for allergy in the next 10 years?

The greatest challenge of allergy is to understand the genetic and environmental basis for the development of the atopic march and to achieve its prevention and/or reversal, even after it has started. There are still several approaches which may be followed: epigenetic interventions, induction of primary or secondary tolerance, IgE regulation.

What will be the next great breakthrough in allergy in the next 10 years?

As indicated above, the greatest breakthrough would be the clinical possibility to prevent or reverse the development of atopy through targeted immunological intervention(s). We have followed that dream for more than 30 years, but the increasing knowledge of the allergic patient's immune system may make it possible within the next 10–20 years.

6

Reference

De Weck A: Memories: Failures and Dreams. Berlin, Pro Business, 2008, vol 1: One life, many dreams.

Bergmann K-C, Ring J (eds): History of Allergy. Chem Immunol Allergy. Basel, Karger, 2014, vol 100, pp 350–352
DOI: 10.1159/000360097

Alfred William Frankland

London, UK

Year of birth
1912

Place(s) of university education
Oxford

Who were your most important teachers in allergology?
Dr. John Freeman, Prof. Tom Platts-Mills

Please list your 5 most important publications

Frankland AW, Augustin R: Prophylaxis of summer hay-fever and asthma; controlled trial comparing crude grass pollen extracts with isolated main protein component. Lancet 1954;i:1055–1057.

Frankland AW, Hughes WH, Gorrill RH: Autogenous bacterial vaccines in treatment of asthma. Br Med J 1955;2:941–944.

Frankland AW: High and low dosage pollen extract treatment in summer hay fever and asthma. Acta Allergol 1955;9:183–187.

Frankland AW, Parish WE: Anaphylactic sensitivity to human seminal fluid. Clin Allergy 1974;4:249–253.

Frankland AW: Latex-allergic children (review). Pediatr Allergy Immunol 1999;10:152–159.

Have you ever had a function as a President and/or Secretary General of an allergological society?
Secretary General of EAACI
President of EAACI
President of the British Society of Allergy & Clinical Immunology
President of Section of Allergy & Immunology, Royal Society of Medicine

Which position has had the greatest impact on your professional life?
Consultant in Charge of the Allergy Department of St. Mary's Hospital, Paddington, London (the largest Allergy Clinic in Europe)

Questions about your professional life

What brought you to allergy?

Chance. As a medical student I had been socially involved with Dr. John Freeman because of his and my interest in a very active shooting club at St. Mary's Hospital. This interest in shooting was one of the reasons Freeman asked Leonard Noon to join him at St. Mary's Hospital in 1906 and also why Freeman asked Sir Almroth Wright to employ Alexander Fleming (penicillin) to come to work at St. Mary's Hospital.

From whom (academic, teacher) did you learn the most?

John Freeman to begin with but I soon disagreed with many of his views. During the last 6 decades there have been so many people that I have learnt from. They include Sir Henry Dale, Rosa Augustin, who also taught me basic immunochemistry, Dr. D.A. Williams (Cardiff), Dr. Egon Bruun (Copenhagen), Prof. Steve Durham (London), Prof. Steve Holgate (Southampton) and Prof. Tom Platt-Mills (USA).

What was your greatest achievement in allergy?

(1) Publishing the first double-blind controlled trial in immunotherapy in an allergic disease in 1954; this paper was followed by many other controlled trials of immunotherapy in seasonal hay fever with or without associated asthma. Also, showing, in 1955, that autogenous bacterial vaccines in so-called infective asthma gave no specific help.

(2) In 1951, starting the pollen count and giving daily records to news media from 1961.

(3) Causing self-induced severe anaphylaxis from an insect *(Rhodnius)* in 1955.

(4) When allergy is immunity gone wrong – investigating human seminal fluid causing anaphylaxis, in 1974.

What was your greatest disappointment?

The Allergy Department not being made part of the Immunology Department when it was eventually formed at my suggestion at St. Mary's Hospital.

What was your most funny experience?

Investigating a woman who was anaphylactically allergic to the semen of the man she wanted to marry. After leaving her husband and children, she admitted that in the subsequent 3 or 4 years she had had many partners. 'I was on the pill and I had no problems with any of them. I am sure it will please you because you always like controls when investigating rare allergic problems, but those controls were not done for your benefit, only mine.' We both laughed.

Who would you list among the top 10 allergists of the world? (Please only mention individuals already deceased.)

Francis Rackemann, who I first met in Paris in 1958 and who I later stayed with at his home in Boston. He is remembered perhaps because of his description of asthma as extrinsic (allergic) or intrinsic. He also said of allergy that we should learn about 'the gun which was loaded and the trigger which fired the charge'. Rackemann was a delightful man and a marvelous host.

Secondly, Jack Pepys. I gave him his first part-time job at St. Mary's Hospital when he arrived from South Africa. He was doing research using guinea pigs, which he was very allergic to! He was always full of new immunological ideas. Even 50 years ago his advice then, as now, should be followed: 'If you are going to use the word "atopy", you must define it and this definition must be immunological and not clinical.'

Thirdly, Carl Prausnitz Giles. Before his seminal report was published in 1921, allergic complaints were considered to be produced by poisons. Freeman referred to allergens as 'idiotoxins' all his life. Prausnitz, internationally known in Europe, finally came to England in 1935 and changed his name to Giles. He was a much-loved general practitioner for the last 5 years of his life. A very humble but a very erudite man.

Who would you list among the top 10 living allergists?

Prof. Steve Durham, Prof. Steve Holgate and Prof. Frank Austen.

What do you see as the greatest problem for allergy in the next 10 years?

There are many problems to overcome before we understand the mechanisms of organ allergic inflammation.

What will be the next great breakthrough in allergy in the next 10 years?

The sequencing of the human genome in 2003 has allowed us to see human genetic variation. Will this information allow a personalized treatment of many complaints, including the symptomatic and specific treatment of systemic disease that allergy represents?

Being involved more than 5 decades ago in purifying and standardizing allergens, our methodology was not very advanced compared with today. The bacteriologists and not the biologists dealt with infection. Stem cell therapy has been tried in over 100 different ailments and now nanomedicine is the process of diagnosing, treating and preventing disease injury using molecular knowledge of the human body.

We will learn more about why some treatments help or harm individuals. We will learn about genes and cells. Specific lifestyle, dietary modifications and prophylactic treatment may be advised before a baby is born, but I suspect what will be found, and what every good clinician knows, is that we may all apparently be similar but in fact are all a little different, leading to treatments that are individualized.

Bergmann K-C, Ring J (eds): History of Allergy. Chem Immunol Allergy. Basel, Karger, 2014, vol 100, pp 353–355
DOI: 10.1159/000360099

Oscar L. Frick

San Francisco, Calif., USA

Year of birth
1923

Place(s) of university education
Cornell University (BA, 1944; MD, 1946)
Stanford University (PhD, 1964)
University of Pennsylvania (MMed Sci, 1960)

Who were your most important teachers in allergology?
Carl Arbesman, Buffalo, N.Y., USA; Bernard Halpern, Paris, France; Sidney Raffel, Stanford, Calif., USA

Please list your 5 most important publications
Frick OL, German DF, Mills J: Developemnt of allergy in children: association with virus infections. J Allergy Clin Immunol 1979;63:228–41.

Frick OL, Brooks DL: Immunoglobulin E antibodies to pollens augmented in dogs by virus vaccines. Am J Vet Res 1983;44:940–945.

Mapp C, Hartiala, Frick OL, Shields RL, Gold WM: Immunologic and physiologic responsiveness in ragweed-sensitized dogs. J Appl Physiology 1986; 61:1467–1474.

Chung KF, Becker AB, Lazarus SC, Frick OL, Nadel JA, Gold WM: Antigen-induced airway hyperresponsiveness and pulmonary inflammation in allergic dogs. J Appl Physiol 1985;58:1347–1353.

Buchanan BB, Yee BC, Ermel R, Frick OL: Thioredoxin-linked mitigation of allergic responses to wheat. Proc Natl Acad Sci USA 1997;94:5372–5377.

Have you ever had a function as a President and/or Secretary General of an allergological society?
American Academy of Allergy and Immunology: President (1977–1978)
International Association of Allergology and Clinical Immunology (now WAO): Secretary General (1985–1991)

Which position has had the greatest impact on your professional life?
American Academy of Allergy and Immunology: President (1977–1978)

Questions about your professional life

What brought you to allergy?
My father's severe angioedema due to milk and a sister with eczema.

6

From whom (academic, teacher) did you learn the most?
Carl Arbesman, Bernard Halpern.

What was your greatest achievement in allergy?
Discovering the association of virus infections and triggering of allergy in infants at risk.

What was your greatest disappointment?
Waiting for the Ishizakas and Johansson to win the Nobel Prize for discovering IgE.

What was your most funny experience?
A stormy boat ride on the gulf of Naples where many got sea sick at a symposium of the Collegium Internationale Allergologicum (CIA).

Who would you list among the top 10 allergists of the world? (Please only mention individuals already deceased.)
Clemens von Pirquet, Karl Prausnitz and Heinz Küstner, Robert Cooke, Zoltan Ovary, Bernard Halpern, Dan Campbell, Frank Dixon, Sir Henry Dale, Tomio Tada, Roy Patterson, Mary Loveless.

Who would you list among the top 10 living allergists?
Kimishige and Terry Ishizaka, Gunnar Johansson, Frank Austen, Alain de Weck[1], Rudi Valenta, Johannes Ring, Gianni Marone, Donata Vercelli, Dean Metcalfe, William Frankland.

What do you see as the greatest problem for allergy in the next 10 years?
Long-term funding for patient care of chronic diseases like asthma, eczema and IBD in the entire world, with more expensive technology for disease treatment.

What will be the next great breakthrough in allergy in the next 10 years?
3D printing of stem cells for organ and cell transplants and producing missing enzymes in various diseases.

[1] Alain de Weck sadly deceased in the course of the preparation of this book in 2013.

Reflections on my career in allergy-immunology

What made me decide on allergy-immunology as a career? My sister had severe eczema and hay fever. In the 1930s, my father developed a severe angioedema, involving the lips, eyes and extremities, which he discovered was due to ingestion of cow's milk. This was before discoveries of antihistamines and corticosteroids. He found that he could 'desensitize' himself by putting increasing numbers of drops of milk on his tongue until he could tolerate two tablespoons of milk. When he exceeded this threshold, he had an attack requiring him to return to baseline, rest for 1 month and restart the drop regimen, like a 'shoots and ladder' game. A similar oral immunotherapy regimen is under investigation today.

In 1950, my pediatric residency chairman discouraged me from going into allergy, which he labeled as 'just witchcraft done by shot doctors'. However, I wanted to determine if allergy had an immunological basis. I was most fortunate in finding enthusiastic mentors in Dr. Carl Arbesman (Buffalo), Dr. Bram Rose, Dr. Alec Sehon, (Montreal), Dr. Sidney Raffel (Stanford) and Dr. Bernard Halpern (Paris). I founded an allergy practice at the University of California in San Francisco and was co-director of a postdoctoral allergy-immunology training program.

My career high point came in 1966 when Kimi Ishizaka asked me for several half-liter serum samples from grass pollen-allergic patients in my practice. I had developed a friendship with Kimi and Terry from previous allergy meetings. That summer I spent 2 months with them in Denver at the Children Asthma Research Institute and Hospital (CARIH). They had discovered that the allergic antibody to ragweed and ovalbumin was located in a column fraction not in fraction IgA but closely adjacent, possibly a new immunoglobulin. With my patients' sera we confirmed that rye grass pollen antibody is in the same immunoglobulin column fraction. Concomitantly, in Sweden, Johansson and Bennich described a new myeloma immunoglobulin, IgND. After exchanging sera, Ishizaka and Johansson confirmed that the new immunoglobulin IgE carried the allergic activity. Johansson subsequently developed the

RAST assay for measuring IgE antibodies applied for clinical use.

Another career highlight occurred in the early 1970s when several national allergy organizations were considering establishing a new Allergy and Immunology Board. A co-sponsoring committee was formed consisting of representatives from the American Academy of Allergy and Immunology, the American College of Allergy and Immunology, the American Medical Association, the American College of Physicians, the American Academy of Pediatrics, and the Clinical Ecology group. As Chairman of the Allergy Section of the American Academy of Pediatrics, I was its representative on the committee. After 2 years of sometimes contentious meetings focusing on whether to train in allergy directly after internship or require Board certification in internal medicine or pediatrics first, a new sub-board of ABIM and ABP was formed in 1972. Dr. Charles Reed and I were elected (he first) as Co-Chairmen of the American Board of Allergy and Immunology.

Later career highlights were service on executive committees of the American Academy of Allergy and Immunology (AAAI), International Association of Allergology and Clinical Immunology (IAACI), and Collegium International Allergologicum (CIA), culminating as President of the AAAI in 1978 and Secretary General of the IAACI from 1980 to 1986. Our postdoctoral training program in allergy and immunology at UCSF trained 96 academic and practicing allergist-immunologists from 1964 through to 1996 when I retired from my pediatric professorship at UCSF. This has been for me a most exciting and enjoyable career that established lasting friendships among colleagues from around the world.

Bergmann K-C, Ring J (eds): History of Allergy. Chem Immunol Allergy. Basel, Karger, 2014, vol 100, pp 356–360
DOI: 10.1159/000360100

Kimishige Ishizaka

Tokyo, Japan

Year of birth
1925

Place(s) of university education
University of Tokyo, School of Medicine (both MD and phD)

Who were your most important teachers in allergology?
Prof. Keizo Nakamura, University of Tokyo
Prof. Dan H. Campbell, California Institute of Technology

Please list your 5 most important publications

Ishizaka K, Ishizaka T, Hornbrook MM: Physicochemical properties of human reaginic antibody. IV. Presence of a unique immunoglobulin as a carrier of reaginic activity. J Immunol 1966;97:75–85.

Ishizaka K, Ishizaka T, Hornbrook MM: Physicochemical properties of reaginic antibody. V. Correlation of reaginic activity with γE globulin antibody. J Immunol 1966;98:840–853.

Ishizaka K, Ishizaka T: Identification of γE antibodies as a carrier of reaginic activity. J Immunol 1967;99:1187–1198.

Tomioka H, Ishizaka K: Mechanisms of passive sensitization. II. Presence of receptors for IgE on monkey mast cells. J Immunol 1971;107:971–978.

Ishizaka T, Ishizaka K: Biology of immunoglobulin E. Prog Allergy 1975;19:60–121.

Have you ever had a function as a President and/or Secretary General of an allergological society?
Collegium International Allergologicum: President (1982–1986)

Which position has had the greatest impact on your professional life?
Professor of Medicine, Johns Hopkins University, School of Medicine (1970–1989)

Questions about your professional life

What brought you to allergy?
When I was accepted at the Medical School of the University of Tokyo in 1944, I was expecting to be a physician in the future. However, I became interested in basic science after I spent the summer vacation in 1946 receiving training on bacteriology from

Prof. Keizo Nakamura at the Institute of Infectious Diseases. He was a bacteriologist but he had a great interest in immunology, and his major research project was the mechanism of anaphylaxis. After the summer vacation, he asked me to translate a book entitled *The Chemistry of Antigens and Antibodies* written by Prof. J.R. Marrack in 1938. As the content of the book was very impressive for me, I became interested in immunochemistry and made up my mind to focus on immunology after graduation from Medical School.

In 1950, the Japanese Society of Allergy was established, and Prof. Nakamura was elected as the President of the Society. As I helped him to organize the first annual scientific meeting of the society, I became acquainted with many allergists in Japan, and had the opportunity to learn problems in allergic diseases.

From whom (academic, teacher) did you learn the most?

I got my lifelong research projects as a postdoctoral fellow of Prof. Dan H. Campbell at the California Institute of Technology from 1957 to 1959. His idea was that antigen-antibody complexes may have biological activities, which are lacking in either antigen or antibody alone, and that the formation of such bioactive complexes in vivo may induce anaphylactic reactions. He explained his idea and asked me to test his hypothesis. When I asked him about the experimental systems to be used, he said: 'That is your business. I gave you a research project. You should decide on appropriate experimental systems to test my hypothesis.'

Fortunately, our studies proved that preformed soluble antigen-antibody complexes induced an increased permeability of guinea pig skin capillaries. Analysis of the antigen-antibody complexes revealed that the bioactive complexes contained two or more antibody molecules, while the complex composed of two antigen molecules and one antibody molecule was inactive. The results suggested to us the possibility that the role of antigen for the formation of bioactive complexes is to bring two antibody molecules into close proximity.

I wondered whether the nature of antigen or the nature of antibody molecules is important for the formation of bioactive antigen-antibody complexes. Dr. Campbell agreed with me to proceed with experiments to answer the question; however, he asked me to form a manuscript of the paper before beginning actual experiments, adding: 'I am not kidding you.' Carl Landsteiner always wrote his manuscript before he began his experiments, and sent the paper for publication as soon as he got actual data. 'You can do it!' It was great advice for me as a professional research scientist. I followed his advice, and wrote a manuscript without any data.

The results of the experiments actually showed that the generation of biological activities by the formation of antigen-antibody complexes depends on the nature of antibody molecules rather than the nature of antigen involved. Further studies showed that aggregated normal rabbit γ globulin, which was prepared using a chemical coupling agent, induced skin reactions in the normal guinea pig and fixed complement.

Terry (Teruko Ishizaka) and I continued the research after we went back to Japan, and proved that the Fc portion of rabbit antibody molecules contained the structures which are essential for the formation of bioactive antigen-antibody complexes. Indeed, polymerized Fc fragment of rabbit γ globulin (IgG) induced skin reactions in the normal guinea pig and fixed complement, whereas neither the polymerized Fab fragment nor monomeric Fc fragment did.

I wondered whether common molecular mechanisms might be involved in both the experimental anaphylaxis in the guinea pig and allergic reactions in humans. At that time, however, no hay fever patient had been reported in Japan. Thus, I visited Prof. Campbell in Pasadena on my way to New York, where the International Congress of Allergology was held in 1961. Following his advice, I accepted an offer from Dr. Sam Bukantz, and moved back to the USA to extend our research to human allergy at the Children's Asthma Research Institute and Hospital (CARIH) in Denver, Colorado. My plan was to investigate the immunochemical mechanisms of allergic reactions in humans by using 'reagin', which had been described by Prausnitz and Küstner in 1921. Retrospectively, I would not have gone into research on the immunochemical mechanisms of human allergy if I had not had the chance to work with Prof. Campbell.

What was your greatest disappointment?

In early 1962, Heremans and Vaerman from Belgium reported that IgA isolated from the serum of atopic patients had skin-sensitizing activity, as determined by the Prausnitz-Küstner (P-K) reaction. Since the results were confirmed by several other investigators, most immunologists and allergists believed that 'reagin' is the IgA antibody against allergen. Thus, I planned to study the mechanisms of reaginic hypersensitivity by using human IgA antibodies. I repeatedly immunized normal type O individuals with 'blood group A substance', and isolated IgA, IgG and IgM in their sera. As each purified immunoglobulin contained much anti-A antibody, as determined by radioimmunoassay, I injected each of the purified immunoglobulin, containing 1–2 μg of anti-A antibody, intracutaneously into non-allergic type O individuals, and challenged the skin sites with 'A substance' 24 h later. However, no erythema-wheal reaction was observed at any of the skin sites.

Thus, we repeated the experiment by Heremans and Vaerman. Indeed, IgA isolated from the serum of ragweed-sensitive hay fever patients contained a high titer of reagin, as determined by the P-K reaction. In view of the fact that anti-A IgA antibodies did not have reaginic activity, I added rabbit antibodies specific for human IgA to the purified IgA fraction of the serum of ragweed-sensitive patients, and removed all IgA in the preparation. To my great surprise, essentially all reaginic activity in the purified IgA fraction remained in the supernatant, indicating that the reaginic activity in the so-called 'pure' IgA preparations was not associated with IgA, but with the other protein which was not detectable by usual immunological methods. Thus, I had to give up our original plan to use IgA antibodies for elucidation of the mechanisms of reaginic hypersensitivity.

The results of the experiments created more difficult problems. After removal of IgA in the purified IgA fraction of the serum of hay fever patients, the concentration of the total human immunoglobulin in the supernatant was 1 μg/ml or less. Yet, the P-K titer of the supernatant was comparable to the titer of the original serum, from which the IgA preparation was obtained. The results suggested that the concentration of the carrier protein of reaginic activity in the original serum was in the order of 1 μg/ml or less. In the 1960s, isolation and physicochemical characterization of the purified protein was the minimal requirement for claiming the presence of the distinct protein. However, our results indicated that several liters of serum from pollinosis patients would be required for isolation of a sufficient amount of the carrier protein of reaginic activity for physicochemical characterization. At this point, I had to give up the strategy.

What was your greatest achievement in allergy?

Our greatest achievement in allergy was 'identification of reagin in vitro, and discovery of a unique immunoglobulin IgE as the carrier protein of reaginic activity'.

Since our experiments indicated that the carrier protein of reaginic activity is a minor component of human serum proteins, I switched our strategy to the preparation of rabbit antibodies specific for the carrier protein. If such antibodies were available, it would be possible to identify 'reagin' in vitro without purification. Thus, we repeatedly immunized rabbits with a reagin-rich fraction of patients' serum, and absorbed the antisera with known human immunoglobulins such as IgG, IgA and IgD. After absorption, the antisera did not show a precipitin band with any of the known human immunoglobulins, nor with a normal human serum. However, addition of the antiserum obtained from one of the rabbits to serum samples of hay fever patients resulted in complete removal of reaginic activity in the patients' sera, indicating that the rabbit antiserum contained the antibodies specific for 'reagin'. By using the rabbit antiserum and radiolabeled allergen, we identified reagin in vitro in 1965. We tentatively called the carrier protein of reaginic activity γE, because I believed that the antibodies detected by our method were responsible for the induction of erythema-wheal reactions.

Detection of γE antibodies in vitro in the serum of hay fever patients by using the anti-γE antibodies and radiolabeled allergen facilitated physicochemical characterization of γE. Similar procedures revealed that γE possessed distinct antigenic determinants, which are lacking in the known immunoglobulins, together with the antigenic determinants in both κ and λ chains, indicating that γE represents a unique immunoglobulin isotype. Based on the physicochemical properties of γE, we spent 6 months isolating the protein from a large quantity of the serum of ragweed-sensitive patients. On a weight basis, reaginic activity of the purified γE was 1,000 times more active than the original serum, and gave positive P-K reactions at a dilution of 1:80,000.

One month later, I received a letter from Dr. Gunnar Johansson and Dr. Hans Bennich in Sweden, and learned that they had obtained an atypical myeloma protein, the physicochemical properties of which were almost identical to those of γE. Subsequent collaboration with them actually showed that our anti-γE reacted with the atypical myeloma protein, while the antibodies specific for the myeloma protein reacted with γE in the serum of ragweed-sensitive patients, indicating that the myeloma protein possessed the antigenic determinants characteristic for γE. Thus, γE was officially designated IgE by the World Health Organization in 1968.

What was your most funny experience?

I happened to suffer from 'atopic dermatitis' as the result of intracutaneous injections of E myeloma protein and anti-IgE antibodies into my forearm. The incident happened after Terry and I had visited Dartmouth University Hospital in Hanover, New Hampshire, in February 1969, to carry out some tests on the E myeloma patient (the second known case). The patient failed to accept passive sensitization with reaginic antibodies for P-K reactions, and reacted only to the intracutaneous injection of a high concentration of anti-IgE. It was also found that his myeloma protein inhibited the passive sensitization of my skin with the serum of a ragweed-sensitive patient for the P-K reaction. As I used myself as a normal control in these experiments, I injected E myeloma protein and anti-IgE into several skin sites of my right forearm.

On our way back to Denver I felt itching on my right forearm and recognized that the skin sites that had received anti-IgE had flared up. By the time we arrived at Denver airport red papules had spread all over my right forearm with intense itching. The next morning, I went to CARIH and showed my forearm to Dr. Elliot Middleton, who was the President of the Institute. He said: 'Oh my God! This is atopic dermatitis! What happened to you?'

The intense itching and papules with erythema lasted for about 1 week, and then gradually subsided. As I had never had an allergic disease before, and I frequently used my forearm for P-K reactions without any trouble, the cause of the dermatitis must have been IgE-anti-IgE complexes formed in my skin.

Who would you list among the top 10 allergists of the world? (Please only mention individuals already deceased.)

Dr. Bram Rose and Dr. Carl Arbesman.

Dr. Rose was Professor of Medicine at McGill University, Montreal, Canada, and Dr. Arbesman was Professor of Medicine at New York State University, Buffalo, USA. When I was at CARIH, Denver, Colorado, both Dr. Rose and Dr. Arbesman had big research and clinical groups for allergy, and physicochemical characterization of reagin was one of the major research projects in both groups. In a sense, we were their competitors, but they helped our studies for several years for the common purpose. Both Dr. Rose and Dr. Arbesman supplied serum samples of ragweed-sensitive patients for our experiments.

Dr. Rose was the President of the International Congress of Allergology, which was held in Montreal in October 1967. I greatly appreciated his invitation to the symposium on reaginic antibodies at the congress as one of the main speakers. I believe that 'γE' was recognized and accepted internationally at that symposium.

As Dr. Arbesman had been interested in detecting 'reagin' using monkeys, we collaborated with his group to prove that γE (IgE) antibodies in the serum of ragweed-sensitive patients can be detected by passive cutaneous anaphylaxis in the monkey. He also tried to reproduce our findings on γE. As his group could not prepare anti-γE, I sent him a small amount of our rabbit antiserum specific for human γE upon his request. Thus, he confirmed that our anti-γE could remove reagin in the serum samples of his patients, and he could detect γE antibodies in the sera by using our anti-γE and radiolabeled ragweed antigen. After my presentation before the International

Congress in Montreal, he made his comments and showed their data to the audience. I believe that his comments convinced the audience of the truth of our conclusion that reagin represents the γE antibodies specific for allergen.

Dr. Arbesman was elected President of the International Congress of Allergology held in London. Just before the Congress, however, he called me by telephone and let me know that he was suffering from cancer. He said that he wished to go to London even if he might die on the way. I still remember the long telephone conversation with him at that time.

What do you see as the greatest problem for allergy in the next 10 years?

In the past 40 years so much knowledge has been gained on the immunological, biochemical and molecular mechanism of allergy and allergic diseases. I greatly appreciate the progress. However, the greatest problem which remains to be solved is the increase of allergy patients, particularly in developed countries. Environmental exposure to microbial products may play a critical role during the maturation of the immune system of children, and modifications of the pattern of microbial exposure of children may be important factors for the prevalence of atopic disorders. Thus, the so-called 'hygiene hypothesis' may partly explain the increase of allergy patients. However, changes in lifestyle may also be an important reason for the increase of patients. Heating or air-conditioning were not available before the end of the Second World War. Changes in lifestyle may have caused epidermal barrier dysfunction. I believe that the greatest problem for allergy in the next 10 years will be finding an effective method for preventing the increase of allergy patients in westernized countries.

Bergmann K-C, Ring J (eds): History of Allergy. Chem Immunol Allergy. Basel, Karger, 2014, vol 100, pp 361–362
DOI: 10.1159/000360103

Lothar Jäger

Jena, Germany

Year of birth
1934

Place(s) of university education
University of Jena

Who were your most important teachers in allergology?
H. Kleinsorge (others are also mentioned below)

Please list your 5 most important publications

Jäger L: Untersuchungen zur Atemregulation beim Asthma bronchiale. Respiration 1968;25:216–231.

Jäger L, et al: Monoclonal antibodies in the standardization of allergens. Allergy Clin Immunol 1989;6:180–193.

Jäger L, et al: Epitopes on allergens; in Ring J, Przybilla B, et al (eds): New Trends in Allergy III. Berlin, Springer, 1991, pp 33–47.

Müller WD, Jäger L, et al: Analysis of human T cell clones reactive with group V grass pollen allergens. Int Arch Allergy Immunol 1994;105:391–396.

Jutel M, Jäger L, et al: Allergen-specific immunotherapy with recombinant grass pollen allergens. J Allergy Clin Immunol 2005;116:608–613.

Jäger L (ed): Klinische Immunologie und Allergie. Jena, Fischer, 1978–1989 (3 German and 1 Russian edition).

Jäger L, Merk H-F: Arzneimittelallergie. Stuttgart, Fischer, 1996.

Jäger L, Wüthrich B (eds): Nahrungsmittelallergien und -intoleranzen. Ulm, Fischer, 1998–2008 (3 German editions).

Have you ever had a function as a President and/or Secretary General of an allergological society?

Society of Clinical and Experimental Immunology (GDR): President and Secretary General (several terms between 1965 and 1991)

INTERASMA: President (1978–1981)

Federation of Asthma Research in Europe (FARE): President (1992–1995)

Which position has had the greatest impact on your professional life?
Head of the Department of Clinical Immunology, University of Jena, Germany

Questions about your professional life

What brought you to allergy?

In the very beginning it was mere chance. I absolved my training in internal medicine at the Medical Policlinic of the University in Jena where the first Unit for Allergy and Asthma in Germany was located. After finishing my training in internal medicine I became head of this unit which I later developed into an independent Department of Clinical Immunology (including Allergy) – consisting of routine and research labs, a ward and an outpatient department.

From whom (academic, teacher) did you learn the most?

My first academic teachers at Jena, H. Kleinsorge and G. Klumbies. Later on I received important immunologic stimuli from A.D. Ado (Moscow), H. Ambrosius (Leipzig), A. de Weck (Switzerland), J. Kalden (Erlangen), F. Melchers (Switzerland) and I. Roitt (London). Clinical stimuli came from K. Hansen and E. Fuchs.

What was your greatest achievement in allergy?

Being convinced that the most important problems in allergic disease can be solved only by means of immunologic approaches, I developed the Unit for Allergy and Asthma into a Department of Clinical Immunology, including research labs, a ward and outpatient department. With this background we improved the analysis of allergens, including control of quality (especially grass pollen, food and selected occupational allergens), the IgE-based diagnosis, the relationship between IgE and T cell epitopes, and – together with others – the first immunotherapy in grass pollinosis with recombinant allergens.

What was your greatest disappointment?

The fact that after my retirement my department was changed to a Department of Immunology without any connection to the clinic.

That the financial problems of public health led to enormous restrictions in the treatment of allergic diseases, hindering the translation of research progress into clinical practice.

Who would you list among the top 10 allergist of the world? (Please only mention individuals already deceased.)

L. Noon and J. Freeman, P. Ehrlich, K. and T. Ishizaka, J. Pepys, K. Hansen, M. Samter.

Who would you list among the top 10 living allergists?

G. Johansson, H. Löwenstein, H. Sampson, A. de Weck[1], J. Ring.

What do you see as the greatest problem for allergy in the next 10 years?

What dominates the process from sensitization to clinical manifestation and how this can be prevented.

What will be the next great breakthrough in allergy in the next 10 years?

Identification of the decisive mechanisms of IgE-mediated sensitization, and improvement of specific immunotherapy.

[1] Alain de Weck sadly deceased in the course of the preparation of this book in 2013.

Bergmann K-C, Ring J (eds): History of Allergy. Chem Immunol Allergy. Basel, Karger, 2014, vol 100, pp 363–364
DOI: 10.1159/000360105

Terumasa Miyamoto

Tokyo, Japan

Year of birth
1930

Place(s) of university education
University of Tokyo, School of Medicine, Japan
Northwestern University, Chicago, Ill., USA

Who were your most important teachers in allergology?
Mary Loveless, USA
Roy Patterson, USA
Yoshio Oshima, Japan

Please list your 5 most important publications

Miyamoto T, et al: Respiratory changes in passively sensitized dogs and monkeys as models of allergic asthma. Am Rev Resp Dis 1968;96:76–88.

Miyamoto T, et al: Allergenic identity between the common floor mite (*Dermatophagoides farinae*, Hughes 1961) and house dust as a causative allergen in bronchial asthma. J Allergy 1968;42:14–28.

Miyamoto T, et al: Physiologic and pathologic respiratory changes in delayed type hypersensitivity reaction in guinea pigs. Am Rev Resp Dis 1971;103: 509–515.

Muranaka M, et al: Adjuvant activity of diesel-exhaust particulates for the production of IgE antibody in mice. J Allergy Clin Immunol 1986;77:616–623.

Okudaira H, Terada E, Yokoyama M, Miyamoto T: IgE-isotype-specific suppressor cells in the mouse: characterization using tetraparental chimera mice of high (DBA/2) and low (SJL) IgE responder embryos. Int Arch Allergy Appl Immunol 1988; 85:462–466.

Have you ever had a function as a President and/or Secretary General of an allergology society?
Japanese Society of Allergology: President (1987)
International Association of Allergology and Clinical Immunology (currently WAO): President (1991–1994)
Japanese Society of Allergology: Chairman, Board of Directors (1994–2000)

Which position has had the greatest impact on your professional life?
Chairman, Board of Directors, Japanese Society of Allergology (1994–2000)

6

Questions about your professional life

What brought you to allergy?

I was working as a resident and research fellow at the National Jewish Hospital (NJH) in Denver, USA, for 4 years from 1956 to 1960, shortly after my graduation from the University of Tokyo. NJH was well known as the institute of tuberculosis and non-tuberculosis chest diseases. About 50 severe cases of asthmatic patients were hospitalized, and I had a good opportunity to take care of those patients.

During that time, Prof. Mary Loveless joined the NJH from Cornell University, New York, and became chairman of the Asthma and Allergy Department for about 1 year. I worked with her and directly received basic knowledge and experience of research techniques.

As a research fellow, I worked with Dr. Solbert Permutt in the cardiopulmonary laboratory at NJH. He later became a professor at Johns Hopkins University. We did various cardiopulmonary physiologic studies in asthmatic patients. Among those, we carried out cardiac catheterization in asthmatic patients to measure pulmonary pressures and O_2 gas pressures, etc. before and during allergen inhalation provocation tests.

I returned to Japan in 1960. Since one of the main clinical and research subjects of my department at the University of Tokyo was traditionally allergy and asthma, I naturally went into that field.

From whom (academic, teacher) did you learn the most?

Mary Loveless, Irving Kass and Yoshio Oshima.

What was your greatest achievement in allergy?

Two years later and independent of R. Voorhorst's discovery, we found that house dust mites were the major elicitors of allergy in house dust. We identified 36 species of house dust mites in house dust. Among them, *Dermatophagoides* carried the major allergen, although house dust mites have immunological cross-reactivity over large or small species of *D. farinae*, and *D. pteronyssinus* showed almost identical allergenicity. Feces showed the identical allergenicity to body. *D. farinae* was the original mite in our study, as we could culture it purely.

We discovered that diesel exhaust particles (DEP) have a kind of adjuvant effect to produce IgE antibody in mouse experiments. A similar effect was also found in humans. This is probably the first finding of the effect of air pollution to promote the prevalence of allergic diseases in the world.

What was your greatest disappointment?

(i) I had a patient with a food-dependent exercise-induced anaphylaxis in 1961. The patient, who had eaten bread and was running to catch the bus, passed out. I asked her to eat the same brand of bread in our presence; however, she did not show any reaction this time, so I abandoned the study. Later, food-dependent exercise-induced anaphylaxis was reported. I was so sorry to have missed the chance to be the first person to report this case in the world.

(ii) During the time of my inhalation provocation studies around 1960, I noticed the late-phase reaction (4–6 h later) following the immediate reaction. Late reactions occurred more often after mold (especially *Candida*) allergen inhalation. However, I did not pay much attention to it. I should have studied this in greater detail around that time to become famous.

Who would you list among the top 10 allergists of the world? (Please only mention individuals already deceased.)

Mary Loveless, Samuel Feinberg, Max Samter, Jack Pepys, Roy Patterson, Richard Farr, Jaques Charpin, Carl Arbesman, Tomio Tada, Yoshio Oshima.

Who would you list among the top 10 living allergists?

Frank Austen, Oscar Frick, Alain L. de Weck[1], S.G.O. Johansson, Johannes Ring, Stephen Holgate, Charles Reed, Albert Sheffer Kimishige, Teruko Ishizaka.

What do you see as the greatest problem for allergy in the next 10 years?

The prevalence of allergic diseases will still increase in the next 10 years, which will be the greatest problem. New effective drugs will be added to treat allergic patients and, consequently, medical expenses will go up.

What will be the next great breakthrough in allergy in the next 10 years?

New effective drugs, especially biological drugs, will be developed and allergic patients will be more easily treated. Tailor-made medicine will develop and the quality of life of patients will improve much more than before. Also, genetic research will improve a great deal and give us insight to understand the basic problems of allergy better than before.

[1] Alain de Weck sadly deceased in the course of the preparation of this book in 2013.

Bergmann K-C, Ring J (eds): History of Allergy. Chem Immunol Allergy. Basel, Karger, 2014, vol 100, pp 365–367
DOI: 10.1159/000360106

Harry Morrow Brown (1917–2013)

Derby, UK

One of the last of the independent researchers?

Reflections

Dr. Harry Morrow Brown was born in Auchterarder, Scotland, in 1917. He qualified with an MB ChB from Edinburgh University in 1939, and he served in the Royal Army Medical Corps from 1939 to 1946, mainly in India. His postgraduate studies in Edinburgh led to an interest in the low sodium rice diet for hypertension, finally resulting in a thesis on 'Adaptation and adaptive dysfunction', which was accepted with commendation for MD in 1950. The main conclusion was that allergies are the most common manifestation of faulty adaptation to the environment, but there was no possibility to develop this concept in 1950. He became a member of the Royal College of Physicians of Edinburgh in 1949 and was elected a Fellow in 1965. He received an Honorary Doctorate from Derby University in 2004, was the first recipient of the BSACI William Frankland Award in 1999 for outstanding services to clinical allergy, and was elected an International Fellow of the American Academy of Allergy in 2006.

After a registrarship with the Medical Professorial Unit in Dundee he specialised in respiratory medicine and was appointed Consultant Chest Physician in Derby in 1953. He inherited a run-down clinic where the major problem was tuberculosis, but nearly all patients were cured by 1956, making the treatment of other respiratory diseases possible.

In 1956, a British Medical Research Council multi-central trial of oral steroids in chronic asthma concluded that steroids were no better than bronchodilators. Morrow Brown could not believe this because he had treated asthmatics with oral steroids with dramatic improvement, and his thesis had been closely concerned with the early development of corticosteroids. In 1956, consultant physicians in the National Health Service had the freedom to conduct clinical trials on their own initiative, so he decided to carry out his own trial and appealed for chronic asthmatics.

Ninety patients were treated with oral steroids. After 3 months, 60 were greatly improved but 30 were unchanged. Suspecting that he was treating two different diseases he began sending sputum to the local laboratory and asking them to look for eosinophils, but none were reported even when he was sure they should be abundant.

This negative finding was also unacceptable, so he decided to look for them himself using the antique Leitz microscope he had used as a student. Developing a rapid wet smear method of looking for eosinophils in the clinic, he discovered that the 60

Harry Morrow Brown sadly deceased in the course of the preparation of this book in 2013.

who had responded to steroids had many eosinophils, while the 30 non-responders had none. These striking findings were published in *The Lancet* in 1958 [1] but attracted no attention whatsoever, even though this was actually the very first study to show that the presence of eosinophils indicates steroid responsiveness. It was many years before sophisticated methods of examining induced sputum confirmed his findings.

The ability to select steroid-responsive patients proved very helpful for clinical management, but Morrow Brown was not satisfied with long-term oral steroids because of their side effects and, thus, became deeply involved in clinical allergy. The result was that from 1958 onwards he built up an allergy research centre, supported by a local charity he founded, and he organised five 'Charles Blackley International Symposia on Clinical Aspects of Allergic Disease' at Nottingham University between 1973 and 1984.

Research was devoted to finding the causative allergens and introducing avoidance or immunotherapy so that oral steroids could be reduced or stopped. A major interest became aerobiology and seasonal allergies, using a spore trap he made himself, so pollen and spore counts became routine [2]. The range of allergic conditions treated expanded to include all body systems, particularly food allergy and eczema.

In 1968, Sir David Jack and his team at Glaxo developed the very first steroid aerosol containing beclomethasone dipropionate (BDP), but trials in Edinburgh concluded that they were ineffective and should be discarded. Fortunately, Dr. Wilfrid Simpson, the Glaxo Medical Director, heard Dr. Morrow Brown talking about eosinophils at a symposium organised by Glaxo. He realised that the Edinburgh investigators might have been treating non-responsive cases of COPD, so he asked him to carry out another trial for which the entry criteria were that all patients had to have eosinophils in their sputum and all trialists had peak flow meters to obtain hard data.

The results were dramatic and BDP aerosols were reprieved from the dustbin within a few months. The results were announced for the first time at the European Congress of Allergology in October 1971, and published in the *British Medical Journal* in 1972 [3], soon to be followed by many confirmatory studies. The first study of BDP in children was published in the following year [4] and finally a long-term survey of BDP in children was published in 1980 [5].

His latest publication on BDP was a letter to the editor of *The Lancet* in 2003 drawing attention to the importance of the change to HFA propellants which enabled the production of an ultra-fine aerosol which could reach the whole bronchial tree for the first time [6]. While appreciating the benefits inhaled steroids have given to patients worldwide, he regrets that this development has enabled any doctor to treat asthma or rhinitis effectively without even thinking about possible allergic causes or having any knowledge of allergy!

Several years ago he produced a very large website (www.allergiesexplained.com) with Bill Frankland acting as editor, containing an account of his researches and clinical experience with allergy since 1958 so that the public can access this information. Good fortune and serendipity have played an important part in his career, supported by a passion for microscopy and personal investigation, and refusal to accept negative findings when they do not fit.

Continuing in consultant practice since retirement from the National Health Service in 1982, he conducted a successful controlled trial of SLIT for hay fever between 1986 and 1989, and a very successful open trial of Acarosan for mite allergy, both published on his website. He developed methods of using the patient's own house dust for skin testing to assess the amount of allergen in the patient's own house dust, and produced several portable air sampling devices in his well-equipped workshop for investigating occupational and environmental asthma. He invented a standardised skin testing needle, a re-breathing bronchial provocation test, and a 'microspoon' to hold the right amount of grass pollen for nasal provocation.

Charles Blackley observed grass pollen grains discharging their granules on exposure to water in 1873. Morrow Brown made a video of this phenomenon and another of motile bacteria in rainwater, which was first seen by Leeuwenhoek in 1670. Until his death in 2011, he continued studies of the inorganic crystals, mostly pleomorphic calcium sulphate, which are found in profusion in the air in certain weather conditions.

References

1 Brown HM: Treatment of chronic asthma with prednisolone: significance of eosinophils in the sputum. Lancet 1958;ii:1245.
2 Brown HM: The relationship of aerobiological data to seasonal allergic symptoms: a review of 27 years' experience. Immunol Allergy Pract 1992;14:318–329.
3 Brown HM, Storey G, George WH: Beclomethasone dipropionate: a new steroid aerosol for the treatment of allergic asthma. Br Med J 1972;1:585–590.
4 Brown HM, Storey G: Beclomethasone dipropionate steroid aerosol in treatment of perennial allergic asthma in children. Br Med J 1973;3:161–164.
5 Brown HM, Bhowmik M, Jackson FA, Thantrey N: Beclomethasone dipropionate aerosols in the treatment of asthma in childhood. Practitioner 1980;224:847–851.
6 Brown HM: A neglected breakthrough in asthma therapy. Lancet 2003;361:433–434.

6

Bergmann K-C, Ring J (eds): History of Allergy. Chem Immunol Allergy. Basel, Karger, 2014, vol 100, pp 368–370
DOI: 10.1159/000360107

Albert K. Oehling

Navaleno, Spain

Year of birth
1928

Place(s) of university education
University of Granada, Spain

Who were your most important teachers in allergy?
Prof. Karl Hansen, Prof. Wilhelm Gronemeyer, Prof. Erich Fuchs and Prof. E Letterer

Please list your 5 most important publications
Gestal J, Oehling A: The nervous system in the regulation of the immune response. I. Experimental contribution to the role of the anterior hypothalamus (in Spanish). Allergol Immunopathol (Madr) 1974;2:169–188.

Gestal J, Oehling A: The nervous system in the regulation of the immune response. III. The posterior hypothalamus and its vital importance in the immune response (in Spanish). Allergol Immunopathol (Madr) 1974;2:307–320.

Gamboa PM, Oehling A, Sanz ML, Castillo JG: Decrease of beta-receptors in asthmatic and rhinitic patient. Allergol Immunopathol (Madr) 1987;15:65–68.

Garcia BE, Sanz ML, Fernandez M, Diéguez I, Oehling A: Value of lgG4 antibodies against foods in atopic-dermatitis. Allergol Immunopathol (Madr) 1990;18:187–190.

Oehling A, Sanz ML, Resano A: Importance of IgG4 determination in in vitro immunotherapy follow-up of inhalant allergens. J Investig Allergol Clin Immunol 1998;8:333–339.

Oehling A: Bacterial infection as an important triggering factor in bronchial asthma. J Investig Allergol Clin Immunol 1999;9:6–13.

Have you ever had a function as a President and/or Secretary General of an allergological society?
International Association of Asthmology (Interasthama): Secretary General (14 years)

International Association of Asthmology (Interasthma): President (1984–1987)

European Foundation of Allergy Research (FARE): President (1980–1983)

International Association of Allergology and Clinical Immunology: President (1990–1991)

International Association of Allergology and Clinical Immunology: President (1994–1998)

Which position has had the greatest impact on your professional life?

Full Professor of Allergology and Clinical Immunology at the Medical School of the University of Navarra in Pamplona, Spain

Director of the Department of Allergology and Clinical Immunology at the University Clinic (Clinica Universidad de Navarra), from 1961 to 1999

Questions about your professional life

What brought you to allergy?

My teacher in internal medicine advised me to pursue a specialization in allergology. His advice came from the influence of Prof. Jimenez Diaz, a pioneer of allergology in Spain. I started in allergic diseases with a small section at the University Hospital of Granada (1955–1957).

From whom (academic, teacher) did you learn the most?

My stay for 1 year (1957) at the Clinic of Prof. Karl Hansen, a pioneer of allergology in Europe, in the Hospital of Lübeck, Germany, was a very important moment in my professional life. After that, I joined his disciple, Prof. Gronemeyer, in the Allergie-Forschungs-Institut und Asthma-Klinik in Bad Lippspringe, Germany (from January 1958 to October 1961). It was precisely there, also with Prof. Erich Fuchs, where I enriched my specialty and I enjoyed the great affection and generosity of both. Equally, I was influenced by the teachings of Prof. Letterer (Tübingen, Germany).

What was your greatest achievement in allergy?

My greatest achievement was introducing allergology to the Medical School of the University of Navarra, as well as the teaching of allergology and clinical immunology as separate subjects in the medical curriculum, with the same importance as cardiology or neurology. This course was taught for 3 months in the school year, and for 28 years I proudly held that role at the university. As a consequence many of my students chose allergology as a specialty. Obtaining recognition in education, as well as the specialist qualification in allergology and clinical immunology, was another great achievement, realized through the committee created by the Spanish Society of Allergology.

What was your greatest disappointment?

In my professional life, my biggest disappointment was that in my years as a member of the Committee on Education in Allergology, and also as its president, I went many times to the presidents of the various national societies of allergology in our association requesting their co-operation in order to create the specialty and to introduce its teaching in medical schools. The result was truly disastrous to such an extent that in some countries the title of the specialty still does not exist. Another disappointment was that our International Association of Allergology, due to etymological unknowns, changed its name to World Allergy Organization (WAO). Here the specialty of allergology (allergologos) was confused with the phenomenon allergy (allos meaning 'different' and ergon meaning 'reaction').

What was your most funny experience?

This is a very difficult question to answer indeed. There have been many satisfactions that we have enjoyed throughout our professional lives. For me, the most important has been the great universal recognition that has reached our department of the University Hospital of Navarra (Clinica Universidad de Navarra) and the many disciples we have had in four continents. The level attained by our publication, *Journal of Investigational Allergology and Clinical Immunology*, also represents an enjoyable experience. Finally, a very valuable experience was that through the many different conferences in which I participated for almost 50 years, I had the opportunity to meet and get on with eminent professionals. Due to that I knew and enjoyed the friendship of many of my colleagues.

Who would you list among the top 10 allergists of the world? (Please only mention individuals already deceased.)

In my memory I think that the top ten allergologists that influenced me the most are the following professors: Hansen, Jimenez Diaz, Halpern, Serafini,

Fuchs, Volfrom, Voorhorst, Sangiorgi, Pepys, Lahoz and Wilken-Jensen.

Who would you Iist among the top 10 living allergists?

Again, I find this question very difficult to answer. It is hard to highlight only ten of the many good allergologists of today. Therefore, in the following list many people will be omitted because of the limited number. In this list should be the professors: Bousquet, Canonica, Vervloet, Bergmann, Ring, Wahn, Kay, Kaplan, Kaliner and Lockey.

What do you see as the greatest problem for allergy in the next 10 years?

I think the low standard of basic research in this field remains a major problem for allergology. This is reflected in the publication of numerous repetitive works on what we already know from what has been previously published. The lack of interest that is given to the teaching of allergology in medical schools is also very worrying.

What will be the great breakthrough in allergy in the next 10 years?

This is a difficult question to answer because it depends on the success of the struggle of the national societies in getting allergology to be considered as a specialty and not as a sub-specialty. On the other hand, it also depends on the existing centers of allergology; they must give more importance to research in the bases and mechanisms of the allergic response. Achieving both outcomes is important and urgent for the future of allergology.

Bergmann K-C, Ring J (eds): History of Allergy. Chem Immunol Allergy. Basel, Karger, 2014, vol 100, pp 371–372
DOI: 10.1159/000360108

Heimo Reulecke

Iffeldorf, Germany

Year of birth
1939

Place(s) of university education
Mainz, Germany, and Stanford, USA

Who were your most important teachers in allergology?
Roger Altounyan, Wolfgang Schmutzler, Karl-Christian Bergmann and Ernst Fuchs

Which position has had the highest impact on your professional life?
Managing Director of Fisons, Germany (1978–1992) and President of Fisons Corp., USA (1992–1995)

Questions about your professional life

What brought you to allergy?
In 1978, after 12 years of activity in Portugal, Indonesia, Thailand and the Philippines, I took over the management of the German establishment of the English group Fisons, based in Cologne. After the re-orientation of the enterprise, the therapeutic potential of a combination of sodium cromoglycate and a bronchial diluting substance became apparent to me. Reproterol could be offered as a combination partner with cromoglycate because I had worked for many years for the manufacturer Asta Medica.

After a long development time the licensing and market launch occurred in 1983. The combination had almost no side effects and, under the name Aarane and Allergospasmin, quickly became the best-selling anti-asthmatic drug in Germany, and later also in Switzerland.

A new concept of treatment requires clarification and new methods in advanced medical training. In the course of years of collaboration with many opinion leaders, Fisons Germany became the synonym for successful advanced doctor training. This culminated in the 'German-German asthma dialogue' after the reunion of Germany, a common idea of Prof. Christian Bergmann and myself. About 20 of the most experienced German pneumologists were involved in this success. This 'united continuing education' was only one example of a successful co-operation between physicians and the pharmaceutical industry, and formed technical and human bridges between the East and West.

'German Lung Day' originated from my demand that asthma patients must bear highly their own responsibility for dealing with their illness. Again, Prof.

Bergmann was the technical competence. Today, the Lung Day has grown to involve between 30,000 and 50,000 visitors, and is the biggest public event in German pneumology. In 1983, the German Pollen Information Service Foundation was initiated and financed by Fisons in co-operation with the German Weather Service and the allergist Dr. Ruppert.

From whom (academic, teacher) did you learn the most?

An unforgettable moment in my professional life in the pharmaceutical industry was my acquaintance with an unusual person, physician, pharmacologist and researcher. Roger Altounyan (1922–1987) was the discoverer of the pioneering substance disodium cromoglycate and the powder inhalation. He suffered severely from asthma and never got tired of taking part in the worldwide meetings of 'his' enterprise, Fisons, and attending congresses to present his ideas for the treatment of asthma.

His charisma was brilliant, his appearance was unpretentious and his knowledge about the connections of asthma and immunology were excellent. All these attributes had to be admired. To have experienced and known him instilled my enthusiasm for the treatment of asthma and allergies.

What was your greatest achievement in allergy, and what was your greatest disappointment?

In 1990, the reunion of Germany brought me, after 12 years of successful management of Fisons, the additional responsibility for the new federal states and the region of Central Europe. In 1992, a career jump occurred when I became the president of Fisons USA. Several years of restructuring the enterprise could not prevent the necessity for the company to be sold. I did not succeed in preventing this, and this is probably the biggest disappointment of my professional activity.

Back in Germany my dream of independence came true. The foundation of the company Pulmopharm in 1997 in Munich was a great challenge. Also, the official licensing and market launch of the inhalation solution TOBI® for patients with cystic fibrosis was a highlight.

Bergmann K-C, Ring J (eds): History of Allergy. Chem Immunol Allergy. Basel, Karger, 2014, vol 100, pp 373–375
DOI: 10.1159/000360111

Václav Špičák

Prague, Czech Republic

Year of birth
1929

Place(s) of university education
Charles University Prague, Pediatric Faculty (1948–1953)

Who were your most important teachers in allergology?
Josef Liška ('father' of allergology in Czechoslovakia), Marie Bělská, Vladimír Zavázal, Jacques Charpin, Bernard Halpern

Please list your 5 most important publications
Špičák V, Vondra V: Asthma bronchiale – od dětství do dospělosti (Asthma from Childhood to Adulthood). Prague, Avicenum, 1988.
Špičák V, Panzner P: Allergology. Prague, Galén, 2004.
Špičák V: Bydlení pro alergiky (Living for Allergic People). Brno, ERA Group, 2003.
Samšiňák K, Dusbabek F, Vobrázková E: Note on the house dust mites in Czechoslovakia. Folia Parasitol 1972;19:383–384.
Barnes P, Godfrey S, Špičák V, Dunitz M: Asthma. London, Dunitz, 1997.
Špičák V, Dab I, Hulhoven R, et al: Pharmacokinetics and pharmacodynamics of cetirizine in infants and toddlers. Clin Pharmacol Ther 1997;61:325–330.
Špičák V: Place des auto-vaccins bactériens dans le traitement des enfants asthmatiques. Med Hyg 1970;28.

Have you ever had a function as a President and/or Secretary General of an allergological society?
EAACI: Vice President (1977–1981)
Czech Society of Allergology and Clinical Immunology: President (1990–2005)
Czech Society of Allergology and Clinical Immunology: Secretary (1964–1968)
Czech Medical Association of Jan Evangelista Purkyne: Secretary General (1989–1993)

Which position has had the greatest impact on your professional life?
Head of the Pediatric Department, Faculty Hospital Bulovka, Prague (1981–1996)
Chairman of the Czech Society of Allergology and Clinical immunology
Member of the expert panel of the WHO-GINA (1992–1995)

Questions about your professional life

What brought you to allergy?
I became an allergist by chance. I always wanted to work always as a pediatrician and I studied at the

Pediatric Faculty of Charles University (1948–1953). In the last year of my studies I was asked by Prof. Švejcar to prepare a seminar on a case report of an allergic child. During the preparation of the seminar I had to go through all the existing knowledge on allergy and I found the topic a fascinating 'detective story'. That was in 1953. It was no wonder that 2 years later pediatric allergy and childhood asthma became the subject of my PhD thesis, and then of my professional life.

From whom (academic, teacher) did you learn the most?

Josef Švejcar (pediatrics), Helena Rašková (pharmacology), Jaroslav Šterzl (immunology), Bernard Halpern (allergy and clinical immunology; one year in his institute in the Hospital Broussais, Paris, 1961) and Josef Liška (practical allergology, specific immunotherapy).

What was your greatest achievement in allergy?

The greatest achievement was perhaps the results of my co-operation with the Czech acarologist Karel Samšiňák in 1972 (regional study: 'House dust mites in flats of asthmatic children and in summer houses' [Folia Parasitol 1979, vol. 26]). However, I consider that my greatest achievement in allergy has been the 42 years of summer camps for children with allergy and asthma (since 1970), including my personal attendance and responsibility without any interruption (the most recent at the time of writing was in July 2013). These camps were our response to the isolation of such children from standard life; they were disqualified from the attendance of summer camps, school trips and sports activities. Their morbidity and school absence was very high, they suffered from asthma attacks with frequent recurrent symptoms, and their physical fitness and social status was low (New trends in therapy and prevention of bronchial asthma, with M. Revenda et al. [Allergol Immunopathol 1977, suppl. IV]; Physical fitness and performance of asthmatic children, with M. Revenda, B. Mrzena [Allergol Immunopathol 1977;5:4]). Today, the attendees of the camp do not have any exercise-induced asthma symptoms any longer and their physical abilities do not differ from healthy children. This is evidence of the successful implementation of the global strategy of asthma treatment in our clinical practice. Thus, the 42 years of our camps served as a unique experiment and provide a view of the history of the care of childhood asthma in our country.

What was your greatest disappointment?

The deaths of asthmatic children before the era of inhaled corticosteroids.

What was your most funny experience?

The Czech society of allergology and clinical immunology has a history stretching over 55 years. My generation of allergologists spent the majority of their carrier under an old politically non-democratic regime which meant, among many problems, limited contact with the world community. As we considered such contact essential, we always worked very hard to overcome these limitations and to participate at international events in allergology. It was even worse after 1968. In this context I especially remember the INTERASMA Congress in Warsaw in 1985. At that time, by chance, the father of one of my patients had a high position at the Ministry of Transport and he managed to rent a special train carriage for 30 allergologists – members of our society. It was fantastic – the carriage offered not only accommodation, but also breakfast and dinner for us. The only funny problem was that on each day of the congress the carriage was parked on a different platform of Warsaw station, sometimes even at a different city station. Sometimes the location of the carriage changed during the day. So imagine that you leave your accommodation at some train station and you find it later in the evening at another location. This story fits the famous sentence of Pierre de Coubertin: 'The most important thing is not winning, but taking part.' This for us was the most important thing – we all took part!

Who would you list among the top 10 allergists of the world? (Please only mention individuals already deceased.)

Pasteur Valery Radot, Carlos Jimenez Diaz, Bernard Halpern, Jacques Charpin, Lino Businco, Jacques Pepys, W.J. Quarles van Ufford, Andrzej Szczeklik, Z. Eriksson-Lihr, A.D. Ado.

Who would you list among the top 10 living allergists?

A. William Frankland, Gunnar Johansson, Alain de Weck[1], Kimishige Ishizaka, Stephen Holgate, Barry Kay, Estelle Simons, Ulrich Wahn, Jean Bousquet, Zdeněk Pelikán, and many others....

What do you see as the greatest problem for allergy in the next 10 years?

Three things: food allergy; mucosal immunity – its role and immunomodulation, allergen immunotherapy and the management of lifestyle.

What will be the next great breakthrough in allergy in the next 10 years?

The results of epigenetics and molecular allergology – way to efficient diagnostic and allergen immunotherapy.

[1] Alain de Weck sadly deceased in the course of the preparation of this book in 2013.

6

7 Allergy Societies and Collections

Bergmann K-C, Ring J (eds): History of Allergy. Chem Immunol Allergy. Basel, Karger, 2014, vol 100, pp 378–379
DOI: 10.1159/000360247

AAAAI
American Academy of
Allergy Asthma
& Immunology
www.aaaai.org

What is the society's complete title/name (and its abbreviation)?

American Academy of Allergy, Asthma & Immunology (AAAAI)

When and where was it established? What were the circumstances?

The AAAAI was founded as the American Academy of Allergy on December 4, 1943, in New York City. However, the roots of this professional association date back to the 1920s with the establishment of two organizations: the Western Society for the Study of Asthma, Hay Fever and Allergic Diseases (west coast of the USA) and the Society for the Study of Asthma and Allied Disorders (east coast of the USA).

Eventual overlap in membership, scientific endeavors and educational objectives led to years of talks about a merger. This finally came to pass when the two organizations joined to form the American Academy of Allergy, creating one strengthened and integrated society. Some say the final impetus was the difficulty in negotiating travel arrangements to attend the meetings of two societies during the war years, but this might have been simply coincidental. Considerable deliberation, debate and negotiation preceded the eventual merger.

The organization's name became the American Academy of Allergy & Immunology in 1982. The name was changed to the American Academy of Allergy, Asthma & Immunology in 1995. These successive changes are reflective of the growth of the specialty.

Who were the founding members of the society and from which medical disciplines did they come (e.g. dermatology, immunology, pulmonology)?

The presidents of the two coastal societies under whose leadership amalgamation was effected were Samuel Feinberg, MD (Western) and Robert Chobot, MD (Eastern). Although Dr. Feinberg served as President of the Western Society, he agreed to step aside and let Dr. Chobot assume the role of President of the American Academy of Allergy. Other members of the original executive committee were: Oscar Swineford Jr. (Vice President), Karl D. Figley (Treasurer), Will Cook Spain (Secretary), Matthew Walzer and Milton Cohen.

The merger of these organizations resulted in a founding membership of 272 physicians. While the initial membership represented the disciplines of internal medicine and immunology, the majority of members were actively pursuing the phenomenon of hypersensitivity. As fundamental knowledge of hypersensitivity mechanisms and clinically translatable information developed, the scope of the Academy's functions broadened.

How many members does the society have today?

The AAAAI membership includes more than 6,800 allergist/immunologists, members of the allied health community, researchers and related health care professionals from the USA, Canada and 72 other countries worldwide. The AAAAI is a democratic organization, with leadership elected by full members and Fellows of the AAAAI.

While led by its Board of Directors, the work of the AAAAI is driven by 7 interest sections, 6 assemblies and 70 committees and task forces. The AAAAI also places a high value on its alliances with related professional societies, patient advocacy organizations, accreditation boards and other organizations.

What is the main emphasis of the society: immunology or allergy?

The AAAAI is dedicated to the advancement of the knowledge and practice of allergy, asthma and immunology for optimal patient care. Thus, the emphasis runs across the breadth of the specialty.

The AAAAI is also home to the Allergy, Asthma & Immunology Education and Research Organization, Inc. (ARTrust™). The mission of the ARTrust is to find treatments and cures for the millions of people suffering from allergies, asthma and other immunologic diseases by supporting education and research.

What are the society's most important prizes and honors?

In addition to lectureships and ARTrust awards, the most prestigious annual awards bestowed by the AAAAI are its Honorary Awards. These include: Allied Health Professionals Recognition Award; Distinguished Clinician Award; Distinguished Layperson Award; Distinguished Service Award; Distinguished Scientist Award; Outstanding Volunteer Clinical Faculty Award; RSLAAIS Leadership Award; Special Recognition Award, and the President's Humanitarian Award.

These awards are presented during the AAAAI Annual Meeting. The Academy's first Annual Meeting in 1944 was a 2-day event with 4 sessions and 23 presentations. Now, more than 7,000 delegates gather annually from around the globe for hundreds of sessions presented throughout 5 days of learning and networking.

What are the names of the society's journals? Which journal is the official organ of the society?

The Journal of Allergy and Clinical Immunology (JACI), the official publication of the AAAAI, began in 1929 with the first edition of *The Journal of Allergy*. Respected worldwide, the *JACI* is the most cited journal in the allergy/immunology specialty.

In 2013, the AAAAI launched *The Journal of Allergy and Clinical Immunology: In Practice*, a publication devoted to presenting the best clinical research and practical management recommendations in allergy/immunology.

Please indicate the Internet address of your society

http://www.aaaai.org

Acknowledgements

Much of this historical review is credited to Sheldon G. Cohen, MD, FAAAAI. Dr. Cohen chronicled the history of the organization within the document: *The American Academy of Allergy: A Historical Review.*

A. Wesley Burks, MD, Chapel Hill, N.C.

7

Bergmann K-C, Ring J (eds): History of Allergy. Chem Immunol Allergy. Basel, Karger, 2014, vol 100, pp 380–382
DOI: 10.1159/000360249

The Asia Pacific Association of Allergy, Asthma and Clinical Immunology (APAAACI) is an association of national societies of allergy and clinical immunology in the Asia-Pacific region. In some areas in the region no formal society exists and in these circumstances the APAAACI accepts membership by individual medical practitioners who have made a significant contribution to the field of asthma, allergy and clinical immunology. As the major professional association for allergy and clinical immunology in the region, the APAAACI has a unique opportunity for advancing education and awareness of allergic disorders and the theory and practice of immunological disease in the most populous and diverse region in the world.

Current member national societies include:

Allergy, Asthma and Immunology Society of Thailand

Allergy and Clinical Immunology Society Singapore

Allergy and Immunology Society Sri Lanka

The Australasian Society of Allergy and Clinical Immunology

The Bangladesh Society of Immunology and Allergy

The Chinese Society of Allergology

The Hong Kong Institute of Allergy

Indian College of Asthma, Allergy and Applied Immunology

The Indonesian Society of Allergy and Immunology

The Japanese Society of Allergology

The Korean Academy of Asthma, Allergy and Clinical Immunology

The Malaysian Society of Allergy and Immunology

The Mongolian Society of Allergology

The Philippine Society of Asthma, Allergy and Immunology

The Taiwan Society of Asthma, Allergy and Clinical Immunology

Individuals from Pakistan and Myanmar are also members.

The Early Years

By the early 1970s, it was evident that the prevalence of allergy-related diseases in the Asia-Pacific region was increasing significantly. However, there were few allergy/immunology specialists to service this need and there was little in the way of data to inform research. Prior to 1982 there had been no regional Asian allergy meeting organised. In 1982, the

Korean/Japanese allergy meeting was organised by Prof. Seok Young Kang (Korea) and Prof. Tatsushi Ishizaka (Japan). This meeting rotated between Korea and Japan on a biennial basis. In 1986, the organising committee decided to expand the meeting by inviting leaders from other Asian nations and the meeting became the West Pacific Symposium of Allergology. Sharing knowledge and experience of allergic disease management between colleagues became a top priority for this group.

In 1986, Prof. Karnen Baratawidjaja (Indonesia) met with Prof. Montri Tuchinda and Prof. Phabillya Phanichyakarn (Thailand) to discuss the possibility of organising a Symposium of Allergology for the region and to discuss the possibility of establishing an Asia-Pacific organisation. Bali was chosen as the venue for this inaugural meeting which was held in 1989.

The Bali meeting was attended by 17 representatives of various societies in the Asia-Pacific region and they are listed below:

Prof. Karnen G Baratawidjaja
Prof. Montri Tuchinda
Prof. Phailboolya Phanichyakarn
Prof. Minoru Okuda
Prof. Terumasa Miyamoto
Prof. Kue-Hsiung Hsieh
Prof. Manuel F. Ferreria
Prof. Lee Sang Yong
Prof. Keven J. Turner
Prof. Ronald S. Walls
Prof. Feng Pao Hsii
Prof. Nasamuddin Bin Abdullah
Prof. Siti Boedina Kresno
Prof. Jcanc Latu
Prof. Suharyono
Prof. Sjamsuridjal
Prof. Santoso Cornain

Those present at the Bali meeting agreed to name the new organisation the Asia Pacific Federation of Allergology and Clinical Immunology Societies (APFAIS). Prof. Baratawidjaja from Indonesia became the first chairman of the APFAIS. The House of Delegates was attended by 15 delegates and 3 observers from the regional countries. At that first meeting constitution bylaws were adopted and it was agreed to have triennial congresses.

In 1992, a combined meeting was held between the newly formed APFAIS and the Japanese and Korean delegates at the 14th International Congress of Allergology and Clinical Immunology in Kyoto, Japan. Also in 1992, during its congress in Bangkok, the name APFAIS was changed to Asian Pacific Association of Allergology and Clinical Immunology and the Bangkok meeting was called the first APAACI Congress. The Bangkok congress is seen as the time of the official establishment of the Asia Pacific Association of Allergology and Clinical Immunology, marking the successful conclusion of a process that had begun in Bali 3 years earlier with the proposal to form a regional association of allergy and immunology specialists. It was at the 7th congress in Bangkok, in 1999, that the name of the regional organisation was updated to the Asia Pacific Association of Allergy, Asthma and Clinical Immunology (APAAACI), the name by which it is known at the present time.

The APAAACI has met every 2–3 years in Taipei (1995), Manila (1998), Sydney (2000), Seoul (2002), Tokyo (2004), Bangkok (2007) and Singapore (2010) since the first congress in Bangkok. Taiwan is hosting the next congress in 2013.

Two notable congresses have been held in conjunction with the World Allergy Organisation (formerly known as the International Congress of Allergology and Clinical Immunology, ICACI). In 2000, Australia hosted the International Congress and this was held in partnership with APAAACI and the Australasian Society of Clinical Immunology and Allergy, and was a great success, heralding an exciting period at the beginning of a new millennium in the fields of allergy and clinical immunology. Prof. Antony Basten was President of the congress and Prof. Constance Katelaris was the Secretary General for that meeting.

The second combined congress with the World Allergy Organisation was held in Bangkok in 2007. Prof. Pakit Vichyanond was the Secretary General for that meeting. In 2010, the APAAACI combined with another regional group, the Asia Pacific Association of Pediatric Allergy, Respirology and Immunology (APAPARI) for a very successful congress in Singapore.

In more recent times, the APAAACI executive has seen the need to expand the work of the organisation. Under Prof. Sang Il Lee's presidency, the APAAACI has commenced its very own regional journal, *Asia Pacific Allergy*. This has gained listing in PubMed. Prof. Sang Il Lee is the first Editor in Chief and he is supported by Associate Editors in Chief – Prof. Constance Katelaris, Prof. Hee Bom Moon and Prof. Akihiro Morikawa (Japan). The managing editors are Dr. Yoon-Seok Chang (Korea) and Dr. Kang Mo Ahn (Korea).

With the commencement of the most recent APAAACI term under the leadership of Prof. Constance Katelaris (President) and Associate Prof. Frank Thien (Secretary General), the APAAACI is entering a new era of endeavour. The work of the organisation has been expanded and now includes the publication of a quarterly newsletter, a new website and creation of a number of working parties to address specific needs within the practice of allergy and immunology.

The objectives of the APAAACI are to:

(1) promote the exchange and progress of knowledge on allergology, asthma and clinical immunology in this region;

(2) promote the study, prevention and treatment of allergy, asthma and immune-related diseases with particular emphasis on problems specific to this region;

(3) promote exchange in training programs between member countries in the region;

(4) promote co-operation in clinical and basic research on allergology, asthma and clinical immunology in this region;

(5) encourage, assist and co-ordinate the development of programs of public information and education in allergology, asthma and clinical immunology;

(6) co-operate with other international organisations in the study of allergology, asthma and clinical immunology, and

(7) foster dissemination of this knowledge through international congresses on allergology, asthma and clinical immunology, and by other means.

APAAACI Journal: *Asia Pacific Allergy*: http://www.apallergy.org

APAAACI website: http://APAAACI.org

Secretariat arinex pty limited: secretariat@apaaaci.org

C.H. Katelaris, Sydney (President)

Bergmann K-C, Ring J (eds): History of Allergy. Chem Immunol Allergy. Basel, Karger, 2014, vol 100, pp 383–387
DOI: 10.1159/000360253

A Brief Introduction to the Collegium Internationale Allergologicum

Any volume on the history of allergy which hopes to convey something about the scientific and interpersonal interactions which have contributed to the development of this field, as well as information about the field's important discoveries and pioneers, should include a brief description of the origins, goals and traditions of the Collegium Internationale Allergologicum (CIA).

The CIA differs from many scientific societies in several respects. From its foundation, the CIA has markedly limited its number of active members. The number was originally 200, but was increased to 250 in 1986, reflecting the increased number of scientists in the allergy community. The aim of the CIA is to gather into the Society for a long period of time, possibly for the remainder of one's professional lifetime, a community of investigators who have exhibited excellence in pursuing a scientific approach to allergy, either in their clinical work with patients and/or in experimental research in the laboratory. Accordingly, members are elected from the worldwide community of productive investigators, working in academia or in the biopharmaceutical sector, who have demonstrated evidence of scientific independence and sustained leadership in allergy, clinical immunology and related fields. New members must be proposed by two CIA members in good standing, and must make a scientific presentation during at least one CIA symposium. The invitation to candidates and other non-members to present work at a CIA symposium must come from a CIA member.

Founding

On October 15, 1954, 48 distinguished physicians and scientists from 18 countries on 6 continents (table 1), and representing different fields of medicine and biological research, gathered in London in order to sign the inaugural document founding the Collegium Internationale Allergologicum, soon to be known under the acronym 'CIA'. Figure 1 shows the signatures of some of the founding members. At that time allergy and immunology had not yet been established as independent scientific and academic disciplines in most countries of the world. However, allergy societies had already been established in some countries. The International Association of Allergy and Clinical Immunology (IAACI, renamed the World Allergy Organization, WAO, in 2000) was founded in 1951. The European Academy for Aller-

Table 1. Founding members of the CIA

	O.G. Bier (São Paulo)
(C)	P. Blamoutier (Paris)
	D. Bovet (Rome)
	C.J.C. Britton (London)
	H. Christensen (Roskilde)
(C)	R.R.A. Coombs (Cambridge)
	Sir H.H. Dale (London)
(C)	H.A.E. van Dishoeck (Leiden)
	R.H.O. Donald (Melbourne)
(VP)	J. Duchaine (Bruxelles)
	J. Freeman (London)
	C. Frugoni (Rome)
	C.P. Giles (Ventnor)
(C)	F. Gross (Basel)
(C)	M.T. Gutman (Jerusalem)
(C)	K. Hansen (Lübeck)
	D. Harley (London)
(T) (P)	C. Jimenez-Diaz (Madrid)
	E.A. Kabat (New York)
(S)	P. Kallós (Helsingborg)
	L. Kallós-Deffner (Helsingborg)
	W. Kaufman (Bridgeport)
	A. Lunedei (Florence)
	W. Löffler (Zurich)
	M. Maekawa (Kyoto)
	J.R. Marrack (Cambridge)
	R.L. Mayer (Summit)
	R. Meier (Basel)
	G. Melli (Milan)
	G. Miescher (Zurich)
	H.R. Olivier (Paris)
	D. Ordman (Johannesburg)
	Z. Ovary (Rome)
	W. Pagel (London)
	G.W. Pickering (London)
	S. Raffel (Stanford)
	Bret Ratner (New York)
	B.M.B. Riley (Sidney)
	C. Rimington (London)
	E. Rothlin (Basel)
	H. Selye (Montreal)
(C)	U. Serafini (Rome)
	M.A. Solari (Buenos Aires)
	R.S. Steel (Sidney)
	A. Stoll (Basel)
	G.L. Waldbott (Detroit)
	J. Waldenström (Malmö)
	F.F. Yonkman (Summit)

P = President; VP = Vice President; T = Treasurer; S = Secretary; C = Council Member.

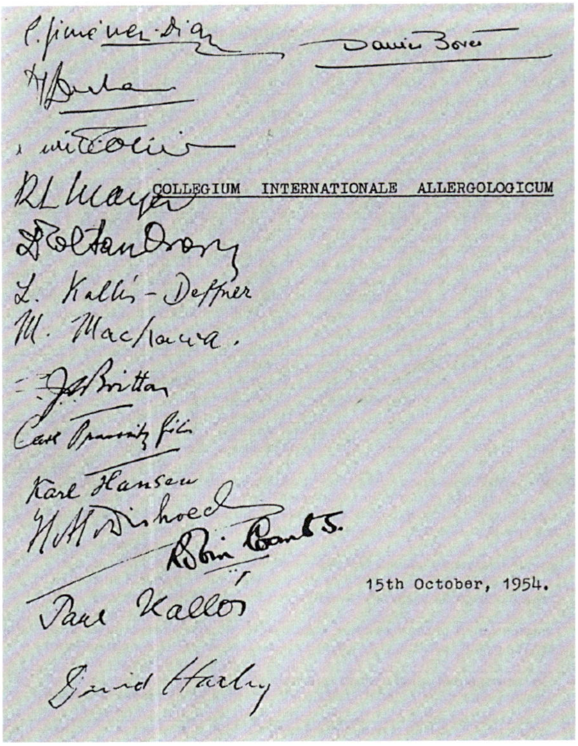

Fig. 1. Signatures of the founding members of the CIA.

gology and Clinical Immunology (EAACI) was established in Florence in 1956, 2 years after the CIA was founded. While such large national and international societies provide great value to the allergy and immunology community, it soon became clear to its early members that the CIA added a distinct but important professional opportunity – providing a mechanism for gathering together a small and collegial group of distinguished scientists in order to communicate effectively about the latest advances in the field.

The founding members were from the UK (10), USA (7), Italy (6), Switzerland (6), Australia (3), Sweden (3) and France (2), and several other countries were represented by one member each. Among the founders is a remarkable collection of famous personalities in medicine and in the emerging field of allergy and clinical immunology: Daniel Bovet, Robin R.A. Coombs, Sir Henry Dale, Carl Prausnitz-Giles, Karl Hansen, Elvin Kabat, Paul and Liselotte Kallós-Deffner, W. Kaufman, W. Löffler, Guido Miescher, Zoltan Ovary, B.M.B. Riley, Hans Selye, Umberto Serafini and Jan G. Waldenström, just to name a few. The founders thus included eminent figures who fundamentally contributed to the development of allergology and clinical immunology worldwide.

During the CIA's first 20 years, Paul Kallós, a clinical immunologist and allergist not affiliated with a university, was the 'moving spirit' running the organization; all those who met him will never forget his charismatic personality, brought to full force as he tried to recruit into the CIA the brightest young allergists from all over the world.

Subsequently, for several decades the group was largely run by Alain de Weck and Peter Dukor. Although there was a succession of presidents and a façade of democracy, it was always clear who, in fact, led the organization. In the tradition of the CIA, the presidents in many cases can be considered to have had largely ceremonial roles, except for the selection of the venues of the meetings and attending to the bureaucratic responsibilities of the organization. However, some of the presidents are remembered for their unusual or endearing individual characteristics. Geoffrey B. West is remembered for the style of his hilarious minutes of the meetings. Kimishige Ishizaka will have a special place in the history of allergy for his role in the discovery of IgE and his dedication to the CIA. Larry Lichtenstein was a devoted and informal president, also unforgettable for his cigars. John Bienenstock followed the Lichtenstein 'informal style' in running the CIA. Gianni Marone courted catastrophe twice, once during the frightening boat ride from Sorrento 'half way' to Capri in 1982, and then again in 2010 when the meeting he organized in Ischia during his presidency almost had to be cancelled because of the eruption of a volcano in Iceland! Johannes Ring is a prominent member of the group of 'informal Presidents' and is particularly gifted as Honorary Historian of the CIA. Stephen Galli has carried on in the style of Geoffrey West in reporting the 'funny minutes' of the meetings, and he and several recent Presidents have made special efforts to increase the diversity of the membership.

The Secretaries of the CIA have done a lot of the CIA's important work and have exerted considerable influence behind the scenes, doing so under the changing titles of 'Executive', 'Honorary' or 'General' Secretary. For example, Paul Kallós (Honorary Secretary from 1954 to 1974) conducted the affairs of the CIA with utmost diplomacy. Subsequently, Alain de Weck (Honorary Secretary from 1974 to 1986) and Peter Dukor (Executive Secretary from 1974 to 1988) were the operating pillars of the CIA. They contributed significantly to the smooth transition of the CIA from a European and slightly British-shaded club into a truly international scientific society. Alain de Weck was certainly one of the most remarkable members of the CIA from the past 40 years. In recognition of his outstanding contributions to the CIA over many years, the membership decided, during the XXVIII meeting held in Ischia in 2010, to initiate the Alain de Weck Travel Grant Program to provide travel grants to young scientists to attend the CIA symposia. Table 2 lists the CIA Officers from its foundation. The history of the CIA is described in much more detail in a book [1], and is also kept alive by a robust oral tradition.

The Concept

Article 1 of the CIA constitution is in essence the 'magna carta' of the CIA, describing the rationale for its existence:

> The Collegium is an international group for the study of scientific and clinical problems in allergy and related branches of medicine and immunology. The Collegium aims to promote the humble spirit of scientific inquiry, friendly cooperation, good fellowship and professional relationship in the field of allergy.

The organization of the CIA should be free of politics and non-scientific influences, the affairs conducted with a minimum of formality and bureaucracy.

Symposia

The primary activities of the CIA are the election of new members and the hosting of scientific symposia which take place every other year. CIA

Table 2. Officers of the CIA

President	
D. Harley	1954–1974
G.B. West	1974–1978
F. Milgrom	1978–1982
K. Ishizaka	1982–1986
A. Sehon	1986–1990
A. de Weck	1990–1994
L. Lichtenstein	1994–1998
J. Bienenstock	1998–2002
J. Ring	2002–2006
G. Marone	2006–2010
S.J. Galli	2010–2014
Vice President (Presidents-Elect)	
J. Duchaine	1954–1970
F. Milgrom	1970–1978
K. Ishizaka	1978–1982
A. Sehon	1982–1986
A. de Weck	1986–1990
L. Lichtenstein	1990–1994
J. Bienenstock	1994–1998
J. Ring	1998–2002
G. Marone	2002–2006
S.J. Galli	2006–2010
S. Holgate	2010–2014
Honorary Secretary	
P. Kallos	1954–1974
A. de Weck	1974–1986
A. Capron	1986–1990
J. Ring	1990–1998
Executive Secretary	
A. Cerletti	1954–1974
P. Dukor	1974–1988
J. Bienenstock	1988–1994
Secretary General	
G. Marone	1998–2002
S.J. Galli	2002–2006
S. Holgate	2006–2010
B. Bochner	2010–2014

meetings are organized by prominent members of the CIA at specially selected sites that represent attractive settings for small meetings that both lack 'parallel sessions' and include substantial amounts of unscheduled time for informal interactions (table 3). Accordingly, CIA symposia have the unique characteristic of providing an atmosphere of friendly collegiality and intimacy that is quite different from that of the crowded meetings of international societies where thousands of participants attend 10–20 parallel sessions. This informal scientific atmosphere is only possible by limiting the number of participants to approximately 250 scientists.

This tradition started with the first meeting in London in 1954, organized by Paul Kallós and David Harley (table 3). Since then, CIA symposia have been organized almost every other year for the last 60 years. Not only are the scientific presentations traditionally of the highest quality, but CIA symposia are among a small number of scientific events in which scientists dare to present even unpublished data. Over its history, the CIA has hosted an outstanding list of special lectures – some of them given by Nobel laureates (after or before they received the prize; in alphabetical order: Luc Montagnier, Erwin Neher, Stanley B. Prusiner and Bengt Samulesson) – and has also hosted the first presentations of many new findings and breakthroughs in the fields of allergy and clinical immunology.

Indeed, the programs and the proceedings of the CIA symposia over more than half a century read like a list of highlights of key discoveries in allergy and clinical immunology, including histamine receptors, the origin, physiology and pathophysiology of mast cells, the discovery of T cell subpopulations, the concept of Th1, Th2 and Th17 cells, IgE and IgE receptors, and the regulation of IgE synthesis, the discovery of leukotrienes and platelet-activating factor, the mechanisms of acquired and innate immunodeficiencies, and novel treatments for allergic and immune disorders.

In addition to the excellence in science, there are certain essential elements that characterize the CIA symposia:

- two honorary lectures (the Carl-Prausnitz lecture and the Paul Kallós lecture);
- one 'relaxing from immunology' lecture (that is enjoyed both by members and accompanying persons);
- a boat ride;
- the reading of the 'funny minutes' of the previous meeting;
- the semi-formal introduction of new members at a gala dinner on the last evening of the meeting.

Table 3. History of CIA symposia

Date	Site	Organizer(s)
1954	London	P. Kallòs, D. Harley
1955	Basel	A. Stoll, E. Rothlin
1957	London	P. Kallós, R.R.A. Coombs
1959	Rome	L. Businco
1962	Freiburg im Breisgau	F. Hahn, H. Gierz, W. Schmutzler
1964	London	G.B. West
1968	Tel Aviv	I. Glazer, M. Feldmann
1970	Montreux	A. de Weck
1972	London	F. Feinberg, J. Pepys, J.L. Turk, G.B. West
1974	Copenhagen	B. Diamant, N. Hjorth, P. Kallós, H. Rorsmann
1976	Heidelberg	K. Rother, H. Gierz, E. Schöpf, G. Till
1978	New Orleans	J. Salvaggio
1980	Constance	P. Dukor, A. de Weck
1982	Sorrento	G. Marone, M. Condorelli, G. Rossi, M. Ricci
1984	Puerto Vallarta (Mexico)	P. Norman, L. Lichtenstein, T. and K. Ishizaka
1986	Gothenburg	L.A. Hanson, N. Lindholm
1988	Martinique	M. and A. Capron
1990	Madeira	S. Holgate, J. Bienenstock
1992	Capri	G. Marone
1994	Nantucket	S.J. Galli, A.L. Sheffer
1996	Fuschl/Salzburg	D. Kraft, J. Ring
1998	Corfu	A. Togias, L. Lichtenstein
2000	Hakone	T. Ishikawa, T. Miyamoto, H. Tomioka
2002	Bermuda	A. Togias, J. Bienenstock
2004	Bornholm	H. Loewenstein, J. Ring
2006	Malta	S. Holgate, B. Kay
2008	Curacao	R. Van Ree, J. Ring
2010	Ischia	G. Marone, M. Triggiani, A. Genovese
2012	Jeja	Y.Y. Kim, S. Galli
2014	Petersberg/Bonn	M. Maurer, H. Behrendt, T. Bieber

The scientific excellence, collegiality and informal atmosphere of the CIA symposia, which have remained essential characteristics from its founding, continue to help to attract to the membership of this organization the best investigators in the field of allergy and clinical immunology.

On behalf of the CIA, the former President (G.M.), the Honorary Historian (J.R.) and the current President (S.J.G.) wish this book great success. It may help interested readers all over the world to gain further insight into the exciting cosmos of allergy and clinical immunology.

CIA website: http://www.ciaweb.org/

Gianni Marone, Naples
Johannes Ring, Munich
Stephen J. Galli, Stanford, Calif.

7

Reference

1 Ring J, de Weck A (ed): CIA – Collegium Internationale Allergologicum: History and Aims of a Special International Community Devoted to Allergy Research, 1954–2006, ed 2. Munich, Urban & Vogel, 2006.

Bergmann K-C, Ring J (eds): History of Allergy. Chem Immunol Allergy. Basel, Karger, 2014, vol 100, pp 388–391
DOI: 10.1159/000360258

EAACI
EUROPEAN ACADEMY OF ALLERGY
AND CLINICAL IMMUNOLOGY

What is the society's complete title/name (and its abbreviation)?

The official name is the European Academy of Allergy and Clinical Immunology (EAACI). The former title of European Academy of Allergology (from 1957) was changed in 1971 to European Academy of Allergology and Clinical Immunology.

When and where was it established? What were the circumstances?

The idea of a closer collaboration on a European level in the field of allergy was suggested for the first time during the 1st European Congress on Allergy, held in Paris from May 31 to June 1, 1950, and was organized by Prof. Valery Radot, Prof. B.N. Halpern and Prof. P. Blamoutier. On that occasion, the representatives of the European Council had the task of organizing the next European Congress. The 2nd European Congress, entrusted to the Danish Society for Allergological Research and organized by Dr. E.B. Salen and Dr. E. Bruun, was held in Copenhagen on May 20–23, 1953. Although both congresses were extremely successful, it was nevertheless evident that a closer co-operation was necessary, not only for organizing important meetings, but also for assuring a continuous exchange of views and information which could be accomplished only through the creation of a specialized European Society. After hard preparatory work, this objective was finally attained during the 3rd European Congress of Allergy, organized in Florence by Prof. A. Lunedei and Prof. U. Serafini in September 1956.

Who were the founding members of the society and from which medical disciplines did they come (e.g. dermatology, immunology, pulmonology)?

As mentioned above, Prof. A. Lunedei and Prof. U. Serafini were the organizers of the 3rd European Congress of Allergy. The name of the Society was The European Academy of Allergy.

Purpose
European co-operation in the field of allergy (training, meetings, research)

Nomination of officers
President: Prof. U. Serafini

Vice Presidents: Dr. E. Bruun, Dr. F.J. Farrerons-Co, Dr. D.A. Williams
Secretary: Dr. W. Quarles van Ufford

Main advisory committee
Prof. Z. Eriksson Lihr
Prof. B.N. Halpern
Prof. K. Hansen
Prof. C. Jimenez Diaz
Prof. A. Lunedei
Prof. Pasteur Valery Radot
Prof. V. Spoujitch

Official journal
Acta Allergologica

Official languages
English, French, German

Place and date of the 4th European Congress
London, 1959

Nomination of honorary members
Sir Henry Dale and Prof. Cesare Frugoni

It was pointed out that the Academy, although accepting individual members, had as its basic object the grouping together of the already existing European societies devoted to the study of allergy, which together had about fifteen hundred members. In addition it was decided that outstanding workers in the field of allergy from countries without a specific society should be invited to join the Academy.

The Academy's constitution and bylaws were drawn up in Utrecht in 1957. Some amendments to them have, however, been made through the years.

A special agreement was reached with *Acta Allergologica*, which became the official organ of the Academy together with the Northern Society of Allergology. Some of the most important works of the Academy have been reported in this journal, such as the proceedings of the Brussels Meeting and of the London and Copenhagen Congresses.

Special attention was given by the various Executive Committees to the organization of congresses and meetings in order to attain the best possible co-ordination of the European activities in the field of allergy.

The Florence Congress was followed by the IV European Congress in London (1959), organized by R.S. McDowall and D.A. Williams; the V European Congress was held in Basel (1962) and was organized by R. Schuppli; the VI European Congress, organized by S. Hellerstrom and S. Krapelien, took place in Stockholm (1965); the VII European Congress was held in Berlin (1968), organized by H. Herxheimer and E. Stresemann; the VIII European Congress was held in Marseille (1971), organized by J. Charpin; the IX European Congress was held in London (1974) and was organized by K.M. Citron and R.S. Bruce Pearson; the X European Congress was held in Prague (1977), organized by Dr. V. Zavazal (President) and Dr. V. Spicak (Scientific Secretary), and lastly the XI European Congress was held in Vienna (1980), organized by Prof. C. Steffen (President) and Dr. H. Ludwig (Secretary).

As the European Congresses, owing to their international character, were held at rather long intervals, annual ('small') meetings were organized between the congresses with the object of improving and updating knowledge in selected fields of allergy and clinical immunology. Here follows a list of the annual meetings held so far: Brussels (1957); The Hague (1958); Belgrade (1959); Barcelona (1960); Berlin (1961); Prague (1962); Bologna (1963); Brussels (1966); Prague (1967); Geneva (1969); Oslo (1972); Pamplona (1973); Rome (1975); Aachen (1976); Athens (1978); Helsinki (1979); Clermont-Ferrand (1981); Funchal (1982).

With regard to the Academy's constitutional aim of 'encouraging and assisting international co-operation among European workers in the field of allergy', special care was given to the formation and function of various committees which were established with the object of developing scientific and practical knowledge in specialized fields.

Ten scientific committees were set up between 1956 and 1959 to deal with such subjects as: Occupational Allergy, Food Allergy, Education in Allergy, Climate and Allergy, Airborne Allergens, Drug Allergy, Standardization, Allergy and Insurances, Pharmacology and Drugs, and Testing Procedures. Several other Committees were added during the period between 1959 and 1962, such as: History and Allergy,

Table 1. EAACI presidents

1956–1959	U. Serafini (Italy)
1959–1962	D.A. Williams (UK)
1962–1965	E. Bruun (Denmark)
1965–1968	H. Herxheimer (Germany)
1968–1971	J. Duchaine (Belgium)
1971–1974	S. Kraepelien (Sweden)
1974–1977	J. Charpin (France)
1977–1980	A.W. Frankland (UK)
1980–1983	J.P. Girard (Switzerland)
1983–1986	C. Molina (France)
1986–1989	M. Debelic (Germany)
1989–1992	A.B. Kay (UK)
1992–1995	F.B. Michel (France)
1995–1998	S.G.O. Johansson (Sweden)
1998–2001	Sergio Bonini (Italy)
2001–2003	Paul van Cauwenberge (Belgium)
2003–2005	Ulrich Wahn (Germany)
2005–2007	Anthony Frew (UK)
2007–2009	Roy Gerth van Wijk (the Netherlands)
2009–2011	Jan Lötvall (Sweden)
2011–2013	Cezmi Akdis (Turkey/Switzerland)

Autoimmunity, Allergy and Nervous System, Allergy and Rheumatism, Pediatric Allergy, and Lung Function Tests. Three workshops were organized in 1962: Physiotherapy, Rehabilitation in Allergic Diseases, and Social Measurements and Allergic Diseases. Some reports by these committees and workshops were published. After a few years, the activity of many committees was discontinued. The *Lexicon Allergologicum* (Johann Ambrosium Barth, Leipzig, 1964) was published with the support of the Academy. It was edited by Dr. J.K. Wilken-Jensen with the valuable collaboration of Dr. J. Duchaine, Dr. W. Gronemeyer, Dr. R.S. Bruce Pearson, Dr. A.W. Frankland, Dr. U. Serafini and Dr. A. Ado, and includes the translation of the principal technical and scientific allergological terms in six languages (English, French, German, Spanish, Italian and Russian). Table 1 provides a list of the EAACI presidents.

How many members does the society have today?

The Academy has 7,400 members from 121 countries and 42 national societies.

What is the main emphasis of the society: immunology or allergy?

Both. The name European Academy of Allergology (1957–1971) was changed to European Academy of Allergology and Clinical Immunology owing to the close relationship between these two fields of study, and also in view of the possibility of establishing co-operation between them.

What are the society's most important prizes and honors?

The EAACI Awards. Since 2005 the Executive Committee has selected the EAACI Award winners for the four categories we have. With these awards the EAACI is honoring scientists and clinicians in the field of allergy and clinical immunology:

- Daniel Bovet Medal for improving treatment and prevention of allergic diseases;
- Clemens von Pirquet Medal for outstanding contributions in clinical research;
- Paul Ehrlich Medal for improving experimental research in allergy/clinical immunology;
- Charles Blackley Medal for the promotion of allergy as a specialty in Europe.

The award ceremony takes place during the opening ceremony of every EAACI Congress. Table 2 lists the winners of each award to date.

What is the name of the society's journal? Which journal is the official organ of the society?

Allergy – the European Journal of Allergy and Clinical Immunology is the official publication of the EAACI and is available online via Blackwell Synergy/Wiley InterScience. It has an impact factor of 6.297 (2nd among 21 allergy journals in 2010). To view abstracts and tables of contents for free (and full texts if you have a subscription) go to Blackwell Synergy/Wiley InterScience.

Pediatric Allergy and Immunology is the official publication of the Pediatric Section of the EAACI and it is also available online via Blackwell Synergy/

Table 2. EAACI awards

	Clemens von Pirquet Medal for Clinical Research	Daniel Bovet Award for Treatment and Prevention	Paul Ehrlich Award for Experimental Research	Charles Blackley Medal for Promotion of the Specialty in Europe
2005	Dietrich Kraft	Bengt Bjorksten	Barry Kay	Alain de Weck
2006	William Frankland	Jean Bousquet	Kurt Blaser	S.G.O. Johansson
2007	Ulrich Müller	Tari Haahtela	Henning Löwenstein	Paul van Cauwenberge
2008	Andrzej Szczeklik	Ulrich Wahn	Stephen Holgate	Sergio Delgiacco
2009	Steve Durham	Bengt Bjorksten	Rudi Valenta	Brunello Wüthrich
2010	Johannes Ring	Hans-Jörgen Malling	Rob Aalberse	Sergio Bonini
2011	Gabrielle Pauli	Erika von Mutius	Gianne Marone	Anthony J. Frew
2012	Glenis Scadding	Arne Höst	Werner Pichler	Roy Gerth van Wijk
2013	Martin K. Church	Claude Molina	Monique Capron	François-Bernard Michel

Wiley InterScience. Its impact factor is 2.874 (8th among 21 allergy journals and 10th out of 107 Pediatric journals in 2010). To view abstracts and tables of contents for free (and full texts if you have a subscription) go to Blackwell Synergy/Wiley InterScience.

Clinical and Translational Allergy is a peer-reviewed open-access journal aiming to provide a platform to publish original research and reviews in the field of allergy. Such articles can be based on clinical, translational or basic research. Commonly known as *CTA*, it is one of several journals in the portfolio of the EAACI and is one of the first open-access journals in this field. Open-access publishing enables free access to all content, thus ensuring a wide dissemination of articles; the electronic format and the optimized manuscript handling process allows a very rapid publication of papers.

CTA is an international journal reaching out far beyond the borders of Europe and invites clinicians and researchers from all countries of the world to contribute. *CTA* publishes original research articles and reviews, as well as EAACI position articles, EAACI Task Force reports and EAACI guidelines.

Please indicate the Internet address of your society

http://www.eaaci.org corporate website

Cezmi Akdis, Davos

7

Bergmann K-C, Ring J (eds): History of Allergy. Chem Immunol Allergy. Basel, Karger, 2014, vol 100, pp 392–393
DOI: 10.1159/000360321

What is the society's complete title/name (and its abbreviation)?

Japanese Society of Allergology (JSA)

When and where was it established? What were the circumstances?

On the occasion of the first meeting of the International Association of Allergy (currently named World Allergy Organization), held in 1951, the preparation for organizing a Japanese society in allergology was initiated. In April of the next year the founding members gathered in Tokyo to agree on the society's regulation. The first official meeting of the JSA was held on October 17–18, 1952, in Tokyo. That was the birth of the Japanese Society of Allergology with 600 participants.

Who were the founding members of the society and from which medical disciplines did they come (e.g. dermatology, immunology, pulmonology)?

The first President of the JSA was Prof. Keizo Nakamura, Bacteriology, Nippon Medical School, Tokyo, Japan.

How many members does the society have today?

10,175 members as of October 31, 2011

What is the main emphasis of the society: immunology or allergy?

Allergy and clinical immunology

What are the society's most important prizes and honors?

The JSA Best Presentation Award, which is given annually to the best presentations selected from all the presentations of the two JSA meetings, the Spring and Autumn meetings.

What is the name of the society's journal? Which journal is the official organ of the society?

Japanese Journal of Allergology (in Japanese)
Allergology International (in English)

Please indicate the Internet address of your society

http://www.jsaweb.jp/ (for the Japanese page)
http://www.jsaweb.jp/modules/en (for the English page)

Kazuo Akiyama, Sagamihara

7

Bergmann K-C, Ring J (eds): History of Allergy. Chem Immunol Allergy. Basel, Karger, 2014, vol 100, pp 394–396
DOI: 10.1159/000360325

SLaai
Sociedad Latinoamericana de Alergia, Asma e Inmunología

What is the society's complete title/name (and its abbreviation)?

Sociedad Latinoamericana de Alergia, Asma e Inmunología (SLAAI) – Latin American Society of Allergy, Asthma and Immunology

When and where was it established? What were the circumstances?

In 1945, a group of allergists recognized the need to unite with a common language and geography and gain international representation by forming a partnership on a scientific basis. That motivated Dr. David M. Gordillo and Dr. Mario Sanchez, Presidents of the Allergy Societies of Mexico and Colombia, respectively, to organize the '1st Seminar of Allergy' and call together doctors from different countries in Latin America. Later, on October 18, 1961, a group of visionary medical doctors was meeting in New York with the firm purpose of enhancing friendship, strengthening scientific collaboration and establishing a scientific society. Among them were Dr. Carlos Canseco González, Dr. Ernesto Méndez, Dr. Mario Sánchez Medina, Dr. José Luis Cortez, Dr. Armando Pérez Lozano and Dr. Foruchman, from Mexico, Colombia, Argentina, Brazil and Venezuela. They signed a document stating the legal constitution of the Latin American Society. This event marked a watershed in the history of allergy in Latin America.

Who were the founding members of the society and from which medical disciplines did they come (e.g. dermatology, immunology, pulmonology)?

The founders of the Latin American Society were allergists from Mexico, Venezuela, Colombia, Brazil, Argentina and Ecuador:

Mexico: Dr. Carlos Canseco, Dr. David Gordillo, Dr. Julio Cueva, Dr. Pérez Martín and Dr. Romero;

Venezuela: Dr. Ortega Tamayo and Dr. Pérez Lozano;

Colombia: Dr. Mario Sánchez, Dr. Zubiria, Dr. Medina and Dr. Baquero;

Brazil: Dr. Croce Negreiros and Dr. Méndez; Argentina: Dr. Mathov and Dr. Raimondo; Ecuador: Dr. Naranjo and Dr. Moreno.

How many members does the society have today?

The SLAAI is an association of 18 member societies of 16 different countries in Latin America. The active members of the SLAAI number 2,418.

Argentina
Sociedad Argentina de Alergia e Inmunopatología
President: Dr. Betina Dwek
http://www.saaei-med.org/

Brazil
Associação Brasileira de Alergia e Imunopatologia
President: Dr. João Negreiros Tebyriçá
http://www.asbai.org.br

Colombia
Asociación Colombiana de Alergia, Asma e Inmunología
President: Dr. Gustavo Cuadros Trillos
http://www.asocaai.com/

Chile
Sociedad Chilena de Alergia e Inmunología
President: Dr. Paola Toche
http://www.scai.cl/

Republica Dominicana
Sociedad Dominicana de Alergia e Inmunología
President: Dr. Antonio J. Castillo

El Salvador
Asociación Salvadoreña de Alergia e Inmunología
President: Dr. María Emilia Castro Mendoza

Ecuador
Sociedad Ecuatoriana de Alergia e Inmunología
President: Dr. Manuel Viteri Acayturri
Sociedad Ecuatoriana de Alergia e Inmunología y Ciencias Afines
President: Dr. Sergio Barba Albán

Spain
Sociedad Española de Alergología e Inmunología Clinica
President: Dr. José María Olaguibel Rivera
http://www.seaic.org

Mexico
Colegio Mexicano de Pediatras Especialistas en Inmunología Clínica y Alergia (COMPEDIA)
President: Dr. Fernando Iduñate Palacio
http://www.compedia.org.mx/
Colegio Mexicano de Inmunología Clínica y Alergia, A.C. (CMICA)
President: Dr. Raúl Humberto Barnica Alvarado
http://www.cmica.org.mx

Panama
Sociedad Panameña de Alergia e Inmunología
President: Dr. Paulo Barrera

Paraguay
Sociedad Paraguaya de Alergia, Asma e Inmunología
President: Dr. Jaime A. Guggiari (h)
http://www.spaai.org.py/

Peru
Sociedad Peruana de Inmunopatología y Alergia
President: Dr. José Mori San Román

Portugal
Sociedade Portuguesa de Alergologia e Imunologia Clínica
President: Dr. Mário Morais de Almeida
http://www.spaic.pt

Uruguay
Sociedad Uruguaya de Alergología e Inmunología
President: Dr. Juan F. Schuhl

USA
Hispanic American Allergy and Immunology Association
President: Dr. Jorge Quel
http://www.haama.org/

Venezuela
Sociedad Venezolana de Alergia e Inmunología
President: Dr. Eliana Rísquez Cupello
http://www.svaai.org.ve/

What is the main emphasis of the society: immunology or allergy?

As a society we have a firm commitment to maintaining the highest levels of excellence amongst all of our members. This is to encourage continued participation at national and international conferences, where members of the Latin American Society present research projects, initiatives, publications, surveys and books with topics in both allergy and clinical immunology.

What are the society's most important prizes and honors?

Traditionally, at every scientific meeting held by the Latin American Society a Memorial Lecture is given and an award is bestowed to founders and shapers of the Latin American Society for their medical and scientific contributions.

What is the name of the society's journal? Which journal is the official organ of the society?

Revista Alergia México

Please indicate the Internet address of your society

http://www.slaai.org

Sandra Nora González Díaz, Monterrey

Bergmann K-C, Ring J (eds): History of Allergy. Chem Immunol Allergy. Basel, Karger, 2014, vol 100, pp 397–401
DOI: 10.1159/000360335

WAO™

WORLD ALLERGY ORGANIZATION

Sixty-two years back, the leaders in allergy from around the world felt the need to establish a professional society for allergy at an international level. This led to the official founding of an organization named the International Association of Allergy (IAA) [later named International Association of Allergology and Clinical Immunology (IAACI) and now World Allergy Organization (WAO)] in Zurich, in 1951. The first President of the IAA was Fred Wittich from the USA (from 1951 to 1955).

As described by Alain de Weck, former President of the IAACI, in his elaboration of the history of the IAACI (published in the *WAO Journal*; http://www.waojournal.org/) at the end of World War II, under the impulse primarily of physicians such as Robert Cooke, Mary Loveless and Fred W. Wittich, and scientists such as Merrill Chase (USA), William Frankland (UK), Pasteur Valéry-Radot (France), Bernard Halpern (France) and Mauricio Rocha e Silva (Brazil), the concept of allergic diseases based on similar pathophysiological mechanisms emerged. These diseases affecting different organs, such as the nose (rhinitis), the lungs (asthma), the skin (urticaria, atopic eczema and contact dermatitis) and the eye (conjunctivitis), or the cardiovascular system (anaphylaxis), were being diagnosed and treated by various medical specialists (dermatologists, internists, otorhinolaryngologists and ophthalmologists). Around 1950, nobody had been primarily or exclusively trained as an allergist. It was the discovery of reaginic antibodies by Prausnitz and Küstner, antigens and antibodies by Landsteiner and Heidelberger, allergens by Blackley and Haurowitz, and sensitized lymphocytes by Chase, that revealed the various underlying clinical phenomena that really created some unity of thinking and provided the emergence of allergy as a medical and scientific discipline.

In the first 2 decades after its establishment, the IAA mainly focused on the organization of triennial congresses, with no other activities in the interim period. However, during the period from 1950 to 1980 there were continuous exchanges between allergy and immunology. During the first IAA congresses, the program comprised of a wide range of topics encompassing not only clinical allergy, but also basic and clinical immunology (fig. 1). This resulted in the change of name of IAA to IAACI, which was officially endorsed at the X International Congress of

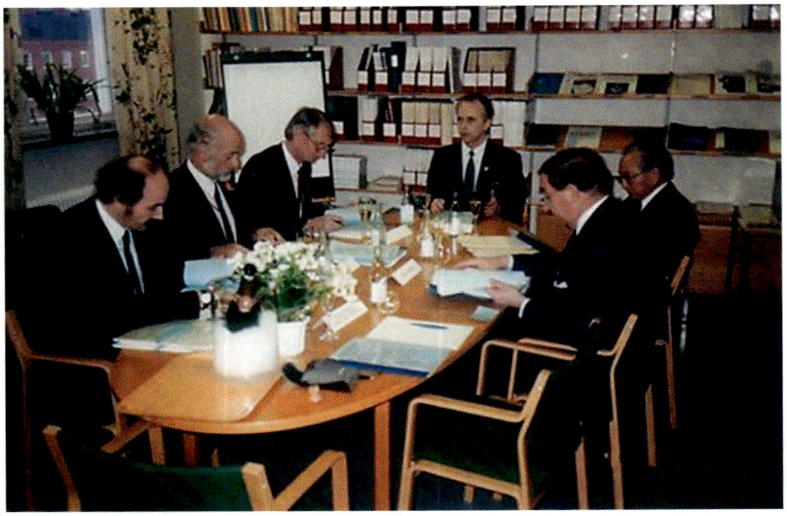

Fig. 1. WAO leaders met in Buenos Aires, December 1987. From left to right: Johannes Ring, John Bienenstock, Denis Stanworth, Gunnar Johansson, Andre Capron, Terumasa Miyamoto.

Allergology and Clinical Immunology in Jerusalem in 1979. One of the leaders who brought the two specialties together was Alain de Weck. He was also instrumental in the establishment of other scientific societies, such as the IUIS (International Union of Immunological Societies) and CIA (Collegium Internationale Allergologicum). During the 1970s and 1980s, there was close collaboration between the IAACI and IUIS which resulted in several common projects, such as allergen standardization – which was also in collaboration with the World Health Organization (WHO).

During the period between 1980 and 1995, the IAACI also pursued, beyond the organization of its triennial congresses, other initiatives based on practical needs and improvements in the practice of allergy. Among the various initiatives were a series of specialized workshops and international studies on house dust mite allergy and the establishment of a committee on Specialty and Training. In the later part of the 1990s, the WAO, the current successor of the IAACI, started to initiate a more active role in the interim period between the congresses, which led to the development of several programs, initiatives and committees. This new vision of the WAO was to optimize allergy care worldwide and serve as a global alliance of allergy and immunology societies with a mission to advance excellence in clinical care, research, education and training. Beginning in 1998, five areas of focus were identified and were put into place: education, communication, global recommendations, research and training. Also in support of this new vision, two important papers were created: the 'Prevention of allergy and allergic asthma (PAAA)', led by Gunnar Johansson and Tari Haahtela in 2004, and 'Revised nomenclature for allergy for global use: report of the nomenclature review committee of the WAO', an initiative to clarify allergy nomenclature spearheaded by Gunnar Johansson in 2003. In addition, beginning in 2003, the WAO decided to hold its congresses biennially.

Today, the WAO has 92 member societies and reaches out to more than 35,000 physicians worldwide. The WAO uses global surveys to collect data used for various purposes, including, but not limited to: needs assessments, consensus documents, guidelines, recommendations and state of allergy commentary. A majority of these global surveys have led to globally disseminated publications. Over the years, the WAO has developed several position papers that have influenced the world of allergy. Among them are position papers on 'The biodiversity hypothesis and allergic disease', 'Maintenance of skills, competencies, and performance in allergy and clinical immunology: time to lay the foundation for a universal approach', 'A guideline for the management of hereditary angioedema', 'WAO diagnosis and rationale for action against cow's milk allergy

(DRACMA) guidelines', 'Speaking a common language in grading subcutaneous immunotherapy systemic reactions: WAO subcutaneous immunotherapy systemic reaction grading system', 'Sublingual immunotherapy: WAO position paper 2009', 'Recommendations for appropriate sublingual immunotherapy clinical trials', 'EAACI/GA^{2}LEN/EDF/WAO guideline: definition, classification and diagnosis of urticaria', 'EAACI/GA^{2}LEN/EDF/WAO guideline: management of urticaria', 'Recommendations for competency in allergy training for undergraduates qualifying as medical practitioners', 'State of world allergy report 2008: allergy and chronic respiratory diseases', 'What is an allergist?', 'Requirements for physician competencies in allergy: key clinical competencies appropriate for the care of patients with allergic or immunologic diseases', 'Recommendations for standardization of clinical trials with allergen-specific immunotherapy for respiratory allergy', 'Allergy practice worldwide'. (A full list of WAO Position Papers and Statements can be found here: http://www.worldallergy.org/definingthespecialty/position_papers_and_statements.php) Several more position papers, statements and consensus documents are being developed currently. These global position papers are circulated to WAO member societies for their input in order to develop a global consensus and also to understand different practices around the world. The WAO is constantly scanning the environment to see where there is a need for other such documents to be developed. In addition, International Consensus (ICON) documents are also being jointly developed with the EAACI, AAAAI and ACAAI as part of a collaborative initiative called ICAALL (International Collaboration in Asthma and Allergy).

Furthermore, the WAO educational initiatives, such as GLORIA (Global Resources in Allergy), seminars and lectures, and the World Allergy Forum (WAF) were developed to bring state-of-the-art, cutting-edge knowledge on specific topics to our members (http://www.worldallergy.org/educational_programs). Also, in an effort to expand the specialty of allergy to emerging regions, the Emerging Societies Program (ESP) was developed, in collaboration with the ACAAI, as an important international outreach program to interact with areas that do not have allergy societies and to offer support in the development of the specialty. More recently, the WAO Allergy Training School (WATS), first held in 2009 in Dubai, has become an important and popular educational initiative of the ESP. Several successful WATS programs, in collaboration with the local societies and the National Ministry of Health, were subsequently held in Hanoi (2010); Moscow (2011); Cancun (2011); Nairobi (2012), and Hyderabad (2012), and will be held in Zimbabwe and Indonesia in 2013.

In 2008, to continue the WAO's growth, a number of 'special committees' were developed as a way to involve more allergists in the WAO and to develop new initiatives. Since 2008, this has further expanded and today we have a total of 30 committees, including these special committees, focusing on different disease areas or areas of interests (http://www.worldallergy.org/wao_societies/committeesandcouncils.php). The WAO has also developed recommendations for undergraduate training in allergy and is in the process of developing curriculum materials to be made available for national societies and for use in medical schools.

One of WAO's flagship initiatives was the development of the *WAO Journal* in 2008 with Johannes Ring as the first Editor-in-Chief and proceeded by the leadership of Lanny Rosenwasser as Editor-in-Chief. The *WAO Journal* is an online-only international journal accessible to all allergists free of charge (www.waojournal.org). The *WAO Journal* publishes monthly postings of original research and review articles and maintains an online archive. This journal is now an open-access journal and is indexed on PubMed Central.

A major endeavor of the WAO was the development of the *WAO White Book on Allergy* (http://www.worldallergy.org/definingthespecialty/white_book.php), which emphasizes the importance of the specialty of allergy, the need for enhanced medical teaching of allergic diseases, and the necessity to provide specialized treatment for the tens of millions of allergy sufferers worldwide. It contains state-of-the-art information on allergy worldwide and is designed as a way to influence government decision makers when considering the distribution of resources among various medical specialties.

Another important initiative deliberated about from 2008 but initiated in 2010 was the WAO International Scientific Conference (WISC). WISC is a theme-based scientific meeting that alternates with and complements the WAO's biennial World Allergy Congress (WAC). The WISC provides a forum for the latest research, reviews of current theory and practice, and hands-on problem-based learning. Participants gain insight into the most effective advances in the diagnosis and management of allergy and asthma. WISC 2010 was held in Dubai with the theme of 'Asthma and its Co-Morbidities' and WISC 2012 was held in Hyderabad, with the theme of 'Severe Allergies, Severe Asthma: New Strategies for Optimal Treatment and Management'. WISC 2014 will be held in Rio de Janeiro, under the leadership of Lanny Rosenwasser, who will be President of the organization for the 2014–2015 term.

The WAC remains one of the major focal points of the WAO. The last WAC was held in Milan in June 2013 in collaboration with European Academy of Allergy and Clinical Immunology (EAACI), and the following WACs will be held in Seoul in 2015, with the Korean Academy of Allergy and Clinical Immunology, and then in the USA in 2018 with the American Academy of Allergy Asthma and Clinical Immunology (AAAAI). At its biennial congress, the WAO confers prestigious awards, such as the Gold Medal Award, Distinguished Service Award, Scientific Achievement Award, Outstanding Clinician Award and the Special Recognition Award. This year the WAO will also confer the Lifetime Achievement Award to Prof. Alain de Weck (posthumously).

The WAO's website, www.worldallergy.org, is a premier global allergy and immunology resource. The site supports, complements and enhances all WAO educational activities, provides essential information for physicians and patients about global allergy and immunology activities in an easily navigable format, and provides links to important allergy and immunology resources across the Web. The WAO website also acts as a portal for online and distance learning, and hosts pages dedicated to specific diseases or target audiences, including patients. The website is continuously redesigned to include online lectures, webinars, CME modules, various forms of educational resources, allergy quiz, WAO news and notes, Presidents' messages, book reviews, resources that contribute to 'defining the specialty', junior members' initiatives, ask the expert, WAO TV, and much more.

Table 1. List of WAO presidents

2012–2013	Ruby Pawankar (Japan)
2010–2011	Richard F. Lockey (USA)
2008–2009	G. Walter Canonica (Italy)
2006–2007	Michael A. Kaliner (USA)
2003–2005	Carlos E. Baena-Cagnani (Argentina)
2000–2003	Allen P. Kaplan (USA)
1997–2000	S.G.O. Johansson (Sweden)
1994–1997	Albert K. Oehling (Spain)
1991–1994	Terumasa Miyamoto (Japan)
1990–1991	Albert K. Oehling (Spain)
1988–1990	Jacques P. Charpin (France)
1985–1988	Alain L. de Weck (Switzerland)
1982–1985	Jack Pepys (UK)
1979–1982	Carl E. Arbesman (USA)
1976–1979	Enrique Mathov (Argentina)
1973–1976	Tiuzi Sindo (Japan)
1970–1973	Max Samter (USA)
1967–1970	Umberto Serafini (Italy)
1964–1967	Bram Rose (Canada)
1961–1964	Carlos Jimenez Diaz (Spain)
1958–1961	Bernard M. Halpern (France)
1955–1958	Samuel M. Feinberg (USA)
1951–1955	Fred Wittich (USA)

Beginning with the first event in July 2005, the WAO has hosted a 'World Allergy Day' in association with the biennial World Allergy Congress. Realizing the need to expand this program and bring greater awareness across the globe, the WAO initiated World Allergy Week (WAW) in 2011 as an annual program of the WAO together with its member societies to raise the awareness of allergic disease, its related disorders, and advocate for the provision of training and resources in the diagnosis, management and prevention of these diseases and asthma. The WAO established the initiative with the vision of bringing together multiple stakeholder groups, including physicians, medical educators, patient advocates, policy makers, the general public and healthcare authorities for an integrated approach to addressing the needs of patients who suffer from allergic diseases and asthma, and those who provide care for them.

The WAO is interacting with several international key organizations, including the United Nations and World Health Organization (WHO) for advocating the cause of allergy as a global health issue, and with regulatory bodies like the European Medicines Agency (EMA) and Food and Drug Administration (FDA) in the USA for harmonization of certain therapeutic areas at a global level. The WAO is in the process of recognizing and naming WAO Centers of Excellence and is actively collaborating with other related organizations in addition to member societies.

While we and some of our predecessors have had the privilege of serving the Organization in various positions leading up to becoming the President of the WAO (table 1), the successful initiatives of the Organization, its vision and direction have been carved and shaped by the dedicated and valuable contribution and collegiality of several colleagues around the world who have served or are serving on the Board of Directors, the various committees and councils, the faculty at conferences, those who have participated in the various initiatives and our 92 member societies. Finally, the life and pillars of strength of the Organization are our WAO staff, to who we owe a lot for their dedication, professionalism and courteousness 'service with a smile'.

Ruby Pawankar, Tokyo (President, WAO)
Giorgio W. Canonica, Genoa (Historian, WAO)

Correspondence to: Prof. Ruby Pawankar
Department of Pediatrics
Nippon Medical School
1-1-5 Sendagi, Bunkyo-ku
Tokyo 113-8603 (Japan)
E-Mail pawankar.ruby@gmail.com
Tel./Fax +81 3 5802 8177

Bergmann K-C, Ring J (eds): History of Allergy. Chem Immunol Allergy. Basel, Karger, 2014, vol 100, pp 402–404
DOI: 10.1159/000360337

AAAAI Archives

Since 1943, the American Academy of Allergy, Asthma & Immunology (AAAAI) has been dedicated to the advancement of the knowledge of allergy, asthma and immunology for optimal patient care. Throughout the decades, the AAAAI has worked to achieve this mission through annual educational meetings, peer-reviewed journals, fellowship and research grants, public education campaigns, practice and policy endeavors, and collaborative workgroup reports, position statements and practice parameters (fig. 1).

Along the way, the AAAAI has accumulated a wealth of historical artifacts and materials that paint a picture of the specialty's past and offer a glimpse at the AAAAI growth and development. In the late 1990s, the AAAAI Board of Directors directed the Academy to create an archive to document and preserve these records. Today, researchers from around the world now tap this extensive archive collection to study both the history of the organization and advances in treating allergic and immunologic diseases.

The AAAAI archives are housed within the Archives Department of the University of Wisconsin-Milwaukee Libraries, located in the state of Wisconsin, USA. These impressive archives consist of 506 boxes, 40 binders, 115 audio files, including oral histories, and 1,186 digital text files, film reels, and historical artifacts. The materials span 15 categories including 70 years of Annual Meeting documents, more than 8 decades of peer-reviewed journals, public education materials and AAAAI business-related records.

Of particular interest are the tins and cartons of early 20th century asthma and allergy treatments (fig. 2, 3). The collection features, for example, a tin of 'Dr. Kinaman's Asthma Remedy' that dates from the turn of the 20th century. While the tin does not list ingredients for the 'asthma remedy', the directions state that a person should place a teaspoonful on a plate, set fire to it and inhale the fumes. The collection also includes cardboard boxes of 'Dr. Guild's Green Mountain Asthmatic Cigarettes' from the 1940s and 'Abbott's Allergenic Extra of Mixed Ragweed Pollen' from the 1950s.

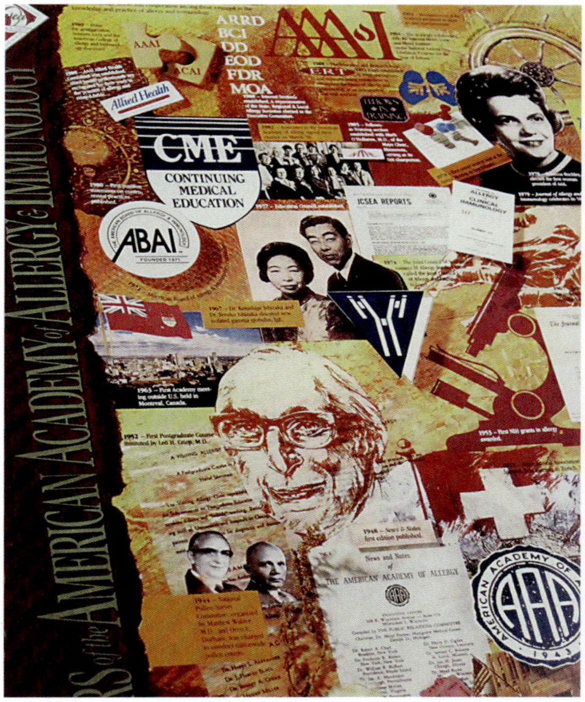

Fig. 1. Cover of the program on the occasion of the 50th anniversary of the American Academy of Allergy and Immunology.

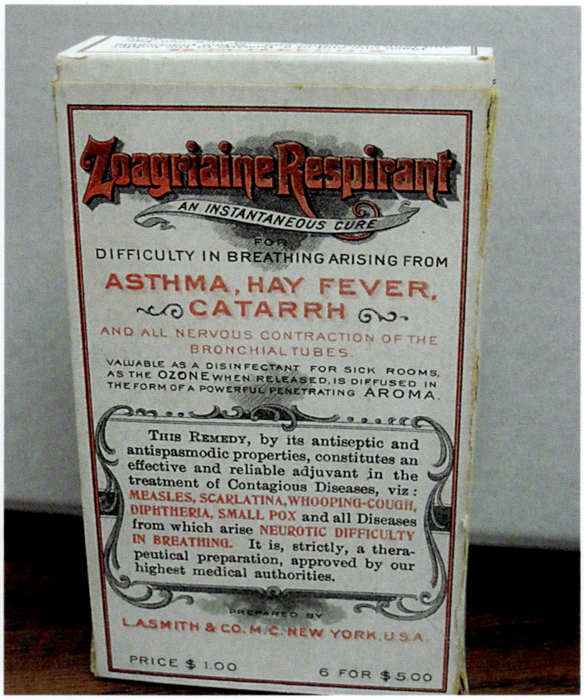

Fig. 2. Zoagriaine Respirant remedy advertised for asthma, hay fever and catarrh from Lasmith and Co. in New York.

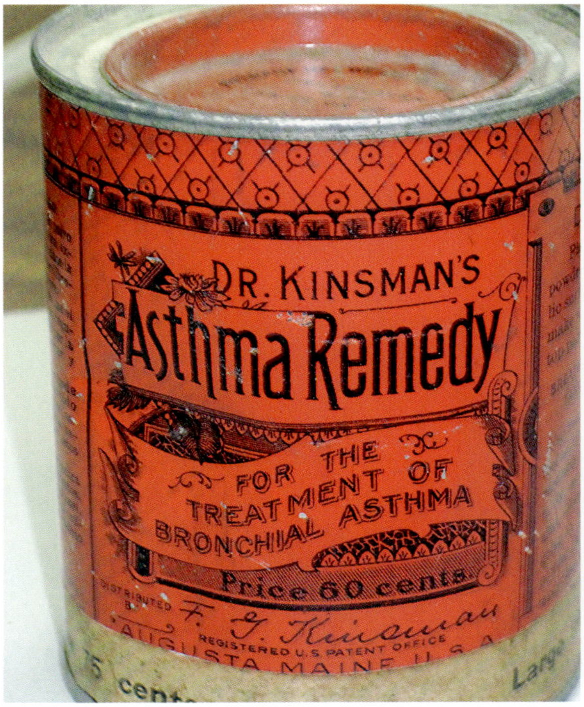

Fig. 3. A box of Dr. Kinsman's Asthma Remedy.

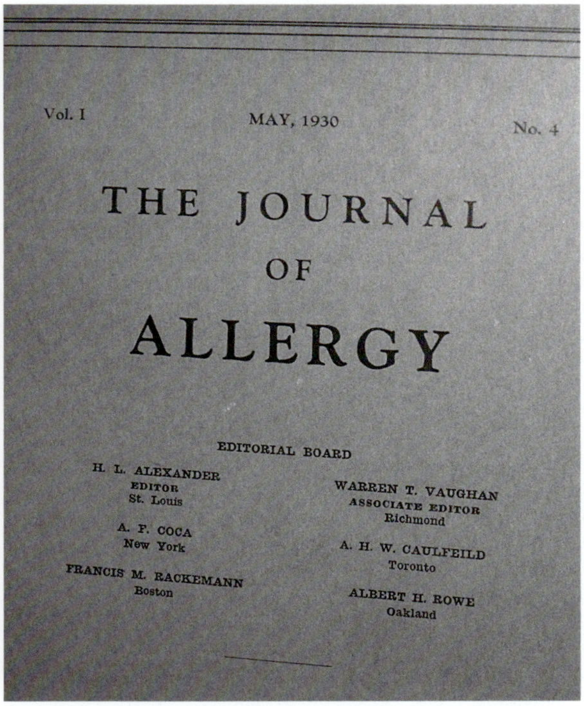

Fig. 4. Title page of the 4th issue of volume 1 of *The Journal of Allergy* from May 1930.

Visitors to the archives can also gain access to the AAAAI's peer-reviewed journal dating back to its inception in 1929, when *The Journal of Allergy and Clinical Immunology* was known simply as *The Journal of Allergy* (fig. 4). A copy from November 1929 (vol. 1, issue 1) gives insight into the allergy issues of interest to physicians in the 1920s. 'The relations of bacterial allergy to scarlet fever' and 'Cedar hay fever', for example, are among the articles listed in the table of contents.

More historical information can be found in the taped oral histories from former AAAAI presidents and other leaders in the specialty. These audio files contain reports of milestones in the history of the organization, the AAAAI's impact on the field of allergy and immunology, and advances in the management and treatment of allergic and immunologic diseases. While the oral histories have restricted access for the lifetime of the participant, persons interested in reading or listening to them can be granted special access by contacting the archivist.

The UW-Milwaukee Libraries Archives Department is open to the public on weekdays. The mailing address is: Archives Department, UWM Libraries, 2311 East Hartford Avenue, PO Box 604, Milwaukee, WI 53201, USA.

Bergmann K-C, Ring J (eds): History of Allergy. Chem Immunol Allergy. Basel, Karger, 2014, vol 100, pp 405–408
DOI: 10.1159/000360343

The Ilya Mechnikov Collection in Riga

One of the most interesting and valuable collections at the Pauls Stradins Museum of the History of Medicine in Riga is that of Ilya Mechnikov (1845–1916), who established the theory related to phagocytosis and studied immunology. The history of the collection is unusual in that it has been cared for by several institutions. After Mechnikov's death in 1916, his second wife, Olga Mechnikova, tried to preserve her husband's scientific heritage and ensure that it would be available to scholars and other interested parties. The Pauls Stradins Museum has held the collection since 1975, and it was first displayed to the public in 1982.

Mechnikov's widow carefully arranged his articles, lectures, research protocols, and extensive correspondence with distinguished scholars and other individuals. This far-sighted work preserved evidence of the famous scientist and his work, and to a certain extent also reflected the development of the natural sciences in the late 19th and early 20th century.

Olga first offered the materials to the Institute Pasteur in Paris, where her late husband had spent the last 29 years of his life and where he was buried. The historical building of the institute, alas, was not appropriate for the composition, and the director, Emile Roux, suggested that it be housed in a new building which was not finished at that time. It appears that this was the reason why Olga Mechnikova contacted one of her late husband's students and good friends, Lev Tarasevich (1868–1929), who suggested that the collection be transported to his Institute of Experimental Therapy and Control of Serums and Vaccines in Moscow, where a museum could be established for that purpose.

Some of the collection was transported from Paris to Moscow in August 1926, but the rest of it remained with Olga until 1935, when some more items were contributed to the museum in Moscow. She herself was the curator of the first exhibition. On September 22, 1926, the scientific council of the State Institute for the People's Welfare heard the unusual

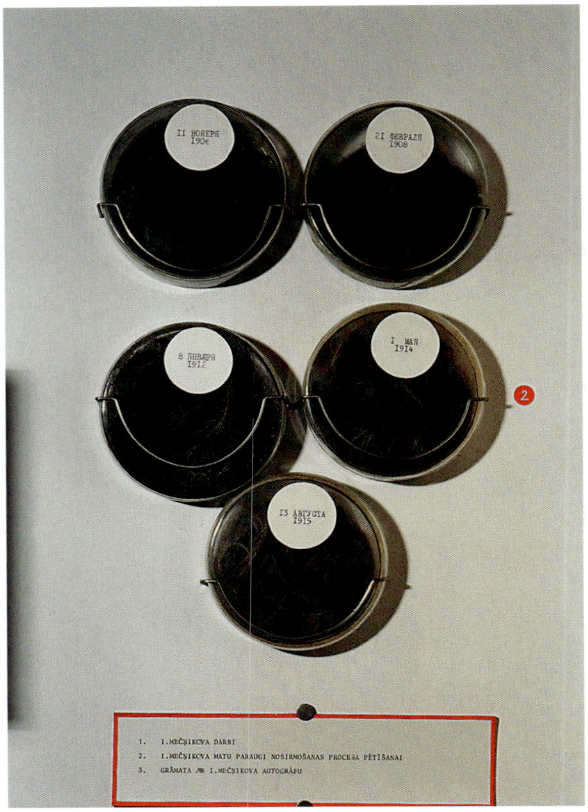

Fig. 1. Ilya Mechnikov's hair samples for his study on graying (1906–1915).

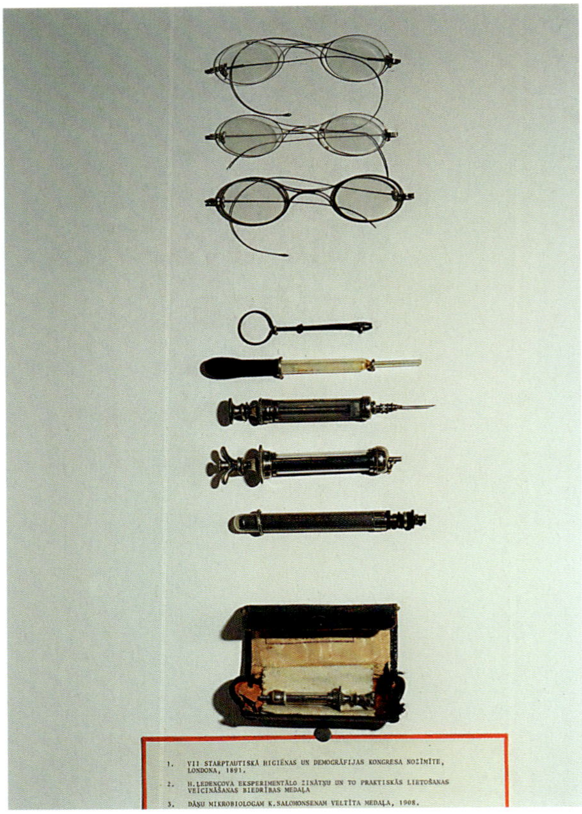

Fig. 2. Personal belongings of Ilya Mechnikov (from top): Mechnikov's glasses, glass tube holder, dropper, injection syringe with needle, injection syringe, syringe metal carry case, syringe leather case.

dedication statement of Mrs. Mechnikova, in which she wrote: 'I think that the collected materials can serve the cultural sector of the history of biology and medicine for half a century to study the working processes of Ilya Mechnikov and remembering him as a man who devoted his entire life to science.' She also expressed the desire that her late husband's materials be kept together, that his correspondence not be published for the time being, and that work on a compendium of Mechnikov's papers should begin.

The museum was opened the next day, and Health Commissioner Nikolai Semashko (1874–1949) invited Olga Mechnikov to become the honorary patroness of the institution. Her partnership with the museum was interrupted by World War II and Olga died in 1944.

Initially the collection was made up of four large groups of materials. The first included print materials which Mechnikov released in various languages, as well as books about him, the work of other scientists, fiction and notes. The second group was made up of handwritten manuscripts and documents, including Mechnikov's notebooks from 1861, research protocols beginning in 1884, manuscripts, lectures, delivered papers, records of an expedition to the steppes of Kalmykia, observations about his own illnesses, correspondence, diplomas and greetings, etc. The third group is iconographic in that it includes paintings, portraits, photographs and illustrations for publications. The fourth and last group contains personal objects owned by Mechnikov (fig. 1, 2) – silver dishes, an inkwell, a pen, work instruments, a

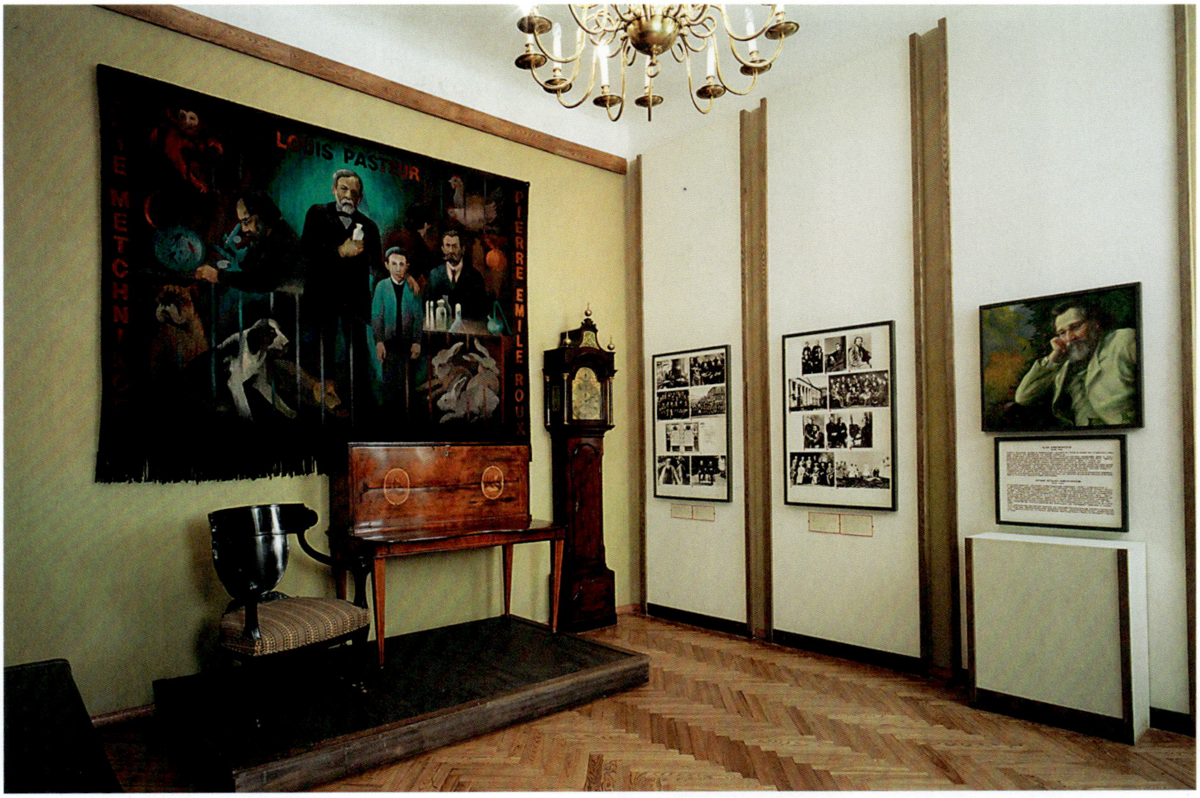

Fig. 3. Part of the interior of the exhibition dedicated to Ilya Mechnikov at the Pauls Stradins Museum of the History of Medicine in Riga (Latvia).

seal, 26 Petri dishes with samples of the scientist's hair, as well as orders and medals which he received during his lifetime.

The museum was split into two parts in 1950. The manuscripts and documents were transferred to the archive of the Soviet Academy of Medical Science, while his personal effects, publications, paintings and photographs became the foundation for a new memorial museum at the Mechnikov Institute for the Scientific Study of Serums and Vaccines near Moscow. The valuable collection remained there until 1965, when it was transferred to the History Department of the Gamaleya Institute of Microbiology and Epidemiology of the Soviet Academy of Medical Science. Annual reports from the department show that the collection was endangered in that there was no room for it, and it did not have a curator. The presidium of the academy voted in 1975 to transfer the collection, except for manuscripts and documents, to the Pauls Stradins Museum of the History of Medicine in Riga so as to preserve the collection and ensure its accessibility (fig. 3).

The received collection included books published by Mechnikov, many of them published with the author's notes, as well as five volumes of scholarly papers published between 1865 and 1916 and, in many cases, dedicated by the author to his wife. Some of the volumes are in ornate covers with the initials of Olga Nikolayevna or Ilya Ilyich Mechnikov. There are also books of fiction, popular magazines from the era, notes and books about the history of art.

The iconographic section of the collection includes valuable paintings by Olga Mechnikova, who was an artist – portraits of her husband, a self-portrait and landscapes (12 canvases in all; fig. 4). The

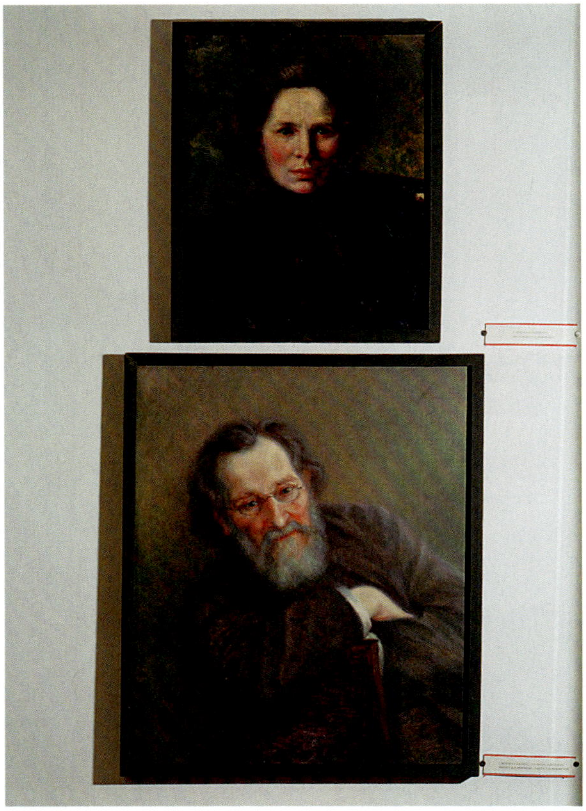

Fig. 4. O. Mechnikova, self-portrait, oi , not dated (above); I. Mechnikov by O. Mechnikova, oil, 1912 (below).

museum also has an outstanding portrait of Ilya Mechnikov that was painted by his wife's teacher, Eugene Carrière (1849–1906), as well as two water color miniature portraits of the scientist's parents by artist M. Vishnevecki (1801–1871).

Of particular value are Mechnikov's orders and medals, including the Nobel Prize which he and Paul Ehrlich received in 1908 for their study of immunology. There is also the Godfrey Copley (1653–1709) Medal from the Royal Society of London, several orders from the French Legion of Order (the class of Knight, Officer and Commander), the 4th class Order of St. Vladimir IV from Russia, and the Japanese Order of the Rising Sun, etc. The Pauls Stradins Museum of the History of Medicine processed and restored all of the exhibits, and they are part of the national collection. Initially they were only displayed at exhibitions of new exhibits, but since 1982 the museum has had a separate memorial hall for Mechnikov. In January 2014, Mechnikov's collection was extended with a new exhibition for the Nobel Prize winners in physiology and medicine.

The Pauls Stradins Museum of the History of Medicine is open daily (except Sundays and Mondays) at Antonijas Street 1, LV–1360 Riga, Latvia. The museum can be found on the Internet at www.mvm.lv. Tel. +371 6722 2914, E-Mail info@mvm.lv.

Juris Salaks, Riga

References

1 Mechnikova ON: Zhizn' Il'i Il'icha Mechnikova. Moscow, Gosudarstvennoe Izdatel'stvo, 1926, p 232.
2 Gosudarstvennyj Nauchnyj Institut Zdravoohranenija (SSSR): Muzej pamjati I.I. Mechnikova. Moscow, Gosmedizdat, 1930, p 71.
3 Ilja Mečnikovs: Sastādīja Aija Dirbe. Riga, Pauls Stradins Museum, 1988.
4 Zalkind S: Ilya Mechnikov: His Life and Work. Honolulu, University Press of the Pacific, 2001, p 212.

8 Online Supplementary Material

Online Supplementary Material

Bergmann K-C, Ring J (eds): History of Allergy. Chem Immunol Allergy. Basel, Karger, 2014, vol 100, pp 410
DOI: 10.1159/000360357

Movie 1: Anaphylaxie et Allergie

In 1901, the Prince of Monaco organized a scientific expedition on his research vessel in the coastal waters of the Azores and Cape Verde islands. Prof. Charles Richet (1850–1935) and Prof. Paul Portier (1866–1962) were aboard and carried out scientific experiments.

They thought (then realized) that an extract from sea anemones was very toxic, with the injection in small laboratory animals already in low tins. After returning to the Pasteur Institute in Paris they decided to continue the experiments in dogs for better interpretation of the reactions. Portier suggested that Richet try an immunization of the animals against the toxin.

The 'core attempt' consisted of a dog called Neptune receiving the second injection (booster) 27 days after the first injection. The reaction to this second injection with a very low dose, which had led to no reaction in a control dog, was dramatic – Neptune broke down!

Portier and Richet had discovered a completely new and unexpected phenomenon to which they gave the name 'anaphylaxis'. The experiments leading to the realization of anaphylaxis are described in the historic film 'Anaphylaxie et Allergie' [see www.karger.com/chial100_movie1] in which the 93-year-old Paul Portier also explains the coinage of the term 'anaphylaxie'.

The film is in color and was recorded in 1956, with a length of about 46 min. After the introduction by Portier the anaphylactic shock of a dog is shown. Afterwards, the principles of allergic reactions, diagnosis and therapy, including hyposensitization, are explained.

K.-C. Bergmann, Berlin

Bergmann K-C, Ring J (eds): History of Allergy. Chem Immunol Allergy. Basel, Karger, 2014, vol 100, pp 411–412
DOI: 10.1159/000360358

Movie 2: World Allergy: The Disease of Civilization

On the occasion of the International Congress of Allergology and Clinical Immunology (ICACI; now called World Allergy Congress) in Stockholm in June 1994, the incoming president, Prof. Alain de Weck, initiated the production of a movie on essential aspects of the history of allergy. The film [see www.karger.com/chial100_movie2] starts with a reflection on history and the presumed first allergic individual, namely Pharaoh Menes from the old dynasty in Egypt, who supposedly died because he was stung by a wasp. However, critical analysis offers an alternative account – that he was killed by a hippopotamus. The movie takes us to the zoo in Monaco and we also learn about the birth of the term anaphylaxis.

Going back in history, the classical questions of Hippocrates about how the patient feels and how to analyze his or her history were for the first time supplemented with regard to allergological questions by Ramazzini, around 1700, who also added a new question regarding the occupation of the patient, thus giving the first description of baker's asthma.

Alain de Weck acts as a guide and interpreter in this movie and gives his often very personal and precisely put thoughts. In a random series of interviews you can see and listen to top researchers, all of whom are regarded as pioneers. Jack Pepys describes the discovery of *Micropolyspora* as the trigger of farmer's lung, seen as 'the needle in a haystack'. The Nobel laureate Bengt Samuelsson describes his discovery of leukotrienes as carriers of the slow-reacting substance of anaphylaxis. Other Nobel laureates to be mentioned in allergy history are Charles Richet, the discoverer of anaphylaxis, Paul Ehrlich, who came up with the first chemotherapeutic agent and with the side-chain theory that gave an impression on T cell receptors, and Daniel Bovet, who invented the first antihistamine.

OSM

Other pioneers giving interviews in the movie include Larry Lichtenstein on the topic of basophils and their releasability, and S.G.O. Johansson, who reflects on the summer of 1965, when he recognized an abnormal electrophoresis pattern in a single patient which turned out to be the first case of IgE myeloma. Terumasa Miyamoto was the first to provide evidence for the role of pollutants in the rising prevalence of allergic diseases, mainly diesel exhaust and cedar pollinosis in Japan. Patrick Holt speculates on the neonatal phase, which is decisive in early life with regard to the development of allergy or tolerance. François Michel stresses the role of allergy in asthma. Bengt Björksten and M. Riikjärf talk about their experience in comparing allergy prevalences between Swedish and Estonian children, and their different lifestyles. Heidrun Behrendt comments on the German comparison study between West and East German children after reunification and the influence of an 'experimentum dictaturae' upon allergy development, as well as the influence of air pollutants on pollen grains in the ambient air.

Finally, Alain de Weck concludes with the question of whether allergy may be the price to be paid for civilization?

Johannes Ring, Munich

List of Illustrations / Figure Credits

p. 42 Fig. 33: Urbach E: Klinik und Therapie der allergischen Krankheiten. Vienna, Wilhelm Maudrich, 1935.
p. 43 Fig. 35: Urbach E: Methodik des Allergennachweises. Munch Med Wochenschr 1933; 80:134.
p. 43 Fig. 37: Copyright KEYSTONE/Science Photo Library/US National Library of Medicine/ Sheldon G. Cohen.

p. 55 Fig. 1: The National Library of Medicine.
p. 56 Fig. 3, 4: Musée océanographique de Monaco.
p. 57 Fig. 5, 6: Musée océanographique de Monaco.
p. 58 Fig. 7: Courtesy of Josef Donnerer.

p. 70 Fig. 1, 2: Bing LU: Outlines of Chinese History. Shanghai, Shanghai Commercial Press, 1914.
p. 70 Fig. 3: The National Library of Medicine.
p. 71 Fig. 4: Deutsches Apotheken-Museum, Heidelberg, Germany.
p. 72 Fig. 5: Wellcome Library, London.
p. 73 Fig. 6: Bibliothèque de l'Académie Nationale de Médecine.
p. 74 Fig. 8: The Bodleian Libraries, The University of Oxford G.A. Staffs 4° 8, 562/563.
p. 74 Fig. 9: Wellcome Library, London.
p. 75 Fig. 10: Wellcome Library, London.
p. 75 Fig. 11: Ruysch F: Opera Omnia. 1721, tome 21.
p. 76 Fig. 12: Amsterdam Museum.
p. 76 Fig. 13: Copyright The Hunterian, University of Glasgow, 2013.
p. 77 Fig. 14, 15: The National Library of Medicine.
p. 77 Fig. 16: Wellcome Library, London.
p. 78 Fig. 17: Charcot JM, Vulpian EFA: Note sur les cristaux particuliers trouvés dans le sang et les viscères d'un sujet leucémique. Gaz Méd (Paris) 1860;7:755.
p. 78 Fig. 18: The National Library of Medicine.
p. 78 Fig. 19: Photograph by Nicola Perscheid, 1906. The National Library of Medicine.
p. 78 Fig. 20: The National Library of Medicine.

p. 84 Fig. 1: Ferdinand Hebra: Atlas der Hautkrankheiten. Vienna, 1864. Leaflet IV, plate 12, fig a: Eczema impetiginosum faciei, Porrigo larvalis Willan (Anton Elfinger).
p. 85 Fig. 2: Collection of the Musée Photographique de l'Hôpital Saint-Louis, ref. 29/605.
p. 86 Fig. 3: Collection of the Musée Photographique de l'Hôpital Saint-Louis, Paris, ref. 3/261. Reproduced in Brocq L: Traité de dermatologie pratique. Paris, Doin, 1907, tome II, p 155.
p. 86 Fig. 4: Collection of the Société française d'histoire de la dermatologie.
p. 87 Fig. 5: Brocq L: Traité élémentaire de dermatologie pratique. Paris, Doin, 1907, tome I, pp 42–43.
p. 88 Fig. 6: Collection of the Société française d'histoire de la dermatologie.
p. 91 Fig. 7: Fitzpatrick et al: Dermatology in General Medicine. New York, McGraw Hill, 1971, p 683. Reproduced with permission.

p. 111 Fig. 2: Wellcome Library, London.
p. 112 Fig. 3: Author's own material.
p. 115 Fig. 4: Modified version of Wüthrich B, Ballmer-Weber BK: Klinik der Nahrungsmittelallergien; in Jäger L, Wüthrich B, Ballmer-Weber B, Vieths S (eds): Nahrungsmittelallergien und -intoleranzen: Immunologie – Diagnostik – Therapie – Prophylaxe, ed 3. Munich, Urban & Fischer, 2008, p 65.
p. 116 Fig. 5: Wüthrich B: Oral desensitization with cow's milk in cow's milk allergy; in Wüthrich B, Ortolani C (eds): Highlights in Food Allergy. Basel, Karger, 1996, pp 236–240.

p. 123 Fig. 1: Jacobi E: Atlas der Hautkrankheiten, ed 3. Berlin, Urban und Schwarzenberg, 1907.
p. 124 Fig. 2: Jacobi E: Atlas der Hautkrankheiten, ed 3. Berlin, Urban und Schwarzenberg, 1907.
p. 127 Fig. 3: Jacobi E: Atlas der Hautkrankheiten, ed 3. Berlin, Urban und Schwarzenberg, 1907.
p. 128 Fig. 4: Jacobi E: Atlas der Hautkrankheiten, ed 3. Berlin, Urban und Schwarzenberg, 1907.

p. 141 Fig. 1: Kaplan AP, Greaves MW: Angioedema. J Am Acad Dermatol 2005;53:373–388.
p. 144 Fig. 2: Fields T, Ghebrehiwet B, Kaplan AP: Kinin formation in hereditary angioedema plasma: evidence against kinin derivation from C2 and in support of 'spontaneous' formation of bradykinin. J Allergy Clin Immunol 1983;72:54–60.
p. 145 Fig. 3: Author's own material.

p. 156 Fig. 1: Author's own material.
p. 158 Fig. 2: Author's own material.
p. 160 Fig. 3: Author's own material.
p. 162 Fig. 4: Author's own material.
p. 163 Fig. 5: Author's own material.

p. 166 Fig. 1a, b: Pincus et al: Properties of structurally restricted antibody to type VIII pneumococcal polysaccharide. J Immunol 1970;104:1149–11544. Copyright The American Association of Immunologists Inc.
p. 166 Fig. 1c, d: Tomioka H, Ishizaka K: Mechanisms of passive sensitization. II. Presence of receptors for IgE on monkey mast cells. J Immunol 1971;107:974. Copyright The American Association of Immunologists Inc.

p. 167 Fig. 2: Adapted from fig. 1 of Kitamura Y, Yokoyama M, Matsuda H, Ohno T, Mori KJ: Spleen colony-forming cell as common precursor for tissue mast cells and granulocytes. Nature 1981;291:159–160.
p. 169 Fig. 3: Author's own material.

p. 174 Fig. 1: Author's own material.
p. 178 Fig. 2: Author's own material.
p. 183 Fig. 3: Author's own material.

p. 194 Fig. 1: Extracted and adapted from Wharton Jones T: The blood-corpuscle considered in its different phases of development in the animal series. Memoir I. Vertebrata. Philosophic Trans Royal Soc London 1846;136:63–87. Plate I, 1st phase.
p. 194 Fig. 2: Extracted and adapted from fig. 1 and 4 in Brewer DB: Max Schultze and the living, moving, phagocytosing leucocytes: 1865. Med Hist 1994;38:91–101.
p. 195 Fig. 3: http://en.wikipedia.org/wiki/File:Paul_Ehrlich_Arbeitszimmer.jpg.
p. 201 Fig. 4: Picture of eosinophil extracted from http://en.wikipedia.org/wiki/File:Eosinophil2.png.

p. 207 Fig. 1: Kaplan AP, Austen KF: A pre-albumin activator of prekallikrein. J Immunol 1970;105:802–811.
p. 207 Fig. 2: Silverberg M, Dunn J, Garen L, Kaplan AP: Autoactivation of human Hageman factor. Demonstration utilizing a synthetic substrate. J Biol Chem 1980;255:7281–7286.
p. 208 Fig. 3: Mandle RJ Jr, Kaplan AP: Hageman factor substrates. Human plasma prekallikrein mechanism of activation by Hageman factor and participation in Hageman factor-dependent fibrinolysis. J Biol Chem 1977;252:6097–6104.
p. 210 Fig. 4: Author's own material.
p. 211 Fig. 5: Author's own material.
p. 212 Fig. 6: Joseph K, Tholanikunnel BG, Kaplan AP: Factor XII-independent cleavage of high-molecular-weight kininogen by prekallikrein and inhibition by C1 inhibitor. J Allergy Clin Immunol 2009;124:143–149.

p. 220 Fig. 1: Author's own material.
p. 221 Fig. 2: Author's own material.

p. 230 Fig. 1: The Society for the Promotion of Palynological Research in Austria. http://www.paldat.org/. Picture credit: H. Halbritter.
p. 230 Fig. 2: Miall LC: History of Biology. London, Watts & Co, 1911.
p. 230 Fig. 3: Oliver FW (ed): Makers of British Botany. Cambridge, Cambridge University Press, 1913.
p. 231 Fig. 4: Grew N: Anatomy of Plants. London, Rawlins, 1682.
p. 231 Fig. 5: Grew N: Anatomy of Plants. London, Rawlins, 1682.

p. 235 Fig. 1: Private collection.
p. 235 Fig. 2: Private collection.
p. 236 Fig. 3: Private collection.
p. 236 Fig. 4: Private collection.

p. 250 Fig. 1: Author's own material.
p. 253 Fig. 2: Author's own material.

p. 262 Fig. 1: Taken from IPR006044 and Becker WM, Schocker F, Petersen A: Allergene der Erdnuss: Struktur und Charakteristika; in Werfel T, Wüthrich B (eds): Nahrungsmittel und Allergie. Munich, Dustri, 2010, pp 156–166.
p. 262 Fig. 2: Modified from fig. 4a in Krause S, Latendorf T, Schmidt H, Darcan-Nicolaisen Y, Reese G, Petersen A, Janssen O, Becker WM: Peanut varieties with reduced Ara h 1 content indicating no reduced allergenicity. Mol Nutr Food Res 2010;54:381–387. Copyright Wiley-VCH Verlag GmbH & Co. KGaA. Reproduced with permission. Allocation of the allergens according to fig. 3 from Schmidt H, Gelhaus C, Latendorf T, Nebendahl M, Petersen A, Krause S, Leippe M, Becker WM, Janssen O: 2-D DIGE analysis of the proteome of extracts from peanut variants reveals striking differences in major allergen contents. Proteomics 2009;9:3507–3521.
p. 263 Fig. 3: Authors' own material.

p. 274 Fig. 1: Behrendt H: Grundlagen der Allergie und mögliche Angriffspunkte für Umweltchemikalien. Allergologie 1989;12:95–99.

p. 279 Fig. 1: Kunsthaus Zürich.
p. 280 Fig. 2: Author's own material.
p. 282 Fig. 3: Author's own material.
p. 283 Fig. 4: Author's own material.
p. 285 Fig. 5: Author's own material.

p. 290 Fig. 1: Oliver G, Schäfer EA: On the physiological action of extract of the suprarenal capsules. J Physiol 1894;16:I–IV.
p. 294 Fig. 2: Dahlström A, Fuxe K: Evidence for the existence of monoamine neurons in the central nervous system. I. Demonstration of monoamines in the cell bodies of brain stem neurons. Acta Physiol Scand 1964;62(suppl 247):1–55.
p. 296 Fig. 3: Dale HH: On some physiological actions of ergot. J Physiol 1906;34:163–206.

p. 298 Fig. 4: Based on Frederiksson R, Lagerström MC, Lundin LG, Schiöth HB: The G-protein-coupled receptors in the human genome form five main families. Phylogenetic analysis, paralogon groups, and fingerprints. Mol Pharmacol 2003,63:1256–1272.
p. 299 Fig. 5: Donated by Brian Kobilka to Wikimedia Commons.

p. 303 Fig. 1: http://www.ultimateitaly.com/peoples/daniel-bovet.html.
p. 303 Fig. 2: Bovet D: Introduction to antihistamine agents and antergan derivative. Ann NY Acad Sci 1950;50:1089–1126. Reproduced with permission.
p. 303 Fig. 3: Reproduced with kind permission by Georges Halpern (son of Bernard Halpern).
p. 304 Fig. 4: Authors' own material.

p. 312 Fig. 1: Copyright ullstein bild - Roger-Viollet/Jacques Boyer.
p. 312 Fig. 2: Copyright ullstein bild - Roger-Viollet.
p. 313 Fig. 3: John E. Bordley by William F. Draper, oil on canvas, 1968. Courtesy of the Alan Mason Chesney Medical Archives of the Johns Hopkins Medical Institutions. Photograph by Aaron Levin.
p. 314 Fig. 4: Private collection.

p. 320 Fig. 6, 7: Wellcome Library, London.

p. 328 Fig. 1: Private collection.
p. 330 Fig. 2: By courtesy of Kåre Meno, ALK.

p. 384 Fig. 1: Private collection.

p. 398 Fig. 1: Private collection.

p. 403 Fig. 1–4: UW-Milwaukee Libraries Archives, Milwaukee, Wisc., USA.

p. 406 Fig. 1: Pauls Stradins Museum of the History of Medicine, Riga. Inv. No. 6481/1A, 6481/4A, 6481/11A, 6481/21A, 6481/24A.
p. 406 Fig. 2: Pauls Stradins Museum of the History of Medicine, Riga. Inv. No. 6476/1A, 6476/2A, 6476/3A, 6511A, 6513A, 6507/1A, 6487A, 6484A, 6486A, 6489A.
p. 407 Fig. 3: Pauls Stradins Museum of the History of Medicine, Riga. Artist: M. Grīnfelde, 1981. Inv. No. LA 11.148.
p. 408 Fig. 4: Pauls Stradins Museum of the History of Medicine, Riga. Inv. No. 6516A, 6493A.

Addendum

The authors and the publisher have made every effort to obtain permission for all copyright-protected material. Any omissions are entirely unintentional. The publisher would be pleased to hear from anyone whose rights unwittingly have been infringed.

Subject Index

ANDREAS VESALIUS

The Fabric of the Human Body

An Annotated Translation of the 1543 and 1555 Editions of "De Humani Corporis Fabrica" by

DANIEL H. GARRISON
MALCOLM H. HAST

with contributions by Vivian Nutton and Nancy Siraisi

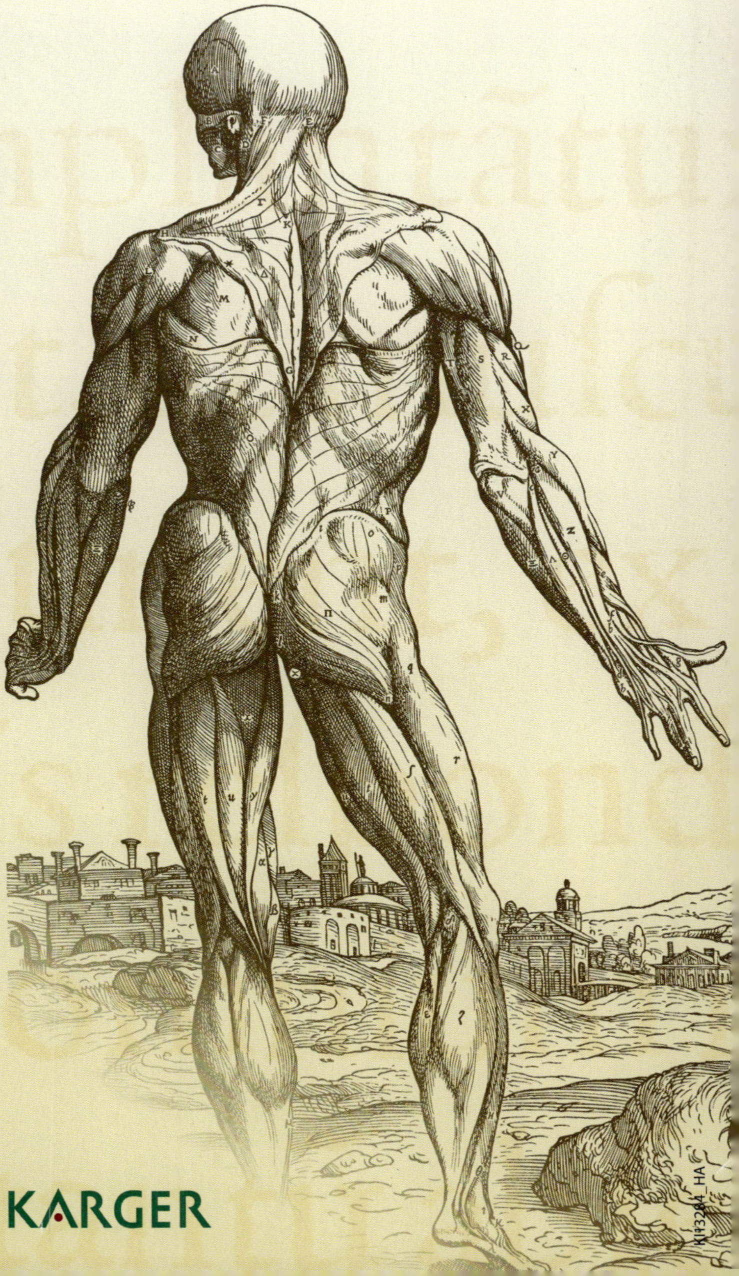

For the first time ever, both editions of Andreas Vesalius' masterpiece "De Humani Corporis Fabrica" are accessible in the English language. They were critically compared and published in a modern layout transforming the Renaissance anatomical atlas for the 21st-century reader. More than 5,000 annotations cover anything from antique sources over Galenic references to the medical and cultural background of Vesalius' time. Also included are Vesalius' handwritten notes for a never published third edition.
To enable the reader and medical student to really study Vesalius' woodcut illustrations, the images were digitally enhanced and often enlarged to feature his painstaking work of marking each pertinent anatomical part with characters. All over Vesalius' descriptive text, the standard Latin *Nomina Anatomica* and *Terminologia Anatomica* provide the reader with the modern medical terminology.

Vesalius, A., The Fabric of the Human Body
An Annotated Translation of the 1543 and 1555 Editions of
"De Humani Corporis Fabrica Libri Septem" by
D.H. Garrison and M.H. Hast
CXX + 1338 p., 340 fig., in two volumes, hard cover, with slip case, 2014
315 x 435 mm / 12 x 17", 16 kg / 35 lbs
ISBN 978-3-318-02246-9

www.karger.com

www.vesalius-fabrica.com

KARGER